AF449258

PLEASE RETURN TO
THE CLAUDE MOORE

Hepatitis B

Contributors

Leonardo Bianchi

Friedrich Deinhardt

Jules L. Dienstag

Robert J. Gerety

Paul V. Holland

Jay H. Hoofnagle

Sten A. Iwarson

Ulrich Junge

R. James Klingenstein

Saul Krugman

Makoto Mayumi

Yuzo Miyakawa

William S. Robinson

Richard E. Sampliner

Leonard B. Seeff

J. Wai-Kuo Shih

Hans-Peter Spichtin

Edward Tabor

Arie J. Zuckerman

Hepatitis B

Edited by

ROBERT J. GERETY
Potomac, Maryland

1985

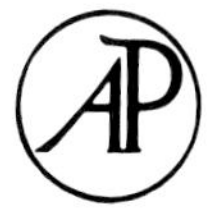

ACADEMIC PRESS, INC.
(Harcourt Brace Jovanovich, Publishers)

Orlando   San Diego   New York   London
Toronto   Montreal   Sydney   Tokyo

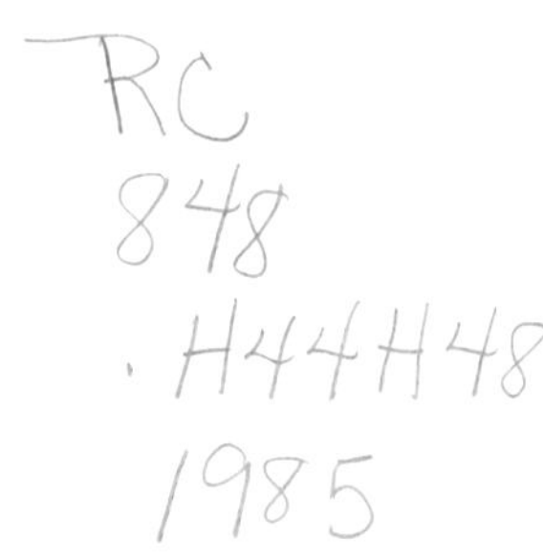RC
848
.H44H48
1985

COPYRIGHT © 1985 BY ACADEMIC PRESS, INC.
ALL RIGHTS RESERVED.
NO PART OF THIS PUBLICATION MAY BE REPRODUCED OR
TRANSMITTED IN ANY FORM OR BY ANY MEANS, ELECTRONIC
OR MECHANICAL, INCLUDING PHOTOCOPY, RECORDING, OR
ANY INFORMATION STORAGE AND RETRIEVAL SYSTEM, WITHOUT
PERMISSION IN WRITING FROM THE PUBLISHER.

ACADEMIC PRESS, INC.
Orlando, Florida 32887

United Kingdom Edition published by
ACADEMIC PRESS INC. (LONDON) LTD.
24–28 Oval Road, London NW1 7DX

Library of Congress Cataloging in Publication Data

Main entry under title:

Hepatitis B.

    Includes index.
    1. Hepatitis B. 2. Hepatitis B--Preventive inocula-
tion. I. Gerety, R. J. [DNLM: 1. Hepatitis B. WC 536
H5333]
RC848.H44H48 1985   616.3'623   84-21539
ISBN 0-12-280672-7 (alk. paper)

PRINTED IN THE UNITED STATES OF AMERICA

85 86 87 88   9 8 7 6 5 4 3 2 1

Contents

5. The Epidemiology of Hepatitis B

ROBERT J. GERETY AND EDWARD TABOR

6. The Acute Manifestations of Hepatitis B Virus Infection

ULRICH JUNGE AND FRIEDRICH DEINHARDT

7. Chronic Hepatitis B

STEN A. IWARSON

8. Follow-Up and Management of Hepatitis B Carriers

RICHARD E. SAMPLINER

9. Therapy of Chronic Hepatitis B

JAY H. HOOFNAGLE

10. Immunopathogenesis of Acute and Chronic Hepatitis B

R. JAMES KLINGENSTEIN AND JULES L. DIENSTAG

11. Hepatitis B Virus and Primary Hepatocellular Carcinoma

EDWARD TABOR

16. Active Immunization/HBsAg Particle Vaccines

ROBERT J. GERETY

17. Active Immunization/Polypeptide and Newer Vaccines

ARIE J. ZUCKERMAN

18. New Technologies

J. WAI-KUO SHIH

Contributors

Numbers in parentheses indicate the pages on which the authors' contributions begin.

LEONARDO BIANCHI (269), Department of Pathology, University of Basel, CH-4003 Basel, Switzerland

FRIEDRICH DEINHARDT (93), Max von Pettenkofer Institute for Hygiene and Medical Microbiology, University of Munich, 8000 Munich 2, West Germany

JULES L. DIENSTAG (221), Gastrointestinal Unit (Medical Services), Massachusetts General Hospital, and the Department of Medicine, Harvard Medical School, Boston, Massachusetts 02114

ROBERT J. GERETY (27, 77, 385), Center for Drugs and Biologics, Office of Biologics Research and Review, Food and Drug Administration, Bethesda, Maryland 20205

PAUL V. HOLLAND (5), Sacramento Medical Foundation Blood Center, Sacramento, California 95816

JAY H. HOOFNAGLE (173), Liver Diseases Section, Digestive Diseases Branch, National Institute of Arthritis, Diabetes, Digestive and Kidney Diseases, National Institutes of Health, Bethesda, Maryland 20205

STEN A. IWARSON (119), Department of Infectious Diseases, University of Göteborg, Östra Hospital, 416 85 Göteborg, Sweden

ULRICH JUNGE (93), Department of Internal Medicine, University of Ulm, D-7900 Ulm, West Germany

R. JAMES KLINGENSTEIN[1] (221), Gastrointestinal Unit (Medical Services), Massachusetts General Hospital, Boston, Massachusetts 02114

SAUL KRUGMAN (1), New York University Medical Center, School of Medicine, New York, New York 10016

MAKOTO MAYUMI (47), Immunology Division, Jichi Medical School, Minamikawachi-Machi, Tochigi-Ken 329-04, Japan

YUZO MIYAKAWA (47), The Third Department of Internal Medicine, Faculty of Medicine, University of Tokyo, Tokyo, Japan

[1]Present address: Newton Wellesley Hospital, Newton, Massachusetts 02160.

WILLIAM S. ROBINSON (319), Division of Infectious Diseases, Stanford University Medical Center, Stanford, California 94305

RICHARD E. SAMPLINER (155), Gastroenterology Section, Veterans Administration Medical Center, and University of Arizona Health Sciences Center, Tucson, Arizona 85723

LEONARD B. SEEFF (353), Gastroenterology/Hepatology Section, Veterans Administration Medical Center, and Georgetown University Medical Center, Washington, D.C. 20422

J. WAI-KUO SHIH[2] (429), Hepatitis Branch, Office of Biologics Research and Review, Food and Drug Administration, Bethesda, Maryland 20205

HANS-PETER SPICHTIN (269), Department of Pathology, University of Basel, CH-4003 Basel, Switzerland

EDWARD TABOR (77, 247, 303), Division of Anti-Infective Drug Products, Office of Biologics Research and Review, Food and Drug Administration, Rockville, Maryland 20857

ARIE J. ZUCKERMAN (413), Department of Medical Microbiology, London School of Hygiene and Tropical Medicine, London WCE 7HT, England

[2]Present address: Department of Transfusion Medicine, Clinical Center, National Institutes of Health, Bethesda, Maryland 20205.

Preface

From the identification of the hepatitis B surface antigen and the hepatitis B virus to the successful cloning of the hepatitis B virus genome, our understanding of this virus and the disease it causes has become more complete. It is only now possible to attempt to write a definitive book on this subject from the discovery of HBsAg to the genetically engineered vaccines to prevent hepatitis B. *Hepatitis B*, like its predecessors *Non-A, Non-B Hepatitis* and *Hepatitis A*, is a comprehensive book covering all aspects of a single virus and the disease it causes. The authors, mainly physicians and doctoral level researchers, write here about their particular area of interest and expertise.

Hepatitis B is intended for physicians (one of the high-risk groups for acquiring the disease), immunologists, microbiologists, virologists, students, and those engaged in health administration throughout the world.

I thank my friends for their truly outstanding contributions to this book, my family (Joan, Andrew, Kathleen, and Nancy) for their support and love, and the staffs of the National Naval Medical Center (especially Drs. Massimiano and Cattau) and the Cancer Surgery Branch of the National Cancer Institute (especially Drs. Rosenberg, Lotze, Andriole, and St. Clair) for their kindness and excellence in a difficult time for me. I also thank my brother Jim for a lifetime of encouragement and friendship.

ROBERT J. GERETY

Chapter 1

Introduction

SAUL KRUGMAN
New York University Medical Center
School of Medicine
New York, New York

The viral etiology of hepatitis was first suggested in 1908 by McDonald, a pathologist. In discussing the cause of acute yellow atrophy (necrosis) of the liver, he stated that "It may well be that the typical condition is only produced when some special virus acts on a previously damaged liver." Convincing evidence of a viral etiology was established by various investigators who conducted human volunteer studies during the 1940s. Studies in Germany (Voegt, 1942), in Palestine (Cameron, 1943), in Great Britain (MacCallum and Bradley, 1944), and in the United States (Havens, 1944) indicated that hepatitis could be transmitted by a nonbacterial, filterable agent. These findings confirmed that a virus was the most likely cause of the hepatitis.

Two types of hepatitis were identified during the 1940s, so-called infectious hepatitis and serum hepatitis. In 1947 MacCallum proposed the terms hepatitis A for infectious hepatitis and hepatitis B for serum hepatitis or homologous serum jaundice. This terminology was proposed because of the striking differences in the epidemiology of the two diseases. For example, hepatitis A was transmitted via the fecal–oral route, either by intimate contact with an infected person or by ingestion of fecally contaminated food or water; parenteral transmission was possible, but it was an unusual occurrence. In addition, hepatitis A occurred after a short incubation period (2–6 weeks). On the other hand, in the 1940s it was thought that hepatitis B was transmitted exclusively by the parenteral route (Havens, 1944).

The first recognized epidemic of hepatitis B, in retrospect, occurred in Bremen, Germany ~100 years ago (Lürman, 1885). Of 1289 shipyard workers who had been inoculated with smallpox vaccine prepared from glycerinated lymph of human origin, 15% became jaundiced several weeks to several months later. It is amazing that epidemics of hepatitis B such as this were not recognized during the eighteenth and early nineteenth centuries. During that era the extensive use of variolation and

1

Copyright © 1985 by Academic Press, Inc.
All rights of reproduction in any form reserved.
ISBN 0-12-280672-7

smallpox vaccine prepared from human lymph must have been responsible for many unrecognized outbreaks of hepatitis B.

During the first half of the twentieth century, outbreaks of "long incubation period" hepatitis were observed in many countries of the world. Infections occurred in patients who attended venereal disease, diabetic, and tuberculosis clinics, in those who received blood transfusions, in children who were inoculated with mumps or measles convalescent serum, and in military personnel who received yellow fever vaccine during World War II. These outbreaks were caused by the use of hepatitis B-contaminated needles, syringes, blood, and blood products. In this regard, it is likely that the human serum contained in the yellow fever vaccine was obtained from an unrecognized hepatitis B carrier.

The Willowbrook studies that were begun in the mid-1950s confirmed and extended previously reported observations of the epidemiology, natural history, and prevention of hepatitis A and hepatitis B (Krugman *et al.*, 1962, 1967). It would have been impossible to acquire much of the new knowledge during the course of these studies if serum enzyme assays were not available. The development of these tests in 1955 provided a marker of hepatitis even in the absence of jaundice.

During the course of our Willowbrook studies in the 1960s, we identified two types of viral hepatitis, each with distinctive clinical, epidemiological, and immunological features (Krugman *et al.*, 1967). One type, designated "MS-1," resembled hepatitis A, and the other, designated "MS-2," resembled hepatitis B. Contrary to the prevailing concept at that time, the MS-2 strain of hepatitis B was infectious orally as well as parenterally, and patients with this infection were shown to be moderately contagious. These findings indicated that hepatitis B could be transmitted from person to person via intimate personal contact. These new epidemiological findings were confirmed when the discovery of Australia antigen and its association with hepatitis B led to the development of specific tests for the identification of hepatitis B infections.

The story of the discovery of Australia antigen and its association with hepatitis B has been well documented in published reports (Blumberg *et al.*, 1965, 1967; Prince, 1968). Extensive studies during the 1960s and 1970s clarified the distribution of the antigen in various population groups and in patients with diseases unrelated to hepatitis B. Seroepidemiological surveys revealed that this antigen was present in the blood of 0.1 to 0.3% of healthy blood donors, in 10 to 20% of persons living in Africa and Asia, in 10 to 15% of patients with leukemia or Hodgkin's disease, in 20 to 30% of institutionalized patients with Down's syndrome, and finally, in ~20% of patients with viral hepatitis.

The demonstration that Australia antigen was associated with viral hepatitis was followed by studies documenting its specific association with hepatitis B (Giles *et al.*, 1969). Later, after Dane and colleagues (1970) identified the so-called Dane particle under the electron microscope, it was demonstrated that the surface component of this particle was immunologically distinct from its core component. The surface component was designated hepatitis B surface antigen (HBsAg). The core component contained endogenous DNA polymerase, double-stranded circular DNA, and two antigens, hepatitis B core antigen (HBcAg) and hepatitis B e antigen (HBeAg).

The accumulated evidence indicated that the Dane particle was, indeed, the hepatitis B virus (HBV), a member of a new family of viruses tentatively called hepadna viruses. The biophysical and biochemical characteristics of HBV, HBsAg, HBcAg, and HBeAg are described in detail in subsequent chapters of this volume.

During the course of our studies on the natural history of hepatitis B in 1970, we developed, by pure serendipity, a crude inactivated hepatitis B vaccine as the direct result of a study designed to determine the effect of heat (boiling for 1 min) on the infectivity of a 1:10 dilution of MS-2 serum in distilled water (Krugman *et al.*, 1970). A previous study had revealed that MS-2 serum contained both HBV and HBsAg. The results of this study indicated that heat treatment appeared to destroy the infectivity of HBV, but much to our surprise the inactivated MS-2 serum proved to be immunogenic. In subsequent studies it was shown that this heat-inactivated serum was immunogenic and partially protective; it possessed the characteristics of an inactivated hepatitis B vaccine (Krugman *et al.*, 1971a). In retrospect, it was clear that the heat-inactivated MS-2 serum was immunogenic because it contained enormous quantities of heat-resistant HBsAg particles. This study indicated that the plasma of HBsAg-positive carriers was a potential source of antigen for hepatitis B vaccine development. The sequence of events that led to the development and subsequent licensure of subunit hepatitis B vaccines is described by Gerety in detail in Chapter 18.

The availability of tests to identify hepatitis B antibodies as well as antigens provided the technology necessary to identify those units of blood that contained antibody to HBsAg (anti-HBs). Hepatitis B immune globulin was prepared from these anti-HBs-positive units. Our preliminary studies (Krugman *et al.*, 1971b) indicated that hepatitis B immune globulin was an effective passive immunizing agent for the prevention or modification of hepatitis B. In addition, its use was associated with passive–active immunization. The results of subsequent studies with hepatitis B immune globulin will be described in detail by Seeff in Chapter 15.

Progress achieved in hepatitis B research during the past 15 years has been phenomenal. The extraordinary developments are described in detail in various chapters of this volume. The virtual explosion of new knowledge has clarified the natural history of the disease as well as the complex characteristics of HBV, its causative agent. It was Dr. John F. Enders who aptly described the birth of this important era in hepatitis research when he stated that "After a long and arid period a new and exhilarating phase in the study of hepatitis has begun. The discovery of Australia antigen came like an unexpected shower on desert soil." The extraordinary consequences of this important development are described in subsequent chapters.

References

Blumberg, B. S., Alter, H. J., and Visnich, S. (1965). *JAMA, J. Am. Med. Assoc.* **191**, 541–546.

Blumberg, B. S., Gersley, B. J., and Hungerford, D. A. (1967). *Ann. Intern. Med.* **66**, 924–931.

Cameron, J. D. A. (1943). *Q. J. Med.* **12**, 139–155.

Dane, D. S., Cameron, C. H., and Briggs, M. (1970). *Lancet 1*, 695–698.

Giles, J. P., McCollum, R. W., Berndtson, L. M., Jr., and Krugman, S. (1969). *N. Engl. J. Med.* **281**, 119–122.

Havens, W. P. (1944). *Proc. Soc. Exp. Biol. Med.* **57**, 206–208.

Krugman, S., Ward, R., and Giles, J. P. (1962). *Am. J. Med.* **32**, 717–728.

Krugman, S., Giles, J. P., and Hammond, J. (1967). *JAMA, J. Am. Med. Assoc.* **200**, 365–373.

Krugman, S., Giles, J. P., and Hammond, J. (1970). *J. Infect. Dis.* **122**, 432–436.

Krugman, S., Giles, J. P., and Hammond, J. (1971a). *JAMA, J. Am. Med. Assoc.* **217**: 41–45.

Krugman, S., Giles, J. P., and Hammond, J. (1971b). *JAMA, J. Am. Med. Assoc.* **218**, 1655–1670.

Lürman, A. (1885). *Berl. Klin. Wochenschr.* **22**, 20–23.

MacCallum, F. O., and Bradley, W. H. (1944). *Lancet 2*, 228–230.

Prince, A. M. (1968). *Proc. Natl. Acad. Sci. U.S.A.* **60**, 814–821.

Voegt, H. (1942). *Muench. Med. Wochenschr.* **89**, 76–79.

Chapter 2

Hepatitis B Surface Antigen and Antibody (HBsAg/Anti-HBs)

PAUL V. HOLLAND
Sacramento Medical Foundation Blood Center
Sacramento, California

I. Introduction

The discovery of reproducible serologic markers in type B viral hepatitis has resulted in enormous progress in our understanding, and now in prevention, of this widespread form of viral hepatitis. Without markers for viral antigens of the hepatitis B virus or the means to identify serological responses to them, research on this disease was difficult, slow, and not very productive (Havens, 1954). The identification of the Australia antigen, which was eventually shown to be hepatitis B surface antigen (HBsAg), ushered in an era of unprecedented gain in our realization of the magnitude, means of transmission, and pathogenesis of hepatitis B. Carriers of hepatitis B virus can usually be identified by the detection of excess viral coat protein, HBsAg, circulating in their plasma (Gocke, 1970). Transmission of hepatitis B from HBsAg carriers can be obviated, and some such individuals now serve as the source of HBsAg used to manufacture a highly efficacious vaccine for prevention of this disease.

The identification of an antibody directed to HBsAg has furthered our understanding of hepatitis B, its transmission, and its prevention. In addition, antibody to HBsAg (anti-HBs) is our best measure of immunity to the hepatitis B virus (HBV). Thus, serologic tests to detect anti-HBs allow us to identify the majority of individuals exposed to HBV and to predict who is or is not immune to this virus, and whether they have been exposed naturally (by infection) or artificially (by vaccination) to HBV/HBsAg. The pattern of antibody response to HBsAg, as well as to other HBV determinants, can also provide an excellent clue to the time of exposure to HBV and its antigens and to the outcome of that exposure.

The purpose of this chapter is to describe HBsAg and anti-HBs. The history, physical characteristics, significance, means of identification, and subtypes of HBsAg will be covered. The antibody response to HBsAg will be similarly presented. Finally, the simultaneous presence of HBsAg and anti-HBs will be discussed along with the possible clinical significance of this uncommon situation.

II. Identification, Characteristics, and Methods of Detection of HBsAg

A. Identification of HBsAg

Utilizing sera from a multitransfused patient with hemophilia and from an Australian aborigine, Blumberg *et al.* (1965) identified a precipitin line by the Ouchterlony technique of double diffusion in agar gel (AGD). The patient with hemophilia appeared to have an antibody in his serum directed against an antigen circulating in the serum of the aborigine, hence the name Australia antigen (Au). Subsequent serological surveys using AGD revealed that Au was rarely present in blood donors in the United States (0.1%), but was common among certain patient populations (e.g., 10% of patients with leukemia). Thus, Au was initially thought to be a marker for leukemia (Blumberg *et al.*, 1965). Subsequent findings of an increased frequency of Au among patients with Down's syndrome who have an increased risk of leukemia, supported this hypothesis (Blumberg *et al.*, 1967). However, the appearance of Au in the serum of a technologist in Dr. Blumberg's lab at the time that this individual developed viral hepatitis, and the occurrence of this same finding in a patient with Down's syndrome who developed hepatitis, provided a better explanation for the identity of Au. Subsequent studies revealed that the Au antigen was found in patients with viral hepatitis, specifically hepatitis B, regardless of whether they had concomitant leukemia, Down's syndrome, or neither. Eventually the name and designation of the Au antigen became HBsAg for the hepatitis B (virus) surface antigen. The solid link between HBsAg and hepatitis B (Prince, 1968) and the reproducibility of assays for the detection of this antigen prompted ever-increasing research into the understanding and control of hepatitis B, with dramatic and gratifying progress.

B. Nature of HBsAg

Subsequent to the epidemiological link between HBsAg and hepatitis B (Prince, 1968), laboratory studies of this antigen revealed its physical characteristics and that it is an integral part of the HBV. Foremost are the morphologic studies of HBsAg. Electron microscopic examination of HBsAg-positive serum revealed virus-like particles (Bayer *et al.*, 1968), most being 22-nm spheres or tubules of varying length, but 22 nm in diameter; however, some particles were 42-nm (Dane *et al.*, 1970), double-shelled spheres (Fig. 1). The smaller spheres, the tubules, and the outer coat of the larger spheres all appeared to be HBsAg. The 42-nm particles had additional constituents including a core antigen (Almeida *et al.*, 1971), DNA polymerase (Kaplan *et al.*, 1973), and a specific viral DNA (Robinson *et al.*, 1974), which make this particle the presumed complete HBV. Immunofluorescence studies of liver tissue from individuals with HBsAg in serum showed cytoplasmic localization of HBsAg within hepatocytes (Lamothe *et al.*, 1976).

Biophysical studies of purified HBsAg reveal a number of characteristics of this particulate material. Most HBsAg has a density of 1.20 g/cm^3 in cesium chloride (1.15–1.17 g/cm^3 in potassium tartrate or sucrose); a smaller portion of HBsAg has a density of 1.39 to 1.40 g/cm^3 (Gerin *et al.*, 1971). The lower density material is only HBsAg, composed of small spheres and tubules; the higher density material appears to be composed of the 42-nm complete virion, or Dane particle (Gerin *et al.*, 1975). Biochemical studies revealed that HBsAg is made up of protein and lipid (Alter and Blumberg, 1966) but that the antigenic determinants are primarily protein (Mishiro *et al.*, 1980); the amino acid composition of HBsAg has been determined (Peterson *et al.*, 1977). Purified HBsAg has a high molecular weight, $\sim 3 \times 10^6$; but the antigenic determinants of HBsAg are expressed on polypeptides of much smaller sizes, for example, 22,000, 27,000, and 49,000 daltons (Mishiro *et al.*, 1980).

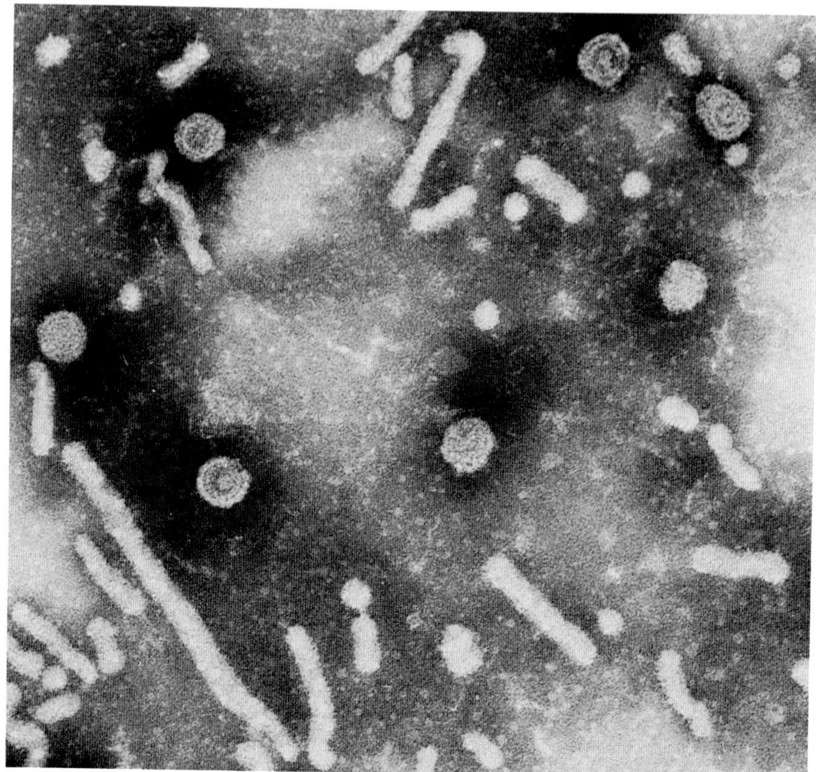

Figure 1. Electron micrograph of HBsAg-positive serum illustrating the 22-nm spheres, 22-nm diameter tubules of various lengths, and the 42-nm double-shelled structures, the Dane particles that are probably complete hepatitis B virions. Stain, 1% phosphotungstic acid ×150,000. (Photo courtesy of Dr. John Gerin, Georgetown University.)

C. Tests for HBsAg

Virtually all tests to detect HBsAg are immunological assays. The original means of identifying HBsAg was double diffusion in agar gel (AGD); for this purpose, sera suspected of containing HBsAg were tested versus human sera containing high levels of anti-HBs (Blumberg *et al.*, 1965). AGD was specific and reproducible but slow and insensitive. While AGD was the method of choice for years because one could compare unknown material to known HBsAg-positive sera and look for lines of identity, it is little used today save for some investigations of subtype specificities using sera with high levels of HBsAg and anti-HBs. Many additional immunological techniques were subsequently adapted to HBsAg detection, especially when it became a requirement to test all blood donors for HBsAg before their blood could be transfused.

TABLE I
Tests for Detection of HBsAg

Least sensitive	Intermediate sensitivity	Most sensitive
Agar gel diffusion	Counterelectrophoresis	Reversed passive hemagglutination
	Complement fixation	Enzyme-linked
	Immunofluorescence	immunosorbent assay
	Platelet agglutination	
	Immune electron	
	microscopy	Radioimmunoassay
	Hemagglutination	
	inhibition	
	Immune adherence	
	Latex agglutination	

1. Types of Tests for HBsAg Detection. Table I lists most of the immunological tests for HBsAg detection. They are ranked in roughly the order that they were developed, and generally from less sensitive to more sensitive techniques. After agar gel diffusion, the "first-generation" test, came a host of "second-generation" tests. These techniques were all more sensitive than AGD and generally took less time to perform. Counterelectrophoresis (CEP), also known as immune electroosmophoresis (IEOP), is the most practical of these tests of intermediate sensitivity. CEP was the test of choice for several years when commercial techniques and reagents first become available for the screening of blood donors for HBsAg.

2. Comparison of Sensitive Tests for HBsAg. The optimal techniques today for HBsAg detection are highly sensitive, specific, rapid, so-called "third-generation" tests. Radioimmunoassay (RIA), enzyme-linked immunosorbent assay (ELISA or EIA), and reversed passive hemagglutination (RPHA) methods are commercially available, simple, and quite reproducible; these have been used most extensively in screening blood donors for HBsAg (Seidl and Trautmann, 1981). Tests of equal or superior sensitivity to these are required to be applied to all blood and blood products intended for transfusion to minimize the risk of transfusion-transmitted HBV (Fine, 1975). Table II compares several techniques for HBsAg detection that are commercially available; it illustrates the abilities of many different laboratories to correctly identify which serum samples are either HBsAg positive or HBsAg negative as part of proficiency testing. Radioimmunoassay procedures are the most sensitive and specific; using RIA techniques, laboratory workers had the greatest proficiency and correctly identified 99.2% of the HBsAg-positive sera and 98.9% of the HBsAg-negative sera (Table II). ELISA techniques were

TABLE II
Comparison of Available Tests for HBsAg Detection[a]

HBsAg method	Number of labs reporting[b]	HBsAg-Positive samples (7) correct responses		HBsAg-Negative samples (3) correct responses	
		Total	%	Total	%
RIA[c]	554	3841/3873	99.2	1594/1611	98.9
RPHA	82	468/572	81.8	240/243	98.8
ELISA	8	54/56	96.4	20/24	83.3
LATEX (third generation)	21	66/147	44.9	57/60	95.0
LATEX (second generation)	5	3/35	8.6	15/15	100
CEP	2	1/14	7.1	6/6	100

[a]Reproduced with permission of the editor and publishers from Keating and Silvergleid, 1981.
[b]Includes Referee labs.
[c]Short incubation procedure not included.

the next most sensitive for HBsAg-positive sera, followed by RPHA techniques. The false positive rate on HBsAg-negative sera was highest for the ELISA test, followed by RPHA.

In another study of proficiency of HBsAg testing performed during the period 1978–1979 using one RIA test, routine blood processing laboratories of the American Red Cross Blood Service Regions found a 2% false-negative rate for HBsAg-positive sera and a 0.6% false-positive rate for HBsAg-negative sera (Nath *et al.*, 1982b). Lot-to-lot variability of the commercial RIA test used in the survey was considered the major cause of these error rates. It was believed that current lots not only had less variability but could detect even lower levels of HBsAg in serum samples. It should be kept in mind, however, that HBsAg testing of thousands of blood donor sera, most of which would be expected to be negative, might not in practice equal the excellent performance achieved during proficiency testing. The RIA test for HBsAg appears to be the most sensitive, reproducible, and objective technique for correctly identifying HBsAg in coded samples by blood banks (Gerety *et al.*, 1975).

While most techniques for HBsAg detection can identify HBsAg carriers because of the high levels of circulating HBsAg in the serum of such individuals, a better comparison of the various third-generation tests is possible when they are used to detect weakly reactive specimens (Pol-

TABLE III

Comparison of Third-Generation HBsAg Test Methods Based on a Proficiency Survey[a]

	Participants reporting correctly (%)		
Test method	All HBsAg-positive samples		Weakly reactive samples (RIA ratio < 15)
	1975–1976	1979–1980	1979–1980
RIA	98.8	96.6	93.1
RIA (30 min)	—	88.9	76.9
ELIA	—	89.2	75.4
RPHA	84.2	75.8	49.2
LATEX[TG]	—	58.2	30.6

[a]Reproduced with permission of the authors from Polesky and Hanson, 1981.

esky and Hanson, 1981). Sera with low levels of HBsAg might represent low-level carriers of HBV or those individuals who are early or late in the course of an acute episode of hepatitis B. Table III compares the results of HBsAg testing over two periods of time with an evaluation of results on weakly reactive samples during the second time period. This comparison again illustrates the superiority of RIA, and shows that even an abbreviated RIA procedure is equal to or better than any of the other commercially available, third-generation tests for HBsAg detection. However, the limited dating period of RIA testing kits and the problems in working with radioisotopes have prompted many laboratories to adopt ELISA procedures, which have neither of these problems yet still have "third-generation" sensitivity.

3. Quantitation of HBsAg. RIA tests have been most extensively utilized to quantitate the amounts of HBsAg in serum samples. One commercial RIA can routinely detect 2 ng/ml of HBsAg subtype **ad** and 6 ng/ml of HBsAg subtype **ay** (see section II,E on HBsAg subtypes). Most tests for HBsAg prepared in the United States appear to be able to detect lower levels of the **ad** subtype of HBsAg than the **ay** subtype. Careful performance of one available RIA test for HBsAg can detect as little as 1 ng/ml of HBsAg/**ad** and 2 ng/ml of HBsAg/**ay**; with a simple rotation modification of this RIA technique, detection levels could be further reduced by one-half (Nath *et al.*, 1981). In some donor serums in which antibody to the hepatitis B core antigen (anti-HBc) was the only marker of exposure to the HBV, the rotation modification of the RIA technique could detect specific, HBsAg positivity not demonstrable by conventional performance of the same RIA test.

4. Specificity of HBsAg Tests. All techniques for HBsAg give some false-positive results. These are primarily due to technical errors, but have also been due to cross-reactive antibodies and antigens (Alter *et al.*, 1972). Before concluding that a serum sample is HBsAg positive after a single test by one method, the test should be repeated. Most false-positive results are not reproducible. If a sample is repeatedly positive in a test for HBsAg, it is probably a true positive. However, to be certain of a true positive test for HBsAg, either of two additional procedures should be utilized. The preferred one is to perform a specificity test (Alter *et al.*, 1973) for HBsAg, that is, to determine that serum with anti-HBs specifically neutralizes the HBsAg in the test sample while a re-agent serum without anti-HBs does not. This technique usually rules out cross-reactive antibodies or antibodies that falsely react on the basis of species specificity. If the same technique as that for HBsAg detection is employed for specificity determination (neutralization against sera with and without anti-HBs), then the sensitivity of that detection system can be effectively used. A second method of determining specificity is to employ a different technique for HBsAg detection, which generally has different reagents. If this second technique is of comparable sensitivity to the first, and the HBsAg result is duplicated, then it is likely that the serum is truly HBsAg positive. The problem with this approach is that the verifying technique may not be as sensitive, and therefore may not detect equally low levels of true HBsAg positivity; to utilize this approach, the verifying technique should be of comparable or increased sensitivity to the screening test for HBsAg.

D. Significance of HBsAg

The finding of HBsAg in the serum of an individual indicates that he has HBV and potentially can transmit it to others (Barker and Murray, 1972). Donor blood that is HBsAg positive can transmit HBV to suscepti-ble recipients (Gocke, 1970; Holland *et al.*, 1973). Testing for HBsAg in blood donors and prevention of transfusion of HBsAg-positive blood or blood products has resulted in a decrease in transfusion associated hep-atitis B and in the associated morbidity and mortality of this disease (Goldfield *et al.*, 1975). HBsAg testing of all blood, blood products, and plasma intended for immediate or subsequent transfusion is a require-ment in the United States (Fine, 1975) and in most countries of the world.

HBsAg is thus *the* marker of an HBV infection, even though the stage of the disease may not be clear without clinical details and additional laboratory test results. Figure 2 illustrates the usual sequence of labora-

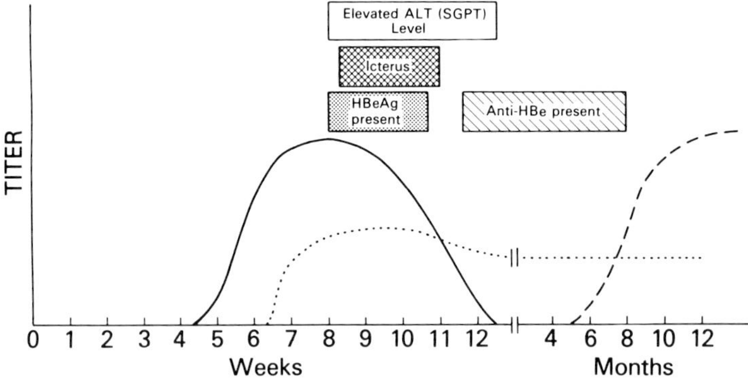

Figure 2. Sequence of laboratory findings and jaundice in an idealized patient with acute hepatitis B virus infection who subsequently recovers. The titers of HBsAg (—), anti-HBs (– – –), and anti-HBc (···) are in arbitrary units; the levels are just indicative of the time of detectability. (Reproduced by permission of the editor and publishers from Keating and Silvergleid, 1981).

tory findings in an idealized case of HBV infection. HBsAg may appear as early as 6 days after exposure to HBV (Krugman *et al.*, 1979), but is generally first detectable by 4 to 8 weeks. HBsAg may be the only indication of an acute hepatitis B infection for days to weeks before clinical symptoms, if any, appear or other markers of infectivity [e.g., antibody to the hepatitis B core antigen (anti-HBc)] are present.

HBsAg is generally present at a high and easily detectable level when a patient is clinically ill with hepatitis B. On occasion, however, HBsAg levels have already begun to decline when the patient is symptomatic; HBsAg may rarely be undetectable by the time the patient seeks medical attention. The surface antigen may persist for a few weeks or for as long as 3 months in patients who eventually recover from their acute HBV infection. If HBsAg persists in a patient's serum for >3 months, there is increased likelihood that the patient is, or will become, chronically infected. If HBsAg is present for >6 months, the likelihood that the individual is and will remain a chronic carrier of HBsAg is very high.

When HBsAg is detected in the serum of an individual, that single determination cannot be used to ascertain the stage of HBV infection. The individual could be in the early, presymptomatic phase of an acute illness, he could be in the midst of an acute episode of hepatitis B, he could be convalescing from an HBV infection, or he could already be a long-term asymptomatic carrier of HBsAg. Asymptomatic carriers of HBsAg might have been infected for years, even since birth. Follow-up studies for clinical evidence of disease, chemical evidence of hepatic inflammation, and for additional serological markers of an HBV infection will usually permit determination of the type and severity of the ongoing hepatitis B infection. In those individuals who are asymptomatic long-term carriers of HBsAg, about two-thirds have some evidence of hepatic dysfunction, such as elevated levels of serum alanine aminotransferase (ALT, SGPT) on one or more occasions (Koretz *et al.*, 1978). Liver biopsy of HBsAg carriers may reveal a spectrum of findings from essentially normal histology (Shrago *et al.*, 1977) to nonspecific, necroinflammatory findings, definitive evidence of chronic persistent or chronic active hepatitis, cirrhosis, and even hepatocellular carcinoma (Viola *et al.*, 1981).

All HBsAg-positive material is potentially infectious for hepatitis B unless treated or inactivated by some means. When the hepatitis B e antigen (HBeAg) is also present along with HBsAg, the material should be considered highly infectious (Alter *et al.*, 1976); however, even when HBeAg is absent or antibody to HBeAg is present (anti-HBe) in HBsAg-positive specimens, they remain infectious for hepatitis B (Shikata *et al.*, 1977). The reason for the increased infectivity of HBsAg-positive material, which is also HBeAg positive, is due to the fact that HBeAg is part of the core of the HBV virion (Neurath and Strick, 1979) and thus identifies specimens with increased numbers of complete viruses (Dane particles).

HBsAg has been detected in other materials besides whole serum and plasma. Virtually all blood components and products prepared from HBsAg-positive serum or plasma can contain HBsAg (Hoofnagle *et al.*, 1976). Unless such material has been adequately heated (e.g., 10 hr at 60°C for albumin preparations) to destroy the associated, complete hepatitis B virions or was prepared by specific, physicochemical techniques (e.g., cold ethanol-fractionated immune globulin preparations), material with HBsAg in it is potentially infectious for hepatitis B (Barker *et al.*, 1970). While the HBsAg in cold ethanol-fractionated, heat-treated albumin is immunogenic and not infectious (Mori *et al.*, 1973), the HBV in HBsAg-positive serum may not be completely inactivated by the same heating process (10 hr at 60°C) (Shikata *et al.*, 1978). The latter may be due to the fact that serum proteins may partially prevent the heat inactivation of HBV in HBsAg-positive serum, or that HBV particles are separated from the majority of HBsAg-positive but noninfectious particles by the cold ethanol-fractionated process of albumin preparation (Shih *et al.*, 1983).

HBsAg has been demonstrated in a variety of human body fluids and secretions. Most of these likely contain HBsAg from associated serum or plasma contamination. Thus, saliva, tears, breast milk, bile duct fluid, and urine from HBsAg-positive individuals may all contain HBsAg and infectious HBV (Scott *et al.*, 1980). Only stool from individuals with HBsAg in their blood does not seem to contain detectable HBsAg (Feinman *et al.*, 1979). Stool from infected individuals has not been shown to reproducibly transmit hepatitis B virus infection (Havens, 1946).

HBsAg is a remarkably stable antigen. Reference preparations retain their reactivity for years (Seagroatt *et al.*, 1982) under a variety of conditions (Schable *et al.*, 1979). HBsAg-positive materials can retain their antigenicity and immunogenicity even when subjected to conditions that inactivate the accompanying HBV (Mori *et al.*, 1973; Szmuness *et al.*, 1980).

E. Subtypes of HBsAg

Particulate HBsAg may possess a number of antigenic subdeterminants (Kim and Tilles, 1971). One, the a specificity, appears to be common to all HBsAg preparations regardless of geographic origin or clinical source. Thus, the a subdeterminant is regarded as a group-reactive, HBsAg specificity (Le Bouvier, 1971). No HBsAg-positive specimen has been found to lack the a determinant. Additional subtype determinants are also present, but not all of these determinants are present on the HBsAg produced by an individual patient infected with HBV. Many HBsAg subdeterminants other than a appear to be "allelic" or mutually exclusive; for example, neither the d and y determinants of HBsAg nor the w and r determinants generally occur together. Thus, the major subtypes of HBsAg appear to be **adw, ayw, adr,** and **ayr** (Holland, 1975). A host of additional subtype determinants have been described, including some that further subdivide the aforementioned w specificity (Couroucé *et al.*, 1976). Many of the subtype determinants plus the proposed subdivisions of HBsAg are shown in Table IV.

At an international workshop held in Paris in 1975, an extensive comparison of HBsAg subtypes and reagents was carried out (Couroucé *et*

TABLE IV
Subtypes of HBsAg

Group determinant	"Allelic" determinants
a	**d-y**
Major subtypes of HBsAg	**w-r**
adw, ayw, adr, ayr	
Additional subtype determinants	
x, n, t, q, Re, j, k	
and designations	
$a_1(w1), a_2{}^1(w2), a_2{}^3(w3), a_3(w4)$	

TABLE V
HBsAg Subtype Designations

Paris workshop designation	Original designation	Major subtype category
P1	a_1yw	**ayw**
P2	$a_2{}^1yw$	**ayw**
P3	$a_2{}^3yw$	**ayw**
P4	a_3yw	**ayw**
P5	ayr	**ayr**
P6	$a_2{}^1dw$	**adw**
P7	a_3dw	**adw**
P8	adr	**adr**
P9	adyw	**adyw**
P10	adywr	**adywr**

al., 1976). A proposed HBsAg subtype nomenclature and the establishment of reference reagent repositories resulted from this conference. While additional subdeterminants have been described since then, and some of the HBsAg workshop categories may have to be split (Couroucé-Pauty and Holland, 1978), the HBsAg designations arrived at then are still useful (Table V).

The important aspects of the subtypes of HBsAg are the following: (a) subtypes of HBsAg exist, are well defined, and indicate heterogeneity of expression of antigenic determinants of different hepatitis B viruses; (b) the subtype of HBsAg remains the same during an acute and/or chronic infection in an individual; (c) the subtype of HBsAg "breeds true" when HBV is transmitted to a susceptible individual (Mosley *et al.*, 1972); (d) the subtype can only elicit antibodies with specificities appropriate to the injected HBsAg or acquired HBV infection (Gold *et al.*, 1974); (e) there is geographic variation in the frequencies of the various subtypes (Holland, 1975); and (f) the subtype may occasionally be a predictor of clinical course (Couroucé-Pauty and Holland, 1978) or type of infection with HBV (Gianotti, 1973; Ishimaru *et al.*, 1976).

Reagents to perform HBsAg subtyping are not generally available. With known subtyped HBsAg preparations, antibody reagents can be developed (e.g., monoclonal antibodies to HBsAg subdeterminants; Shih *et al.*, 1980) or identified (Couroucé *et al.*, 1976). Tests for HBsAg detection can be modified to perform subtyping of HBsAg (Holland *et al.*, 1972).

Subtyping of HBsAg, while potentially useful, is rarely indicated or necessary. Vaccines prepared from purified, inactivated HBsAg (Szmuness *et al.*, 1980) generally elicit antibody to the group-reactive determinant (anti-HBs with anti-**a** specificity). Thus, inclusion of more than one subtype of HBsAg does not seem to be important in the preparation of hepatitis B vaccine; cross-immunity to HBV bearing HBsAg/**adw** will be elicited by an HBsAg/**ayw** vaccine and vice versa through the antibody response to the common **a** determinant in chimpanzees (Murphy *et al.*, 1974) and in humans (Szmuness *et al.*, 1982).

III. Antibody to HBsAg (Anti-HBs)

Anti-HBs is specific antibody directed against HBsAg (one or more of its subdeterminants). Anti-HBs is generally an IgG antibody, and appears after exposure to HBsAg in the form of vaccine or following recovery from infection with HBV (Lander *et al.*, 1972). Anti-HBs generally appears within a few weeks after HBsAg is cleared from the circulation, thus during the early convalesent phase of an acute HBV infection. In some patients, however, anti-HBs may not appear for many months after resolution of the HBV infection (McMahon *et al.*, 1981); if anti-HBs has not appeared by 1 year following recovery from HBV infection, or 1 month after a booster hepatitis B vaccine injection, it will not likely appear subsequently (Hoofnagle *et al.*, 1978).

The usual appearance of anti-HBs following HBV infection is depicted in Fig. 2; the appearance of anti-HBs after vaccination with hepatitis B vaccine is discussed in detail in Chapter 18. Up to 20% of individuals recovered from a hepatitis B infection (Barker *et al.*, 1973), and 5–15% of those injected with hepatitis B vaccine may never produce anti-HBs (Szmuness *et al.*, 1980). While those individuals recovered from HBV infection without production of anti-HBs are probably immune to reinfection (Kerlin *et al.*, 1979), most who do not respond to vaccine with the production of anti-HBs appear to still be susceptible to infection with hepatitis B virus (Szmuness *et al.*, 1980). Anti-HBs is the best predictor of immunity to HBV, whether the antibody is produced after natural infection or in response to the HBsAg in vaccine. Once produced, anti-HBs generally persists for years (Barker *et al.*, 1973).

A. Tests to Detect Anti-HBs

The test methods used initially to detect HBsAg could all be utilized for detection of anti-HBs. However, the first- and second-generation test methods for HBsAg were in general even less sensitive for detecting anti-HBs. Only individuals with a high titer of anti-HBs and animals hyperimmunized to HBsAg have anti-HBs detectable by tests such as agar gel diffusion, CEP, and complement fixation. The passive hemagglutination test for anti-HBs was the first method that had both good sensitivity and specificity (Vyas and Shulman, 1970). While the passive hemagglutination test was for years the mainstay of anti-HBs detection, its function has been largely supplanted by even more sensitive techniques such as enzyme immunoassay and radioimmunoassay methods. Currently, RIA tests are the most widely used for anti-HBs detection because of their commercial availability and high sensitivity and specificity (Nath *et al.*, 1982b).

Like all immunological tests, those for anti-HBs detection can be both falsely negative and falsely positive. Errors in performance of anti-HBs tests can result in either false-positive or false-negative results; false-positive results more often result from nonspecificity of the tests for anti-HBs (Nath *et al.*, 1982a). About 4% of all individuals with a positive test for anti-HBs demonstrated by RIA are nonspecifically positive (Nath *et al.*, 1982a). The possibility that the anti-HBs result is falsely positive is enhanced when the test indicates a low level of anti-HBs reactivity; almost half of the positive reactions with a sample-to-negative control (S/N) ratio <10 prove to be nonspecific (Nath *et al.*, 1982a), even though a test is considered positive (by definition) when the S/N is >2.1. Most nonspecific positive results for anti-HBs will not repeat as positive. Before a positive test for anti-HBs is presumed to be specific and indicative of immunity to the hepatitis B virus, the test should be reproducibly positive and preferably shown to be specific (especially if the S/N ratio is low). To be certain that anti-HBs is indeed specific, a neutralization test using pooled HBsAg-positive serum should be performed and compared to results with HBsAg-negative serum in an identical anti-HBs detection method. Alternatively, the individual with presumed anti-HBs should be tested for antibody to the hepatitis B core antigen (anti-HBc). If the latter test is also positive, then it is likely that the anti-HBs test is indeed specific and indicative of exposure and immunity to the hepatitis B virus. Detecting anti-HBc in a serum containing HBsAg is another method to verify that the positive test result for HBsAg is specific. With a commercial RIA procedure for anti-HBs, it can be shown that ~8% of American blood donors have anti-HBs (Holland *et al.*, 1980); thus they have been exposed to the hepatitis B virus despite a negative history of overt viral hepatitis.

B. Significance of Anti-HBs

The presence of anti-HBs in an individual's serum indicates that he has been exposed to HBsAg either in the form of hepatitis B vaccine or by infection with the hepatitis B virus; for the latter, it also means that he has recovered from the infection. Without a history of viral hepatitis, the presence of specific anti-HBs in an individual who has not received vaccine means he has had an inapparent infection with the hepatitis B virus at some time in his life. Further, anti-HBs almost always indicates that an individual is immune to infection by HBV (Szmuness *et al.*, 1980; Trepo and Prince, 1976). Only in a few instances has prior anti-HBs not protected against subsequent exposure to HBsAg-positive inocula (Barker *et al.*, 1972). In such situations, the apparent anti-HBs may have represented a false-positive result (Nath *et al.*, 1982a), or an unusually high HBV load, (such as that in a whole unit of HBsAg-positive blood) may have temporarily neutralized the anti-HBs (Trepo and Prince, 1976). Alternatively, the subtype specificity of the anti-HBs may not have been directed against that of the HBV in the HBsAg-containing material (Brandt *et al.*, 1980). For all intents and purpose, anti-HBs is the protective antibody to the hepatitis B virus whether it resulted from exposure to vaccine or from an overt or inapparent HBV infection.

Individuals with anti-HBs have virtually always recovered from their HBV infection and are no longer infectious for hepatitis B. One proof that individuals with anti-HBs no longer have hepatitis B virus in their blood has come from studies of donated blood. Blood donors with anti-HBs do not carry an increased risk of transmitting HBV when compared to blood donors without anti-HBs (Aach *et al.*, 1974). Thus, anti-HBs in a blood donor indicates that he has completely recovered from HBV infection and that he is no longer infectious. Another proof is the finding that the frequency of HBV infections in infants born to mothers with anti-HBs is not increased (Drucker *et al.*, 1981).

Blood donors with anti-HBs can be used as a source of plasma from which a high-titered immunoglobulin preparation for passive prophylaxis of hepatitis B can be produced. Hepatitis B immune globulin (HBIG) is an example of such a high-titered immune globulin preparation. HBIG contains high levels of anti-HBs (generally >1:100,000 titer by passive hemaglutination assay or RIA) and variable, but usually lower, levels of anti-HBc. HBIG can provide effective passive protection against HBV in several situations (see Chapter 17). HBIG has also effectively inactivated HBV in a coagulation factor concentrate (Tabor *et al.*, 1980).

An individual with anti-HBs without a history of either hepatitis or vaccination with HBsAg should be considered immune to hepatitis B. Provided the anti-HBs is specific, such an individual would not require either active immunization against HBV or passive prophylaxis with HBIG even if exposed to a different subtype of HBV.

C. Subtype Specificity of Anti-HBs

After exposure to HBsAg (vaccine or natural infection), individuals who develop anti-HBs respond generally to the **a** subdeterminant of HBsAg (Gold *et al.*, 1974). Thus, most anti-HBs contains anti-**a**. Individuals may also produce antibody (anti-HBs) to other subdeterminants of HBsAg. These additional anti-HBs responses, in addition to those to the **a** specificity, are rarely as strong or as persistent as the response to the **a** subdeterminant (Holland, 1975). Anti-**d**, and even less commonly anti-**w**, may form in response to exposure to HBsAg/**adw**; but fewer individuals seem to produce anti-**y** or anti-**r** after exposure to **ayw** and **adr**, respectively. Identifying anti-HBs with more than anti-**a** specificity is usually not necessary; finding anti-**d** or anti-**y** along with an anti-**a** response is primarily of use in epidemiological studies. When anti-HBs does not have anti-**a** specificity, for example, only anti-**d** or anti-**y** activity, an individual may be susceptible to another subtype of HBV (Koziol *et al.*, 1976) or actively coinfected with HBV with a different subtype of HBsAg (Le Bouvier *et al.*, 1976). The lack of formation or persistence of anti-**a** has been postulated as one of the mechanisms for the occasional finding of simultaneous HBsAg and anti-HBs (Brandt *et al.*, 1980), where the HBsAg is of one subtype and the anti-HBs is directed against a subdeterminant not on that antigen (Koziol *et al.*, 1976).

IV. Simultaneous HBsAg and Anti-HBs

On occasion, HBsAg and anti-HBs are present simultaneously in the serum of a patient or apparently healthy blood donor. This may be a real finding (both HBsAg and anti-HBs tests are specifically positive), or one or the other test for antigen or antibody may be falsely positive (Grangeot-Keros *et al.*, 1982). In various series, the frequency of simultaneous anti-HBs in HBsAg-positive individuals is generally ~1% but has been reported to be as high as 10% (Couroucé-Pauty and Holland, 1978). In those series in which there is a high frequency of simultaneous HBsAg plus anti-HBs in the same serum, it is likely that one or the other test is falsely positive (Vyas *et al.*, 1977).

There are a number of situations in which specific HBsAg and anti-HBs appear to be present at the same time (Couroucé-Pauty and Holland, 1978). In most of these situations, the HBsAg is of one subtype, for example, **adw,** and the anti-HBs is directed against a subdeterminant not present on the co-occurring HBsAg, for example, anti-**y**. Individuals who are HBsAg carriers of one subtype may be subsequently exposed to

HBV of a different subtype; they may mount an anti-HBs response to a subdeterminant of the latter without producing anti-**a**. More commonly, it appears that after exposure to HBV, a patient will respond just with anti-HBs to the **d** or **y** subdeterminant, or that the antibody to this subdeterminant will persist and the anti-**a** response will not (Brandt *et al.*, 1980). Then, on exposure to HBV again (e.g., to HBsAg/**adw**), anti-**y** present from a prior infection is not protective. Thus, the test for HBsAg (due to **adw** subtype) may be specifically positive at the same time and in the same serum specimen as is the test for anti-HBs (due to anti-**y**). Additionally, patients acutely infected with HBV who have HBsAg present in their blood cannot produce anti-HBs with anti-**a** specificity, but this is rarely demonstrable unless tests for immune complexes are used. For example, with a newly developed solid phase RIA method for HBsAg bound to IgM, complexes of HBsAg–anti-HBs may be measured in patients with acute hepatitis B infections; persistence of these complexes for >4 weeks generally identified individuals in whom chronic liver disease developed (Careoda *et al.*, 1982). Where passive prophylaxis with HBIG has failed to prevent an HBV infection, simultaneous, exogenous anti-HBs might be briefly present with endogenous HBsAg; this also is rarely, if ever, a cause of simultaneous HBsAg and anti-HBs.

V. Summary

Hepatitis B surface antigen (HBsAg) and its corresponding antibody (anti-HBs) were the first, reproducible, serological markers identified for a viral hepatitis agent. The antigen and antibody are specific for hepatitis B infections. HBsAg is viral coat protein of the HBV; this antigen can be identified in the serum and secretions of acutely and chronically HBV-infected individuals by a variety of sensitive and specific immunological techniques. HBsAg is usually the first indication of HBV infection, preceding by weeks or months other laboratory evidence of hepatitis B and any clinical signs or symptoms of the disease. HBsAg may be the only indicator of a long-term, asymptomatic carrier state for individuals with a chronic hepatitis B infection. HBsAg, when suitably purified from the plasma of HBsAg-positive carriers, has been shown to provide a safe, immunogenic, and effective vaccine for prevention of hepatitis B infections (see Chapter 18).

Anti-HBs can be detected by a variety of specific, sensitive, immunological techniques. This antibody, almost exclusively of the IgG class, may be produced by individuals in response to infection with the HBV (with or without clinical illness) or after immunization with the hepatitis B vaccine whether prepared from HBsAg-positive plasma or by recombinant DNA technology (Scolnick *et al.*, 1984). Thus, anti-HBs indicates exposure to HBsAg by vaccination or prior infection with the HBV. Anti-HBs in an individual almost always indicates that the person is immune to infection by HBV if the antibody is produced endogenously. Immune globulin preparations rich in anti-HBs can provide temporary, passive prophylaxis after acute exposure to HBsAg-positive materials in those susceptible to HBV infection (those with no anti-HBs of their own). The exogenously acquired anti-HBs does not provide complete protection, is temporary, and most often works by modifying the severity of the HBV infection (not by preventing it).

Serological tests may indicate the simultaneous presence of anti-HBs in some HBsAg-positive individuals. While these uncommon results may indicate exposure to two different subtypes (presumably strains) of HBV/HBsAg, more likely either the HBsAg test or the anti-HBs test is falsely positive. Specificity testing for HBsAg should be performed before concluding that the HBsAg positivity is true and hence that the individual is a carrier of the hepatitis B virus. Similarly, specificity testing for anti-HBs should be performed before concluding that an individual is immune to hepatitis B and (a) need not receive hepatitis B vaccine to stimulate active immunity to this virus and/or (b) need not receive HBIG for temporary passive prophylaxis after acute exposure to HBV.

References

Aach, R. D., Alter, H. J., Hollinger, F. B., Holland, P. V., Lander, J. J., Melnick, J. L., and Weiler, J. M. (1974). *Lancet 2*, 190–193.

Almeida, J., Rubenstein, D., and Stott, E. (1971). *Lancet 2*, 1225–1227.

Alter, H. J., and Blumberg, B. S. (1966). *Blood* **27**, 297–309.

Alter, H. J., Polesky, H. F., and Holland, P. V. (1972). *J. Immunol.* **108**, 358–369.

Alter, H. J., Holland, P. V., Purcell, R. H., and Gerin, J. L. (1973). *Blood* **42**, 947–957.

Alter, H. J., Seeff, L. B., Kaplan, P. M., McAuliffe, V. J., Wright, E. C., Gerin, J. L., Purcell, R. H., Holland, P. V., and Zimmerman, H. J. (1976). *N. Engl. J. Med.* **295**, 909–913.

Barker, L. F., and Murray, R. (1972). *Am. J. Med. Sci.* **263**, 27–33.

Barker, L. F., Shulman, N. R., Murray, R., Hirschman, R. J., Ratner, F., Diefenbach, W. C. L., and Geller, H. (1970). *JAMA, J. Am. Med. Assoc.* **211**, 1509–1512.

Barker, L. F., Peterson, M. R., and Murray, R. (1972). *Prog. Immunobiol. Stand.* **5**, 89–94.

Barker, L. F., Peterson, M. R., Shulman, N. R., and Murray, R. (1973). *JAMA, J. Am. Med. Assoc.* **223**, 1005–1008.

Bayer, M. E., Blumberg, B. S., and Werner, B. (1968). *Nature (London)* **218**, 1057–1059.

Blumberg, B. S., Alter, H. J., and Visnich, S. (1965). *JAMA, J. Am. Med. Assoc.* **191**, 541–546.

Blumberg, B. S., Gerstley, B. J. S., Hungerford, D. A., London, W. T., and Sutnick, A. I. (1967). *Ann. Intern. Med.* **66**, 924–929.

Brandt, K. H., Katchaki, J. N., Bronkhorst, F. B., and Meinders, A. E. (1980). *Neth. J. Med.* **23**, 233–236.

Careoda, F., de Franchis, R., Monforte, A. D., Vecchi, M., Rossi, E., Primignani, M., Palla, M., and Dioquardi, N. (1982). *Lancet 2*, 358–360.

Couroucé, A. M., Holland, P. V., Muller, J. Y., and Soulier, J. P. (1976). *Proc. Int. Workshop HBs Antigen Subtypes,* pp. 1–158.

Courouce-Pauty, A.-M., and Holland, P. V. (1978). *In* "Viral Hepatitis" (G. N. Vyas, S. N. Cohen, and R. Schmid, eds.), pp. 649–654. Franklin Institute Press, Philadelphia, Pennsylvania.

Dane, D. S., Cameron, C. H., and Briggs, M. (1970). *Lancet 1*, 695–698.

Drucker, J., Barin, F., Chiron, J. P., Coursaget, P., and Goudeau, A. (1981). *Lancet 2*, 259.

Feinman, S. V., Berris, B., Rebane, A., Sinclair, J. C., Wilson, S., and Wrobel, D. (1979). *J. Infect. Dis.* **140**, 407–410.

Fine, S. D. (1975). *Fed. Regist.* **40**, 29706–29712.

Gerety, R. J., Hoofnagle, J. H., Mitchell, F. D., Barker, L. F., and Meyer, H. M. (1975). *Am. J. Clin. Pathol.* **63**, 573–580.

Gerin, J. L., Holland, P. V., and Purcell, R. H. (1971). *J. Virol.* **7**, 569–576.

Gerin, J. L., Faust, R. M., and Holland, P. V. (1975). *J. Immunol.* **115**, 100–105.

Gianotti, F. (1973). *Arch. Dis. Child.* **48**, 794–799.

Gocke, D. J. (1970). *Vox Sang.* **19**, 327–331.

Gold, J. W., Alter, H. J., Holland, P. V., Gerin, J. L., and Purcell, R. H. (1974). *J. Immunol.* **112**, 1100–1106.

Goldfield, M., Black, H. C., Bill, J., Srihongse, S., and Pizzuti, W. (1975). *Am. J. Med. Sci.* **270**, 335–342.

Grangeot-Keros, L., Lambert, T., Dubreuil, P., Briantais, M. J., and Pillot, J. (1982). *Vox Sang.* **42**, 160–163.

Havens, W. P., Jr. (1946). *J. Exp. Med.* **83**, 441–447.

Havens, W. P., Jr. (1954). *Nat. Acad. Sci.-Natl. Res. Counc., Publ.* **322**, 93–99.

Holland, P. V. (1975). *Am. J. Med. Sci.* **270**, 161–164.

Holland, P. V., Purcell, R. H., Smith, H., and Alter, H. J. (1972). *J. Immunol.* **109**, 420–425.

Holland, P. V., Alter, H. J., Purcell, R. H., Walsh, J. J., Morrow, A. G., and Schmidt, P. J. (1973). *In* "Australia Antigen" (J. E. Prier and H. Friedman, eds.), pp. 191–203. University Park Press, Baltimore, Maryland.

Holland, P. V., Golosova, T., Szmuness, W., Ketiladze, E., Purcell, R., Budnitskaya, P., Gerety, R., Vorozhbieva, T., Harley, E., Burlev, V., Alter, H. J., Margolina, A., and Lubashevskaya, E. (1980). *Transfusion (Philadelphia)* **20**, 504–510.

Hoofnagle, J. H., Gerety, R. J., Thiel, J., and Barker, L. F. (1976). *J. Lab. Clin. Med.* **88**, 102–113.

Hoofnagle, J. H., Seeff, L. B., Bales, Z. B., Gerety, R. J., and Tabor, E. (1978). *In* "Viral Hepatitis" (G. N. Vyas, S. N. Cohen, and R. Schmid, eds.), pp. 219–242. Franklin Inst. Press, Philadelphia, Pennsylvania.

Ishimaru, Y., Ishimaru, H., Toda, G., Baba, L., and Mayumi, M. (1976). *Lancet 1*, 707–709.

Kaplan, P. M., Greenman, R. L., and Gerin, J. L. (1973). *J. Virol.* **12**, 995–1005.

Keating, L. J., and Silvergleid, A. J. (eds.) (1981). "Hepatitis: A Technical Workshop." Am. Assoc. Blood Banks, Washington, D.C.

Kerlin, P., Ashcavi, M., Redeker, A., Peters, R., and Jones, M. (1979). *Gastroenterology* **77,** A–22.

Kim, C. Y., and Tilles, J. G. (1971). *J. Infect. Dis.* **123,** 618–628.

Koretz, R. L., Lewin, K. J., Rebhun, D. J., and Gitnick, G. L. (1978). *Gastroenterology* **75,** 860–863.

Koziol, D. E., Alter, H. J., Kirchner, J. P., and Holland, P. V. (1976). *J. Immunol.* **117,** 2260–2263.

Krugman, S., Overby, L. R., Mushahwar, I. K., Ling, C.-M., Frosner, G., and Deinhardt, F. (1979). *N. Engl. J. Med.* **300,** 101–106.

Lamothe, F., Laurencin-Piche, J., and Cote, J. (1976). *Gastroenterology* **71,** 102–108.

Lander, J. J., Holland, P. V., Alter, H. J., Chanock, R. M., and Purcell, R. H. (1972). *JAMA, J. Am. Med. Assoc.* **220,** 1079–1082.

Le Bouvier, G. L. (1971). *J. Infect. Dis.* **123,** 671–675.

Le Bouvier, G. L., Capper, R. A., Williams, A. E., Pelletier, M., and Katz, A. F. (1976). *J. Immunol.* **117,** 2262–2264.

McMahon, B. J., Bender, T. R., Berquist, K. R., Schreeder, M. T., and Harpster, A. P. (1981). *J. Clin. Microbiol.* **14,** 130–134.

Mishiro, S., Imai, M., Takahashi, K., Machida, A., Gotanda, T., Miyakawa, Y., and Mayumi, M. (1980). *J. Immunol.* **124,** 1589–1593.

Mori, Y., Momose, M., Nakano, Y., and Ata, S. (1973). *Vox Sang.* **25,** 235–239.

Mosley, J. W., Edwards, V. M., Meihaus, J. E., and Redeker, A. G. (1972). *Am. J. Epidemiol.* **95,** 529–535.

Murphy, B. L., Maynard, J. E., and Le Bouvier, G. L. (1974). *Intervirology* **3,** 378–381.

Nath, N., Fang, C. T., and Dodd, R. Y. (1981). *Transfusion (Philadelphia)* **21,** 457–461.

Nath, N., Fang, C. T. and Dodd, R. Y. (1982a). *Transfusion (Philadelphia)* **22,** 300–301.

Nath, N., Fang, C. T., Pielech, M., Lawson, W., and Dodd, R. Y. (1982b). *Vox Sang.* **43,** 105–112.

Neurath, A. R., and Strick, N. (1979). *J. Gen. Virol.* **42,** 645–649.

Peterson, D. L., Roberts, I. M., and Vyas, G. N. (1977). *Proc. Natl. Acad. Sci. U.S.A.* **74,** 1530–1535.

Polesky, H. F., and Hanson, M. (1981). *In* "Hepatitis: A Technical Workshop" (L. J. Keating and A. J. Silvergleid, eds.), pp. 15–34. Am. Assoc. Blood Banks, Washington, D.C.

Prince, A. M. (1968). *Proc. Natl. Acad. Sci. U.S.A.* **60,** 814–821.

Robinson, W. S., Clayton, D. A., and Greenman, R. L. (1974). *J. Virol.* **14,** 384–391.

Schable, C. A., Barbaree, J. M., Bond, W. W., Murphy, B. L., Berquist, K. R., Favero, M. S., and Maynard, J. E. (1979). *J. Biol. Stand.* **7,** 293–299.

Scolnick, E. M., McLean, A. A., West, D. J., McAleer, W. J., Miller, W. J., and Buynak, E. B. (1984). *JAMA, J. Am. Med. Assoc.* **251,** 2821–2815.

Scott, R. M., Snitbhan, R., Bancroft, W. H., Alter, H. J., and Tingpalapong, M. (1980). *J. Infect. Dis.* **142,** 67–71.

Seagroatt, V., Ferguson, M., MaGrath, D. I., Schild, G. C., and Cameron, C. H. (1982). *Lancet 2,* 391–392.

Seidl, S., and Trautmann, L. (1981). *Blood Transfus. Immunohaematol.* **24,** 319–335.

Shih, J. W.-K., Cheung, H. L., Holland, P. V., and Gerety, R. J. (1983). *Gastroenterology* **84,** 1397.

Shih, J. W.-K., Cote, P. J., Dapolito, G. M., and Gerin, J. L. (1980). *J. Virol. Methods* **1,** 257–273.

Shikata, T., Karasawa, T., Abe, K., Uzawa, T., Suzuki, H., Oda, T., Imai, M., Mayumi, M., and Moritsugu, Y. (1977). *J. Infect. Dis.* **136,** 571–576.

Shikata, T., Karasawa, T., Abe, K., Takahashi, K., Mayumi, M., and Oda, T. (1978). *J. Infect. Dis.* **138,** 242–244.

Shrago, S. S., Auslander, M. D., and Gitnick, G. L. (1977). *Arch. Pathol. Lab. Med.* **101,** 648–651.

Szmuness, W., Stevens, C. E., Harley, E. G., Zang, E. A., Oleszko, W. R., William, S. C., Sadovsky, R., Morrison, J. M., and Kellner, A. (1980). *N. Engl. J. Med.* **303,** 833–841.

Szmuness, W., Stevens, C. E., Harley, E. J., Zang, E. A., Alter, H. J., Taylor, P. E., DeVera, A., Chen, G. T. S., Kellner, A., and the Dialysis Vaccine Trial Study Group (1982). *N. Engl. J. Med.* **307,** 1481–1486.

Tabor, E., Aronson, D. L., and Gerety, R. J. (1980). *Lancet 2*, 68–70.

Trepo, C. G., and Prince, A. M. (1976). *Ann. Intern. Med.* **85,** 427–430.

Viola, L. A., Barrison, I. G., Coleman, J. C., Paradinas, F. J., Fluker, J. L., Evans, B. A., and Murray-Lyon, I. M. (1981). *Lancet 2*, 1156–1159.

Vyas, G. N., and Shulman, N. R. (1970). *Science* **170,** 332–333.

Vyas, G. N., Roberts, I., Peterson, D. L., and Holland, P. V. (1977). *J. Lab. Clin. Med.* **89,** 428–432.

Chapter 3

Hepatitis B Core Antigen and Antibody (HBcAg/Anti-HBc)

ROBERT J. GERETY
Center for Drugs and Biologics
Office of Biologics Research and Review
Food and Drug Administration
Bethesda, Maryland

I. Introduction

Electron microscopic studies of sera containing hepatitis B surface antigen (HBsAg) reveal three characteristic morphological forms of this antigen. They are small spherical particles ~22 nm in diameter, elongated tubules or filaments 22 nm in diameter and variable in length, and the larger hepatitis B virus (HBV) particles 42 nm in total diameter; each HBV particle has a 27-nm electron-dense core. The 27-nm core particles

Copyright © 1985 by Academic Press, Inc.
All rights of reproduction in any form reserved.
ISBN 0-12-280672-7

[hepatitis B core antigen (HBcAg)] can be released from within the HBV by detergent treatment (Almeida *et al.*, 1971). On electron microscopic examination of thin sections of liver tissue obtained during acute or chronic hepatitis B from either experimentally infected chimpanzees or naturally infected humans, 27-nm HBcAg particles can be seen in the nuclei of infected hepatocytes (Barker *et al.*, 1974). HBcAg particles have been purified from hepatocyte nuclei and from intact HBV by ultra-centrifugation, and shown to be specifically associated with hepatitis B and to be antigenically distinct from other HBV-associated antigens. Specific antibodies to HBcAg (anti-HBc) develop early during acute hepatitis B and persist for long periods in persons convalescent from hepatitis B; anti-HBc is present in all individuals with chronic hepatitis B (Barker *et al.*, 1974; Hoofnagle *et al.*, 1973). Serological tests have been developed to detect both IgM anti-HBc, which appears early in acute hepatitis B, and IgG anti-HBc, which appears late in disease or during recovery and persists beyond convalescence. IgM anti-HBc may also persist in some persons with chronic hepatitis B.

Fluorescein-labeled anti-HBc is capable of localizing HBcAg in the nuclei of infected hepatocytes, while antibody to HBsAg (anti-HBs) can localize HBsAg in the cytoplasm of the same or different liver cells (Brzosko *et al.*, 1973; Hoofnagle *et al.*, 1978a). Similarly, these antibodies aggregate their corresponding antigen particles and not the alternative particles (Almeida *et al.*, 1971; and see below).

Two distinct populations of HBcAg have been identified and separated by ultracentrifugation on the basis of their discrete densities. The heavier HBcAg particles (1.36 g/cm^3) contain DNA and HBV-specific DNA polymerase, while the lighter particles do not (Kaplan *et al.*, 1976). DNA polymerase activity in serum is directly related to the number of infectious HBV contained in that serum.

Within HBcAg particles resides a unique, partially double-stranded, circularized DNA and both a DNA polymerase activity and a phosphokinase activity. A major polypeptide of HBcAg has been shown to be ~19,000 daltons (Hruska and Robinson, 1977). Details regarding the biology and biochemistry of HBV including the DNA and enzyme activities residing within the HBcAg are discussed in detail in Chapter 15. When treated with 2-mercaptoethanol and SDS or pronase, HBcAg immunological reactivity is converted into that of another HBV-associated antigen (HBeAg), which circulates free in the serum of acutely infected and some chronically infected individuals. The exact chemical and immunological relationship between HBcAg and HBeAg is discussed in detail in Chapter 4.

II. Early Studies

A. Identification

Almeida *et al.* (1971), using immunoelectron microscopy, were the first to demonstrate the presence of HBcAg/anti-HBc in hepatitis B. They disrupted intact HBV with Tween-80 to expose the inner HBcAg. Serum from a patient obtained during convalescence from hepatitis B was shown to react with the inner, core component (HBcAg) but not with the outer, surface component (HBsAg). Serum obtained prior to infection with HBV did not react with either HBsAg or HBcAg; serum from a hemophiliac reacted with both of these antigens. On the basis of these studies, Almeida *et al.* postulated the existence of an antibody response in hepatitis B directed against the internal, core component of HBV. Substantiation of the duality of antibody responses in hepatitis B came from immunofluorescence studies that demonstrated two distinct immunological staining patterns in liver biopsies, one directed against a cytoplasmic antigen (HBsAg) and one directed against a nuclear antigen (HBcAg) (Barker *et al.*, 1973; Brzosko *et al.*, 1973). Finally, complement fixation and radioimmunoassay (RIA) (Hoofnagle *et al.*, 1973) techniques have demonstrated the regular occurrence of anti-HBc in hepatitis B.

B. Isolation

HBcAg particles were initially isolated from the liver of a chimpanzee who died during the acute phase of experimentally induced hepatitis B while being treated with cyclophosphamide (Markenson *et al.*, 1975; Barker *et al.*, 1974). This animal circulated HBsAg for 11 weeks until its death (resulting from pneumonitis and sepsis). Liver function tests had been normal, and liver histology at necropsy revealed only minimal lymphocytic infiltrates in the portal areas with hepatocyte necrosis. On electron microscopy, numerous HBcAg particles were seen in the nuclei of hepatocytes (Fig. 1). The liver was removed at necropsy, frozen and thawed twice, homogenized in a Waring blender, and diluted in hypotonic saline. Particulate material was removed by low-speed centrifugation (1,500 rpm for 30 min) and the HBcAg concentrated by high-speed centrifugation (28,000 rpm for 2 hr). The resuspended pellet from this ultracentrifugation contained 27-nm HBcAg particles by electron microscopy (Fig. 2); this HBcAg preparation was used to develop complement fixation (CF) tests to detect both HBcAg and anti-HBc. To further purify this antigen, the HBcAg preparation was layered on a continuous ce-

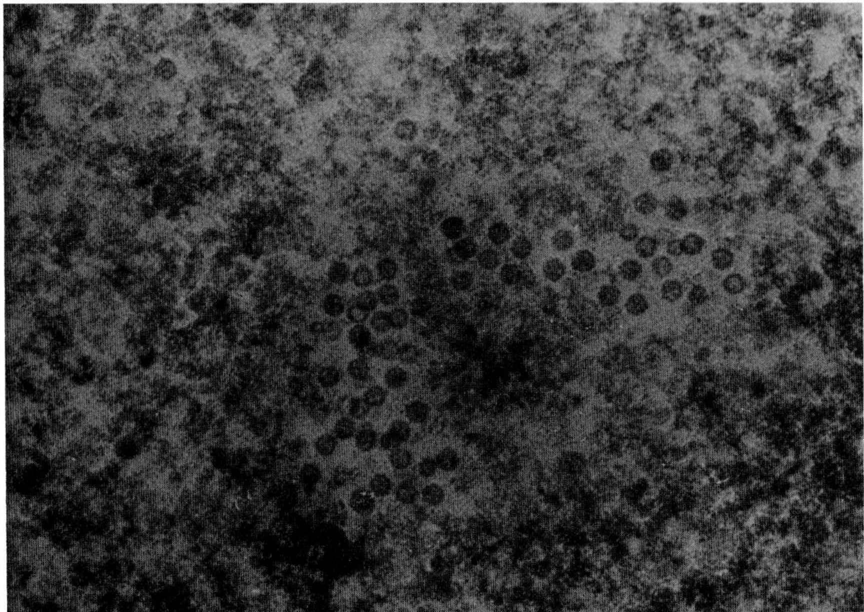

Figure 1. Twenty-seven-nm HBcAg particles visible by electron microscopy in the nucleus of a hepatocyte from a chimpanzee experimentally infected with HBV (×25,000).

sium chloride gradient (density 1.2–1.5 g/cm³) and centrifuged at 23,000 rpm for 16 hr. HBcAg banded at a density of 1.32 g/cm³ and was found by radioimmunoassay to be free of both chimpanzee serum components and chimpanzee liver antigens by agar gel diffusion and complement fixation.

C. Immune Responses in Guinea Pigs

Antibody and delayed cutaneous hypersensitivity responses to the two particulate hepatitis B antigens (HBsAg and HBcAg) were studied in guinea pigs (Gerety *et al.*, 1974). HBsAg was purified from plasma of an asymptomatic human HBsAg carrier by a series of two isopycnic and one rate zonal ultracentrifugations in cesium chloride. Hartley guinea pigs were inoculated subcutaneously with 0.1 cm³ of various dilutions of either plasma-derived HBsAg or liver-derived HBcAg emulsified in complete Freund's adjuvant. The animals were bled at 13 days and their sera tested for anti-HBs, for anti-HBc (Hoofnagle *et al.*, 1973), for antibodies to normal chimpanzee serum by counterelectrophoresis and agar gel diffusion, and for antibodies to control liver homogenate from an uninfected chimpanzee by both complement fixation and counterelectrophoresis.

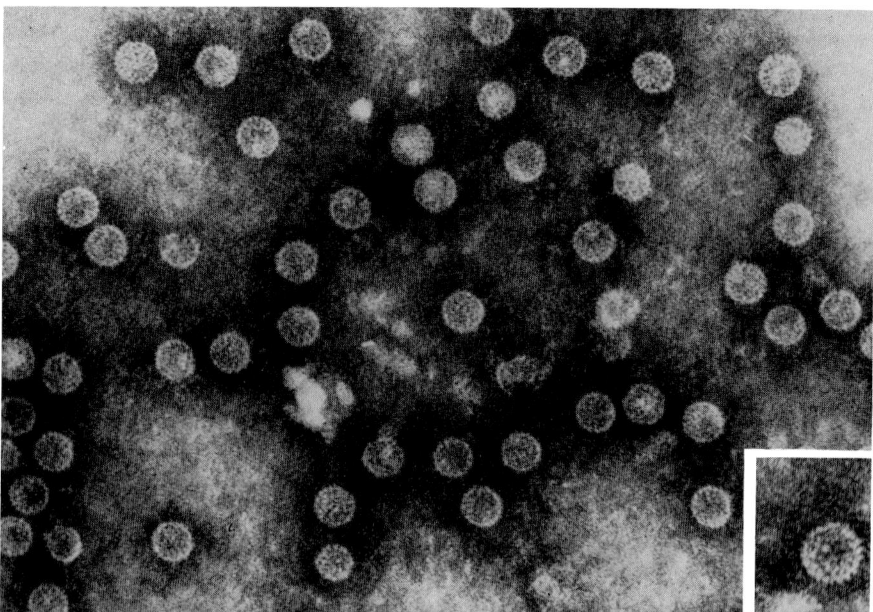

Figure 2. Purified HBcAg particles obtained at a density of 1.32 g/cm³ in CsCl. The purity of the preparation and the morphology of the core particles are shown. The average diameter of the particles is 27 nm; occasional particles are only 20 nm in diameter (×230,000). The inset shows a single core particle at a higher magnification (×350,000). Here the distinctive subunit construction of HBcAg is visible. (From Barker *et al.*, 1974.)

On day 14, the animals were skin-tested with either purified HBsAg and its control antigen (normal human serum diluted 1:50) or with purified HBcAg and its control antigen (uninoculated chimpanzee liver prepared identically to the HBcAg antigen by ultracentrifugation). Skin tests were read at 24 hr; positive responses were those that possessed 10 mm of induration or greater in excess of control reactions. A subset of animals were skin tested with both HBsAg and HBcAg.

Both antigens appeared capable of inducing antibody responses without any apparent cross-reactivity. Little or no delayed skin reactivity to HBsAg could be elicited in HBsAg-immunized guinea pigs, however. Animals immunized with HBsAg developed anti-HBs and no anti-HBc; they showed no skin reactivity to HBcAg. Guinea pigs immunized with HBcAg developed anti-HBc and delayed skin reactivity to HBcAg in the absence of anti-HBs or skin reactivity to HBsAg. Hyperimmunization of guinea pigs with each of these antigens produced only anti-HBs in HBsAg-immunized animals and only anti-HBc in HBcAg-immunized animals.

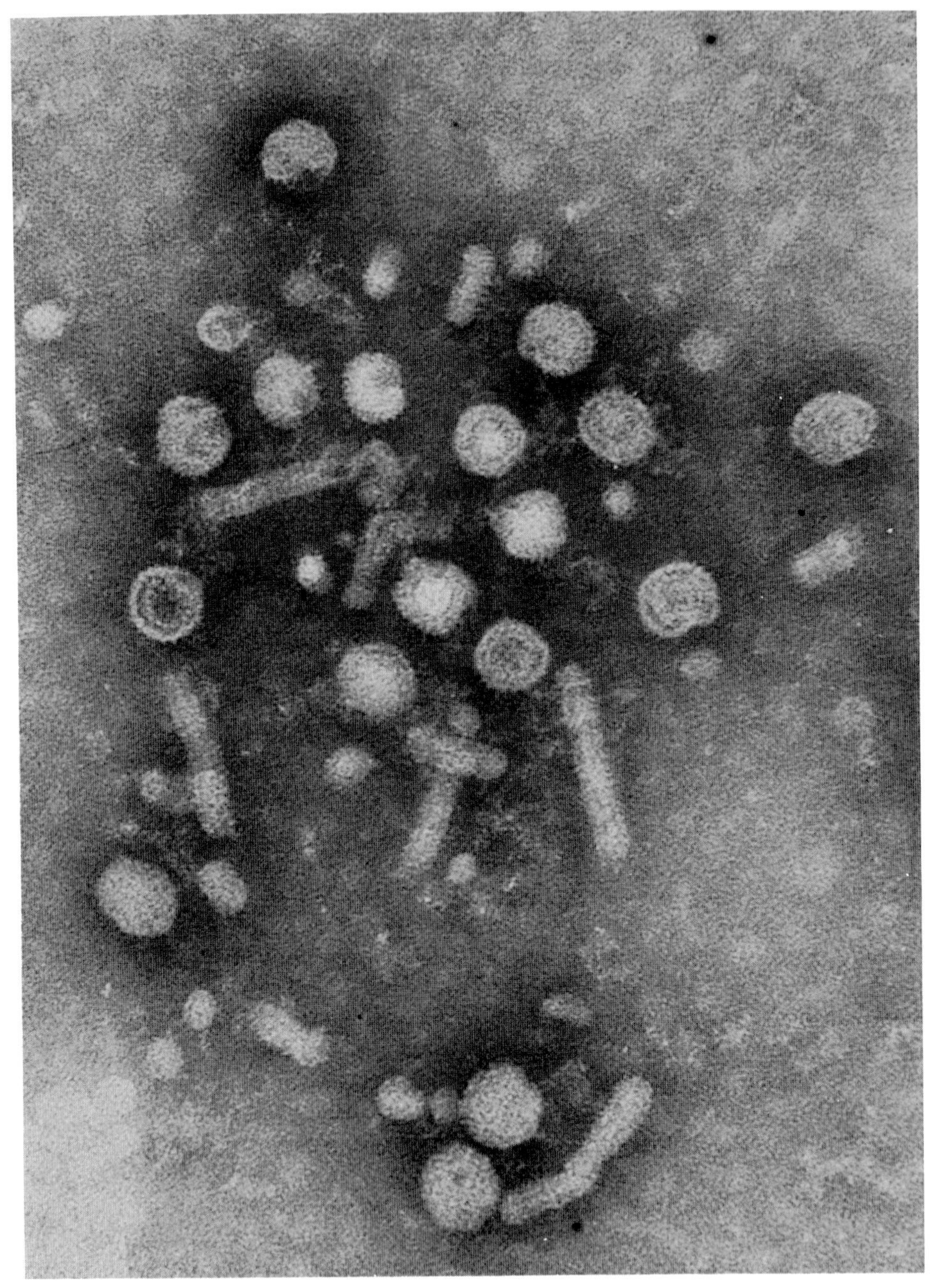

D. Immunoelectron Microscopic Studies

The specificity of the antibody responses elicited by either HBsAg or HBcAg was demonstrated by Almeida using immunoelectron microscopy (Almeida *et al.*, 1971) (Figs. 3 and 4). HBV-rich, HBsAg-positive serum was treated with Tween-80 and reacted with various animal antisera. When guinea pig anti-HBs was allowed to react with disrupted HBV particles, antibody was seen attached to the outer surface of the HBV, but no antibody was seen attached to the inner, core particles. When guinea pig anti-HBc was allowed to react with these disrupted HBV particles, antibody was seen attached to the inner, core component but not to the outer, surface component. When 27-nm core particles purified from the liver of an infected chimpanzee were reacted with hyperimmune chimpanzee anti-HBs, no agglutination or antibody coating of particles was seen. When chimpanzee anti-HBc was reacted with purified HBcAg preparations, particles were aggregated and coated with antibody. Additional experiments using antisera raised in guinea pigs and rabbits confirmed the immumological identity of the internal component of HBV and the 27-nm core particle purified from liver (Fig. 5) (Barker *et al.*, 1974).

E. Fluorescence Microscopic Studies

Confirmation of the morphological and immunological distinction between HBsAg and HBcAg came from immunofluorescence staining patterns seen in infected liver cells using sera containing anti-HBs, anti-HBc, or both of these antibodies. Barker *et al.* (1973) described the cytoplasmic localization of HBsAg in hepatocytes of a chronically infected chimpanzee using fluorescein-conjugated anti-HBs. Using a similar technique, HBcAg was localized in the nuclei of hepatocytes in liver biopsies from experimentally infected chimpanzees. Serial dilutions of anti-HBc, when reacted with human liver biopsy material from patients with hepatitis B, produced exclusively nuclear fluorescence. This nuclear fluorescence could not be removed by preincubation of the anti-HBc with HBsAg in concentrations capable of blocking cytoplasmic (HBsAg) fluorescence elicited with anti-HBs.

In a study of liver biopsies from chimpanzees with experimentally

---

Figure 3. Serum containing all morphological forms of HBsAg including HBV with their internal HBcAg. Anti-HBc has been added but no agglutination is visible as HBcAg is an internal antigen in "untreated" serum. All particles remain dispersed and uncoated (×230,000). (Courtesy of J. D. Almeida.)

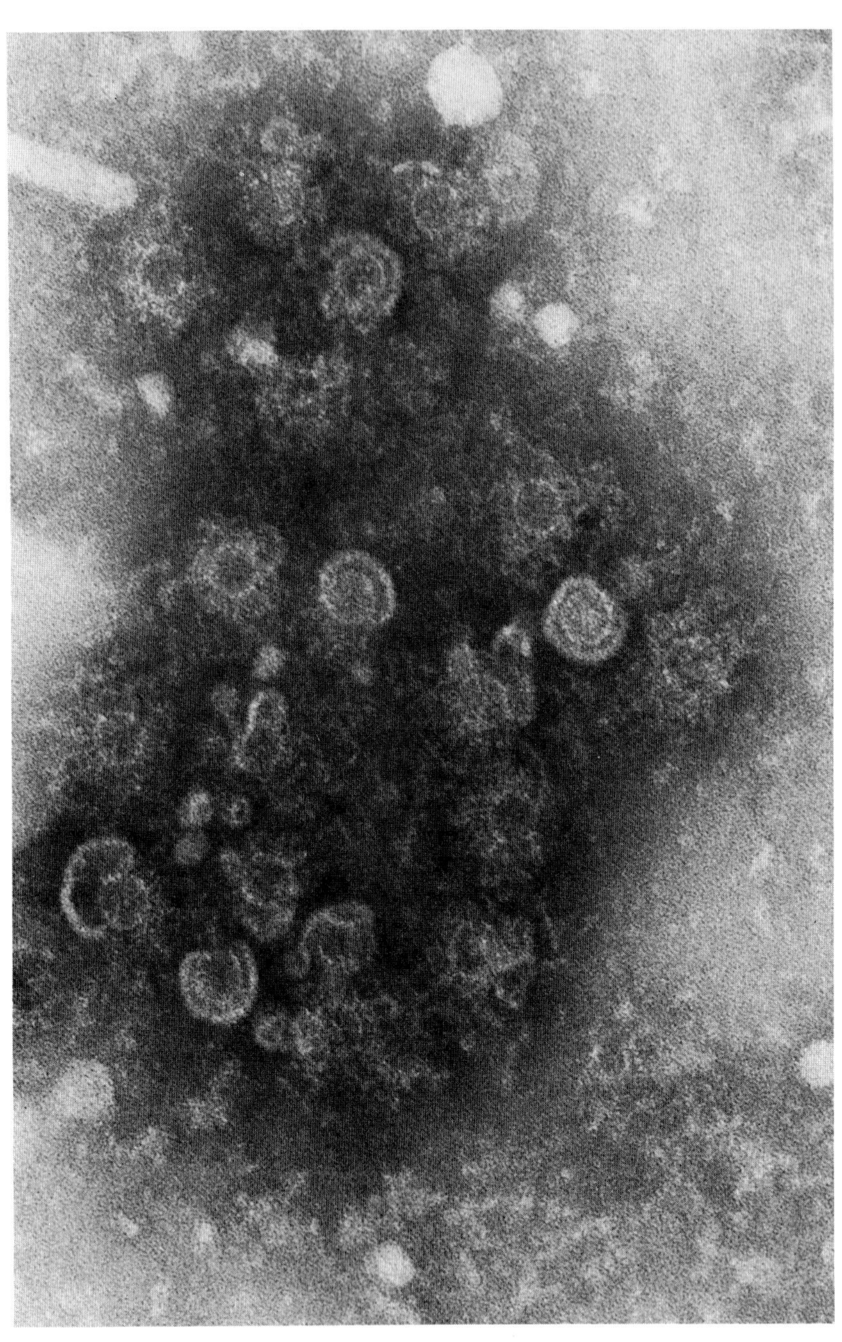

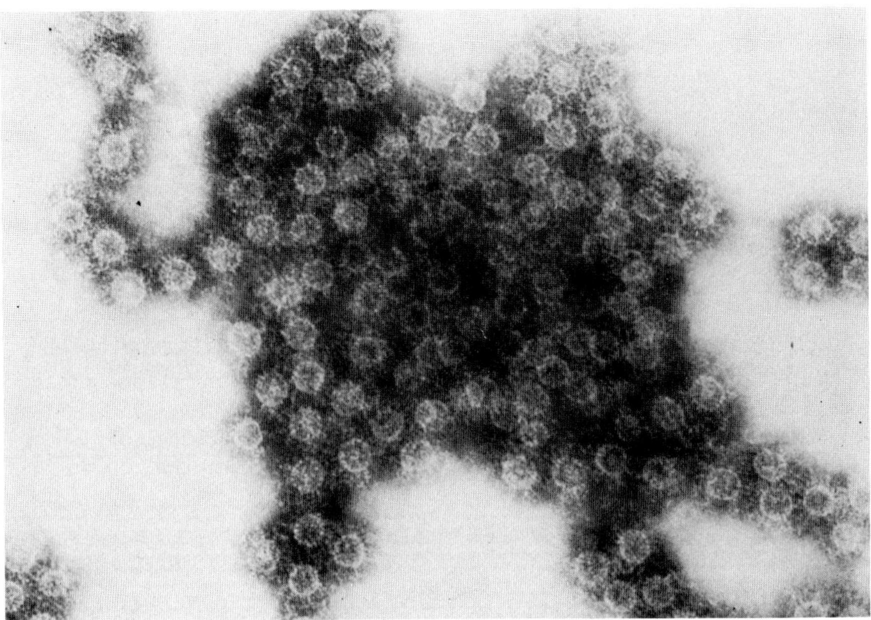

Figure 5. Reaction seen following the addition of anti-HBc to purified HBcAg particles (×158,000). The same antiserum failed to agglutinate HBsAg particles. (From Barker *et al.*, 1974.)

induced hepatitis B (Hoofnagle *et al.*, 1978a), immunofluorescence for HBsAg and HBcAg appeared early in the course of the infection, shortly after the first appearance of HBsAg in the serum and well before the onset of elevated serum aminotranserase activity and light microscopic histopathological changes of hepatitis in liver biopsies. The immunofluorescence usually disappeared at the time of peak serum aminotransferase activities and liver cell morphological changes, but before the disappearance of serum HBsAg. The pattern of reactivity—whether predominantly HBsAg or HBcAg or both—remained constant over the course of the infection for any one chimpanzee and did not appear to be correlated with either the clinical severity of the hepatitis or the presence or absence of hepatitis Be antigen. The occurrence of peak serum aminotransferase activities and clinical disease at the time of disappearance or diminution of hepatic HBsAg and HBcAg expression is consistent

Figure 4. Anti-HBc has been added to HBV particles that have been disrupted by detergent treatment. Antibody has not agglutinated the morphological forms of HBsAg, but can be seen attached to the internal component of the disrupted HBV particles (×230,000). (Courtesy of J. D. Almeida.)

with the concept that tissue injury in hepatitis B is not the result of a direct cytopathic effect of the virus, but is more likely the result of an indirect, host-mediated effect involved in the immune clearance of viral antigens.

III. Physical and Chemical Characterization

A. Ultracentrifugation Studies

HBcAg purified from hepatocyte nuclei from the liver of an experimentally infected chimpanzee banded at 1.30 to 1.32 gm/cm^3 in CsCl in an ultracentrifuge (Barker *et al.*, 1974). The absence of electron-dense centers in these HBcAg particles revealed by the electron microscope, however, suggested that these HBcAg particles did not contain nucleic acid, and that HBcAg particles with nucleic acid would band at a higher density. Indeed, when HBcAg particles were later purified by detergent release from intact serum-derived HBV, two discrete populations of HBcAg particles were identified on the basis of their different densities in an ultracentrifuge in CsCl (Kaplan *et al.*, 1976). The less dense particles had a density of ~1.30 gm/cm^3, similar to the liver-derived HBcAg particles described earlier by Barker *et al.* (1974). The more dense, nucleic acid-bearing particles had a density of 1.36 gm/cm^3; these particles have been shown to contain HBV DNA.

B. Chemical Characterization

Polypeptides derived from the less dense (1.30 gm/cm^3) HBcAg particles as well as the more dense particles (1.36 gm/cm^3) purified either from serum (HBV) or from the nuclei of infected hepatocytes have been chemically characterized by a number of investigators (Budkowska *et al.*, 1979; Hruska and Robinson, 1977; Takahashi *et al.*, 1979). In all of these studies, the major polypeptide component of HBcAg (usually designated P19) was found to be between 16,000 and 19,000 daltons. The amino acid sequence of this polypeptide has been deduced from the nucleotide sequence corresponding to the portion of the HBV genome that codes for HBcAg (Tiollais *et al.*, 1981). This polypeptide, composed of 183 to 185 amino acids, is usually represented by two segments. The initial 140 amino acid residues of the amino-terminal end of the polypeptide exhibit a protamine-like structure with repeating arginines separated by serine and proline (Nakano *et al.*, 1976). It is this latter segment that probably is involved in binding to the HBV DNA molecule. In addition to the major polypeptide described above, several minor polypeptides with molecular weights between 35,000 and 200,000 daltons have been identified by investigators studying HBcAg.

C. Associated Nucleic Acid and Enzyme Activities

Within the HBcAg particles resides the genome of the HBV. This genome consists of a double-stranded, circular DNA of which one strand is always incomplete (see Chapter 15). The total genome of HBV has been cloned and sequenced. Systems for the expression of HBcAg in prokaryotic as well as eukaryotic cells have been developed. HBcAg has been synthesized in *Escherichia coli* by the insertion of cloned HBV DNA contained in a plasmid vector. HBcAg in crude bacterial extracts of these *E. coli* has been used in both radioimmunoassays and enzyme immunoassays to detect anti-HBc (F. Dienhardt, personal communication).

A DNA-dependent DNA polymerase specific for HBV is located within the HBV core particles. Its presence correlates directly with the number of infectious HBV in a given serum. This DNA polymerase has provided a specific marker for HBV infectivity in serum, and has been used effectively to monitor the effects of experimental therapies used to treat patients with chronic hepatitis B (see Chapter 10).

A protein phosphokinase activity has also been described associated with HBcAg particles (Albin and Robinson, 1980). It has been shown that this protein phosphokinase phosphorylates the major peptide (P19) of HBcAg (see Chapter 15).

IV. Relationship to HBeAg/Anti-HBe

HBcAg is found in serum only within HBV particles; it has never been detected free in serum during either acute or chronic hepatitis B. Alternatively, HBeAg is found free in serum, and until recently it was not thought to be present within the core of HBV particles. Each of these antigens, however, has been shown to be directly correlated with the amount of infectivity in a given serum.

In 1979, Takahashi *et al.* detected HBeAg activity in a solublized preparation of HBcAg particles treated with 2-mercaptoethanol and SDS. With the appearance of the HBeAg activity, there was a loss of detectable HBcAg. Furthermore, polypeptides extracted from this HBcAg preparation on SDS gels by electrophoresis exhibited HBeAg activity. Similarly, Neurath and Strick (1979) treated HBcAg with 3 *M* sodium thiocyanate and obtained monomeric HBeAg, while Budkowska *et al.* (1979) treated liver-derived HBcAg with 2-mercaptoethanol and SDS to release HBeAg activity. Ohori *et al.* (1979) treated intact HBV with Sarkosyl to release HBeAg activity from high-density particles only. With the appearance of HBeAg activity, there was no loss of HBcAg activity, however.

Studies involving the purification of HBeAg (Blanchy *et al.*, 1980; Katz *et al.*, 1980; Tedder and Bull, 1979) revealed that HBeAg is a small polypeptide of 17,000 to 20,000 daltons with an affinity for IgG molecules. The molecular weight of HBeAg is obviously similar to that of HBcAg. A study by MacKay *et al.* (1981) attempted to answer the question of whether HBeAg is a unique component of HBV core particles or whether it is a derivative of HBcAg. In this study, HBcAg synthesized in *E. coli* carrying a plasmid containing only the HBcAg gene of HBV was studied. Once again, HBcAg produced by plasmid-containing *E. coli* was converted to HBeAg by proteolytic degradation under dissociating conditions utilizing SDS, pronase E, and 2-mercaptoethanol. These data appear to confirm at the molecular level that HBeAg is related to and most likely derived from HBcAg. The authors hypothesized that HBcAg not bound within the core of HBV may be sensitive to proteolysis in plasma or liver resulting in the conversion of HBcAg to HBeAg (MacKay *et al.*, 1981).

V. Tests to Detect HBcAg/Anti-HBc

A. HBcAg

Tests to detect HBcAg have been developed. These tests include sophisticated methods such as immunoelectron microscopy (IEM), radioimmunoassay (RIA), and immunofluorescence (IF), as well as less sensitive counterelectrophoresis (CEP). Tests to detect HBcAg, however, are restricted to studies of liver biopsy material, HBcAg particles purified from infected liver cells, and sera of chronic hepatitis B patients after detergent treatment to release HBcAg from within HBV. Tests for HBcAg can thus be used to identify sera with high concentrations of HBV or liver tissue suitable for extraction of HBcAg for use in *in vitro* tests to detect anti-HBc. Tests for HBcAg, however, are seldom used to diagnose hepatitis B since this internal antigen is not present in serum except as the internal, normally unavailable antigen within HBV.

B. Anti-HBc

Tests to detect anti-HBc include CEP, complement fixation (CF), and RIA. In 1974, Budkowska *et al.* described a CEP test which detected anti-

HBc in the sera of 40 patients with hepatitis B. The specificity of this antigen–antibody reaction was confirmed when EM analysis of the immunoprecipitin lines revealed HBcAg particles agglutinated by anti-HBc present in the patients' sera being tested. The disadvantages of CEP, a method known not to be particularly sensitive when used to detect antibody, include the relatively large amount of HBcAg required and its limited sensitivity.

CF also requires a large amount of HBcAg, but has the advantage over CEP of not requiring highly purified HBcAg (Hoofnagle *et al.*, 1973). Using CF, anti-HBc was detected in 1% of volunteer blood donors, 8% of paid blood donors, 13% of hemophiliacs, and 100% of chronic hepatitis B carriers (Hoofnagle *et al.*, 1973). Thus, this CF test documented the universal presence of anti-HBc coexisting with infectious HBV in the sera of all hepatitis B carriers.

RIA has the advantage of greatly increased sensitivity over CEP and CF. The available competitive-inhibition RIA adds the advantage of utilizing extremely small quantities of HBcAg. In competitive-inhibition RIA, anti-HBc in tested sera interferes with (competes with) a preformed sandwich consisting of HBcAg–anti-HBc–radiolabeled HBcAg. A direct comparison between CF and RIA for anti-HBc detection was accomplished by Gerety *et al.* in 1978, who tested sera from 129 patients with hemophilia A. Using CF, 27% had anti-HBc; using RIA, 81% had anti-HBc; 78% also had anti-HBs.

Recently, a direct RIA test to detect anti-HBc was described (W. H. Gerlich, personal communication, 1983). In this test, flexible microtiter plates were coated with HBcAg; test sera and finally ^{32}P-labeled HBcAg, were added. The ^{32}P labeling of HBcAg is accomplished by using the endogenous protein phosphokinase activity of HBV. A direct RIA has obvious advantages over competitive-inhibition RIAs with regard to specificity. The sensitivity of this direct RIA has been reported to be 10 times greater than that of a competitive-inhibition assay.

VI. Clinical and Immunological Significance

A. Anti-HBc

Of persons with acute hepatitis B, 90–95% will have HBsAg detectable in their serum when they first present themselves for medical assistance; this leaves 5–10% of acute hepatitis B undiagnosable by HBsAg testing (Hoofnagle *et al.*, 1978b; Kryger *et al.*, 1982; Lemon *et al.*, 1981). If there is a delay in seeking medical assistance, the percentage of undiagnosable

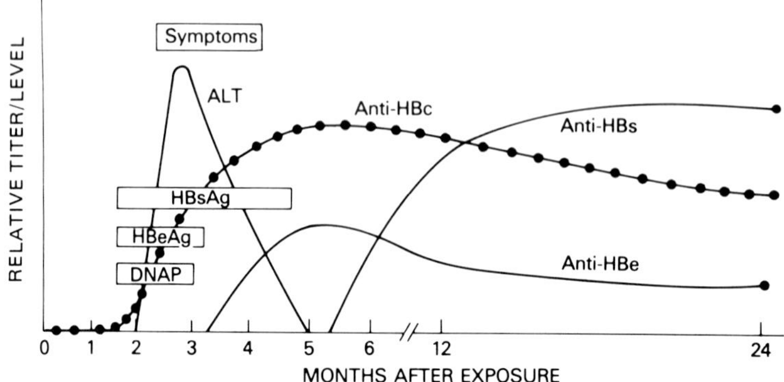

Figure 6. Serological responses in acute hepatitis B. Note the persistence of anti-HBc (and anti-HBe and anti-HBs) long after recovery. ALT, serum aminotransferase activity; HBsAg, hepatitis B surface antigen; HBeAg, hepatitis B e antigen; DNAP, hepatitis B specific DNA polymerase; anti-HBc, antibody to HBcAg; anti-HBs, antibody to HBsAg; anti-HBe, antibody to HBeAg.

acute hepatitis B cases increases proportionately to the delay. In virtually all acute hepatitis B cases, however, anti-HBc is present just after the appearance of HBsAg, during the period when HBsAg persists, and after HBsAg clears (in acute hepatitis B with recovery) (Fig. 6). In addition, anti-HBc is present in virtually all patients with chronic hepatitis B (Fig. 7). If anti-HBc is present during acute hepatitis B and during chronic hepatitis B, why is not anti-HBc used to diagnose hepatitis B? This is because anti-HBc is also present during convalescence and long after recovery from HBV infection (here it usually coexists with the antibody

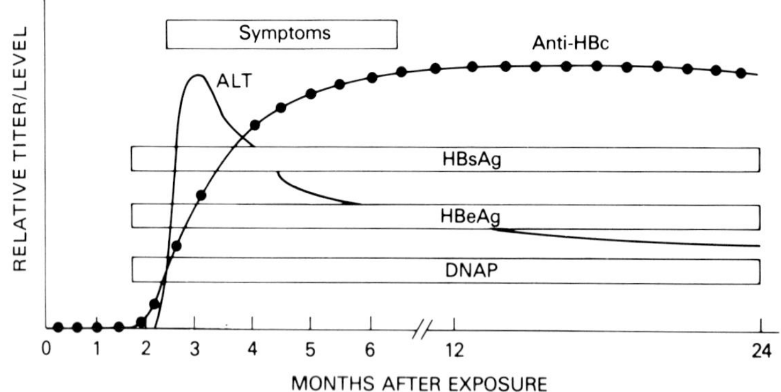

Figure 7. Serological responses in chronic hepatitis B. Note the persistence of anti-HBc (and the absence of anti-HBs) when HBsAg/HBeAg/DNAP all persist. (Abbreviations are explained in Fig. 6.)

TABLE I
Serodiagnostic Profiles in Hepatitis B[a]

| | Serological reactivity | | | Most likely |
Pattern	HBsAg	Anti-HBc	Anti-HBs	diagnosis(es)
1	+	−	−	Early acute hepatitis B (prior to symptoms)
2	+	+	−	Acute hepatitis B
	+	++[b]	−	Chronic hepatitis B
3	−	+	+	Recovered from hepatitis B
4	−	+	−	Long after hepatitis B
	−	++[b]	−	Convalescence in a "low level" chronic hepatitis B carrier
5	−	−	+	Long after hepatitis B
			+ or ++[b]	Immunization with HBsAg (i.e., vaccine)

[a]Adapted from Hoofnagle et al., 1978a.
[b]High titer.

of recovery and immunity, anti-HBs) (Fig. 6). Serodiagnostic profiles can be very complicated but have been summarized adequately in Hoofnagle et al. (1978a) and Overby et al. (1982) (see also Table I).

As early as 1974, it was shown that anti-HBc was a sensitive indicator of past or ongoing HBV replication (Hoofnagle et al., 1974). In addition, it was proposed that detection of anti-HBc in the absence of either HBsAg or anti-HBs might indicate ongoing hepatitis B virus infections in which there were subdetectable levels of serum HBsAg. This proposal remains attractive, although it is clear that persons possessing this serological profile are not usually infectious. Indeed, chimpanzees inoculated with such sera have never contracted hepatitis B (R. J. Gerety, unpublished data).

To screen blood donors for anti-HBc in the absence of either HBsAg or anti-HBs has been proposed as a means to prevent the few cases of hepatitis B (~1%) that occur in recipients of blood transfusions despite testing all donor blood for HBsAg. This proposal is based on retrospective studies suggesting that this serological profile is associated with the transmission of hepatitis B to recipients of their blood (Hoofnagle et *al.*, 1978c). Early data provided by the TTV Study Group indicated that hepatitis B occurred in 14% of recipients of anti-HBc-positive blood, compared to <1% of recipients of blood also positive for anti-HBs (Rakela *et al.*, 1980). Clearly, many blood donors with anti-HBc alone do not circulate infectious HBV in their blood; most have recovered from HBV infection and no longer have detectable anti-HBs.

Stevens *et al.* (1981) reported that 27% of recipients of blood containing anti-HBc developed non-A, non-B hepatitis in their study, while only 8% of recipients of blood negative for anti-HBc did so. This has lead some to suggest that anti-HBc testing of prospective blood donors could reduce the incidence of posttransfusion non-A, non-B hepatitis. The results of Stevens *et al.* most likely reflect the epidemiological association between HBV and the non-A, non-B hepatitis agents and the known proclivity of the latter agent to produce asymptomatic, chronic infections. Screening blood donors for anti-HBc would clearly also identify those immune to hepatitis B, a group that represents a significant percentage of donors in many areas and blood centers and whose plasma is used to make hepatitis B immune globulin.

B. IgM Anti-HBc

Tests to detect anti-HBc of the IgM subclass have been proposed and discussed for use in the differential diagnosis of acute versus chronic hepatitis B, in differentiating acute non-A, non-B hepatitis in those with preexisting chronic hepatitis B, and in providing a prognosis to patients with chronic hepatitis B. Chau *et al.* (1983) found that if a specific test for IgM anti-HBc was used (serum diluted 1:5000 prior to testing to eliminate false positives due to persistent low-level IgM anti-HBc long after acute hepatitis B), they could effectively separate acute from chronic hepatitis B infections. Their data confirm that high titers of IgM anti-HBc persist in acute hepatitis B for only a few months, but that low-titer IgM anti-HBc may persist long beyond acute HBV infection. Others, however, have not been so successful in differentiating between acute and chronic hepatitis B cases on the basis of IgM anti-HBc alone (Gerlich *et al.*, 1980; Lemon *et al.*, 1981; Roggendorf *et al.*, 1981).

Testing for IgM anti-HBc has also been used to differentiate between patients with acute hepatitis B and those with concurrent chronic hepatitis B and acute non-B hepatitis (Feinman *et al.*, 1982; Widell *et al.*, 1982). In patients with chronic hepatitis B, the titers of IgM anti-HBc are usually low. As a result, investigators were able to report that IgM anti-HBc correlated with high levels of HBV replication (Roggendorf *et al.*, 1981), with the biological activity of chronic hepatitis B (Feinman *et al.*, 1982), and even with the presence of hepatocellular carcinoma (Roggendorf *et al.*, 1981).

C. HBcAg

Anti-HBc is common in hepatitis B. It is present in the sera of all cases of acute hepatitis B, in all cases of chronic hepatitis B, and in all cases of recently recovered from hepatitis B. Anti-HBc is directly related to HBV replication and coexists with infectious HBV in serum. It is passively transferred via the placenta to newborns of hepatitis B carriers and does not provide immunity to these newborns. Given these facts, it is difficult to make a case for anti-HBc participating in immunity against hepatitis B.

It is not difficult, however, to make a good case for the participation of cell-mediated immune responses to HBcAg in protection against or recovery from hepatitis B. Anti-HBs alone, as we know, can be sufficient to prevent HBV infection, but what terminates the infection once established in the liver? Judging from passive immunization studies, extremely large volumes of high-titer anti-HBs serum, plasma, or globulin do not alter fulminant hepatitis B or chronic HBV infections. HBsAg appears not capable of inducing good cell-mediated immune response either in laboratory animals (Gerety *et al.*, 1974) or in humans (J. H. Hoofnagle, personal communication). This leaves cell-mediated immune responses to HBcAg as responsible for the termination of hepatitis B infections. Can these responses prevent hepatitis B? Tabor and Gerety (1984) recently reported that immunization with HBcAg in Freund's adjuvant either modified or prevented hepatitis B in chimpanzees first immunized and then challenged intravenously with infectious HBV. HBcAg, for a variety of reasons, has been overlooked as an immunogen (vaccine component) in hepatitis B. When further studies are completed using genetically derived HBcAg, the role of this antigen in immunity against hepatitis B will be clear. At that time, HBcAg, in addition to HBsAg (current vaccines), may represent the vaccine of the future against hepatitis B.

References

Albin, C., and Robinson, W. S. (1980). *J. Virol.* **34**, 297–302.
Almeida, J. D., Rubenstein, D., and Stott, E. J. (1971). *Lancet 2*, 1225–1227.
Barker, L. F., Chisari, F. V., McGrath, P. P., Dalgard, D. W., Kirschstein, R. L., Almeida,

J. D., Edgington, T. S., Sharp, D. G., and Peterson, M. R. (1973). *J. Infect. Dis.* **127,** 649–662.

Barker, L. F., Almeida, J. D., Hoofnagle, J. H., Gerety, R. J., Jackson, D. R., and McGrath, P. P. (1974). *J. Virol.* **14,** 1552–1558.

Blanchy, B., Hantz, O., Vitvitsky, L., and Trepo, C. (1980). *J. Med. Virol.* **5,** 39–46.

Brzosko, W. J., Madalinski, K., Krawczynski, K., and Nowoslawski, A. (1973). *J. Infect. Dis.* **127,** 424–428.

Budkowska, A., Walicka, B., Domaniewska, G., and Brzosko, W. J. (1974). *N. Engl. J. Med.* **290,** 1489–1490.

Budkowska, A., Kalinowska, B., and Nowoslawski, A. (1979). *J. Immunol.* **123,** 1415–1416.

Chau, K. H., Hargie, M. P., Decker, R. H., Mushawar, I. K., and Overby, L. R. (1983). *Hepatology (N.Y.)* **3,** 142–149.

Feinman, S. V., Overby, L. R., Berris, B., Chau, K., Schable, C. A., and Maynard, J. E. (1982). *Hepatology (N.Y.)* **2,** 795–799.

Gerety, R. J., Hoofnagle, J. H., Barker, L. F. (1974). *J. Immunol.* **113,** 1223–1228.

Gerety, R. J., Tabor, E., Hoofnagle, J. H., Mitchell, F., and Barker, L. F. (1978). *In* "Viral Hepatitis" (G. N. Vyas, S. N. Cohen, and R. Schmid, eds.), pp. 121–138. Franklin Inst. Press, Philadelphia, Pennsylvania.

Gerlich, W. H., Lüer, W., Thomssen, R., and the Study Group for Viral Hepatitis of the Deutsche Forschungsgemeinshaft (1980). *J. Infect. Dis.* **142,** 95–101.

Hoofnagle, J. H., Gerety, R. J., and Barker, L. F. (1973). *Lancet* 2, 869–873.

Hoofnagle, J. H., Gerety, R. J., Ni, L. Y., and Barker, L. F. (1974). *N. Engl. J. Med.* **290,** 1336–1340.

Hoofnagle, J. H., Michalak, T., Nowoslawski, A., Gerety, R. J., and Barker, L. F. (1978a). *Gastroenterology* **74,** 182–187.

Hoofnagle, J. H., Seeff, L. B., Bales, Z. B., Gerety, R. J., and Tabor, E. (1978b). *In* "Viral Hepatitis" (G. N. Vyas, S. N. Cohen, and R. Schmid, eds.), pp. 219–242. Franklin Inst. Press, Philadelphia, Pennsylvania.

Hoofnagle, J. H., Seeff, L. B., Bayles, Z. B., Zimmerman, H. J., and the Veterans Administration Hepatitis Cooperative Study Group (1978c). *N. Engl. J. Med.* **298,** 1379–1383.

Hruska, J. F., and Robinson, W. S. (1977). *J. Med. Virol.* **1,** 119–131.

Kaplan, P. M., Ford, E. C., Purcell, R. H., and Gerin, J. L. (1976). *J. Virol.* **17,** 885–893.

Katz, D., Melnick, J. L., and Hollinger, F. B. (1980). *J. Med. Virol.* **5,** 87–100.

Kryger, P., Aldershvile, J., Mathiesen, L. R., Nielsen, O., and the Copenhagen Hepatitis Acuta Programme (1982). *Hepatology* **2,** 50–53.

Lemon, S. M., Gates, N. L., Simms, T. E., and Bancroft, W. H. (1981). *J. Infect. Dis.* **143,** 803–809.

MacKay, P., Lees, J., and Murray, K. (1981). *J. Med. Virol.* **8,** 237–243.

Markenson, J. A., Gerety, R. J., Hoofnagle, J. H., and Barker, L. F. (1975). *J. Infect. Dis.* **131,** 79–87.

Nakano, M., Tobita, T., and Ando, T. (1976). *Int. J. Pept. Protein Res.* **8,** 565–578.

Neurath, A. R., and Strick, N. (1979). *J. Gen. Virol.* **42,** 645–649.

Ohori, H., Onodera, S., and Ishida, N. (1979). *J. Gen. Virol.* **43,** 423–427.

Overby, L. R., Ling, C.-H., Decker, R. H., Mushawar, I. K., and Chau, K. (1982). *In* "Viral Hepatitis" (W. Szmuness, H. J. Alter, and J. E. Maynard, eds.), pp. 169–182. Franklin Inst. Press, Philadelphia, Pennsylvania.

Rakela, J., Mosley, J. W., Aach, R. D., Gitnick, G. L., Hollinger, F. B., Stevens, C. E., and Szmuness, W. (1980). *Gastroenterology* **78,** 1318.

Roggendorf, M., Deinhardt, F., Frösner, G. G., Scheid, R., Bayerl, B., and Zachoval, R. (1981). *J. Clin. Microbiol.* **13,** 618–626.

Stevens, C. E., and the Transfusion-Transmitted Viruses Study Group (1981). *Transfusion (Philadelphia)* **21,** 607.

Tabor, E., and Gerety, R. J. (1984). *Lancet 1,* 172.

Takahashi, K., Akahane, Y., Gotanda, T., Miashiro, T., Imai, M., Miyakawa, Y., and Mayumi, M. (1979). *J. Immunol.* **122,** 275–279.

Tedder, R. S., and Bull, F. G. (1979). *Clin. Exp. Immunol.* **35,** 380–389.

Tiollais, P., Charnay, P., and Vyas, G. N. (1981). *Science* **213,** 406–411.

Widell, A., Hansson, B. G., Lofgren, B., Moestrup, T., Norkrans, G., Johnsson, T., and Nordenfelt, E. (1982). *Acta Pathol. Microbiol. Scand.* **90,** 79–84.

Chapter 4

Hepatitis B e Antigen and Antibody (HBeAg/Anti-HBe)

YUZO MIYAKAWA
The Third Department of Internal Medicine
Faculty of Medicine
University of Tokyo
Hongo, Tokyo, Japan

MAKOTO MAYUMI
Immunology Division
Jichi Medical School
Minamikawachi-Machi
Tochigi-ken, Japan

I. Introduction

Curiosity has often led to important discoveries in the history of medical research. In an Ouchterlony immunodiffusion plate, Magnius and Espmark (1972) gazed not only between two wells each containing HBsAg or anti-HBs, but also between two wells both containing HBsAg.

47

Copyright © 1985 by Academic Press, Inc.
All rights of reproduction in any form reserved.
ISBN 0-12-280672-7

Precipitin lines were observed and they designated the antigen as HBeAg. Thus, HBeAg was added to the scene 7 years after the discovery of HBsAg by Blumberg *et al.* (1965) and 1 year after Almeida and co-workers (1971) introduced HBcAg. It is not clear why Magnius and Espmark picked the letter e to denote the new hepatitis B-associated antigen they discovered, although we understand that they had to avoid the letters which had already been assigned to represent the antigenic determinants encountered in HBV infection, such as **a, c, d, r, w, x,** and **y**.

HBeAg entered the picture as something very important both clinically and epidemiologically, but its nature remained desperately uncertain. Due to its ambiguous character, HBeAg was once compared to an elephant (which starts with the letter e) being touched by seven blindfolded men. Someone thought that e stood for enigmatic. At present, 12 years after the discovery of HBeAg, we know that HBeAg represents the antigenic determinants of a nucleopeptide (P19) coded for by the genome of HBV. Indeed, the disclosure of the nature and implications of HBeAg accomplished in the past 12 years is a typical example of the manner in which a most challenging problem has been solved by means of multidisciplinary efforts and international cooperation among the many scientists.

II. What Is HBeAg?

A. Detection of HBeAg

Despite its undisputed practical value, the exact nature of HBeAg remained ambiguous for quite some time. Until recently, it was not clear whether HBeAg was specified by the genome of HBV, or if it rather represented the product of a specific response of the host to HBV. This was attributable, to a considerable extent, to the lack of sensitive and specific methods to detect HBeAg. For the first 5 years after the discovery of HBeAg, immunodiffusion had remained as the sole method to detect it. This method is neither sensitive nor objective; the results are subject to the eyes of beholders. Moreover, sera presumed to contain HBeAg sometimes revealed more than one line against anti-HBe reagents, which were interpreted as the subspecificities of HBeAg such as e_1, e_2, and e_3 (Williams and Le Bouvier, 1976; Trepo *et al.*, 1978). This, of course, added more to the mystique of HBeAg.

In 1977, a hemagglutination method was introduced for the detection of HBeAg/anti-HBe with a sensitivity 300-fold higher than that of immunodiffusion (Takahashi *et al.*, 1977). After 1978, RIAs and enzyme immunoassays were developed one after another with a sensitivity more than 1,000-fold higher than that of immunodiffusion (Fields *et al.*, 1978b; Miyakawa *et al.*, 1979; Mushahwar *et al.*, 1981; Smith and Tedder, 1981; Mushahwar and Overby, 1981). These sophisticated methods were quite helpful in understanding the nature of HBeAg.

Immunodiffusion has remained a good method for evaluating the difference in antigenicity. In their early studies, Magnius and Espmark (1972) reported that HBeAg was antigenically different from HBsAg or its subtypic specificities. Takahashi *et al.* (1976) presented evidence for the antigenic distinction between HBeAg and HBcAg (Fig. 1).

B. Association of HBeAg with Serum Proteins

Evidence for the host specificity of HBeAg has been presented repeatedly. Early circumstantial evidence was that of an index-case–contact-case pair, a setting in which HBV of the same strain and virulence was presumed to have infected both cases; HBeAg was found in the serum of

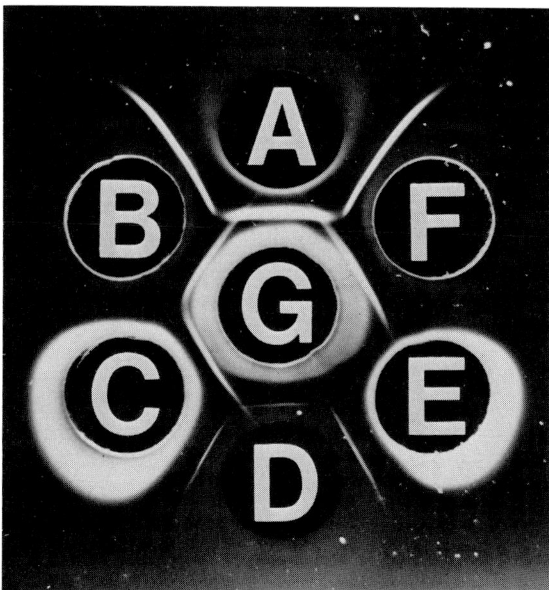

Figure 1. Immunodiffusion pattern showing nonidentity of the HBeAg/anti-HBe, HBcAg/anti-HBc, and HBsAg/anti-HBs systems. A, anti-HBs; B, C, and F, anti-HBe (HBsAg and anti-HBc present also); D, purified HBcAg; E, anti-HBc; G, HBcAg (HBsAg and anti-HBc present also). (From Takahashi *et al.*, 1976.)

one but not in that of the other (Perrillo *et al.*, 1977). Since HBeAg was not necessarily transmitted with HBV infection, Villarejos *et al.* (1978) thought it to be a nontransmissible product or the specific individual response of hosts. Vyas *et al.* (1977) suggested that HBeAg was an isozyme of lactic dehydrogenase. A more direct approach to connect HBeAg with host proteins was attempted by Neurath and Strick (1977), who proposed that HBeAg was idiotypic determinants on antibodies that were formed in response to HBV infection. Further, Fields *et al.* (1978a) suggested it had properties analogous to those of a dimer of IgG. In contradiction to their view, however, HBeAg was detected in the serum of an HBsAg-positive patient with agammaglobulinemia (Chadwick *et al.*, 1978).

Since HBeAg was also found in the serum of chimpanzees experimentally infected with HBV (Aikawa *et al.*, 1978; Tabor *et al.*, 1980a), it would likely represent proteins of nonhuman origins. Failure to detect HBeAg in any sera from 22 patients with posttransfusion hepatitis of non-B origin stood in support of the view that it could be specified by the HBV genome and was not a product of the host raised in response to hepatic injury (Smith *et al.*, 1976). The attempts to clarify the nature of HBeAg, indeed, have given rise to a number of conflicting views.

C. Free and IgG-Bound Forms of HBeAg

Takahashi *et al.* (1978a) reported finding two entities exhibiting HBeAg activity in serum that were different physiocochemically as well as immunologically (Table I). The most conspicuous difference between these two entities was the association of IgG with the large molecular weight HBeAg (Fig. 2). Both "free" small HBeAg and "IgG-bound" large HBeAg gave a line of identity against the well-characterized anti-HBe reagent by immunodiffusion.

The nature of IgG associated with the large molecular weight HBeAg is not yet clear. Large HBeAg may represent either an antigen–antibody complex, that is, HBeAg bound with corresponding antibodies or a result of another protein–protein interaction. There is some circumstantial evidence to support the immune complex nature of large molecular weight HBeAg. Takahashi *et al.* (1979b) observed a shift from small to large molecular weight HBeAg in the serum of individuals infected with HBV either acutely or chronically. Furthermore, in the serum of a chimpanzee experimentally infected with HBV, free HBeAg appeared first. Later, IgG-bound HBeAg emerged, constituting a gradual shift from the free to the IgG-bound form of HBeAg. Finally, IgG-bound HBeAg ac-

TABLE I

Physicochemical Properties of Small and Large Molecular Weight HBeAg in Serum

	Small MW HBeAg	Large MW HBeAg
1.33 M $(NH_4)_2SO_4$	Soluble	Insoluble
Molecular size	$<$ IgG	$>$ IgG
Electrophoretic mobility	α region	$\beta-\gamma$ region
Isoelectric point	4.8	5.7
Association with IgG	No	Yes

counted for all HBeAg activity detectable in the serum; it later disappeared, to be replaced by anti-HBe. This sequence of events, taken together with the electron microscopic observations indicating an immune complex nature of HBeAg (Stannard *et al.*, 1982), appears to imply a possible association of HBeAg and antibody in the large molecular weight HBeAg. Solid evidence has not been obtained in support of this view, however. It has not been possible so far to obtain molecules with antibody activity by dissociating large molecular weight HBeAg.

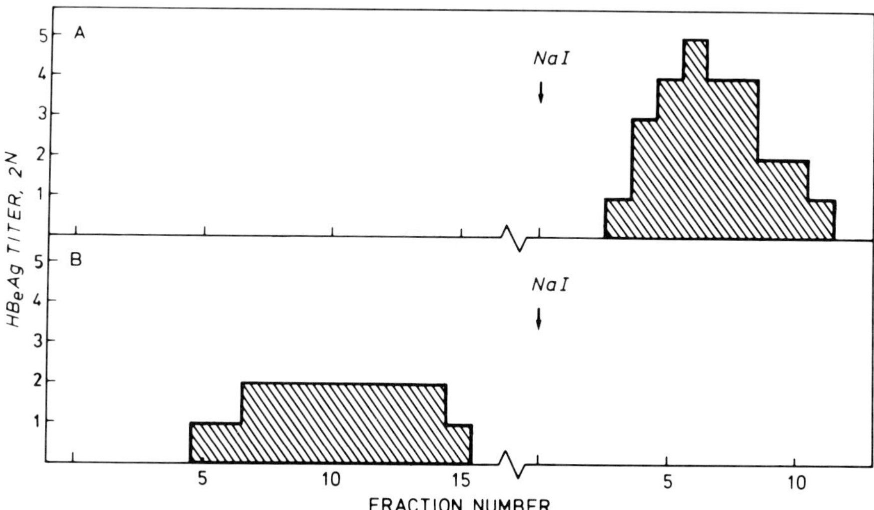

Figure 2. Affinity chromatography of large (A) and small (B) molecular HBeAg on a column of anti-IgG. Shaded areas represent HBeAg activity determined by reversed passive hemagglutination. The arrow indicates the start of elution with 3 M NaI. Large molecular weight HBeAg was trapped on the column and then eluted, while small molecular weight HBeAg just passed through it. (From Takahashi *et al.*, 1978a.)

D. Association of HBeAg and Markers of Dane Particles

HBeAg occurs in the serum of some persons who carry HBsAg. In the serum of other HBsAg-positive persons, anti-HBe is found. There are HBsAg-positive sera that do not show any detectable reactivity of either HBeAg or anti-HBe, depending on the phase of infection as well as on the sensitivity of the methods used to detect HBeAg/anti-HBe.

Dane particles, presently accepted as HBV (Dane *et al.*, 1970), have immunological and biochemical tags, such as HBcAg (Almeida *et al.*, 1971) and HBsAg-associated DNA polymerase (Kaplan *et al.*, 1973). Sera containing HBeAg display a high activity of HBsAg-associated DNA polymerase and HBcAg, contrasting with anti-HBe-positive sera, which show neither activity (Nordenfelt and Kjellen, 1975; Takahashi *et al.*, 1976; Imai *et al.*, 1976). Free DNA capable of annealing to a copy of Dane particle DNA has been found in HBsAg-positive sera containing HBeAg, but rarely in those containing anti-HBe (Werner *et al.*, 1977). Furthermore, Dane particles were detected in large numbers by electron microscopic observations of HBeAg-positive sera, but not (or rarely) in anti-HBe-positive sera (Okada *et al.*, 1976). Dane particles, even when found in anti-HBe-positive sera (Sheikh *et al.*, 1975), were mostly defective, unlike complete ones seen in HBeAg-positive sera (Alberti *et al.*, 1978). Since HBeAg in the serum indicates a high concentration of HBV, HBeAg-positive sera are naturally assumed to contain a high titer of HBsAg (Chien and Vyas, 1978; Sasaki *et al.*, 1979; Nath *et al.*, 1980). These observations provided circumstantial evidence for the close relationship between HBeAg and Dane particles, and helped identify highly infectious sera.

The close association of HBeAg with HBcAg holds true at the tissue level also. HBcAg (Murphy *et al.*, 1976) as well as Dane particles (Kamimura *et al.*, 1981), was detected in liver biopsies from HBsAg carriers with HBeAg in their sera, but not from those with circulating anti-HBe.

E. Localization of HBeAg in Dane Particles

Owing to its apparent close association with Dane particles, HBeAg was inferred to represent the DNA polymerase of HBV, but this turned out not to be the case (Neurath and Strick, 1976). Using immunofluorescence, Trepo *et al.* (1976) reported finding HBeAg in the cytoplasm of hepatocytes infected with HBV. Their findings, however, were soon contradicted by the reports of others who found HBeAg in the nucleus of hepatocytes (Arnold *et al.*, 1977; Yoshizawa *et al.*, 1979).

Neurath *et al.* (1976) announced that Dane particles were precipitated when they had been incubated with anti-HBe employing an immune electron microscopic method. Their findings were so convenient in explaining the apparent lack of infectivity and absence of Dane particles in HBsAg-positive sera containing anti-HBe that they were quoted repeatedly in subsequent papers (Norkrans *et al.*, 1976; Okada *et al.*, 1976). However, two other groups could not reproduce their results (Gerin *et al.*, 1978; Takahashi *et al.*, 1978b). Taken together with the infectivity, albeit at a low level, in some HBsAg-positive sera containing anti-HBe (Berquist *et al.*, 1976; Shikata *et al.*, 1977), it may be concluded that no antigenic sites are available on the surface of Dane particles that react with anti-HBe.

Lam *et al.* (1977) treated Dane-rich material with 0.5% Tween 80 and detected the release of HBeAg by rheophoresis. Since Dane particles were disrupted with their cores exposed by the treatment, this suggested that HBeAg was present between the surface and core of Dane particles. Similarly, Vnek *et al.* (1979) detected HBeAg preferentially in association with Dane particles among variable morphological forms of HBsAg. They noticed that HBeAg activity was potentiated by prior treatment of the Dane particles with Tween 80. Furthermore, when a rabbit was immunized with purified Dane particles, it produced anti-HBe in addition to anti-HBs and anti-HBc (Takahashi *et al.*, 1980). These observations strongly indicated that HBeAg was cryptically present in Dane particles.

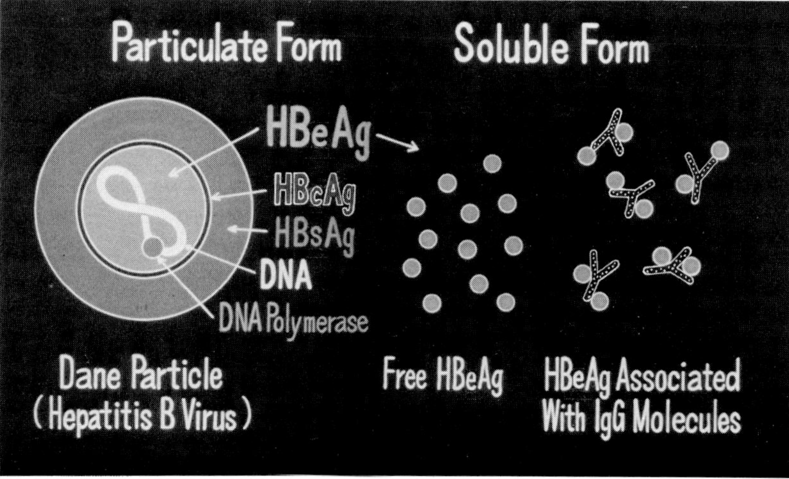

Figure 3. Variable forms of HBeAg in the serum. HBeAg exists in the core of Dane particles and also occurs both free and in association with IgG.

The exact relationship between HBeAg and HBV was uncovered by obtaining polypeptides with HBeAg activity from the cores of Dane particles. Takahashi *et al.* (1979a) purified cores of Dane particles and treated them with 2-mercaptoethanol and sodium dodecylsulphate (SDS). They obtained two major polypeptides with molecular sizes of 19,000 (P19) and 45,000 daltons (P45). Both of them displayed strong antigenicity of HBeAg, but not of HBcAg using conventional test methods. Budkowska *et al.* (1977) obtained a polypeptide of 17,000 daltons from the cores of Dane particles. Hruska and Robinson (1977) demonstrated a polypeptide of 19,000 daltons, and Neurath *et al.* (1978) reported a polypeptide with an apparent molecular size of 16,000 ± 500 daltons. These polypeptides could have been the same as P19, although none of them were tested for HBeAg activity.

Variable forms of HBeAg in serum are schematically illustrated in Fig. 3.

F. Relationship of HBeAg and HBcAg at the Molecular Level

Takahashi *et al.* (1981) purified P19 to homogeneity from cores of Dane particles, and inoculated it into a rabbit. The rabbit produced anti-HBc in addition to anti-HBe (Fig. 4). Thus, although P19 failed to reveal HBcAg activity by conventional assay methods, it was capable of eliciting anti-

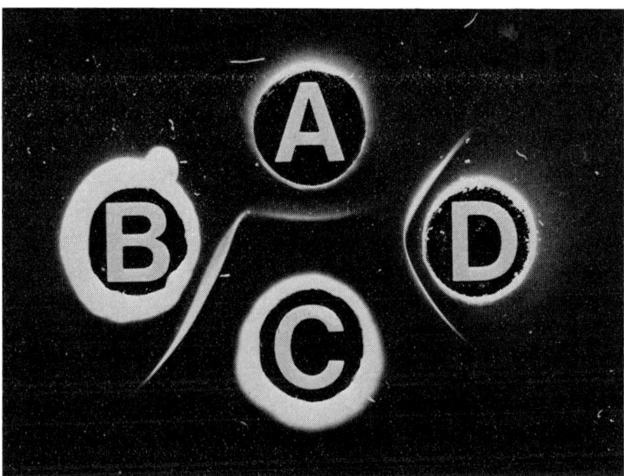

Figure 4. Ouchterlony double-immunodiffusion analysis of a rabbit antiserum raised against P19. A, rabbit anti-P19; B, anti-HBe (anti-HBc and HBsAg also present); C, HBeAg (anti-HBc and HBsAg also present); D, purified hepatitis B core particles. Two precipitin lines are seen, which can be identified as HBeAg line (between A and C, also B and C) and HBcAg line (between A and D, also C and D). (From Takahashi *et al.*, 1981.)

HBc in animals. When P19 was analyzed for its amino acid composition, it was strikingly similar to that of a polypeptide deduced from the nucleotide sequence of HBV DNA (Pasek *et al.*, 1979). This polypeptide is coded for by 549 base pairs, which would produce a molecule of 183 amino acid residues with a calculated molecular size of 21,042 daltons. Undoubtedly, this gene, originally assigned to HBcAg (Pasek *et al.*, 1979), is coding for P19.

In the intact core, P19 appears to be arranged in such a manner that the portion bearing HBcAg is exposed on the surface while HBeAg portions are buried inside. The weight of the core of a Dane particle (a sphere with a diameter of 27 nm and a specific gravity of 1.35 g/cm^3) is 1.3×10^{-17} g. Subtracting from it the presumed weight of DNA and DNA polymerase with estimated molecular sizes of 2×10^6 (Robinson *et al.*, 1974) and 1×10^5 daltons, respectively, and dividing the balance by the weight of P19, the core of a Dane particle is considered to contain approximately 300 P19 molecules.

Imai *et al.* (1982) obtained monoclonal antibodies that recognized two distinct antigenic determinants of HBeAg and designated them as HBeAg/a and HBeAg/b. Ferns and Tedder (1984) also identified two distinct epitopes on HBeAg by monoclonal antibodies. Both HBeAg/a and HBeAg/b were detected on P19. It appears that P19 bears only one each of HBeAg/a and HBeAg/b, since in a solid-phase radioimmunoassay P19 can be sandwiched between anti-HBe/a and anti-HBe/b to allow its detection, but not between two anti-HBe/a's or two anti-HBe/b's.

When small and large molecular weight HBeAg in serum were purified and subjected to electrophoresis in SDS polyacrylamide gel, they gave rise to a polypeptide with a molecular size of 15,500 daltons (P15.5) that bore HBeAg determinants. There was a substantial difference in the molecular size between P15.5 purified from serum and P19 derived from Dane particle cores. When cores of Dane particles were prepared in the presence of proteolytic enzymes, a condition presumed to peel off their protein coat, and then treated with detergent in a reducing condition, however, they gave rise to P15.5 (Takahashi *et al.* 1980).

P19 derived from Dane particle cores and P15.5 from HBeAg in the serum have been further characterized immunochemically (Table II). Takahashi *et al.* (1983) obtained monoclonal antibodies directed to two different epitopes on the core of Dane particles that were designated as HBcAg/α and HBcAg/β. They looked for these two HBcAg determinants and two antigenic determinants of HBeAg, HBeAg/a and HBeAg/b, on P19 and P15.5 by means of their capacity of being sandwiched between two monoclonal antibodies, one of which was fixed on

TABLE II
Immunochemical Properties of P19 and P15.5 as well as Small and Large Molecular Weight HBeAg
Occurring in the Serum[a]

	Antigenic determinants				Molecular size (amino acid residues)	Association with plasma protein
Preparations	HBeAg/a	HBeAg/b	HBcAg/α	HBcAg/β		
Nucleopeptides						
P19	+	+	+	+	21,042 (183)	None
P15.5	+	+	+	−	16,770 (149)	None
HBeAg in the Serum						
Small MW	+	+	−	−	∼ 100,000	Albumin α-Antitrypsin
Large MW (IgG-bound)	+	+	−	−	∼ 300,000	Anti-HBc/α

[a]Nucleopeptides of HBV and HBeAg in serum were tested for antigenic determinants of HBeAg and HBcAg by the solid-phase radioimmunoassay with monoclonal antibodies. Molecular sizes estimated from the nucleotide sequence of HBV DNA or by the elution position in gel filtration, as well as the association with various plasma proteins, are also shown.

a solid-phase support and the other labeled with radioiodine. P19 displayed all of the four antigenic determinants. The presence on P19 of only one antigenic determinant for each specificity was verified by the failure in sandwiching P19 between two monoclonal antibodies of homologous specificity.

By digestion with carboxypeptidase A, the C-terminal amino acid sequence of P15.5 was determined to be -Thr-Thr-Val-Val. The identical sequence of four amino acid residues was found on the gene coding for P19 on HBV DNA, irrespective of three different subtypes (Galibert *et al.*, 1979; Pasek *et al.*, 1979; Valenzuela *et al.*, 1979; Ono *et al.*, 1983). Taken together with its amino acid composition and molecular size, P15.5 is deduced to represent a part of P19 that has been truncated of 34 amino acid residues from its C-terminus. P15.5 bore HBeAg/a, HBeAg/b, and, in addition, one of the determinants present on the surface of core particles, HBcAg/α. Both large and small molecular weight HBeAg occurring in the serum revealed one each of HBeAg/a and HBeAg/b (Table II); they did not show an HBcAg/α determinant, despite the fact that P15.5 is contained in both of them (Takahashi *et al.*, 1980). On the basis of these results, HBcAg/α of P15.5 would be cryptically present in small as well as large molecular weight HBeAg in the serum. P15.5 bound to the IgG fraction obtained from human serum that tested positive for anti-HBc but negative for anti-HBe (Takahashi *et al.*, 1983). HBcAg/α determinant in the large molecular weight HBeAg, therefore, could be occupied by anti-HBc/α. This is a reasonable assumption because essentially all HBeAg-positive sera contain anti-HBc in high titers and both anti-HBc/α and anti-HBc/β are detectable in most human anti-HBc. IgG in the large molecular weight HBeAg, therefore, would be anti-HBc of a restricted specificity.

In view of the association of small molecular weight HBeAg with plasma proteins, such as albumin (Takahashi *et al.*, 1980; Yamada *et al.*, 1981) and α-antitrypsin (S. Kishimoto *et al.*, unpublished observations), HBcAg/α of P15.5 would be masked also. The association of such plasma proteins with P15.5 is by no means haphazard. They bind to P15.5 in such a manner as to cover the HBcAg/α determinant without blocking the binding of HBeAg/a or HBeAg/b determinant with antibody.

The designation of HBcAg was originally assigned based on the availability of its antigenic determinants on the surface of Dane particle cores (Almeida *et al.*, 1970). Similarly, HBeAg was defined by the antigenicity detectable by the corresponding antibody at the outset (Magnius and Espmark, 1972). Later, HBcAg and HBeAg became accepted to represent substances with the respective antigenicity. The fact, as it evolves, is that HBcAg and HBeAg are antigenic determinants of the nucleopeptide of HBV, P19; the distinction between HBcAg and HBeAg determinants of P19 is made by their availability, or their lack of availability, on the surface of Dane particle cores. Despite the presence of an HBcAg/α determinant in HBeAg occurring in the serum (containing P15.5), it is not available for detection with the corresponding antibody due to its association with plasma proteins, either by antigen–antibody complex formation (large molecular weight HBeAg) or another type of protein–protein interaction (small molecular weight HBeAg). Although the conventional usage of HBcAg and HBeAg has its practical advantages, these designations do not appear to be appropriate any longer. HBcAg and HBeAg, as well as immune responses of the host against them, would be better defined in terms of individual antigenic determinants of P19 and the host response against it.

III. Epidemiology of HBeAg

Essentially all HBsAg-positive sera are expected to contain either HBeAg or anti-HBe. Some HBsAg-negative sera, most of which are positive for anti-HBs and/or anti-HBc, contain anti-HBe, but usually not HBeAg. HBeAg can be detected in sera containing HBsAg of any of the subtypes. In early studies with immunodiffusion as the sole method to detect HBeAg/anti-HBe, as many as one-half of HBsAg-positive sera did not show either HBeAg or anti-HBe. With the advent of more sensitive techniques, it is now possible to classify HBsAg-positive sera as either HBeAg or anti-HBe positive at a frequency as high as 90% (Mushahwar *et al.*, 1981), 96% (Fields *et al.*, 1978b), and 98% (Dow *et al.*, 1980; Gotanda *et al.*, 1982). There are HBsAg-positive sera that do not reveal HBeAg or anti-HBe even by the most sensitive methods, however. They are mostly sera with low HBsAg activity (Nath *et al.*, 1980), or those obtained during seroconversion from HBeAg to anti-HBe. Rare sera show both HBeAg and anti-HBe activities; such sera are probably obtained in the course of seroconversion from HBeAg to anti-HBe.

The presence of HBeAg and anti-HBe in HBsAg-positive sera may be influenced by multiple factors including immune competence, ethnic and socioeconomic differences of the host who harbors HBV, and the host's age and sex. In early studies, Magnius and Espmark (1972) reported a high prevalence of HBeAg in patients on maintenance hemodialysis (18/23 or 78%). Since then, their observation has been repeatedly confirmed. Miller *et al.* (1978) noted 16 of 24 (68%) HBsAg-positive patients on hemodialysis were positive for HBeAg. Patients who had received transplants and were under immunosuppressive therapy showed a high prevalence of HBeAg also (50/70 or 71%; Ettenger *et al.*, 1980). The prevalence of HBeAg was particularly high among homosexuals [129/210 (61.4%); Szmuness *et al.*, 1981], with their known disordered immunoregulation (Mildvan *et al.*, 1982). Among mentally retarded patients, the prevalence of HBeAg was much higher in those with Down's syndrome [20/51 (39.2%)] than in those without [4/39 (10.3%); Szmuness *et al.*, 1981].

There is a wide regional variation in the prevalence of HBeAg among asymptomatic carriers of HBsAg. HBeAg was not detected in any of a total of 61 asymptomatic carriers in Sweden, Denmark, and England, while anti-HBe was found in 50 (82%) (Magnius and Espmark, 1972; Skinhøj *et al.*, 1976; Elefthériou *et al.*, 1975). Although the test was carried out by immunodiffusion, a high prevalence of anti-HBe in these sera substantiated the low prevalence of HBeAg in these populations. In contrast, HBeAg was more prevalent among asymptomatic carriers in other countries, such as Taiwan (5–20%) and Japan (18.5%), as well as among Alaskan Eskimos (34%) (Stevens *et al.*, 1975; Sasaki *et al.*, 1979; Maynard *et al.*, 1976). The differences among these populations are ascribable, at least partly, to ethnic differences. In France, the prevalence of HBeAg was found to be much lower in French (4.2%) than in people of other origins (23.7%) (Richer *et al.*, 1977). Similarly, in Denmark HBeAg was detected in only 2/48 compared with 40/58 Vietnamese refugees (Aldershvile *et al.*, 1980). In addition, the prevalence of HBeAg may well be influenced by socioeconomic status, sanitary conditions, and other as yet unidentified factors. In the United States, Tabor *et al.* (1980b), by using agar gel immunodiffusion found HBeAg in 31/200 (15%) of paid donors who carried HBsAg, compared with only 11/200 (5%) of HBsAg-positive volunteer donors. Even among Eskimos of the same age group (10–19 years), the prevalence of HBeAg was much higher in those living on the east coast (12/15) than those living on the west coast of Greenland (1/9) (Aldershvile *et al.*, 1980).

In acute HBV infection, HBeAg appears in the circulation simultaneously with HBsAg, before elevation of serum transaminases (Magnius *et al.*, 1975; Tabor *et al.*, 1980a). Among the three antibodies against HBV-associated antigens, anti-HBc appears first and then anti-HBe, both during the period when HBsAg is circulating (Aikawa *et al.*, 1978). Anti-HBs becomes detectable as the last antibody after HBsAg has disappeared from the circulation. This order of anti-HBc, anti-HBe, and anti-HBs is maintained in both humans and chimpanzees acutely infected with HBV. The seroconversion from HBeAg to anti-HBe during HBsAg positivity may also take place in persons who are persistently infected with HBV. Ohbayashi *et al.* (1976) found a decreasing frequency of HBeAg and an increasing frequency of anti-HBe with age among HBsAg carriers in Japan. Their observation was extended to a larger series of 6,342 asymptomatic HBsAg carriers by Sasaki *et al.* (1979) and also in 268 asymptomatic carriers in Taiwan (Liaw *et al.*, 1984). Such a gradient with age, however, would require a setting in which the HBV carrier state is established at an early age of life; these data were not always reproduced by others. Couroucé-Pauty and Plançon (1978) observed a fluctuating prevalence of HBeAg and a decreasing, rather than increasing, prevalence of anti-HBe with age in a French population. As proposed by Hyland and Shanley (1983), the age-specific prevalence of HBeAg among carriers of HBsAg may not be uniform worldwide. It forms a smooth decreasing gradient with age in districts where HBsAg is acquired at birth or early in life (e.g., Asian countries). In contrast, in communities where a larger proportion of HBsAg infection occurs later in life (e.g., Western countries), the adult population may exhibit a higher HBeAg prevalence. Sasaki *et al.* (1979) found HBeAg slightly but significantly more often in male donors than in female donors (19.1 versus 16.7%) compared with anti-HBe, which was detected a little less frequently in males than in females (49.6 versus 53.1%).

In addition to serum, HBeAg has been detected in body fluid such as a pleural effusion (which also contained HBsAg) (Tabor *et al.*, 1977). HBeAg has been found also in saliva, urine, and feces in which HBsAg are also detected, provided that HBeAg is present in the corresponding sera. The presence of HBeAg in cord sera has been a matter of controversy; early reports did not detect HBeAg in cord sera (Gerety and Schweitzer, 1977; Yanagida *et al.*, 1979). Recently, however, Arakawa *et al.* (1982) reported detecting "IgG-bound" large HBeAg in cord sera. It is intriguing that "free," small HBeAg could not be found in cord sera, although it was present in maternal sera. IgG-bound HBeAg may be transmitted through the placenta along with IgG, which is specifically transported into the fetal circulation. Among macromolecules in the serum of mothers, only IgG appears to be transmitted into the fetal circulation with a concentration gradually approaching or even exceeding that in maternal serum (Gitlin *et al.*, 1964). The receptor for IgG, but not for other plasma proteins, is detectable in placental tissue (Gitlin and Gitlin, 1973).

IV. HBeAg/Anti-HBe and Infectivity of HBsAg-Positive Blood

The close association between HBeAg and infectivity of HBsAg-positive blood was evident from the outset. Magnius and Espmark (1972) noted a high prevalence (78%) of HBeAg in the sera of HBsAg-positive patients on maintenance hemodialysis who were known to possess high levels of infectivity (Garibaldi *et al.*, 1973). In contrast, anti-HBe was frequently found in the sera of asymptomatic carriers. Astonishingly, 10 apparently healthy carriers with anti-HBe had donated 95 blood units, none of which were implicated in the reported cases of posttransfusion hepatitis (Magnius *et al.*, 1975). The close association of HBeAg in the serum with Dane particles, as well as with their immunological and biochemical markers (HBcAg and HBsAg-associated DNA polymerase) provided support for the view that HBeAg indicated a high level of infectious HBV.

The association of HBeAg and infectivity, however, is not absolute. This is naturally assumed since HBeAg does not represent a complete HBV virus, but a viral nucleoprotein released from hepatocytes infected with HBV; the presence of HBeAg in the serum indirectly indicates a high concentration of HBV. It must be remembered that even anti-HBe-positive sera are infectious. Berquist *et al.* (1976) injected four chimps with 5 ml each of HBsAg-positive serum containing anti-HBe; one contracted hepatitis B. The difference in infectivity between HBeAg- and anti-HBe-positive sera, both of which contain HBsAg, is therefore quantitative rather than qualitative. Shikata *et al.* (1977) titrated HBeAg-positive and anti-HBe-positive sera, both containing a comparably high titer of HBsAg. As little as 10^{-8} ml of HBeAg-positive serum transmitted HBV infection to a chimp. As for anti-HBe-positive serum, 1 ml could transmit HBV infection, while 10^{-2} ml failed to do so. The difference in infectivity between these two sera, therefore, was >1,000,000-fold.

Alter *et al.* (1976) studied, after accidental needle-stick exposure, the correlation between HBeAg in HBsAg-positive inocula and transmission of hepatitis B to recipients negative for anti-HBs. Out of 18 who received HBeAg-positive inocula, as many as 14 (78%) developed hepatitis B; none of 12 who received HBeAg-negative inocula became infected. HBeAg indicates a high risk of HBV infection in household contacts, too. Hepatitis was contracted by a spouse who had married an asymptomatic carrier seropositive for HBeAg shortly after their marriage (Ohbayashi *et al.*, 1977). When spouses of HBeAg-positive carriers were tested, 22 of 26 (85%) were found to be positive for either HBsAg or anti-HBs, while such markers of HBV infection were detected only in 12 of 46 (26%) spouses of anti-HBe-positive carriers (Miyakawa and Mayumi, 1978). A similar high exposure rate among spouses of HBeAg-positive carriers, higher than that among those of anti-HBe-positive carriers (78 versus 25%), was observed in a prospective study (Perrillo *et al.*, 1979).

Perinatal transmission of HBV from infected mothers to their babies is a significant route of HBV transmission, especially since such babies develop a persistent carrier state and provide a reservoir for the further spread of HBV in the community. In addition, they themselves may develop a spectrum of hepatic diseases ranging from chronic hepatitis to hepatocellular carcinoma later in their lives (Ohbayashi *et al.*, 1972). Okada *et al.* (1976) followed 10 babies born to HBeAg-positive carrier mothers, and found that all of them developed a persistent carrier state within 12 months after birth, while none of 7 babies born to anti-HBe-positive carrier mothers developed persistent HBV infections. Beasley *et al.* (1977) found that 17 of 20 (85%) carrier mothers positive for HBeAg by immunodiffusion transmitted HBV to their babies, while 13 of 42 (31%) HBeAg-negative mothers did so. The point may be realized, from the results of these two studies, that in early studies when insensitive immunodiffusion tests were used to detect HBeAg, the high infectivity of HBeAg-positive sera was most prominently revealed when they were compared with anti-HBe-positive sera (from which HBeAg was presumed to be excluded). The infectivity of HBeAg-positive sera was less impressive when compared with HBeAg-negative sera (in some of which HBeAg might have been present at undetectable levels).

Stevens *et al.* (1979) confirmed and extended the observation of Okada *et al.* (1976). They determined HBeAg by RIA in carrier mothers in Taiwan and looked at its correlation with persistent HBV infections in their babies. They observed that 40 of 47 (85%) babies born to HBeAg-positive mothers developed persistent HBsAg, compared with none of 14 born to anti-HBe-positive mothers. HBeAg in the sera of mothers with acute hepatitis B also indicated the transmission of the HBV carrier state to their babies (Tong *et al.*, 1981). HBV infection was occasionally contracted by babies born to anti-HBe-positive mothers, but the infection was only transient and a persistent carrier state was never established (Gerety and Schweitzer, 1977; Schweitzer *et al.*, 1975; Stevens *et al.*, 1979; Shiraki *et al.*, 1980). Since the persistent infection is much more serious to the babies as well as to the community, HBeAg or anti-HBe in the sera of carrier mothers expecting babies is a matter of utmost concern.

The presence of HBeAg or anti-HBe in inocula has to be taken into account when the efficacy of immunoprophylaxis is to be evaluated (Alter *et al.*, 1976; Mayumi and Miyakawa, 1978). Immunoprophylaxis of HBV infection in both horizontal and mother-to-baby transmission has been attempted, with equivocal results in studies in which the HBeAg/anti-HBe status of inocula or mothers was not specified (Grady and Lee, 1975; Dosik and Jhaveri, 1978). The results of such studies should be reevaluated in light of the high infectivity of HBeAg-positive inocula and mothers. Recently, a number of efficacious immunoprophylactic procedures, involving the use of both hepatitis B immune globulin and vaccine, have been proposed for preventing the transmission of the HBV carrier state from HBeAg-positive mothers to their offspring (Tada *et al.*, 1982; Beasley *et al.*, 1983; Wong *et al.*, 1984).

The correlation between HBeAg and infectivity in HBsAg-positive sera is particularly high when HBeAg is detected by insensitive methods such as immunodiffusion, the infection ensuing in approximately 80% of the recipients both in needle-stick and mother-to-baby transmission. It may not come as a surprise that the correlation between HBeAg and infectivity becomes less close when a sensitive method, such as RIA, is used to detect HBeAg, which enables the detection of HBeAg even in sera with low infectivity (Werner and Grady, 1982). In other words, all HBeAg-positive sera are not equally infectious. The amount of HBeAg may directly relate to the replication of HBV and infectivity.

Lindenschmidt *et al.* (1984) detected DNA polymerase in 95% of sera that showed HBeAg at a dilution of at least 1:50, in contrast to only 5% of sera with an HBeAg titer of 1:25 or less. Their view goes along with the report of Masuko *et al.* (1985), who followed the staff members in a dialysis unit after accidental needle-stick exposure to blood determined to be HBeAg-positive by RIA. Despite injection with hepatitis B immune globulin within 48 hours after the exposure, 11 of 56 (20%) contracted the HBV infection. There were 37 inocula determined HBeAg-positive by immunodiffusion also, including 10 of the 11 that transmitted infection. HBsAg-associated DNA polymerase activity in the 11 inocula was significantly higher than that in the remaining 45 (log cpm 3.27 ± 0.57 versus 2.09 ± 1.19, $p < .001$).

V. HBeAg/Anti-HBe in Acute and Chronic Liver Disease

Some patients with acute hepatitis B do not recover completely, and go on to later develop chronic disease. Nielsen *et al.* (1974) proposed the predictive value of HBeAg for chronicity in acute hepatitis B. They reported observing progression to chronic hepatitis or cirrhosis in 11 of 19 (58%) patients with acute hepatitis B who were seropositive for HBeAg. Norkrans *et al.* (1976) supported their view by detecting HBsAg for a significantly longer period in patients with HBeAg than in those without HBeAg. The predictive value of HBeAg for chronicity, however, has been seriously questioned by a number of investigators. Thamer *et al.* (1976) followed 11 patients with acute hepatitis B who were seropositive for HBeAg, but could find progression to chronic liver disease in only 1 of them. Fay *et al.* (1977) found HBeAg in 15 of 159 (9%) patients who showed early resolution, as well as in 8 of 18 (44%) of those whose hepatitis became chronic. In their series, therefore, HBeAg in acute hepatitis B indicated chronicity correctly in 35% (8/23), but led to an erroneous prognosis more often [65% (15/23)].

It has become apparent that detection of HBeAg in actue hepatitis B was dependent on when and how often serum samples were drawn for the test; the specimens obtained early in the course of illness tended to be positive for HBeAg more frequently than those obtained later. Gibson and Ruparelia (1977) found an overall prevalence of 13.6% HBeAg in patients with acute hepatitis B, but positivity was 40% within the first week of jaundice. The ubiquitous presence of HBeAg in acute HBV infection was demonstrated by following prospectively the sera of persons at high risk of HBV infection for markers of HBV infection. Aikawa *et al.* (1978) found HBeAg early in the period of HBsAg positivity in all seven medical personnel who contracted acute hepatitis B. Three of them seroconverted to anti-HBe during the observation period. They observed also the seroconversion from HBeAg to anti-HBe in a chimpanzee experimentally infected with HBV. Werner and Blumberg (1978) followed 28 patients in a dialysis unit who converted to HBsAg positive, and detected HBeAg in sera of all 28 during the first week of HBsAg positivity, including 19 in whom HBsAg was present only transiently. On the basis of these observations, HBeAg is invariably present, albeit transiently, in the serum of patients with acute hepatitis B. The detectability of HBeAg in a given case is entirely dependent on the time when serum is taken and the sensitivity of methods used to detect it.

Nevertheless, the *persistence* of HBeAg in acute hepatitis B may have prognostic value. Norkrans *et al.* (1979) reported that all patients developing chronic hepatitis had HBeAg in the serum for more than a year after the onset of illness. In contrast, 12 patients with a normal course of illness kept HBeAg only for 3 to 9 weeks. Similarly, Aldershvile *et al.* (1980) noticed the association between the persistence of HBeAg for longer than 10 weeks after the onset of symptoms and the development of chronic hepatitis B. No evidence was presented to substantiate an acute HBV infection in any of their cases, however. There remains a possibility that the patients who develop a persistent HBV infection in their series could have been infected long before the episode of acute hepatitis. Such an episode could have been any of the following: (1) a flare-up of infection in asymptomatic carriers; (2) an acute exacerbation of their chronic hepatitis B; or (3) an acute non-A, non-B hepatitis superimposed on a persistent HBV infection. Such possibilities would have been excluded by determining IgM anti-HBc in the serum, proving an acute HBV infection (Lemon *et al.*, 1981).

Realdi *et al.* (1980) studied 116 patients with HBsAg-positive, biopsy-proven, chronic liver disease in Italy. They found a higher prevalence of HBeAg (61%) in chronic active hepatitis without cirrhosis than in chronic active hepatitis with cirrhosis (12%). They also reported a reciprocal prevalence of anti-HBe in these two groups of patients (9 versus 36%). Although seroconversion to anti-HBe was always associated with a striking reduction in virus replication, it did not always indicate a good prognosis since it often occurred in individuals who developed cirrhosis. A high prevalence of anti-HBe in patients with HBsAg-positive cirrhosis and hepatocellular carcinoma has been noted by others also (Eleerhériou *et al.*, 1975).

Under these circumstances, one wonders if the seroconversion from HBeAg to anti-HBe is a good or bad sign. In actuality, the seroconversion may have to be evaluated, depending on the stage where the patient stands. At a time not so far from acquiring the infection, loss of HBeAg may indicate the resolution of active illness, while the development of anti-HBe may not be taken as a favorable sign once cirrhosis has developed in subsequent later stages of infection.

Hoofnagle *et al.* (1981) followed 25 patients with chronic hepatitis B in the United States, most of whom were presumed to have been healthy until they acquired HBV infection in adulthood. They observed a seroconversion from HBeAg to anti-HBe in 13, concurrently with or heralded by a fall in serum transaminase levels and loss of detectable HBsAg-associated DNA polymerase activity; none of these patients developed cirrhosis. The 12 patients who remained HBeAg positive continued to have elevated serum transaminase levels; 2 of them developed cirrhosis. If seroconversion implies a good prognosis, its therapeutic induction might be worthwhile as well. Corticosteroids, given for a short period and then withdrawn, could induce seroconversions in some patients with chronic hepatitis B along with a decrease in serum transaminase levels (Hoofnagle, 1982). Liaw *et al.* (1983) made observations that might be relevant to the therapeutic effect of such a short-term corticosteroid therapy. They found that a spontaneous seroconversion to anti-HBe in chronic hepatitis B was preceded, in most cases, by bouts of elevated serum transaminase levels during the 3 months before the clearance of HBeAg. An exacerbation of hepatitis, reflecting the rebound of withdrawing corticosteroid, may trigger the seroconversion. Loss of HBeAg with or without seroconversion to anti-HBe may not necessarily indicate persistent remission of active hepatitis. Davis *et al.* (1984) reported the return of HBeAg in serum, accompanied by reactivated hepatitis, in 7 or 25 (28%) patients within 1 year of loss of HBeAg. The majority (14/25) of their patients were homosexuals with known disordered immunoregulation (Mildvan *et al.*, 1982), who are reasonably assumed to have contracted the infection later in their lives. Their observations, therefore, may not be extended to patients in districts where most persistent carriers acquire the infection very early in their lives.

All in all, HBeAg and anti-HBe are not to be taken frankly as sinister and auspicious signs, respectively, even in persistent HBV infection. This is naturally assumed, inasmuch as by far most carriers of HBV with HBeAg in the serum are asymptomatic clinically, and the great majority of patients with HBsAg-positive hepatocellular carcinoma are positive for anti-HBe in the serum. Nonetheless, there are clinical settings, such as chronic active hepatitis, where a good correlation is observed between HBeAg and clinicopathological activities of the disease. Moreover, the seroconversion may help evaluate the efficacy of therapeutic trials, typified by the short-term steroid therapy. Indeed, such a potentially hazardous therapy, if tailored to a clinically acceptable form, would be valuable until a good method to terminate the persistent HBV infection can be worked out.

VI. HBeAg and Membranous Glomerulonephritis

In previous sections, several lines of evidence were presented regarding the clinical implications of HBeAg. These included HBeAg as a marker of infectivity and a prognostic indicator in hepatic diseases. The significance of HBeAg in these settings, however, is indirect; HBeAg is not infectious by itself, nor is there any solid evidence for its role in the pathogenesis of hepatitis B. Direct evidence for the pathognomonic role of HBeAg was demonstrated in nephritis rather than in hepatitis.

There has been a strong association between HBV infection and membranous glomerulonephritis in children in Japan. Takekoshi *et al.* (1978) noted that among 163 children with pathological proteinuria and/or hematuria, 11 who were diagnosed as membranous glomerulonephritis at biopsy all proved to be persistent carriers of HBV. In contrast, among the remaining 152 with other types of glomerular lesions, only 7 (4.6%) were found to be HBV carriers. HBsAg was not detected, however, in any glomeruli of 9 of 11 on whom immunofluorescent studies were performed. Their observation was confirmed in Taiwan by the study of Hsu *et al.* (1983), who diagnosed membranous glomerulonephritis in 14 of 63 children with primary glomerular disease. Among the 14 with membranous glomerulonephritis, all 13 tested were positive for HBsAg in the serum.

In two patients in their series from whom materials were available, HBeAg was detected in a diffuse granular fashion along glomerular capillary walls, in a pattern similar to the deposition of IgG and C3 (Takekoshi *et al.*, 1979). In the serum of these two patients, "IgG-bound" large HBeAg was detected. The presence of HBeAg in association with IgG both in the circulation and in tissue substantiated the view that immune complexes involving HBeAg induced membranous glomerulonephritis in these cases. Furthermore, by means of monoclonal antibody (Imai *et al.*, 1982) conjugated with fluorescein, HBeAg was stained in immune depositis in the glomeruli from cases of membranous glomerulonephritis who carried HBsAg together with HBeAg, demonstrating the etiological role of HBeAg (Miyakawa and Mayumi, 1982).

Maggiore *et al.* (1981) has cast a serious doubt on the specificity of immunofluorescent staining for HBV-associated antigens in glomerular immune deposits of persons who carry HBV, because of the cryoglobulin which contains an antiglobulin activity of IgM class that is frequently identified in their circulation. Glomerular immune deposits of these patients, especially of IgM class, stained by fluoresceinated anti-HBs were not specific since they were abolished by using anti-HBs F(ab')$_2$ fragments in place of fluoresceintated whole anti-HBs. HBeAg in glomerular immune deposits of patients with membranous glomerulonephritis who carry HBV, however, has been verified in a specific manner. Hirose *et al.* (1984) stained HBeAg by F(ab')$_2$ fragments of monoclonal anti-HBe labeled with fluorescein in immune deposits from 10 of 16 carriers of HBV with membranous glomerulonephritis

Seroconversion from HBeAg to anti-HBe in patients with HBsAg-positive membranous glomerulonephritis was accompanied by the remission of nephritis, further reinforcing the role of HBeAg in their disease. Ito *et al.* (1981) investigated the correlation of circulating HBeAg and disease activity in six patients with membranous glomerulonephritis who carried HBsAg persistently. Four of these had active illness at the time of biopsy, while the remaining two were already in remission. HBV markers in the serum and immunopathological findings in the kidney were markedly different between these two groups of patients. In the serum of the four with gross proteinuria, HBeAg was found along with HBsAg and anti-HBc. In the serum of two without proteinuria, however, anti-HBe but not HBeAg was found. In the kidney of four with proteinuria, numerous electron-dense deposits were identified on and within the glomerular basement membranes. In addition, diffuse granular depositions of HBeAg were detected along glomerular capillary walls in a pattern similar to the deposition of immunoglobulins and C3. In contrast, HBeAg was not detected in the kidneys of two patients who were in remission. Electron microscopic observations of glomeruli from these two patients revealed numerous electron-lucent areas replacing electron-dense deposits, suggesting regression of the disease process. Nagata *et al.* (1981) followed an HBsAg-positive boy with membranous glomerulonephritis by obtaining serial renal biopsies, and observed that immune complexes involving HBeAg disappeared as the patient went into clinical remission. Collins *et al.* (1983) also described a 29-year-old man in whom granular deposition of HBeAg was observed along glomerular capillary walls.

Although the association of HBsAg with membranous glomerulonephritis has long been observed, the identity of the responsible antigen has remained a matter of controversy (Levy and Kleinknecht, 1980). At least 15 groups of investigators have reported finding HBsAg in immune deposits in the glomeruli of 25 of 48 patients, 1 group found HBcAg in deposits of 14 of 23 patients, and 4 groups were not able to detect HBsAg in deposits of any of 22 patients who carried HBsAg. Of particular interest is the deposition of HBcAg reported by one group. Ślusarczyk *et al.* (1980) reported observing HBcAg in immune deposits of 14 of 23 cases of membranous glomerulonephritis who carried HBsAg, and proposed the causative role of HBcAg. In the light of present knowledge concerning the relationship between HBcAg and HBeAg, the antigen they found might well have been HBeAg rather than HBcAg. They used two kinds of fluoresceinated anti-HBc reagents to stain immune deposits in the glomeruli. One anti-HBc was derived from pooled human sera positive for anti-HBc, which most likely contained anti-HBe as well. The other reagent was obtained by immunizing guinea pigs with hepatitis B core particles. Since core particles contain P19, which possesses the immunogenicity of both HBeAg and HBcAg (Takahashi *et al.*, 1981), this antiserum should have contained anti-HBe in addition to anti-HBc.

The etiological role of HBeAg in membranous glomerulonephritis of persons infected with HBV, as well as the clinical remission following seroconversion from HBeAg to anti-HBe, may shed some light on the therapeutic strategy for this disease. Currently, a variety of immunosuppressive therapies are applied to patients with membranous glomerulonephritis with equivocal efficacy. Probably patients with HBeAg-mediated membranous glomerulonephritis would better be *not* treated with steroids and immunosuppressive agents, lest these should inadvertently retard the natural seroconversion to anti-HBe, thereby preventing spontaneous remission of the disease.

VII. HBeAg and the Receptor for Polymerized Human Serum Albumin

Factors that agglutinate sheep red blood cells (SRBC) coated with polymerized human serum albumin (poly-HSA) have been identified in sera from patients with hepatic disorders, including those containing HBsAg, and ascribed to antibodies directed to poly-HSA (Lenkei *et al.*, 1974). Imai *et al.* (1979) reported that HBsAg particles are directly involved in the agglutination of SRBC coated with poly-HSA. All HBsAg-positive sera comparable in HBsAg titers are not equally reactive with SRBC coated with poly-HSA, however. HBsAg-positive sera containing HBeAg display reactivity with poly-HSA in much higher titers than those containing anti-HBe (Imai *et al.*, 1979; Neurath and Strick, 1979; Hansson and Purcell, 1979).

Dane particles, as well as tubular and spherical HBsAg particles with a diameter of 22 nm that had been obtained from HBeAg-positive plasma, were shown to be capable of binding to poly-HSA in electron microscopic observations (Imai *et al.*, 1979). In contrast, 22-nm HBsAg particles derived from anti-HBe-positive plasma did not bind to poly-HSA. On the basis of these observations, the receptor for poly-HSA is postulated to be on Dane, tubular, and spherical HBsAg particles. HBV infection can be divided into HBeAg and anti-HBe phases, because the presence of HBeAg or anti-HBe in the serum has a crucial bearing on the biology of HBV as well as on the clinicopathological status of hosts (Miyakawa and Mayumi, 1982; Hoofnagle, 1983). This view may be extended to a molecular level in HBsAg, because HBsAg polypeptides produced in the HBeAg phase are different from those produced in the anti-HBe phase in terms of the receptor for poly-HSA.

The polyalbumin receptor on HBsAg particles is species specific because it binds to polymerized albumins from humans and chimpanzees, both of which are susceptible to HBV, but not to polymerized albumins from the other animals lacking susceptibility to HBV, such as marmoset, rabbit, horse, guinea pig, rat, and mouse. This appears to suggest a role of polyalbumin receptor in the presumed hepatotropism of HBV, because hepatocytes also bear the receptor for poly-HSA (Lenkei *et al.*, 1977; Trevisan *et al.*, 1982; Thung and Gerber, 1983). Albumin polymers may appear in the circulation as the consequence of molecular aging. Hepatocytes will catch poly-HSA on their surface, which, in turn, would seize Dane particles with the receptor to initiate the infection.

The polyalbumin receptor of HBsAg particles is of protein nature, since it is labile to digestion with proteolytic enzymes. HBsAg particles derived from HBeAg-positive plasma had a density higher than those co-occurring with anti-HBe. When they were treated with pronase, their density was reduced to that of those co-occurring with anti-HBe, with the concomitant loss of the receptor (Imai *et al.*, 1979).

When 22-nm HBsAg particles were treated with detergent and a reducing agent, minor polypeptides with estimated molecular sizes of 31,000 and 35,000 daltons appeared (Machida *et al.*, 1983), in addition to the major polypeptide of HBsAg, P22, and its glycosylated form, P27 (Peterson *et al.*, 1977). Those polypeptides were designated P31 and P35 (the glycosylated form of P31). Similar HBsAg polypeptides have also been described by Stibbe and Gerlich (1982). HBsAg particles harvested in the HBeAg phase carried P31 and P35 several times more abundantly than those in the anti-HBe phase (Machida *et al.*, 1983). The receptor for poly-HSA was borne by both P31 and P35, but not by P22 or P27. The species specificity of the receptor was maintained in P31 and P35. They bound to polymerized albumins from humans and chimpanzees, but not to polymerized albumins from the other animals not susceptible to HBV.

Since P31 shared the C-terminal amino acid sequence with P22, it was considered to be composed of P22 plus an additional amino acid sequence on its N-terminus. P31 had the N-terminal amino acid of methionine. On the HBV DNA, there is a region called pre-*S* upstream to the gene *S* which encodes P22 (Tiollais *et al.*, 1978). The 55th amino acid residue from the N-terminus of P22 is methionine. The putative polypeptide composed of P22 and the 55 amino acid residues in the region pre-*S* would make a polypeptide of 281 residues with a molecular size of approximately 31,000 daltons, the amino acid composition of which is very similar to the values determined for P31. Since P22 was devoid of the receptor, the amino acid sequence of 55 residues encoded by the region pre-*S* was highly suspected of carrying the polyalbumin receptor.

A small polypeptide with an amino acid composition very close to that of the 55 residues in the region pre-*S* was liberated from P31 by the treatment with cyanogen bromide (Machida *et al.*, 1984). The peptide showed reactivity with polmerized albumins from only humans and chimpanzees. There remains little doubt about the receptor for poly-HSA being borne by the sequence of 55 amino acid residues coded for by a part of the region pre-*S*.

At least two applications may be conceived for the pre-*S* polypeptide bearing the receptor for poly-HSA. Pontisso *et al.* (1983) determined the polyalbumin receptor in HBsAg-positive sera and found that in a longitudinal study it correlated with the prognosis of type B hepatitis. The receptor was found to be more predictive than HBeAg, because most HBeAg-positive patients with a low initial titer of the receptor seroconverted to anti-HBe. Okamoto *et al.* (1985) obtained monoclonal antibody against the synthetic peptide of 19 amino acid residues, representing a part of the 55-amino acid (pre-*S*) polypeptide. They chose the peptide because its amino acid sequence displayed a high local hydrophilicity (Hopp and Woods, 1978) and was commonly expressed by HBV DNA, irrespective of different subtypes (Galibert *et al.*, 1979; Pasek *et al.*, 1979; Valenzuela *et al.*, 1979; Ono *et al.*, 1983). A hemagglutination assay has been developed by means of SRBC coated with the monoclonal antibody to the synthetic pre-*S* peptide for detecting HBsAg particles with the receptor in serum. The assay is convenient for the detection of HBsAg particles with the receptor (i.e., containing P31 and P35). The conventional hemagglutination method for detecting polyalbumin receptor that employs SRBC coated with poly-HSA is nonspecific because it gives positive results by antibodies to poly-HSA frequently present in the sera of patients with various hepatic disorders (Lenkei *et al.*, 1974).

Antibodies against the poly-HSA receptor would efficiently block the infection with HBV, inasmuch as the receptor is implicated in the hepatotropism of HBV. By this inference, there is a possibility of using the pre-*S* peptide, as well as synthetic peptides representing its parts, as a hepatitis B vaccine. A strong antigenicity of the pre-*S* peptide has been demonstrated both in humans and experimental animals (Vyas *et al.*, 1983; Okamoto *et al.*, 1985).

VIII. Conclusions

Once again, the truth when uncovered was simple. HBeAg turned out to be the major constituent of the nucleocapsid of HBV. In actuality, HBeAg represents the antigenic determinant(s) of a nucleopeptide (P19) coded for by the genome of HBV that expresses the antigenicity of HBcAg also. This polypeptide, when assembled by *E. coli* with the plasmid harboring its gene, tends to form a sphere resembling the core of HBV (Cohen and Richmond, 1982). P15.5, representing a part of P19, appears in the circulation in association with plasma proteins such as IgG and albumin.

Some questions remain unanswered, however. What triggers the seroconversion from HBeAg to anti-HBe, and why do HBV disappear from the circulation after the switch to anti-HBe despite a continuing HBV infection in the liver? How is HBeAg associated with plasma proteins in the circulation? These questions will be addressed before long by continued efforts with the advent of modern techniques, such as the recombinant gene encoding P19 and monoclonal antibodies directed to its epitopes. Experiments with hepadna viruses in animals will help answer them also. In the meantime, the knowledge accumulated during the pursuit of HBeAg may be extended to the study of other hepatitis viruses such as non-A, non-B agents, which are increasingly coming to the fore as HBV is being prevented by effective measures including hyperimmune globulin and vaccine.

References

Aikawa, T., Sairenji, H., Furuta, S., Kiyosawa, K., Shikata, T., Imai, M., Miyakawa, Y., Yanase, Y., and Mayumi, M. (1978). *N. Engl. J. Med.* **298**, 439–441.
Alberti, A., Diana, S., Scullard, G. H., Eddleston, A. L. W. F., and Williams, R. (1978). *Gastroenterology* **75**, 869–874.

Aldershvile, J., Skinhøj, P., Frosner, G. G., Black, F., Deinhardt, F., Hardt, F., and Nielsen, J. O. (1980). *J. Infect. Dis.* **142,** 18–22.

Almeida, J. D., Rubenstein, D., and Stott, E. J. (1971). *Lancet 2,* 1225–1227.

Alter, H. J., Seeff, L. B., Kaplan, P. M., McAuliffe, V. J., Wright, E. C., Gerin, J. L., Purcell, R. H., Holland, P. V., and Zimmerman, H. J. (1976). *N. Engl. J. Med.* **295,** 909–913.

Arakawa, K., Tsuda, F., Takahashi, K., Ise, I., Naito, S., Kosugi, E., Miyakawa, Y., and Mayumi, M. (1982). *Pediatr. Res.* **16,** 247–250.

Arnold, W., Nielsen, J. O., Hardt, F., and Meyer zum Bueschenfelde, K. H. (1977). *Gut* **18,** 994–996.

Beasley, R. P., Trepo, C., Stevens, C. E., and Szmuness, W. (1977). *Am. J. Epidemiol.* **105,** 94–98.

Beasley, R. P., Hwang, L., Lee, G. C., Lan, C., Roan, C., Huang, F., and Chen, C. (1983). *Lancet 2,* 1099–1102.

Berquist, K. R., Maynard, J. E., and Murphy, B. L. (1976). *Lancet 1,* 1026–1027.

Blumberg, B. S., Alter, H. J., and Visnich, S. (1965). *JAMA, J. Am. Med. Assoc.* **191,** 541–546.

Budkowska, A., Shih, J. W.-K., and Gerin, J. L. (1977). *J. Immunol.* **118,** 1300–1305.

Chadwick, R. G., Thomas, H. C., and Sherlock, S. (1978). *Lancet 1,* 616–617.

Chien, D. Y., and Vyas, G. N. (1978). *N. Engl. J. Med.* **299,** 1253–1254.

Cohen, B. J., and Richmond, J. E. (1982). *Nature (London)* **296,** 677–678.

Collins, A. B., Bhan, A. K., Dienstag, J. L., Colvin, R. B., Haupert, G. T., Mushahwar, I. K., and McLuskey, R. T. (1983). *Clin. Immunol. Immunopathol.* **26,** 137–153.

Couroucé-Pauty, A.-M., and Plançon, A. (1978). *Vox Sang.* **34,** 231–238.

Dane, D. S., Cameron, C. H., and Briggs, M. (1970). *Lancet 1,* 695–698.

Davis, G. L., Hoofnagle, J. H., and Waggoner, J. G. (1984). *Gastroenterology* **86,** 230–235.

Dosik, H., and Jhaveri, R. (1978). *N. Engl. J. Med.* **298,** 602–603.

Dow, B. C., MacVarish, I., Barr, A., Crawford, R. J., and Mitchell, R. (1980). *J. Clin. Pathol.* **33,** 1106–1109.

Elefthériou, N., Thomas, H. C., Heathcote, J., and Sherlock, S. (1975). *Lancet 2,* 1171–1173.

Ettenger, R. B., Tong, M. J., Landing, B. H., Mosley, J., Malekzadeh, M. H., Pennisi, A. J., Uittenbogaart, C. H., Jordan, S. C., Wright, H., and Fine, R. N. (1980). *J. Pediatr. (St. Louis)* **97,** 550–553.

Fay, O., Tanno, H., Roncoroni, M., Edwards, V. M., Mosley, J. W., and Redeker, A. G. (1977). *JAMA, J. Am. Med. Assoc.* **238,** 2501–2503.

Ferns, R. B., and Tedder, R. S. (1984). *J. Gen. Virol.* **65,** 899–908.

Fields, H. A., Bradley, D. W., Davis, C. L., and Maynard, J. E. (1978a). *Infect. Immun.* **20,** 792–803.

Fields, H. A., Bradley, D. W., Davis, C. L., Murphy, B. L., Schable, C. A., and Maynard, J. E. (1978b). *J. Immunol.* **121,** 930–935.

Galibert, F., Mandart, E., Fittousi, F., Tiollais, P., and Charnay, P. (1979). *Nature (London)* **281,** 646–650.

Garibaldi, R. A., Forrest, J. N., Bryan, J. A., Hanson, B. F., and Dismukes, W. E. (1973). *JAMA J. Am. Med. Assoc.* **225,** 384–389.

Gerety, R. J., and Schweitzer, I. L. (1977) *J. Pediatr. (St. Louis),* **90,** 368–374.

Gerin, J. L., Shih, J. W.-K., McAuliffe, V. J., and Purcell, R. H. (1978). *J. Gen. Virol.* **38,** 561–566.

Gibson, P. E., and Ruparelia, K. (1977). *J. Clin. Pathol.* **30,** 925–927.

Gitlin, D., Kumate, J., Urrusti, J., and Morales, C. (1964). *J. Clin. Invest.* **43,** 1938–1951.

Gitlin, J. D., and Gitlin, D. (1973). *Pediatr. Res.* **7,** 290.

Gotanda, T., Imai, M., Sano, T., Oinuma, A., Nomura, M., Miyakawa, Y., and Mayumi, M. (1982). *J. Immunol. Methods* **51,** 347–353.

Grady, G. F., and Lee, V. A. (1975). *N. Engl. J. Med.* **293,** 1067–1070.

Hansson, B. G., and Purcell, R. H. (1979). *Infect. Immun.* **26,** 125–130.

Hirose, H., Udo, K., Kojima, M., Takahashi, Y., Miyakawa, Y., Miyamoto, K., Yoshizawa, H., and Mayumi, M. (1984). *Kidney Int.* **26,** 338–341.

Hoofnagle, J. H. (1982). *In* "Viral Hepatitis" (W. Szmuness, H. J. Alter, and J. E. Maynard, eds.), pp. 573–583. Franklin Inst. Press, Philadelphia, Pennsylvania.

Hoofnagle, J. H. (1983). *Gastroenterology* **84,** 422–424.

Hoofnagle, J. H., Dusheiko, G. M., Seeff, L. B., Jones, E. A., Waggoner, J. G., and Bales, Z. B. (1981). *Ann. Intern. Med.* **94,** 744–748.

Hopp, T. P., and Woods, K. R. (1981). *Proc. Natl. Acad. Sci. U.S.A.* **78,** 3824–3828.

Hruska, J. F., and Robinson, W. S. (1977). *J. Med. Virol.* **1,** 119–131.

Hsu, H.-C., Lin, G.-H., Chang, M.-H., and Chen, C.-H. (1983). *Clin. Nephrol.* **20,** 121–129.

Hyland, C. A., and Shanley, B. C. (1983). *Lancet 2,* 1140–1141.

Imai, M., Tachibana, F. C., Moritsugu, Y., Miyakawa, Y., and Mayumi, M. (1976). *Infect. Immun.* **14,** 631–635.

Imai, M., Yanase, Y., Nojiri, T., Miyakawa, Y., and Mayumi, M. (1979). *Gastroenterology* **76,** 242–247.

Imai, M., Nomura, M., Gotanda, T., Sano, T., Tachibana, K., Miyamoto, H., Takahashi, K., Toyama, S., Miyakawa, Y., and Mayumi, M. (1982). *J. Immunol.* **128,** 69–72.

Ito, H., Hattori, S., Matsuda, I., Amamiya, S., Hajikano, H., Yoshizawa, H., Miyakawa, Y., and Mayumi, M. (1981). *Lab. Invest.* **44,** 214–220.

Kamimura, T., Yoshikawa, A., Ichida, F., and Sasaki, H. (1981). *Hepatology* **1,** 392–397.

Kaplan, P. M., Greenman, R. L., Gerin, J. L., Purcell, R. H., and Robinson, W. S. (1973). *J. Virol.* **12,** 995–1005.

Lam, K. C., Tong, M. J., and Rakela, J. (1977). *Infect. Immun.* **16,** 403–404.

Lemon, S. M., Gates, N. L., Simms, T. E., and Bankroft, W. H. (1981). *J. Infect. Dis.* **143,** 803–809.

Lenkei, R., Mota, G., Dan, M. E., and Laky, M. (1974). *Rev. Roum. Biochim.* **11,** 271–276.

Lenkei, R., Onica, D., and Ghetie, V. (1977). *Experientia* **33,** 1046–1047.

Levy, M., and Kleinknecht, C. (1980). *Nephron* **26,** 259–265.

Liaw, Y. F., Chu, C. M., Su, I. J., Huang, M. J., Lin, D. Y., and Chang-Chien, C. S. (1983). *Gastroenterology* **84,** 216–219.

Liaw, Y. F., Chu, C. M., Lin, D. Y., Sheen, I. S., Yang, C. Y., and Huang, M. J. (1984). *J. Med. Virol.* **13,** 385–391.

Lindenschmidt, E.-G., Granato, C. F. H., Salefsky, C., Laufs, R., and Henning, H. (1984). *Klin. Wochenschr.* **62,** 231–237.

Machida, A., Kishimoto, S., Ohnuma, H., Miyamoto, H., Baba, K., Oda, K., Nakamura, T., Miyakawa, Y., and Mayumi, M. (1983). *Gastroenterology* **85,** 268–274.

Machida, A., Kishimoto, S., Ohnuma, H., Baba, K., Ito, Y., Miyamoto, H., Funatsu, G., Oda, K., Usuda, S., Togami, S., Nakamura, T., Miyakawa, Y., and Mayumi, M. (1984). *Gastroenterology* **86,** 910–918.

Maggiore, Q., Bartolomeo, F., L'Abbate, A., and Misefari, V. (1981). *Kidney Int.* **19,** 579–586.

Magnius, L. O., and Espmark, J. Å. (1972). *J. Immunol.* **109,** 1017–1021.

Magnius, L. O., Lindholm, A., Lundin, P., and Iwarson, S. (1975). *JAMA, J. Am. Med. Assoc.* **231,** 356–359.

Masuko, K., Mitsui, T., Iwano, K., Yamazaki, C., Aihara, S., Baba, K., Takai, E., Tsuda, F., Nakamura, T., Miyakawa, Y., and Mayumi, M. (1985). *Gastroenterology* **88,** 151–155.

Maynard, J. E., Barrett, D. H., Murphy, B. L., Bradley, D. W., Berquist, K. R., and Bender, T. R. (1976). *J. Infect. Dis.* **133,** 339–342.

Mayumi, M., and Miyakawa, Y. (1978). *N. Engl. J. Med.* **299**, 46–47.

Mildvan, D., Mathur, U., Enlow, R. W., Romain, P. L., Winchester, R. J., Colp, C., Singman, H., Adelsberg, B. R., and Spigland, I. (1982). *Ann. Intern. Med.* **96**, 700–704.

Miller, D. J., Williams, A. E., Le Bouvier, G. L., Dwyer, J. M., Grant, J., and Klatskin, G. (1978). *Gastroenterology* **74**, 1208–1213.

Miyakawa, Y., and Mayumi, M. (1978). *In* "Viral Hepatitis" (G. N. Vyas, S. N. Cohen, and R. Schmid, eds.), pp. 193–201. Franklin Inst. Press, Philadelphia, Pennsylvania.

Miyakawa, Y., and Mayumi, M. (1982). *In* "Viral Hepatitis" (W. Szmuness, H. J. Alter, and J. E. Maynard, eds.), pp. 183–194. Franklin Inst. Press, Philadelphia, Pennsylvania.

Miyakawa, Y., Tsuda, F., Akahane, Y., and Mayumi, M. (1979). *Vox Sang.* **36**, 307–311.

Murphy, B. L., Peterson, J. M., Smith, J. L., Gitnick, G. L., Auslander, M. O., Berquist, K. R., Maynard, J. E., and Purcell, R. H. (1976). *Infect. Immun.* **13**, 296–297.

Mushahwar, I. K., and Overby, L. R. (1981). *J. Virol. Methods* **3**, 89–97.

Mushahwar, I. K., McGrath, L. C., Drnec, J., and Overby, L. R. (1981). *Am. J, Clin. Pathol.* **76**, 692–697.

Nagata, K., Fujita, M., Aoyama, R., Miyakawa, Y., Yoshizawa, H., and Mayumi, M. (1981). *Int. J. Pediatr. Nephrol.* **2**, 103–108.

Nath, N., Fang, C. T., Fields, H. A., Doto, I. L., and Maynard, J. E. (1980). *J. Med. Virol.* **6**, 179–184.

Neurath, A. R., and Strick, N. (1976). *Intervirology* **7**, 356–359.

Neurath, A. R., and Strick, N. (1977). *Proc. Natl. Acad. Sci. U.S.A.* **74**, 1702–1706.

Neurath, A. R., and Strick, N. (1979). *Intervirology* **11**, 128–132.

Neurath, A. R., Trepo, C., Chen, M., and Prince, A. M. (1976). *J. Gen. Virol.* **30**, 277–285.

Neurath, A. R., Huang, S.-N. and Strick, N. (1978). *J. Gen. Virol.* **39**, 91–101.

Neurath, A. R., Kent, S. B. H., and Strick, N. (1984). *Science* **224**, 392–395.

Nielsen, J. O., Dietrichson, O., and Juhl, E. (1974). *Lancet* 2, 913–915.

Nordenfelt, E., and Kjellen, L. (1975). *Intervirology* **5**, 225–232.

Norkrans, G., Magnius, L., and Iwarson, S. (1976). *Br. Med. J.* **1**, 740–742.

Norkrans, G., Frosner, G., and Iwarson, S. (1979). *Scand. J. Gastroenterol.* **14**, 289–293.

Ohbayashi, A., Okochi, K., and Mayumi, M. (1972). *Gastroenterology* **62**, 618–625.

Ohbayashi, A., Matsuo, Y., Mozai, T., Imai, M., and Mayumi, M. (1976). *Lancet* 2, 577–578.

Ohbayashi, A., Nakamura, Y., Matsuo, Y., Miyakawa, Y., Baba, K., and Mayumi, M. (1977). *Lancet* 1, 433.

Okada, K., Kamiyama, I., Inomata, M., Imai, M., Miyakawa, Y., and Mayumi, M. (1976). *N. Engl. J. Med.* **294**, 746–749.

Okamoto, H., Imai, M., Usuda, S., Tanaka, E., Tachibana, K., Mishiro, S., Machida, A., Nakamura, T., Miyakawa, Y., and Mayumi, M. (1985). *J. Immunol.* **134**, 1212–1216.

Ono, Y., Onda, H., Sasada, R., Igarashi, K., Sugino, Y., and Nishioka, K. (1983). *Nucleic Acid Res.* **11**, 1747–1757.

Pasek, M., Goto, T., Gilbert, W., Zink, B., Schaller, H., MacKay, P., Leadbetter, G., and Murray, K. (1979). *Nature (London)* **282**, 575–579.

Perrillo, R. P., Gelb, L. D., Milligan, W. H., Wellinghoff, W., and Aach, R. D. (1977). *J. Infect. Dis.* **136**, 117–121.

Perrillo, R. P., Gelb, L., Campbell, C., Wellinghoff, W., Ellis, F. R., Overby, L., and Aach, R. D. (1979). *Gastroenterology* **76**, 1319–1325.

Peterson, D. L., Roberts, I. M., Vyas, G. N. (1977). *Proc. Natl. Acad. Sci. U.S.A.* **74**, 1530–1534.

Pontisso, P., Alberti, A., Bortolotti, F., and Realdi, G. (1983). *Gastroenterology* **84**, 220–226.

Realdi, G., Alberti, A., Rugge, M., Bortolotti, F., Rigoli, A. M., Tremolada, F., and Ruol, A. (1980). *Gastroenterology* **79**, 195–199.

Richer, G., Phaneuf, D., Boisvert, F., Guévin, R., and Viallet, A. (1977). *Can. Med. Assoc. J.* **116**, 757–759.

Robinson, W. S., Clayton, D. A., and Greenman, R. L. (1974). *J. Virol.* **14**, 384–391.

Sasaki, T., Hattori, T., and Mayumi, M. (1979). *Vox Sang.* **37**, 216–221.

Schweitzer, I. L., Edwards, V. M., and Brezina, M. (1975). *N. Engl. J. Med* **293**, 940.

Sheikh, N. E., Woolf, I. L., Galbraith, R. M., Eddleston, A. L. W. F., Dymock, I. W., and Williams, R. (1975). *Br. Med. J.* **4**, 252–253.

Shikata, T., Karasawa, T., Abe, K., Uzawa, T., Suzuki, H., Oda, T., Imai, M., Mayumi, M., and Moritsugu, Y. (1977). *J. Infect. Dis.* **136**, 571–576.

Shiraki, K., Yoshihara, N., Sakurai, M., Eto, T., and Kawana, T. (1980). *J. Pediatr. (St. Louis)* **97**, 768–770.

Skinhøj, P., Cohn, J., and Bradburne, A. F. (1976). *Br. Med. J.* **1**, 10–11.

Ślusarczyk, J., Michalak, T., Nazarewicz-de Mezer, T., Krawczyński, K., and Nowoslawski, A. (1980). *Am. J. Pathol.* **98**, 29–39.

Smith, A. M., and Tedder, R. S. (1981). *J. Virol. Methods* **3**, 1–11.

Smith, J. L., Murphy, B. L., Auslander, M. O., Maynard, J. E., Schalm, S. S., Summerskill, H. J., and Gitnick, G. L. (1976). *Gastroenterology* **71**, 208–209.

Stannard, L. M., Lennon, M., Hodgkiss, M., and Smuts, H. (1982). *J. Med. Virol.* **9**, 165–175.

Stevens, C. E., Beasley, R. P., Tsui, J., and Lee, W.-C. (1975). *N. Engl. J. Med.* **292**, 771–774.

Stevens, C. E., Naurath, R. A., Beasley, R. P., and Szmuness, W. (1979). *J. Med. Virol.* **3**, 237–241.

Stibbe, W., and Gerlich, W. H. (1982). *J. Virol.* **123**, 436–442.

Szmuness, W., Neurath, A. R., Stevens, C. E., Strick, N., and Harley, E. J. (1981). *Am. J. Epidemiol.* **113**, 113–121.

Tabor, E., Russell, R. P., Gerety, R. J., Barker, L. F., Hillis, W. D., and Jackson, D. R. (1977). *Gastroenterology* **73**, 1157–1159.

Tabor, E., Frosner, G., Deinhardt, F., and Gerety, R. J. (1980a). *J. Med. Virol.* **6**, 91–99.

Tabor, E., Goldfield, M., Balack, H. C., and Gerety, R. J. (1980b). *Transfusion (Philadelphia)* **20**, 192–198.

Tada, H., Yanagida, M., Mishina, J., Fujii, T., Baba, K., Ishikawa, S., Aihara, S., Tsuda, F., Miyakawa, Y., and Mayumi, M. (1982). *Pediatrics* **70** 613–619.

Takahashi, K., Imai, M., Tsuda, F., Takahashi, T., Miyakawa, Y., and Mayumi, M. (1976). *J. Immunol.* **117**, 102–105.

Takahashi, K., Fukuda, M., Baba, K., Imai, M., Miyakawa, Y., and Mayumi, M. (1977). *J. Immunol.* **119**, 1556–1559.

Takahashi, K., Imai, M., Miyakawa, Y., Iwakiri, S., and Mayumi, M. (1978a). *Proc. Natl. Acad. Sci. U.S.A.* **75**, 1952–1956.

Takahashi, K., Yamashita, S., Imai, M., Miyakawa, Y., and Mayumi, M. (1978b). *J. Gen. Virol.* **38**, 431–436.

Takahashi, K., Akahane, Y., Gotanda, T., Mishiro, S., Imai, M., Miyakawa, Y., and Mayumi, M. (1979a). *J. Immunol.* **122**, 275–279.

Takahashi, K., Miyakawa, Y., Gotanda, T., Mishiro, S., Imai, M., and Mayumi, M. (1979b). *Gastroenterology* **77**, 1193–1199.

Takahashi, K., Imai, M., Gotanda, T., Sano, T., Oinuma, A., Mishiro, S., Miyakawa, Y., and Mayumi, M. (1980). *J. Gen. Virol.* **50**, 49–57.

Takahashi, K., Imai, M., Nomura, M., Oinuma, A., Machida, A., Funatsu, G., Miyakawa, Y., and Mayumi, M., (1981). *J. Gen. Virol.* **57**, 325–330.

Takahashi, K., Machida, A., Funatsu, G., Nomura, M., Usuda, S., Aoyagi, S., Tachibana, K., Miyamoto, H., Imai, M., Nakamura, T., Miyakawa, Y., and Mayumi, M. (1983). *J. Immunol.* **130**, 2903–2907.

Takekoshi, Y., Tanaka, M., Shida, N., Satake, Y., Saheki, Y., and Matsumoto, S. (1978). *Lancet 2*, 1065–1068.

Takekoshi, Y., Tanaka, M., Miyakawa, Y., Yoshizawa, H., Takahashi, K., and Mayumi, M. (1979). *N. Engl. J. Med.* **300**, 814–819.

Thamer, G., Gmelin, K., and Kommerell, B. (1976). *Lancet 2*, 577.

Thung, S. N., and Gerber, M. A. (1983). *Liver 3*, 290–294.

Tiollais, P., Charnay, P., and Vyas, G. N. (1981). *Science* **213**, 406–411.

Tong, M. J., Thursby, M., Rakela, J., McPeak, C., Edwards, V. M., and Mosley, J. W. (1981). *Gastroenterology* **80**, 999–1004.

Trepo, C., Vitvitski, L., Neurath, R., Hashimoto, N., Schaefer, R., Nemoz, G., and Prince, A. M. (1976). *Lancet 1*, 486.

Trepo, C., Hantz, O., Vitvitski, L., Chevallier, P., Williams, A., Lemaire, J. M., and Sepetjian, M. (1978). *In* "Viral Hepatitis" (G. N. Vyas, S. N. Cohen, and R. Schmid, eds.), pp. 203–209. Franklin Inst. Press, Philadelphia, Pennsylvania.

Trevisan, A., Gudat, F., Guggenheim, R., Krey, G., Dürmüller, U., Lüond, G., Düggelin, M., Landmann, J., Tondelli, P., and Bianchi, L. (1982). *Hepatology* **2**, 832–835.

Valenzuela, P., Grey, P., Quiroga, M., Zaldivar, J., Goodman, H. M., and Rutter, W. J. (1979). *Nature (London)* **280**, 815–819.

Villarejos, V. M., Anderson-Visona, K., and Canales, J. S. (1978). *Am. J. Trop. Med. Hyg.* **27**, 286–289.

Vnek, J., Prince, A. M., Trepo, C., Williams, A. E., Mushahwar, I. K., Ling, C. M., and Overby, L. R. (1979). *J. Med. Virol.* **4**, 187–199.

Vyas, G. N., Peterson, D. L., Townsend, R. M., Damle, S. R., and Magnius, L. O. (1977). *Science* **198**, 1068–1070.

Werner, B. G., and Blumberg, B. S. (1978). *Ann. Intern. Med.* **89**, 310–314.

Werner, B. G., and Grady, G. F. (1982). *Ann. Intern. Med.* **97**, 367–369.

Werner, B. G., O'Connell, A. P., and Summers, J. (1977). *Proc. Natl. Acad. Sci. U.S.A.* **74**, 2149–2151.

Williams, A., and Le Bouvier, G. (1976). *Bibl. Haematol. (Basel)* **42**, 71–75.

Wong, V. C. W., Ip, H. M. H., Reesink, H. W., Lelie, P. N., Reerink-Brongers, E. E., Yeung, C. Y., and Ma, H. K. (1984). *Lancet 1*, 921–926.

Yamada, E., Ohori, H., and Ishida, N. (1981). *J. Gen. Virol.* **55**, 75–86.

Yanagida, M., Horiguchi, S., Fujii, T., Okada, K., Nakao, C., Ishikawa, S., Miyakawa, Y., Baba, K., and Mayumi, M. (1979). *J. Pediatr. (St. Louis)* **95**, 76–77.

Yoshizawa, H., Itoh, Y., Simonetti, J. P., Takahashi, T., Machida, A., Miyakawa, Y., and Mayumi, M. (1979). *J. Gen. Virol.* **42**, 513–519.

Chapter 5

The Epidemiology of Hepatitis B

ROBERT J. GERETY AND EDWARD TABOR
Center for Drugs and Biologics
Office of Biologics Research and Review
Food and Drug Administration
Bethesda, Maryland

I. Introduction

Hepatitis B virus (HBV) infection is endemic in many parts of the world, where transmission occurs from infected mothers to their infants, from close contact within and outside of the family, and perhaps from hematophagous insects and incisions associated with initiation rites. Chronic infections provide a human reservoir. In developed countries, HBV infections occur sporadically. They are transmitted mainly by percutaneous means (blood transfusions, plasma derivative therapy, and occupational exposure to patients' blood), but also occasionally by nonpercutaneous means by intrafamilial contact and from mother to infant. Rapid technological developments have led to a dramatic reduction in the number of posttransfusion hepatitis B cases. Nevertheless, transmission at a lower incidence by blood transfusions has continued. Transmission by plasma derivatives like clotting factor concentrates continues to be a problem, but recently developed virus inactivation procedures have been successfully applied to these products to reduce the risk of HBV transmission following their use.

77

Copyright © 1985 by Academic Press, Inc.
All rights of reproduction in any form reserved.
ISBN 0-12-280672-7

HBV has an ability to produce chronic infections in from 5 to 10% of infected adults and in a significantly higher percentage of infected infants and children, which has provided HBV with a significant human reservoir; current estimates indicate that there are >200 million chronic carriers worldwide. Severe long-term consequences can result from or are associated with chronic hepatitis B, including chronic active hepatitis, cirrhosis, and primary hepatocellular carcinoma (PHC). Figure 1 illustrates the worldwide distribution of chronic HBsAg carriers and the association between chronic hepatitis B and PHC. Existing vaccines can prevent HBV infection (and its sequelae) when administered prior to exposure, but are expensive and not currently available to all who would benefit from them. Hepatitis B vaccines produced by genetic engineering techniques should be less expensive and more readily available to those most in need of vaccination. No means exist currently to "cure" the >200 million hepatitis B carriers that exist worldwide.

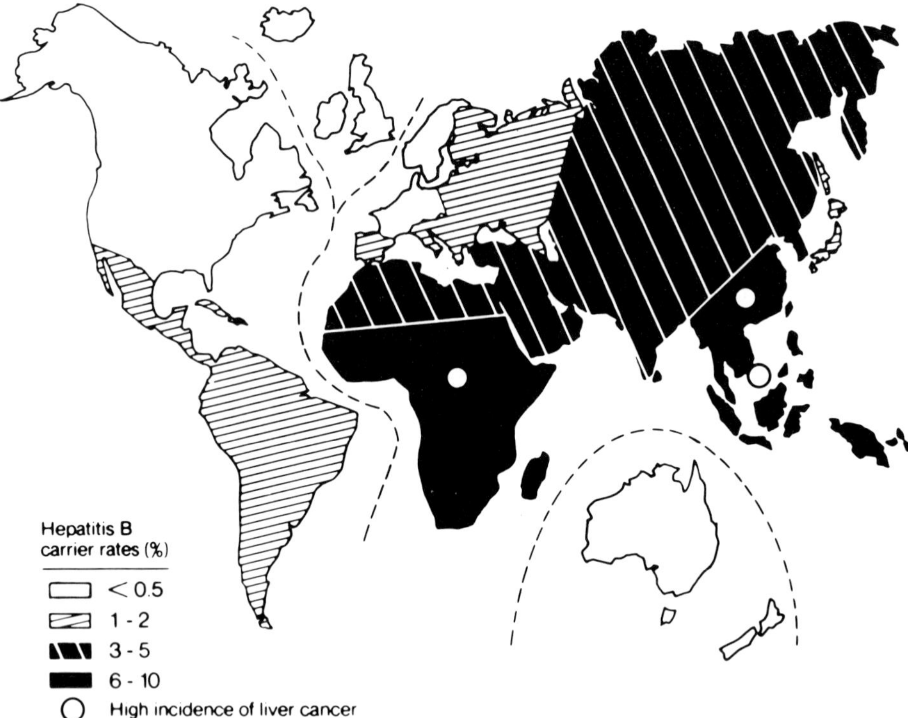

Figure 1. Worldwide prevalence of hepatitis B carriers. (Adapted from Szmuness *et al.*, 1981.)

II. Worldwide Prevalence

Extensive serological surveys have documented that HBV is distributed worldwide with extensive transmission occurring even among persons in geographically isolated populations. Most serological surveys have only reported the prevalence of HBsAg positivity alone (Fig. 1). While such data adequately identify those capable of transmitting HBV infection (chronic carriers), they underestimate the frequency of HBV transmission in a given population by 10- to 20-fold, since the majority of infected persons clear HBsAg. Nevertheless, HBsAg prevalences in developed countries in the West are low (<1%). Intermediate prevalences are seen in eastern and southern Europe, South America, northern Africa, and the Soviet Union (2–10%), while prevalences in southern Africa and southeastern Asia reach 50% in isolated populations (Gust, 1981; Szmuness *et al.*, 1981). HBsAg prevalences, however, can vary dramatically within countries, as is exemplified by the low prevalences among New Zealanders of European origin and the high prevalences among the Maoris living in New Zealand (Gust, 1981). Similar disparities in prevalences of HBV seropositivity have been described among different groups in Zambia (Tabor *et al.*, 1984) and the Gambia (Whittle *et al.*, 1983).

While the modes of transmission of HBV in low prevalence areas appear to be largely percutaneous (Section IV), in high prevalence areas HBV can be effectively transmitted from infected mothers to their infants. In some regions, this mechanism accounts for a high percentage of HBV infections. In other areas of the world, HBV infections are most often acquired later in childhood by either nonpercutaneous or by inapparent percutaneous mechanisms. Stevens *et al.* (1975) and Beasley *et al.* (1977) clearly demonstrated that mother-to-infant HBV transmission is common in Taiwan, especially among infants born to HBeAg-positive mothers. In contrast, Prince *et al.* (1981), and later Whittle *et al.* (1983) and Tabor *et al.* (1984), showed that mother-to-infant transmission of HBV does not appear to occur to any great extent in Africa. Instead, transmission in these areas as well as in Nigeria (Tabor and Gerety, 1979) takes place not at birth, but during childhood. Whittle *et al.* (1983) interpreted their data to indicate transmission from sibling to sibling as a major mode of acquisition of infection, while Tabor *et al.* (1984) concluded that horizontal transmission of HBV infection observed in Zambia was not transmitted among household members but originated outside the household.

III. U.S. Surveillance Data

Viral hepatitis is the second most frequently reported infectious disease in the United States (Centers for Disease Control 1981). Two surveillance systems managed by the Centers for Disease Control provide information about hepatitis in the United States; the states and territories report cases according to the type of hepatitis, the age of the patients, and the date of occurrence. More complete data are obtained from a separate Viral Hepatitis Surveillance Program, which is voluntary and includes information relating to risk factors associated with cases, as well as more complete serological test data. Other serological surveys of HBsAg and anti-HBs prevalences among adults in the United States suggest a much higher attack rate of HBV infection than reported, perhaps 3- to 10-fold higher. This discrepancy, however, is at least partially explained by the fact that HBV infections are commonly subclinical and therefore are neither recognized nor reported. Approximately 60,000 cases of hepatitis are reported each year in the United States; 18,000 (~8 per 100,000 population) are hepatitis B (Centers for Disease Control, 1981). Hepatitis B occurs more frequently among those that are 15–44 years of age, among males, and among Caucasians (Table I).

The frequency of hepatitis B cases differs by state and territory. The highest frequency of hepatitis B cases occurs among east and west coast states, in Alaska and in Tennessee, Indiana, and Colorado (>8 cases per 100,000 population) (Fig. 2). The lowest frequency of reported hepatitis B cases occurs in the north central states and in Puerto Rico and the Virgin Islands (0–3.9 cases per 100,000 population).

Although risk factors for the acquisition of hepatitis B are discussed more fully in Section IV, some data relating to reported cases of hepatitis B and their possible source is worthy of mention here. Contact with a person with hepatitis B, illicit percutaneous drug use, and other potential percutaneous exposures to blood are among those factors most often associated with reported cases of hepatitis B. Although on the average 8% of those reported to have hepatitis B were employed in occupations defined as high risk for the acquisition of HBV infection, this factor accounted for up to 18% of reported cases in some states. Similarly, on an average 6% of hepatitis B cases reported were in male homosexuals; the proportion of male homosexuals among reported cases of hepatitis B in some states was as high as 21%, however.

It has been estimated that the number of HBsAg carriers in the United States approaches 1,000,000 and increases by 8,000–16,000 new carriers each year. Data indicate that the prevalence of HBsAg among first-time

TABLE I
Distribution of Cases of Hepatitis B in the United States by Age,
Sex, and Race[a]

Parameter		Approximate percentage of reported cases
Age (years)	< 5	0.6
	5–9	0.7
	10–14	0.7
	15–19	11.1
	20–29	47.9
	30–39	18.6
	40–49	8.1
	50–59	5.8
	> 60	6.3
Sex	Male	62.7
	Female	37.3
Race	Caucasian	71.2
	Black	20.5
	Other	8.3

[a]From Centers for Disease Control, 1981.

blood donors roughly parallels the frequency of hepatitis B cases in the various regions of the United States (Dodd *et al.*, 1982) (Fig. 3).

Szmuness *et al.* (1981) studied HBsAg carriers identified among volunteer blood donors in New York, and provided valuable epidemiologic data concerning these carriers. They were more often male, nonwhite, born outside of the United States, and not Jewish. They more often belonged to lower socioeconomic groups with a poor education and a low annual income. Compared to controls, they more often had a history of hepatitis or of tattooing. Among all populations tested for HBsAg, Szmuness *et al.* (1981) found that only 0.4% of volunteer blood donors were HBsAg positive; this figure was 14.9% HBsAg positive for dialysis patients (Table II).

Fifty percent of hepatitis B cases reported in the United States each year are among persons in categories designated as high risk for the acquisition of hepatitis B (Section IV). Vaccination of all high-risk individuals in the United States, therefore, could prevent half of all cases of hepatitis B and half of all new chronic infections (4,000–8,000 carriers per year).

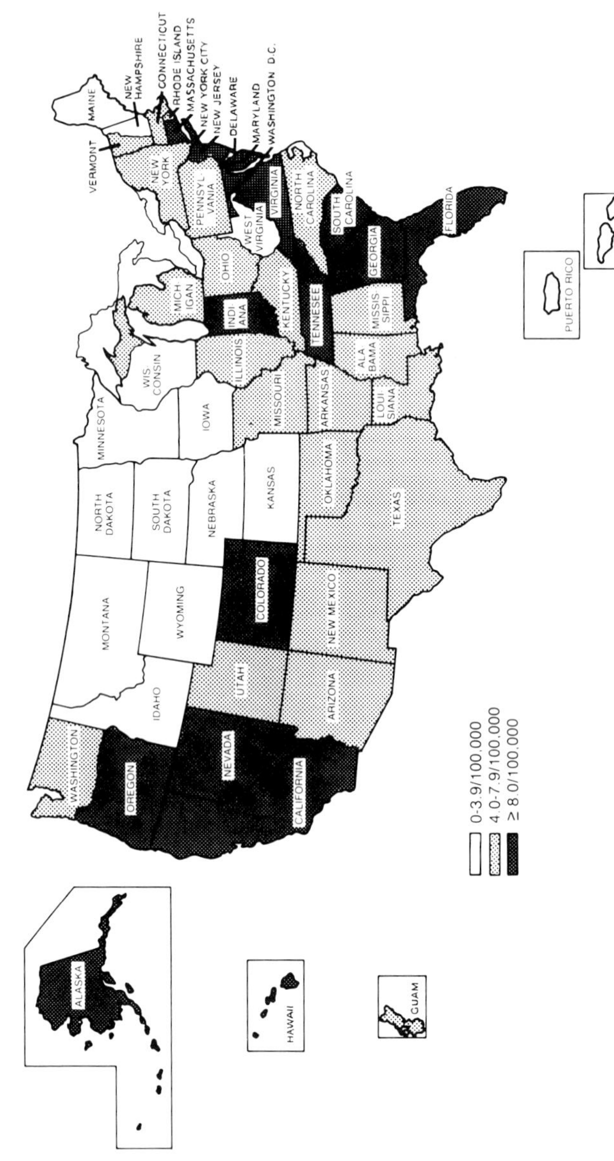

Figure 2. Reported cases of hepatitis B by state or territory (1980).

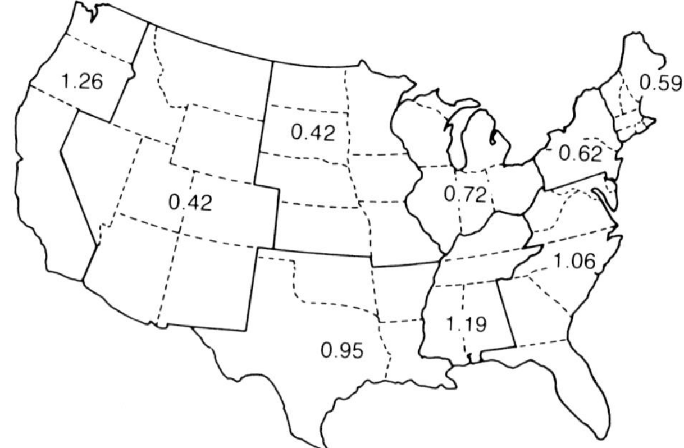

Figure 3. HBsAg detection rates among blood donors (number positive/100,000 donors) in nine geographical regions in the United States.

IV. Risk Factors for Acquisition of Infection and for the Development of Chronicity

A variety of risk factors related to percutaneous as well as to nonpercutaneous exposures to HBV are associated with the acquisition of infection. These include lower socioeconomic status, maternal infection, contact with acutely or chronically infected persons, residence in institutions, and employment as a health care worker (physician, dentist, oral hygienist, and ward or laboratory personnel) who handles blood or body fluids from patients. Table III lists the relative risk of acquisition of HBV infection by job category among health care workers. Other risk

TABLE II
Prevalence of HBsAg Among Selected Populations in New York[a]

Population	Number tested	HBsAg positive (%)
Volunteer blood donors	2163	0.4
Hospital patients	185	0.4
Dialysis staff	659	1.4
Dialysis patients	1288	14.9
Male homosexuals	3000	5.1
Intravenous drug users	321	2.8
Mentally retarded	612	10.5
Chinese–Americans	666	9.3

[a]Adapted from Szmuness et al., 1981.

TABLE III
Relative Risk for the Acquisition of Hepatitis B among Health Care Workers[a]

Standardized prevalence[b]	Occupational category
27	Medical technologists
26	Blood bank, dialysis, and morgue technologists
19	EKG and pulmonary technicians
18	Attending MDs
18	Clinical lab technicians
17	Dentists
17	RNs and anesthetists
17	OR and surgical technicians
15	Aides and orderlies
15	Administrative assistants
15	Laundry, housekeeping and central supply employees
13	Laboratory assistants
13	Inhalation therapists
13	Food service workers
12	Chemists and microbiologists
12	Radiology and nuclear medicine technicians
11	LPNs and LVNs
11	Cytology and other technologists
11	Building maintenance employees
10	Hygienists and therapists ("other")
10	Social workers and dieticians
10	Clerical workers
9	Research technicians
9	Dental hygienists
9	Administrators
6	Pharmacists and assistants

[a]Expressed as standardized prevalence of serological positivity for HBV-related markers.

[b]Compared to a control population where the prevalence was 4–6%. (Source: Centers for Disease Control).

factors include hospitalization, receipt of either blood or a high-risk plasma derivative (Section IV,A,2) or the use of illicit intravenous drugs. The presence in a household of an HBsAg carrier increases the risk that others in that household will be infected, regardless of the relationship between the carrier and the other household members (Bernier *et al.*, 1982). In one study of 422 household contacts of 157 adult chronic carriers conducted by Bernier *et al.*, the HBsAg prevalence was 6.8-fold higher and the anti-HBs prevalence 2.7-fold higher among household contacts of carriers than among controls living in similar households without carriers. In addition to confirming that person-to-person modes of transmission are important for the spread of HBV infection within households, the data from this study suggested that mother-to-infant transmission accounts for the higher HBsAg carrier prevalence, while unidentified types of contact best explained the increased prevalence of anti-HBs. An increased risk of acquisition of HBV infection from persons acutely ill with hepatitis B has also been documented. In a study by Koff *et al.* (1977), 23% of exposed spouses or sexual partners acquired HBV infections from acutely ill persons. This risk, unlike that among contacts of chronic carriers, appeared to be confined to spouses or sexual partners of cases. This lack of risk of transmission during acute hepatitis B except by intimate (sexual) contact is consistent with the lack of transmission of hepatitis B to patients by health care personnel with acute hepatitis B (Gerber *et al.*, 1977).

Transmission of HBV infection by chronic carriers to susceptible persons can also occur by percutaneous means, including blood transfusions, needles shared by users of illicit intravenous drugs, tattooing, acupuncture, or hematophagous insects. Inapparent percutaneous transmission may also occur via shared tooth brushes or razors, or exposure to weeping cutaneous lesions on chronically infected individuals. Bernier *et al.* (1982) found that contacts within households with chronic carriers who had exudative skin lesions had significantly higher rates of HBV infections than those with contacts with carriers lacking such lesions.

Although oral transmission is not believed to play a significant role in the spread of HBV infection, it may occur in certain circumstances. The finding of HBsAg in a number of body fluids other than blood suggests that spread may sometimes occur by means of exposure to saliva, urine, breast milk, semen, cerebrospinal fluid, pleural effusion fluid, or vaginal secretions, even in the absence of detectable blood (Spiegel *et al.*, 1980; Tabor *et al.*, 1977; Villarejos *et al.*, 1974). Hepatitis B has been experimentally transmitted to gibbons by ingestion of saliva from a carrier (Bancroft *et al.*, 1977) and to chimpanzees by the inoculation of semen from human HBsAg carriers (Alter *et al.*, 1977). The spectrum of possible nonpercutaneous or inapparent percutaneous routes of infection may explain why the vast majority of individuals having HBV serological markers have no history of previous blood transfusions.

A. Percutaneous Exposure

1. Transmission by Blood Transfusion. Prior to the introduction of serological testing for HBsAg, as many as 60% of posttransfusion hepatitis cases were hepatitis B (Alter *et al.*, 1975a). As a result of the requirement by federal regulation to test all blood and plasma donations for HBsAg by sensitive techniques in the United States, the percentage of hepatitis B has been reduced to 11–13% of cases of posttransfusion hepatitis (Aach *et al.*, 1978; Alter *et al.*, 1975b), or ~1.7% of all blood recipients (Aach *et al.*, 1978). Since 1977, all blood intended for transfusion in the United States has been required by federal regulations to also be labeled "paid" or "volunteer", according to its source. This requirement is based on the observation that more than twice as many recipients of HBsAg-negative units of blood from paid donors develop HBV infection as compared to those receiving HBsAg-negative blood from volunteer donors (Goldfield *et al.*, 1975). This labelling of blood units is believed to have had a substantial impact on the incidence of hepatitis B following transfusions, augmenting the impact of screening for HBsAg.

2. Transmission by Clotting Factor Concentrates. Infusion of plasma derivatives such as clotting factor concentrates presents a particularly high risk for the transmission of HBV. The plasma pools used in the manufacture of these products include 1,000–10,000 liters of human plasma each, and therefore have a good chance of containing a unit of plasma with a level of HBV that is below the limit of detectability by testing for HBsAg. A plasma sample that is negative for HBsAg may theoretically contain as many as 1000 infectious doses of HBV per milliliter (Tabor *et al.*, 1983). Such plasma units probably represent ~1% of all plasma donations (Aach *et al.*, 1978). Inclusion of such plasma units in a 10,000-liter pool could result in up to 10^8 infectious doses of HBV per pool, or up to 10 infectious doses per milliliter.

Transmission of HBV by some antihemophilic factor (AHF) lots and factor IX complex (Factor IX) lots manufactured after the introduction of screening for HBsAg has been documented. Scaroni *et al.* (1980) found HBV serological markers in 93% of 29 hemophiliacs (27 with hemophilia A; two with hemophilia B) who ranged in age from 2 to 9 years. Gomperts *et al.* (1981) found HBV serological markers in 5 of 7 hemophiliacs born after 1975 who had been treated only with AHF. Gerety *et al.* (1980) found HBV serological markers in 29 of 34 (85%) hemophiliacs <10 years of age, and Norkans *et al.* (1981) described two patients infected by AHF manufactured after 1975. The overall prevalence of HBV serological markers among hemophiliacs continues to range from 81 to 95% (Hasiba *et al.*, 1977; Spero *et al.*, 1978; Preston *et al.*, 1978; Gerety *et al.*, 1980).

It appears that not all AHF and Factor IX lots transmit HBV. Between 5 and 19% of hemophiliacs have no HBV serological markers (Hasiba *et al.*, 1977; Spero *et al.*, 1978; Preston *et al.*, 1978; Gerety *et al.*, 1980). Wyke *et al.* (1979) identified four lots of AHF that did not transmit HBV infection to any of five susceptible hemophiliacs. Although in our current understanding of hepatitis B one must conclude that seronegative hemophiliacs have not had previous HBV infections, it is conceivable that some were previously infected but no longer had detectable HBV serological markers.

Newly diagnosed hemophiliacs who receive AHF or Factor IX for the first time are at a particularly high risk for acquiring HBV infection. Factor IX has also been used in some patients who do not have a documented deficiency of this clotting factor, which has caused great concern among those familiar with its HBV risk.

When hemophiliacs have chronic hepatitis B and chronic elevations of serum alanine aminotransferase (ALT) activity, liver biopsies often reveal either chronic active hepatitis (CAH), chronic persistent hepatitis (CPH), or postnecrotic cirrhosis. The percentage of the total number of hemophiliac carriers who develop CAH or CPH is not known. However, since nearly all hemophiliacs are infected by HBV at some time and 2–5% become chronic carriers with chronic elevations in ALT activity, the percentage of all hemophiliacs with CAH or CPH associated with HBV is at least 2%.

Other derivatives of pooled human plasma are not associated with any risk of HBV transmission. Immune globulin (IG, immune serum globulin, or gamma globulin), when manufactured by the cold ethanol fractionation method of Cohn from plasma that has been screened for HBsAg, does not transmit HBV infections. Both albumin and plasma protein fraction, when heated at 60°C for 10 hr during or subsequent to manufacture, are also free of any risk of transmitting HBV as a result of this heating procedure (Gerety and Aronson, 1982).

The development of methods to inactivate HBV in AHF and Factor IX, in conjunction with the judicious use of hepatitis B vaccine, will eventually reduce or eliminate HBV infections among hemophiliacs. Methods used to inactivate or to reduce infectious HBV in AHF and Factor IX include heating at 60°C for 10 hr after stabilization with glycine and saccharose (Heimburger *et al.*, 1980, 1981), heating at 60°C for 10 hr in the lyophilized state (Rubinstein, 1981), treating with β-propiolactone plus ultraviolet irradiation (Prince *et al.*, 1980) and adding globulin containing high titers of anti-HBs (Tabor *et al.*, 1980a,b). Physical removal of HBV from pools of human plasma, based on the hydrophobic attraction of the lipid-containing HBsAg for an octanoic acid hydrazide–Sepharose 4B column, has also been accomplished (Einarsson *et al.*, 1981). It is expected that products with less risk of HBV infection will soon be available to be used by all hemophiliacs.

3. Other. Table IV shows that the majority of hepatitis B cases reported in the United States result from a variety of percutaneous ex-

TABLE IV
Percutaneous Acquisition of Hepatitis B in the United States[a]

Source	Reported cases (%)
Employed in medical/ dental settings	8
Employed in dialysis/transplant unit	2
Blood transfusion	4
Hospitalization	14
Surgery	7
Dental procedure	14
Illicit intravenous drug use	12
Other percutaneous exposure	15

[a]From Centers for Disease Control, 1981.

posures in addition to the transfusion of blood or the infusion of a plasma derivative. A significant percentage of cases is related either to employment in health care fields (10%) or to hospitalization and surgical procedures during hospitalization (21%).

B. Nonpercutaneous Exposure

1. Sexual. Sexual transmission of HBV infection has been documented to occur, although other types of close contact cannot be ruled out as the actual mechanism of transmission. The prevalence of HBV serological markers is higher among spouses of carriers than in other household members (Bernier *et al.*, 1982); the attack rate of HBV infection in spouses or sexual contacts of persons with acute hepatitis B can reach 23% (Koff *et al.*, 1977). Male homosexuals have also been documented to have high prevalences of HBV serological markers. Six percent of reported cases of hepatitis B in the United States have been in male homosexuals.

2. Mother-to-Infant Transmission. HBV infection from an acutely or chronically infected mother to her infant appears to be a major means to acquire HBV infection and to maintain a reservoir of HBsAg carriers in some parts of the world (Stevens *et al.*, 1975; Beasley *et al.*, 1977) but not in others (Tabor and Gerety, 1979; Tabor *et al.*, 1984; Whittle *et al.*, 1983). Transmission from a chronically infected mother to her infant occurs with a frequency approaching 90% if the mother is HBeAg positive; anti-HBe in the mother's serum suggests either that transmission of infection to her infant will not occur or that it will occur with a low frequency (Gerety and Schweitzer, 1977; Tong *et al.*, 1981). These observations as well as those of incubation periods of infections in infants are consistent with HBV exposure occurring during delivery and when there are higher titers of HBsAg and HBV in the mother's serum. Once infected during the perinatal period, >90% of these infants remain chronic carriers (see Section IV,C). Transmission from acutely infected mothers to their infants occurs only if the acute maternal infection occurs during the third trimester of pregnancy.

3. Other. It is sometimes difficult to distinguish between nonpercutaneous transmission of HBV infection and inapparent percutaneous transmission. Both mechanisms may be active in settings such as households or among children not in the same household in underdeveloped countries or lower socioeconomic areas where there are one or more carriers. Although mouth-to-mouth transmission may be important, transmission also occurs via serous exudates from skin ulcers of carriers, via hematophagous insects, or via inadequate sterilization of reusable syringes and needles (Brown *et al.*, 1984; Favero, 1980).

C. Chronicity

In the early 1970s it was recognized that HBV infection early in life was a major risk factor for the development of chronic HBV infections (Gerety *et al.*, 1974; Krugman and Giles, 1973; Schweitzer *et al.*, 1972). The percentage of infected newborns that became carriers approached 100%; this figure ranged from 29 to 40% among children overseas infected by HBV during childhood (Gerety *et al.*, 1974).

Additional risk factors for chronicity include immune defects and perhaps male sex (males more often become carriers), race, or genetic factors not yet clearly understood. The subtype of HBsAg appears not to be related to either disease severity or to chronicity (Gerety *et al.*, 1975).

V. Prevention

Prevention of hepatitis by specific immune globulin and/or vaccine is discussed in detail in Chapters 15 and 16. To develop an effective prevention program, the epidemiology of the acquisition of HBV infection in a given area must first be determined. If mother-to-infant transmission is either significant or predominant, prevention must be targeted to newborns, and implemented at birth in the delivery room or shortly thereafter (Beasley *et al.*, 1977, 1983a,b; Stevens *et al.*, 1975). If, however, mother-to-infant transmission is uncommon, and horizontal transmission accounts in large part for HBV infections, the age of acquisition should be determined by epidemiological studies such as those conducted by Tabor and co-workers (Tabor and Gerety, 1979; Tabor *et al.*, 1984) and Whittle *et al.* (1983). If HBV infections are acquired during early childhood as in Nigeria (Tabor and Gerety, 1979), prophylaxis should be administered during the early postnatal period. If HBV infections occur most frequently in later childhood, prophylaxis can effectively be administered to preschool children.

VI. Conclusions

The modes of transmission of HBV infections vary throughout the world, with percutaneous transmissions predominating in developed countries and nonpercutaneous or inapparent percutaneous transmission predominating in underdeveloped countries. Mother-to-infant transmission is an important means of HBV transmission in some areas like southeast Asia, while apparently being uncommon in western Africa. No means currently exist to "cure" chronically infected persons, but effective preexposure prevention of HBV infection by vaccine or vaccine plus hyperimmune globulin (HBIG) are available. Some data suggest that hepatitis B vaccine may also effectively prevent HBV infection when administered after exposure to HBV. Data on the epidemiological circumstances of HBV infection in a given area or country, including age of acquisition, are essential to develop an effective prevention program.

References

Aach, R. D., Lander, J. J., Sherman, L. A., Miller, W. V., Kahn, R. A., Gitnick, G. L., Hollinger, F. B., Werch, J., Szmuness, W., Stevens, C. E., Kellner, A., Weiner, J. M. and Mosley, J. W. (1978). *In* "Viral Hepatitis" (G. N. Vyas, S. N. Cohen, and R. Schmid, eds.), pp. 383–396. Franklin Inst. Press, Philadelphia, Pennsylvania.

Alter, H. J., Purcell, R. W., Holland, P. V., Feinstone, S. M., Morrow, A. G., and Moritsugu, Y. (1975a). *Lancet 2*, 838–841.

Alter, H. J., Holland, P. V., and Purcell, R. H. (1975b). *Am. J. Med. Sci.* **270**, 329–334.

Alter, H. J., Purcell, R. H., Gerin, J. L., London, W. T., Kaplan, P. M., McAuliffe, V. J., Wagner, J., and Holland, P. V. (1977). *Infect. Immun.* **16**, 928–933.

Bancroft, W. H., Snitbahn, R., Scott, R. M., Tingpalapong, M., Watson, W. T., Tanticharoenyos, P., Karwacki, J. J., and Srimarut, S. (1977). *J. Infect. Dis.* **135**, 79–85.

Beasley, R. P., Trepo, C., Stevens, C. E., and Szmuness, W. (1977). *Am. J. Epidemiol.* **105**, 94–98.

Beasley, R. P., Hwang, L.-Y., Lee, G. C.-Y., Lan, C.-C., Roan, C.-H., Huang, F.-Y., and Chen, C.-L. (1983a). *Lancet 1,* 1099–1102.

Beasley, R. P., Hwang, L.-Y., Stevens, C. E., Lin, C.-C., Hsieh, F.-J., Wang, K.-Y., Sun, T.-S., and Szmuness, W. (1983b). *Hepatology (N.Y.)* 3, 135–141.

Bernier, R. H., Sampliner, R., Gerety, R. J., Tabor, E., Hamilton, F., and Nathanson, N. (1982). *Am. J. Epidemiol.* **116,** 199–211.

Brown, P., Breguet, G., Smallwood, L., Ney, R., Moerdowo, R. M., and Gerety, R. J. (1984). *Am. J. Trop. Med.* (in press).

Centers for Disease Control (1981). *Morbid. Mortal. Week. Rep.* **32,** 23ss–30ss.

Dodd, R. Y., Nath, N., Bastiaans, M. J., and Barker, L. F. (1982). *In* "Viral Hepatitis" (W. Szmuness, H. J. Alter, and J. E. Maynard, eds.), pp. 145–155. Franklin Inst. Press, Philadelphia, Pennsylvania.

Einarsson, M., Kaplan, L., Nordenfelt, E., and Miller, E. (1981). *J. Virol. Methods* **3,** 213–228.

Favero, M. S. (1980). *In* "Manual of Clinical Microbiology" (E. H. Lennette, A. Balows, W. J. Hansler, Jr., and J. P. Truant, eds.), pp. 952–959. Am. Soc. Microbiol., Washington, D.C.

Gerber, M. A., Lewin, E. B., Gerety, R. J., and Le, C. (1977). *J. Pediatr. (St. Louis)* **91,** 120–123.

Gerety, R. J., and Aronson, D. L. (1982). *Transfusion (Philadelphia)* **22,** 347–351.

Gerety, R. J., and Schweitzer, I. L. (1977). *J. Pediatr. (St. Louis)* **90,** 368–374.

Gerety, R. J., Hoofnagle, J. H., Markenson, J. A., and Barker, L. F. (1974). *J. Pediatr. (St. Louis)* **84,** 661–665.

Gerety, R. J., Hoofnagle, J. H., Nortman, D. F., and Barker, L. F. (1975). *Gastroenterology* **68,** 1253–1260.

Gerety, R. J., Eyster, M. E., Tabor, E., Drucker, J. A., Lusch, C. J., Prager, D., Rice, S. A., and Bowman, H. S. (1980). *J. Med. Virol.* **6,** 111–118.

Goldfield, M., Black, H. C., Bill, J., Srihongse, S., and Pizzuti, W. (1975). *Am. J. Med. Sci.* **270,** 335–342.

Gomperts, E. D., Lazerson, J., Berg, D., Lockhart, D., and Sergis-Davenport, E. (1981). *Am. J. Hematol.* **11,** 55–59.

Gust, I. D. (1981). *In* "Viral Hepatitis" (W. Szmuness, H. J. Alter, and J. E. Maynard, eds.), pp. 129–143. Franklin Inst. Press, Philadelphia, Pennsylvania.

Hasiba, U., Spero, J. A. and Lewis, J. H. (1977). *Transfusion (Philadelphia)* **17,** 490–499.

Heimburger, N., Schwinn, H., and Mauler, R. (1980). *Gelben Hefte* **20,** 165–174.

Heimburger, N., Schwinn, H., Gratz, P., Luben, G., Kumpe, G., and Herchenhan, B. (1981). *Arzneim. Forsch.* **31,** 619–622.

Koff, R. S., Slavin, M. M., Lorna, R. N., Connelly, J. D., and Rosen, D. R. (1977). *Gastroenterology* **72,** 297–300.

Krugman, S., and Giles, J. P. (1973). *N. Engl. J. Med.* **288,** 755–760.

Norkrans, G., Widell, A., Teger-Nilsson, A. C., Kjellman, H., Frösner, G., and Iwarson, S. (1981). *Vox Sang.* **41,** 129–133.

Preston, F. E., Triger, D. R., Underwood, J. C. E., Bardham, G., Mitchell, V. E., Stewart, R. M., and Blackburn, E. K. (1978). *Lancet 2,* 592–611.

Prince, A. M., Stephan, W., Brotman, B., and van den Ende, M. C. (1980). *Thromb. Haemostasis* **44,** 138–142.

Prince, A. M., White, T., Pollock, N., Riddle, J., Brotman, B., and Richardson, L. (1981). *Infect. Immun.* **32,** 675–680.

Rubinstein, A. (1981). *Thromb. Haemostasis* **46,** 339 (abstr.).

Scaroni, C., Cancellieri, V., Carnelli, V., Moroni, G. A., and Angeli, M. (1980). *Lancet 2,* 537–538.

Schweitzer, I. L., Wing, A., McPeak, C., and Spears, R. L. (1972). *JAMA, J. Am. Med. Assoc.* **220**, 1092–1095.

Spero, J. A., Lewis, J. H., Van Thiel, D. H., Hasiba, U., and Rabin, B. S. (1978). *N. Engl. J. Med.* **298**, 1373–1379.

Spiegel, R. J., Tabor, E., Pizzo, P. A., and Gerety, R. J. (1980). *Med. Pediatr. Oncol.* **8**, 115–118.

Stevens, C. E., Beasley, R. P., Tsui, J., and Lee, W.-C. (1975). *N. Engl. J. Med.* **292**, 771–774.

Szmuness, W., Harley, E. J., Ikram, H., and Stevens, C. E. (1981). *In* "Viral Hepatitis" (W. Szmuness, H. J. Alter, and J. E. Maynard, eds.), pp. 297–320. Franklin Inst. Press, Philadelphia, Pennsylvania.

Tabor, E., and Gerety, R. J. (1979). *J. Pediatr. (St. Louis)* **95**, 647–650.

Tabor, E., Russell, R. P., Gerety, R. J., Barker, L. F., Hillis, W. D., and Jackson, D. J. (1977). *Gastroenterology* **73**, 1157–1159.

Tabor, E., Aronson, D. L., and Gerety, R. J. (1980a). *In* "Immunoglobulins: Characteristics and Uses of Intravenous Preparations" (B. M. Alving and J. S. Finlayson, eds.), pp. 133–135. U.S.DHHS, Bethesda, Maryland.

Tabor, E., Aronson, D. L., and Gerety, R. J. (1980b). *Lancet 2*, 68–70.

Tabor, E., Purcell, R. H., London, W. T., and Gerety, R. J. (1983). *J. Infect. Dis.* **147**, 531–534.

Tabor, E., Bayley, A. C., Cairns, J., Pelleu, L., and Gerety, R. J. (1984). *J. Med. Virol.* (in press).

Tong, M. J., Thursby, M., Rakela, J., McPeak, C., Edwards, V. M., and Mosley, J. W. (1981). *Gastroenterology* **80**, 999–1004.

Villarejos, V. M., Visoná, K. A., Gutiérrez, A., and Rodriguez, A. (1974). *N. Engl. J. Med.* **291**, 1375–1378.

Whittle, H. C., Bradley, A. K., McLauchlan, K., Ajdukiewicz, A. B., Howard, C. R., and Zuckerman, A. J. (1983). *Lancet 1*, 1203–1206.

Wyke, R. J., Tsiquaye, K. N., Thornton, A., White, Y., Portman, B., Das, P. K., Zuckerman, A. J., and Williams, R. (1979). *Lancet 1*, 520–524.

Chapter 6

The Acute Manifestations of Hepatitis B Virus Infection

ULRICH JUNGE
Department of Internal Medicine
University of Ulm
Ulm, West Germany

FRIEDRICH DEINHARDT
Max von Pettenkofer Institute
for Hygiene and Medical Microbiology
University of Munich
Munich, West Germany

Copyright © 1985 by Academic Press, Inc.
All rights of reproduction in any form reserved.
ISBN 0-12-280672-7

I. Introduction

Hepatitis B is a major clinical problem; the disease is often severe and prolonged, it has a tendency to become chronic, it is associated with cirrhosis and hepatocellular carcinoma, and no specific therapy exists. Infection with hepatitis B virus (HBV) can lead to different forms of disease: inapparent infection, acute disease of different severities, or persistent infection, with or without chronic liver disease. The incidence of persistent HBV infections varies somewhat in different parts of the world, and is particularly high in some areas of Africa and Asia. The difference in incidence of persistent infections is due partly to genetic factors but also to the age at which infection occurs, that is, infection very early in life (newborn or the first years of life) tends to lead more frequently to a chronic HBV carrier state than does infection occurring later in life. In Western (industrialized) societies, ~45% of all HBV infections result in acute disease, and 1% has a fatal outcome. Chronic infections develop in 5%, and the remaining 50% of all cases of hepatitis B follow an asymptomatic course.

This chapter is limited to a discussion of the diagnosis and clinical aspects of acute hepatitis B and inapparent HBV infections. Chronic HBV infections are covered in Chapters 7 and 8.

II. General Clinical Picture of Acute Viral Hepatitis B

Infection with HBV is not associated with any typical clinical picture, but like infections with other hepatitis viruses, it produces a spectrum of different clinical and laboratory manifestations. The severity of disease ranges from inapparent infection to lethal fulminant hepatitis.

A. Prodromes

The clinical course of acute hepatitis B is usually the same as that of hepatitis A or non-A, non-B hepatitis, although the onset of disease tends to be more insidious than that of hepatitis A. First symptoms are usually noticed 3–4 days before jaundice, but some patients have symptoms up to 14 days earlier.

Lassitude, weakness, and anorexia are the most common prodromes. Anorexia usually progresses towards evening, and patients find food repugnant; food smells may cause nausea. Impaired gustatory acuity and perversion of taste and smell sensations sometimes contribute to the anorexia, and cause patients to lose the desire to smoke or drink alcohol. Vomiting can occur but it is usually mild and not protracted. Constipation or diarrhea are observed in about one-fourth of patients. Abdominal discomfort or right upper abdominal pain is common. All these digestive symptoms result in an average weight loss of 2 to 4 kg. Flu-like symptoms with slight temperature elevation are common, and are usually accompanied by malaise, mild headache, and myalgia. Myalgia and arthralgia without clinical signs are early symptoms in 10–30% of patients with acute hepatitis B (Gocke, 1975; Koff, 1978; Stewart *et al.*, 1978). In one-third of these patients, an urticarial or maculopapular rash, most frequently involving the lower extremities, appears concurrently with joint symptoms, and like them disappears when icterus develops. This syndrome is thought to be caused by immune complexes (Alpert *et al.*, 1971) (see Section VII,A).

B. Icteric Form of Disease

1. Symptoms, Clinical Signs, and Morphological Diagnosis. One to several days before jaundice develops, the urine turns brownish. With the development of icterus, prodromal symptoms like arthralgia, myalgia, and fever subside but lassitude, weakness, anorexia, and right upper abdominal pain may persist or even progress. Jaundice is detected best in the conjunctivae or in the oral mucosa (soft palate), and it may persist for a few days or weeks. Prolonged jaundice occurs particularly in hepatitis B (Stewart *et al.*, 1978) and among older women. Even after many months of jaundice, complete recovery may occur. Depending on the intensity of the icterus, patients have light-, grey-, or yellow-colored stools. During the first signs of icterus, mild and transient itching is common. A few patients suffer from severe pruritus during the early stage of disease, especially in cholestatic-type hepatitis.

Drowsiness, irritability, querulousness, and insomnia are signs of impending hepatic coma, but are also seen early in the disease in ~10% of patients with typical viral hepatitis. The prospect of a protracted illness with possible chronic sequelae, isolation, and inactivity are understandable reasons for concern, but fear and depression are often inappropriate to the situation and may persist until convalescence.

The liver is usually palpable, slightly increased in size (12–14 cm at the midclavicular line) with a smooth, tender edge but with almost normal consistency. Percussion of the right hypochondrium causes pain. The spleen is palpable in ~20% of patients. The posterior cervical lymph nodes may be enlarged; spider angiomata and palmar erythema are not infrequent but disappear in convalescence and do not indicate chronic liver disease. Ascites has been observed in severe acute hepatitis B (Viola *et al.*, 1983).

In typical viral hepatitis, hepatic scintiscanning reveals a diffuse, non-homogenous uptake pattern, mild hepatomegaly, and an enlarged spleen in 20–30% of patients. Ultrasound findings are just as non-specific. Hepatitis serology and laboratory values, especially serum aminotransferase activities together with the clinical findings, are so characteristic that liver biopsy is only indicated in protracted disease when the development of chronic hepatitis is suspected.

III. Clinical Pathology of Acute Viral Hepatitis B

The activities of serum alanine aminotransferase (ALT) and aspartate aminotransferase (AST) are the most valuable laboratory parameters for the diagnosis of acute viral hepatitis and for monitoring its course. Serum transaminase activities rise during the prodromal phase of illness, usually preceding icterus by 8–10 days, and reach peak levels within 10 days (Schmidt and Schmidt, 1983). In acute hepatitis, peak serum transaminase activities are characteristically high, and vary between 500 and 3000 U/liter, ALT activity usually being higher than AST. The height of the serum transaminase activity is not always closely related to the amount of liver cell damage. Activities as high as 2000 U/liter were found in asymptomatic household contacts (Koff and Galambos, 1982), and low levels are an ominous prognostic sign in fulminant hepatitis. Transaminase levels in hepatitis B decrease more slowly than in hepatitis A, and a plateau is more commonly observed. A second rise of transaminase activity of variable duration is not uncommon in hepatitis A or non-A, non-B hepatitis, but is rare in hepatitis B (Schmidt and Schmidt, 1983).

Slight elevations of alkaline phosphatase activities in early disease are usual, but peak activities do not usually exceed twice the normal values, except in cholestatic-type hepatitis (see Section V,B). The relationship of serum transaminase activity to alkaline phosphatase activity has diagnostic importance because patients with cholestatic icterus do not have AST levels >500 U/liter (Schmidt and Schmidt, 1984). The more sensitive gamma glutamyl transpeptidase (GGT) is generally elevated to 5–10 times the normal value. The GGT/AST (or ALT) quotient is ≤1 (Schmidt and Schmidt, 1983).

Glutamate dehydrogenase (GLDH) is a mitochondrial enzyme released from damaged hepatocytes. In acute hepatitis, GLDH activity does not usually exceed 50 U/liter, but is very high (up to 1000 U/liter) in hypoxic or toxic liver damage. With the aid of GLDH, it is possible to differentiate acute viral hepatitis from other liver damage that is accompanied by elevated serum aminotransferase activities; the AST plus ALT/GLDH quotient is >40 in virus hepatitis, <20 in intra- and extrahepatic cholestasis, and <5 in acute circulatory disturbances of the liver (Schmidt and Schmidt, 1983).

Serum bilirubin elevations range widely, and reflect not only hepatocellular damage but also the degree of cholestasis and hemolysis. In uncomplicated viral hepatitis, peak values do not exceed 12 mg/dl, and return to normal within 2–4 weeks (Koff and Galambos, 1982). If serum bilirubin remains elevated, an atypical form of hepatitis should be suspected. As in cholestasis, 60–80% of the total bilirubin is glucuronidated. Bilirubin can be detected in the urine several days before jaundice develops, but bilirubinuria is not closely related to the serum concentration. Bilirubinuria is observed in patients with anicteric hepatitis (Koff *et al.*, 1967); on the other hand, late in the course of icteric hepatitis, the urine may not contain bilirubin despite elevated serum bilirubin (Koff and Galambos, 1982). The reason for this disparity is not known.

Like aminotransferases activity, serum bile acids are increased in viral hepatitis, and remain elevated until complete recovery occurs. Bile acids correlate most with bilirubin but not with aminotransferases or cholestatic enzymes, and are not significantly higher in acute than in chronic hepatitis (Matern and Gerok, 1979), so that bile acid levels provide no diagnostic information in acute viral hepatitis. Serum levels of iron may rise to twice normal values and usually return to normal within 4 weeks (Schmidt and Schmidt, 1983).

Serum electrophoresis usually reveals a normal distribution of serum proteins. In severe and/or prolonged cases of acute hepatitis, γ globulin may reach elevated levels without indicating a transition to chronic hepatitis. Low serum albumin (<2.5 g/dl) and high γ globulin (>3.5 g/dl) indicate a chronic form of hepatitis that should be examined further by liver biopsy. Quantitation of immunglobulin usually reveals elevation of IgM, which is higher in hepatitis A than in hepatitis B or non-A, non-B, but large variations in IgM values prevent their use for identifying the type of hepatitis.

During a normal course of acute hepatitis B, clotting factors show few changes. A decrease of hepatic clotting factors (especially II, V, VII, X, and antithrombin III) indicates a severe form of hepatitis with liver damage. Thus, a regular check of prothrombin time allows early detection of the transition to fulminant hepatitis, in which the prothrombin time is prolonged to a multiple of normal values (Deutsch, 1965: Lechner *et al.*, 1977). Factor VIII can be elevated more than threefold (Poller, 1978). Complement levels tend to be low in the early stages of disease because immune complexes bind complement and synthesis decreases (Kosmidis and Leader-Williams, 1972). Cholinesterase generally remains within the normal range.

Some time after peak aminotransferase activity, raised serum concentrations of α-fetoprotein (AFP) (up to 500 ng/ml) are seen in 30 to 40% of patients with acute viral hepatitis (Kew *et al.*, 1973: Bloomer *et al.*, 1975). Although AFP does not seem to correlate closely with tissue damage, highest concentrations (up to 5000 ng/ml) are seen in some cases of fulminant hepatitis (Alpert and Feller, 1978). The mechanism and significance of these AFP elevations are uncertain, but they probably do not reflect normal liver regeneration. As in other liver diseases, carcinoembryonic antigen (CEA) can be slightly elevated (Molnar and Gitnick, 1977). In uncomplicated acute viral hepatitis, lipoproteins and serum lipids exhibit only minor changes. There is a decrease in the α lipoproteins, an increase in β lipoproteins, and a reduction in lecithin–cholesterol acyltransferase (LCAT) activity (Gione *et al.*, 1971; McIntyre, 1978). In severe disease, especially in fulminant hepatitis, a marked reduction of esterified cholesterol is observed, which is related to the reduction of LCAT activity (Jones, 1979).

The erythrocyte sedimentation rate is high in the preicteric stage, falls to normal with the appearance of icterus, fluctuates thereafter until recovery (Vahrman, 1971), and has no diagnostic value. Hematocrit and hemoglobin concentrations usually remain within normal limits, although the survival of erythrocytes is shortened in a high percentage of patients (Enk and Friss, 1971). Frank Coombs' test-positive hemolytic anemia is a rare complication (Kirel, 1961). In glucose-6-phosphatase dehydrogenase deficiency, hemolysis can occur (Chan and Todd, 1975). Granulocyte counts fall without reaching severe leukopenic levels (Havens and Marck, 1946). With the appearance of jaundice, the number of leukocytes returns to normal, due to an absolute and relative increase of lymphocytes. In 5 to 28% of patients, atypical lymphocytes (virocytes) resembling those seen in infectious mononucleosis appear, but do not usually exceed 10% of cells (Koff and Galambos, 1982). T Lymphocytes in the peripheral blood are decreased (Wicks, 1975), and granulocyte function may be impaired in about half of the patients (Saunders *et al.*, 1978). Rare, severe hematological complications can occur (see Section VII,J).

IV. Virological Diagnosis of Acute Hepatitis B Virus Infection

An HBV infection can be diagnosed specifically by demonstrating HBV or its constituent parts and/or the development of antibodies to HBV antigens.

A. Direct Identification of Hepatitis B Virus Particles and Their Constituents

Hepatitis B virus particles (Dane particles), HBsAg, and core particles can be demonstrated by immune electron microscopy in liver or serum during the latter part of the incubation period (Bianchi and Gudat, 1983). Although electron microscopic studies have added greatly to our knowledge of the structure of HBV and its appearance and localization during infection, electron microscopy is not a technique for routine diagnosis, and the constituents of HBV can be demonstrated better by biochemical, molecular biological, or immunological techniques.

B. Biochemical Detection of Hepatitis B Virus

The DNA polymerase of HBV can be identified in the sera of apparent and inapparent acute cases and in some chronic cases of hepatitis B (Overby, 1983). Its presence is a reliable marker for the infectivity of a given serum; that is, a serum containing HBV DNA polymerase must always be considered infectious because the polymerase indicates the presence of complete HBV particles. However, the absence of DNA polymerase is no guarantee of lack of infectivity, because the polymerase is not very stable and the test systems are not sensitive enough to detect low concentrations ($<10^4$ to 10^5 infectious doses) of HBV. There is a reasonable correlation between the presence in serum of hepatitis B e antigen (HBeAg) and the DNA polymerase, whereas sera with low concentrations of HBeAg are only weakly reactive for DNA polymerase or even negative (nonreactive) (Siegert *et al.*, 1979).

C. Molecular Biological Detection of Hepatitis B Virus

The technique added most recently to our diagnostic armamentarium is the identification of viral infections by demonstration of viral nucleic acids in cells, body fluids, or excretions. This technique was developed after the entire genome of HBV had been identified, mapped, and cloned (Robinson, 1983). Cloned HBV DNA produced in plasmids or phages, in *E. coli,* or in other bacterial cells can be prepared in quantities sufficient for isolation and radioactive labeling by nick translation. Such DNA can then be used as a probe for identifying HBV DNA by molecular hybridization in tissues or fluids (Kam *et al.,* 1982; Blum *et al.,* 1983; Harrison *et al.,* 1983; Burrell *et al.,* 1984). Hybridization can be performed by established techniques allowing a detailed molecular hybridization *in situ* on tissue sections or by fixing DNA from fluids to nitrocellulose filter membranes and subsequently hybridizing on the filter (spot hybridization). With hybridization *in situ,* the exact location of the HBV DNA in the tissue is identified, whereas spot hybridization is a simple and rapid test for the presence of HBV DNA in large numbers of samples. Spot hybridization, however, is less accurate than detailed molecular DNA analysis for identifying the physical nature and completeness of the HBV DNA in the test material. Nevertheless, spot hybridization can detect as little as 0.05–0.1 pg (10^{-13} g) of HBV DNA and can usually detect HBV in serum during the acute stage of hepatitis B. In most cases, strong reactions are observed, corresponding to 5–10 pg or even more of HBV DNA in as little as 5–10 μl of test sample. However, the quantities of detectable HBV DNA vary considerably among patients, and no exact data about the earliest appearance of HBV DNA (probably during the late incubation period), the amounts present during various stages of the disease and the time of its disappearance from the circulation (i.e., disappearance of HBV particles in the normal course of an acute hepatitis B) are yet available.

In the past, it has been assumed that the presence of HBeAg indicates a high degree of infectivity but that development of antibodies to HBeAg (anti-HBe) indicates a substantial reduction in infectivity, although sera positive for HBsAg and anti-HBe can clearly be infectious. This agrees with the identification of HBV DNA, even though in small amounts, in such sera (Lieberman *et al.,* 1983). Hybridization techniques have not been used widely yet for routine identification of HBV, but their use should be evaluated further, particularly for testing the infectivity of sera and for studies on the state of HBV during persistent infections.

D. Immunological Detection of HBV Antigens and Antibodies

Testing for HBV antigens and antibodies will be discussed together because the techniques are the same (for review, see Overby, 1983). A variety of immunological methods such as complement fixation, passive hemagglutination, gel diffusion, counterelectrophoresis, latex agglutination, and others have been used in the past, but in general these methods have been replaced by radio- or enzyme immunoassays. Reversed passive agglutination tests, although less sensitive, are still used in some countries for large-scale screening for HBsAg because these tests are cheaper, and gel diffusion is still sometimes used to analyze HBsAg or HBeAg subtypes. The determination of HBsAg subtypes, however, is irrelevant in diagnosing individual cases, and is only interesting for epidemiological studies or determination of cross-immunity between different subtypes. Such determinations have become particularly important for evaluating the cross-protection of immunity induced with monovalent hepatitis B vaccines, that is, vaccines containing only one HBsAg subtype (Jilg *et al.*, 1984). The differentiation of HBeAg subtypes also has only research interest, and is not used to diagnose individual cases of hepatitis.

The determination of HBsAg and antibodies to HBcAg (anti-HBc) IgG and IgM by sensitive methods is the most important procedure in diagnosing acute cases of hepatitis B. The course of appearance and clearing of various HBV markers during an uncomplicated HBV infection is given in Fig. 1. HBsAg usually becomes detectable in the serum 1–2 weeks before the first symptoms appear, but HBsAg may already be demonstrable in the serum 10–14 days after infection and 6–10 weeks before onset of disease (Krugman *et al.*, 1979). The highest HBsAg concentrations are reached during the early phase of disease, and they decline thereafter to nondetectable levels within a few weeks. An early sign for the establishment of a carrier state is the failure of the HBsAg level to diminish within 2–3 weeks to 50% of the concentration measured at the height of the disease.

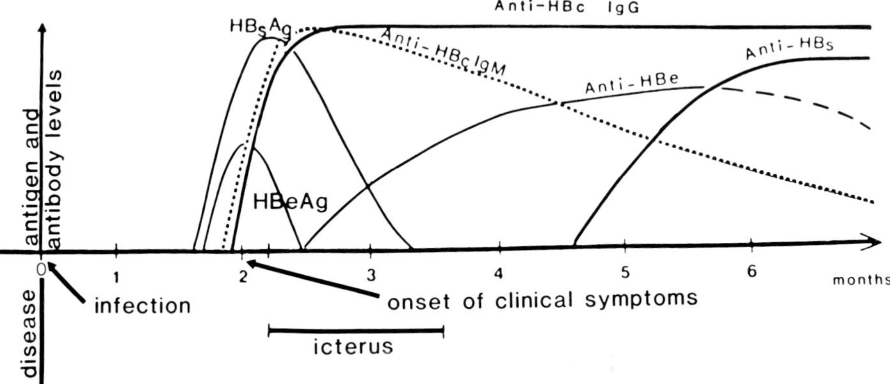

Figure 1. General course of an acute hepatitis B infection.

The presence of HBsAg alone does not allow discrimination between acute disease or a carrier state, and these two possibilities can be distinguished best by measuring anti-HBc IgM and anti-HBc IgG. Anti-HBc IgM appears very early during the acute disease, rises rapidly, and persists with gradually falling titers for 6 to 12 months (the period of detection depends on the sensitivity of the test system). Even in chronic active hepatitis, anti-HBc IgM is found in low to medium titers ($<10^{-2}$), whereas anti-HBc IgG is usually present in higher titers ($>10^{-3}$). In contrast, anti-HBc IgG rises slower during the acute disease so that a high anti-HBc IgM with a lower anti-HBc IgG is diagnostic of acute hepatitis B. Even if HBsAg is undetectable, because the serum may have been obtained too late in the disease or as in some cases because HBsAg is never detectable once disease has begun, the difference between anti-HBc IgM and IgG levels allows a diagnosis to be made (Roggendorf *et al.*, 1981).

HBeAg appears in the serum at about the onset of disease or shortly before, and generally disappears before HBsAg. Persistence of HBeAg for several weeks after the height of the disease indicates the possibility of a longer persistence of HBV and transition to a carrier state. In most instances, anti-HBe becomes detectable shortly (1–2 weeks) after the disappearance of HBeAg, and it usually persists for several (3–6) years. Presence of HBeAg also indicates a high infectivity of the blood, but even after anti-HBe has formed blood must still be considered infectious as long as HBsAg has not been cleared and anti-HBs has developed. Anti-HBs appears weeks to months (up to 6 months) after HBsAg has disappeared and persists for years, in many cases lifelong. Presence of anti-HBs indicates immunity, and cross-immunity exists between the various HBsAg subtypes because all subtypes have a common determinant (a). Today, reliable RIA and ELISA methods are available for measuring all HBV markers discussed above; care must be taken to minimize the interference caused by rheumatoid factor in the serum, which can lead to false-positive results. Low or borderline positive results should be verified as these may be nonspecific. Unfortunately, standardization of the various tests and universal reporting of results in international units or microgram amounts of antigens has not yet been achieved, and efforts to establish international standards and consistent and comparable reporting of results have a high priority.

E. Delta Agent

The δ agent is a defective virus, needing HBV as a helper; it can reproduce only in cells infected with HBV (for review, see Rizzetto, 1983; Verme *et al.*, 1983). Simultaneous infection with HBV and δ virus induces a typical hepatitis that is sometimes but not always more severe than infection with HBV alone. In contrast, infection of an HBV carrier with δ virus often leads to exacerbation of the HBV infection with the development of a severe and not seldom fulminant hepatitis. In diagnosing a case of hepatitis in areas where δ virus is prevalent, testing for δ antigen and antibodies by RIA or ELISA tests should be included. The δ antigen is sometimes present in the serum only for a limited period, and antibodies to the δ antigen (anti-δ) also do not seem to persist permanently. Nevertheless, during or in the period after acute hepatitis B, δ virus markers can be detected if δ virus was involved in the infection.

V. Different Clinical Forms of Hepatitis B

A. Inapparent and Anicteric

Infection with HBV can occur without disease and without symptoms, and even without marked elevation of serum aminotrasferase activity. These inapparent infections occur unnoticed unless a patient is tested regularly for HBsAg and/or anti-HBs. Among homosexual men, 53 of 122 HBV infections occurred without ALT elevations (Szmuness *et al.*, 1980). In one study (Seeff *et al.*, 1977), 2204 blood recipients were tested regularly for ALT levels and serological markers of HBV infection; of this group, 13 developed icteric hepatitis B, 39 developed anicteric hepatitis B, and another 288 (13.1%) developed serological evidence of HBV infection without disease. Thus, only 1 in 26 HBV infections was icteric! A similar rate (1:10–1:30) of icteric to nonapparent hepatitis has been reported in the older literature on posttransfusion hepatitis (which included, of course, non-A, non-B hepatitis) (Shimizu and Kitamoto, 1963; Hampers *et al.*, 1964; Creutzfeldt *et al.*, 1966). Anicteric hepatitis B produces symptoms and laboratory changes like the icteric form; it runs the same course but seems to become more frequently chronic. The reported incidence of inapparent anicteric hepatitis B seems to be less frequent than in HAV infections of children and in non-A, non-B virus infections (Koff *et al.*, 1967; Seeff *et al.*, 1977). Inapparent or anicteric hepatitis B with a tendency toward chronicity is the usual course in patients on dialysis or receiving immunosuppressive treatment (see Section VI,B,C).

B. Cholestatic-Type

Laboratory signs of slight cholestasis are common in acute hepatitis B. In some cases, however, cholestasis is the predominant feature. Patients with this rare, usually benign cholestatic-type hepatitis B suffer from itching and prolonged jaundice. Serum transaminase activities are in the same range as in typical hepatitis, but bilirubin is usually higher and peak alkaline phosphatase activity may reach three times normal values. Cholesterol is elevated and LP-X demonstrable (Schmidt and Schmidt, 1983). Although the course of cholestatic-type hepatitis is usually more severe and more prolonged than usual icteric hepatitis, full recovery is the rule.

C. Fulminant

Hepatitis B virus infection can cause massive liver necrosis, resulting in acute hepatic failure with a lethality of >70%. Fortunately, <1% of all patients with acute hepatitis B develop this fulminant hepatitis, which is characterized by progressive jaundice, hepatic coma, foetor hepaticus, shrinkage of the liver, and hemorrhagic diatheses. Prothrombin time is low, serum ammonia levels elevated, and the serum transaminase activity may decrease when the disease runs a deleterious course. As in all cases of acute liver failure, hypoglycemia, hypokalemia, and respiratory alkalosis occur; hyponatremia, and acidosis are late, prefinal events. Functional renal failure (hepatorenal syndrome), hypotension, acute pancreatitis, cerebral edema, gastrointestinal hemorrhage, and bacterial sepsis are major complications (Horak, 1983). Symptoms of fulminant hepatitis may be present from the beginning of disease or develop during the course of what appears to be usual hepatitis B. Over half of the fatal cases of fulminant hepatitis during World War II died within 10 days of the onset of symptoms (sometimes even before jaundice developed), and three-fourths died within 3 weeks (Lucke and Mallory, 1946).

Each of the hepatitis viruses can cause fulminant hepatitis with similar courses and prognoses (Mathiesen *et al.*, 1980; Gimson *et al.*, 1983), and there are no clinical or prognostic differences between these different forms of fulminant viral hepatitis (Gimson *et al.*, 1983). The frequency of HBsAg-positive fulminant hepatitis varies in different geographic areas between 17 and 61.6% of all non-drug-induced cases of acute liver failure (Horak, 1983). Fulminant hepatitis B seems to be even more frequent than reported, because HBsAg may be cleared faster in this form of hepatitis (Tabor *et al.*, 1976, 1981; Trepo *et al.*, 1976) than in regular hepatitis B, and high levels of anti-HBc IgM are the only signs of HBV infection in up to 80% of all patients with fulminant hepatitis B (Shimizu *et al.*, 1983).

Simultaneous infection with the δ agent seems to increase liver necrosis and favor the development of fulminant hepatitis B: δ markers were more frequent in patients with fulminant (39%) than with ordinary acute hepatitis B (19%) (Smedile *et al.*, 1982), and serological markers for acute δ agent infection (anti-δ IgM) were positive among 33.8% of patients with fulminant hepatitis B, compared to 4.2% of patients with acute hepatitis B (Govindarajan *et al.*, 1984).

VI. Acute Hepatitis B in Special Circumstances

A. Pregnancy

In the western world, viral hepatitis during pregnancy follows the same clinical course and has the same biochemical and serological features, and prognosis as in nonpregnant women (Koff and Galambos, 1982). In developing countries of the Middle East (Gelpi, 1970), Asia (Borhanmanesh *et al.*, 1973), and Africa (Christie, 1976), hepatitis in the last trimester of pregnancy is more severe and deleterious for mother and infant, possibly due to the mother's impaired nutritional status. Pregnancy itself does not enhance susceptibility for HBV infection.

Whereas hepatitis in the first and second trimester does not affect the fetus [the rate of malformations and miscarriages is the same as in healthy women (Siegel, 1966, 1973)], the infant is at some risk when infection occurs in the last trimester. It is uncertain whether the rate of stillbirths is increased, but babies born to mothers with acute hepatitis B in the third trimester have an earlier gestational age and lower birth weights (Schweitzer, 1973).

If acute hepatitis B occurs shortly before or after delivery, the baby is very likely to be infected; ~80% of such babies become HBsAg positive. The rate of transmission of hepatitis B from HBsAg-carrier mothers depends on the race and the presence of HBeAg. Whereas 30–70% of babies in East Asia become HBsAg positive, only ~10% become infected in Europe or North America (Stevens and Szmuness, 1980). The risk of vertical transmission is very high (97%) in HBeAg-positive carrier mothers, but vertical transmission has also been described in carriers without HBeAg (31%) and even in carriers with anti-HBe (21%) (Beasley *et al.*, 1977; Gerety and Schweitzer, 1977; Stevens and Szmuness, 1980).

Although transplacental transmission is possible, it would have to be the exception since the peak incidence of HBsAg in infants born to carrier mothers occurs at 3 months. HBsAg was not detected in cord blood, but was detected in the gastric juice of 96% of newborns from HBsAg-positive mothers (Stevens *et al.*, 1975); thus transmission from leaks across the placenta during labor and/or delivery and birth canal exposure to maternal secretions or blood appear to be the most common routes of infection (Lee *et al.*, 1978). The few infants not infected during delivery are highly likely to become infected postnatally from HBsAg-positive mothers (Beasley and Hwang, 1983). Given these circumstances it is not surprising that preterm ceasarian section does not protect the infant (Giraud *et al.*, 1975).

B. Patients and Staff of Dialysis Units

Patients and nursing staff in hemodialysis units are at high risk of becoming infected with HBV. In the United States, 80% of dialysis units were contaminated with HBV (Garibaldi *et al.*, 1973), and 57% of hemo-dialyis patients had serological evidence of HBV infection (Szmuness *et al.*, 1974; Gahl *et al.*, 1979). Patients usually have a markedly less severe disease; whereas 85–100% of the nursing staff had icteric disease, 60–70% of the patients were anicteric, and many of them had clinically inapparent infections (Kaboth *et al.*, 1971). However, uremic patients are at risk because they frequently become HBsAg- or DNA polymerase-positive carriers, with no or only mild disease but with histological signs of chronic persistent and chronic active hepatitis (Galbraith *et al.*, 1976).

Strict hygienic measures, and separation of HBsAg-positive patients and nursing staff from patients without serological markers of HBV infection, can reduce the rate of hepatitis B in dialysis units drastically (Public Health Laboratory Service Survey, 1976).

C. Immunocompromised Patients

HBV infection is common among recipients of kidney transplants, with a reported incidence of HBs-antigenemia of ~20% (Schimmelpfennig, 1981). Most recipients become infected during the pretransplant period while on hemodialysis. HBV infection *de novo* by the transplant itself (Wolf *et al.*, 1979), during posttransplantation dialysis or by blood transfusions is much less common than continued viral expression and reactivation of HBV replication under immunosuppressive therapy (Dusheiko *et al.*, 1983). The rejection rate of kidney transplants has not been shown to be related to the presence or absence of HBsAg; reports on the association between HBV infection and rejection rates are conflicting (Schimmelpfennig, 1981).

Reappearance of HBsAg in the serum of HBsAg-negative, anti-HBc-positive patients after immunosuppressive drug therapy begins has been reported (Nagington *et al.*, 1977; Villa *et al.*, 1981), and reactivation of a persistent HBV infection has also been documented in anti-HBe-positive HBsAg carriers after cancer chemotherapy (Hoofnagle *et al.*,

1982) and immunosuppression (Dusheiko *et al.*, 1983). HBV infection in immunosuppressed HBsAg-positive patients is usually persistent, with no or few symptoms or laboratory changes. Liver biopsies, however, show progression from chronic persistent to chronic active hepatitis (Degos *et al.*, 1980) with active viral replication (HBcAg is seen in almost all hepatocytes) (Bianchi and Gudat, 1983). Besides these usually anicteric, asymptomatic chronic HBV infections, rare cases of acute fulminant hepatitis B in transplant recipients under immunosuppression occur (Dusheiko *et al.*, 1983).

VII. Acute Hepatitis B as a Generalized Disease

A. Immune Complex Disorders

Serum sickness syndrome, vasculitis, glomerulonephritis, and mixed cryoglobulinemia are thought to be due, at least in part, to immune complexes containing HBV antigens.

1. Serum Sickness Syndrome. Approximately 15 to 20% of patients have joint and skin manifestations resembling serum sickness during the preicteric phase of acute hepatitis B. These serum sickness syndromes are usually mild, lasting for only a few days, and are unrelated to the severity of liver damage. Several skin lesions (see Section VII,B), joint symptoms (see Section VII,D), Raynauds' phenomenon, angioneurotic edema, and subcutaneous nodules are related to immune complexes containing HBsAg (Cosgriff and Arnold, 1976; Duffy *et al.*, 1976; Krugman and Gocke, 1978).

2. Mixed Cryoglobulinemia. Mixed cryoglobulinemia, a disease with symptoms of weakness, purpura, and vasculitis involving primarily the small vessels and glomerulonephritis, has been linked to HBV. HBsAg and anti-HBs were found in the sera of 24–71% of patients with mixed cryoglobulinemia and in the cryoprecipitates of 10–70% (Levo *et al.*, 1977; Bombardieri *et al.*, 1979; Galli and Invernizzi, 1981). Most of these patients had evidence of mild liver disease. It is still unclear whether HBV infection is the primary etiological factor or whether hepatitis B occurred secondarily.

3. Glomerulonephritis. Membranoproliferative or membranous glomerulonephritis associated with nephrotic syndromes has been described in patients, especially children, with persistent HBs-antigenemia and usually mild protracted or chronic hepatitis B (Combes *et al.*, 1971). Deposits of HBsAg (Combes *et al.*, 1971; Brzosko *et al.*, 1974), HBcAg (Slusarczyk *et al.*, 1980), and HBeAg (Takekoshi *et al.*, 1979) together with immunglobulins and complement components, were shown to be distributed along the glomerular basement membrane. Although there is little doubt that immune complexes containing HBV antigens can cause glomerulonephritis, the importance and frequency of this etiology is unclear: a high prevalence of serological HBV markers was observed in children with nephrotic syndrome in some countries (Takekoshi *et al.*, 1978; Kleinknecht *et al.*, 1979) but not in others (Hirsch *et al.*, 1981; Rashid *et al.*, 1981) (see also Chapter 4).

4. Vasculitis. An association of persistent HBV infection and necrotizing vasculitis (periarteritis nodosa) has been observed (Gocke *et al.*, 1970). As many as 40% of these patients had HBV markers, and it was estimated that perhaps 1 in 500 HBV infections may be linked with arteritis nodosa (Gocke, 1975). An etiological role of HBV seems likely, because HBsAg, together with complement components and IgM, has been detected in walls of involved vessels and in cryoprecipitates (Drüeke *et al.*, 1980; Krugman and Gocke, 1978). There is, however, no consistent relationship between onset, severity, and activity of the liver disease and the vasculitis, which may occur with acute or chronic hepatitis B and may be self-limited despite continuing HBs-antigenemia (Sergent *et al.*, 1976).

B. Skin

Several skin lesions are seen in HBV infections: erythematous-macular, maculopapular, or urticarial exanthema lasting days or weeks, purpuric eruptions, and exanthema resembling erythema multiforme (Krugman and Gocke, 1978; Weiss *et al.*, 1978). These lesions may be caused by immune complexes. Infantile papular acrodermatitis (Gianotti–Crosti syndrome) is a rare, nonpruritic, papular-erythematous rash on the face and the extremities in conjunction with lymphadenopathy. It is associated with acute anicteric hepatitis B in children, and is seen mainly in Italy (Gianotti, 1973) and Japan (Ishimaru *et al.*, 1976). Neither HBV antigens nor vasculitis was detected in these skin lesions (Castellano *et al.*, 1978; Gianotti, 1978).

C. Muscle

Muscle pain is observed in the preicteric phase in 10 to 20% of patients with acute hepatitis B (Gocke, 1975; Koff, 1978; Stewart *et al.*, 1978). The association reported between HBV infection and polymyalgia rheumatica (Bacon *et al.*, 1975) was not supported by subsequent studies based on a larger series of patients (Elling *et al.*, 1980).

D. Joints

Besides joint pain in the preicteric stage without other physical signs occurring in 10 to 20% of patients with hepatitis B, frank arthritis resembling acute rheumatoid arthritis is seen in some patients; these manifestations are symmetric, and involve shoulders, elbows, knees, ankles, and the small joints of the hands. This form of arthritis responds to acetylsalicylate therapy, and permanent joint sequelae do not occur (McCarthy and Ormiste, 1973; Duffy *et al.*, 1976; Krugman and Gocke, 1978).

E. Heart and Chest

Involvement of the heart and chest in the course of acute viral hepatitis has been described (Bell, 1971; Nagaratnam *et al.*, 1971). Different pathological changes of the ECG were seen in 17.3% of 1634 patients with acute hepatitis (Maretic and Kuze-Capar, 1970), but these abnormalities disappeared completely with resolution of the acute hepatitis. In fulminant hepatitis, cardiac abnormalities such as extrasystoly, bradycardia, and cardiac arrest are seen in almost all patients (Weston *et al.*, 1976). Pathological findings at autopsy included fatty degeneration of the myocardium, petechial bleeding, pericardial effusion, dilatation of the left ventricle, and edema of the subendocardial myocardium. These changes are thought to be caused by metabolic disturbances arising from liver failure, rather than by viral damage of the heart muscle. Pleural effusion (Gross and Gerding, 1971) and pulmonary fibrosis (Lynne-Davies and Sproule, 1967) associated with acute hepatitis have also been reported.

F. Gastrointestinal Tract

In acute hepatitis, inflammatory reactions of the gastric duodenal and jejunal mucosa have been seen in biopsies (Astaldi *et al.*, 1964; Conrad *et al.*, 1964; Sheehy *et al.*, 1964), but these reactions disappear as patients recover from hepatitis. Whether these changes exceed in intensity those seen in normal controls is controversial (Palmer, 1951; Kudzma *et al.*, 1969). Steatorrhea in acute hepatitis has been reported (Modai and Theodor, 1970), and seems to result from diminished bile flow rather than from damage to the gastrointestinal mucosa.

G. Pancreas

HBsAg has been detected in bile and pancreatic juices (Hoefs *et al.*, 1980). In another hepadna virus infection (duck hepatitis B), viral DNA synthesis was demonstrated in the pancreas of Pekin ducks (Halpern *et al.*, 1983), so it is not surprising that acute pancreatitis has been reported, especially in patients with subacute and fulminant hepatitis B (Achord, 1968; Gillespie, 1973).

H. Kidney

In acute hepatitis, minor histological lesions without clinical symptoms seem to be present in all patients, and these disappear with resolution of the liver disorder (Conrad *et al.*, 1964). Clinically relevant are the "immune complex"-type renal lesions (see Section VII,A,2,3 and Chapter 4), and renal failure which is an ominous, preterminal symptom in fulminant hepatitis B.

I. Nervous System

Neurological complications in the course of acute hepatitis consist of disturbed sensitivity and paraesthesia, and depressed nerve conduction velocities (Davison *et al.*, 1972). Cranial nerve involvement (Mandal and Allbeson, 1972) and impaired smell and taste sensation (Henkin and Smith, 1971) have been described. These neurological changes resolve with improvement of the hepatitis. Persistent neurological abnormalities are seen in connection with immune complexes in chronic hepatitis B.

J. Hematology

Agranulocytosis (Dische and Golding, 1957), thrombocytopenia (Jones and Evans, 1951), pancytopenia (Hagler *et al.*, 1975), or aplastic anemia (Sears *et al.*, 1975) are rare complications in acute hepatitis, occurring 1 week to several months after the onset of the disease. These dangerous sequelae seem to be extremely rare in hepatitis B, because in one study of a large group of such patients none was HBsAg positive (Hagler *et al.*, 1975.

VIII. Treatment

No therapeutic measures prevent liver cell necrosis, suppress inflammatory activity, stimulate liver regeneration, or enhance virus elimination, so the natural course of acute hepatitis B cannot be influenced.

Fortunately, hepatitis B is normally a self-limited, benign disease, and the treatment of acute hepatitis B consists in preventing clinical deterioration.

A. Restriction of Activity

Controlled studies in otherwise healthy young patients with acute viral hepatitis have shown that strict bed rest and prolonged confinement do not influence the outcome of acute hepatitis (Chalmers *et al.*, 1955). On the other hand, it has been reported that vigorous exercise in the preicteric and severe icteric stages resulted in clinical deterioration (Repsher and Freebern, 1969). It is now accepted that in the acute phase patients should not be confined strictly to bed but may be as active as their symptoms allow. Strenuous exercise, however, must be avoided until the recovery phase.

B. Diet

No diet or any nutritional restriction should be forced upon patients, because in a well-nourished population the course of acute hepatitis B cannot be altered by any dietary measures (Leone *et al.*, 1954; Smith and Merigan, 1983). There is also little evidence to support a complete alcohol restriction. Although large amounts of ethanol are deleterious to any liver, infusion of 80 mg ethanol/kg body weight during the icteric stage did not cause increased aminotransferase activities (Galambos, 1963), and drinking habits of soldiers did not influence the outcome of viral hepatitis (Gardner *et al.*, 1949). Similar data have been reported from chimpanzee studies (Tabor *et al.*, 1978). Regular intake of large amounts of alcohol must be avoided, because excessive drinking soon after the resolution of jaundice was followed by hepatitis relapse (Damodaran and Hartfall, 1944), and liver damage is more severe in those HBsAg carriers who regularly drink alcoholic beverages (Villa *et al.*, 1982).

C. Drugs

1. Glucocorticoids. Although they may cause an initial rapid decline in both serum bilirubin and serum aminotransferase activities, glucocorticoids seem to be of no benefit in acute hepatitis B and may even be harmful. Glucocorticoids do not alter the length of the disease, and relapses after cessation of therapy are frequent; side effects may also be harmful (Blum *et al.*, 1969; Stutz *et al.*, 1969). There is evidence that steroids increase the rate of chronic liver disease (Stutz *et al.*, 1969; Laverdant *et al.*, 1978). In controlled studies, glucocorticoids did not influence the time of HBs-antigenemia (Greenberg *et al.*, 1981; Ware *et al.*, 1981). In fulminant hepatitis, glucocorticoids did not improve the clinical situation, but their side effects rather increased mortality (Ware *et al.*, 1974; Gregory *et al.*, 1976; Redeker *et al.*, 1976; Randomized Trial of Steroid Therapy in Acute Liver Failure, 1979; Acute Hepatic Failure Study Group, 1979).

2. Immune Globulin. Immune globulin (Gellis, 1945) as well as hyperimmune serum with very high titers of anti-HBs are of no value in treating either ordinary acute hepatitis B or fulminant hepatitis B (Eisenburg *et al.*, 1975; Acute Hepatic Failure Study Group, 1977).

3. Antiemetics. In the early phase of acute hepatitis, nausea may require antiemetic treatment, and metoclopramide seems to be the drug of choice. It increases the rate of gastric emptying, and unlike phenothiazines it does not affect hepatic excretory function.

4. Estrogens. Estrogens do not aggravate the course of viral hepatitis; the severity of acute hepatitis B is the same in users and nonusers of oral contraceptives (Schweitzer *et al.*, 1975).

5. Drugs of Unproved Effectiveness. Transfer factor is able to transfer cellmediated immunity to a specific antigen from a sensitized donor to a nonresponsive individual. It was hoped that this therapy might enhance virus elimination and prevent chronic hepatitis, but no difference was found in a prospective, randomized, double-blind trial of transfer factor therapy versus a placebo in 29 patients with acute hepatitis B (Ellis-Pegler *et al.*, 1977).

Levamisole is a nonspecific immunostimulant. Compared to a placebo, levamisole enhanced HBsAg clearance and recovery from acute hepatitis B in one study (Par *et al.*, 1977), but further controlled studies of this effect are needed.

Cyanidanol is a naturally occurring flavinoid which has a hepatotropic effect against a number of hepatotoxic agents in experimental animals (Conn, 1983). Studies in acute viral hepatitis showed a slightly more rapid fall in serum bilirubin and transaminase activities (Conn, 1983; Piazza *et al.*, 1983). A faster elimination of HBsAg in acute hepatitis B was observed in one study (Conn, 1983), but this was not confirmed in a larger study (Schomerus *et al.*, 1984).

Interferons are natural cell products that play a role in the host defense mechanisms against viral disease by inducing the production of an antiviral protein by the cell and by enhancing the host's immune response. Interferon from leukocytes or fibroblasts has been tried, mainly in chronic HBV infection (Smith and Merigan, 1983). In 16 patients with acute virus hepatitis, an increase of the interferon serum concentration was observed, but not in 5 of 6 cases with fulminant hepatitis B. In none of these 6 patients could interferon production by mononuclear cells be induced. Interferon was given to 5 of these patients; 3 survived. The use of interferon in the early phase of a severe acute hepatitis has been proposed; its efficacy, however, has not been shown (Levin and Hahn, 1982).

Virazole (Ribavirin) is a nucleotide which has antiviral activity *in vitro* against several RNA and DNA viruses. A more rapid decrease of serum transaminase activity and bilirubin was reported in patients treated with this drug, but the data were insufficient to judge whether the drug really influences spontaneous recovery from hepatitis B (Ayrosa-Galvao and Castro, 1977).

References

Achord, J. L. (1968). *JAMA, J. Am. Med. Assoc.* **205,** 837–840.
Acute Hepatic Failure Study Group (1977). *Ann. Intern. Med.* **86,** 272–277.
Acute Hepatic Failure Study Group (1979). *Gastroenterology* **76,** 1297.
Alpert, E., and Feller, E. R. (1978). *Gastroenterology* **74,** 856–858.
Alpert, E., Isselbacher, K. J., and Schur, H. P. (1971). *N. Engl. J. Med.* **285,** 185–189.
Astaldi, G., Grandini, U., Poggi, C., and Strosselli, E. (1964). *Am. J. Dig. Dis.* **9,** 237–245.
Ayrosa-Galvao, P. A., and Castro, J. O. (1977). *Ann. N.Y. Acad. Sci.* **284,** 278–283.
Bacon, B. A., Doherty, S. M., and Zuckerman, A. J. (1975). *Lancet 2,* 476–478.
Beasley, R. P., and Hwang, L. Y. (1983). *J. Infect. Dis.* **147,** 185–190.
Beasley, R. P., Trepo, C., and Stevens, C. E. (1977). *Am. J. Epidemiol.* **105,** 94–98.
Bell, H. (1971). *JAMA, J. Am. Med. Assoc.* **218,** 387–392.
Bianchi, L., and Gudat, F. G. (1983). *In* "Viral Hepatitis: Laboratory and Clinical Science" (F. Deinhardt and J. Deinhardt, eds.), pp. 335–382. Dekker, New York.
Bloomer, J. R., Waldmann, T. A., McIntire, K. R., and Klatskin, G. (1975). *Gastroenterology* **68,** 342–350.
Blum, A. L., Stutz, R., Haemmerli, U. O., Schmid P., and Grady, G. F. (1969). *Am. J. Med.* **47,** 82–92.
Blum, H. E., Stowring, L., Figus, A., Montgomery, C. K., Haase, A. T., and Vyas, G. N. (1983). *Proc. Natl. Acad. Sci. U.S.A.* **80,** 6685–6688.
Bombardieri, S., Paoletti, P., Ferri, C., Di Munno, O., Fornai, E., and Giutini, C. (1979). *Am. J. Med.* **66,** 748–756.
Borhanmanesh, F., Haghighi, P., and Hekmat, K. (1973). *Gastroenterology* **64,** 304–312.
Brzosko, W. J., Krawczynski, K., Nazarewicz, T., Morzycka, M., and Nowoslawski, A. (1974). *Lancet 2,* 477–481.
Burrell, C. J., Gowans, E. J., Rowland, R., Hall, P., Jilbert, A. R., and Marmion, B. P. (1984). *Hepatology (N.Y.)* **4,** 20–24.
Castellano, A., Schweitzer, R., Tong, M. J., and Omata, M. (1978). *Arch. Dermatol.* **114,** 1530–1532.

Chalmers, T. C., Eckhardt, R. D., Reynolds, W. E., Cigarroa, J. G., Jr., Deane, N., Reifenstein, R. W., Smith, C. W., and Davidson, C. S. (1955). *J. Clin. Invest.* **34,** 1163–1235.

Chan, T. K., and Todd, D. (1975). *Br. Med. J.* **1,** 131–133.

Christie, A. B. (1976). *Lancet* 2, 827–829.

Combes, B., Stastny, P., Shorey, J., Eigenbrodt, E. H., Barrera, A., Hull, A. R., and Carter, N. W. (1971). *Lancet* 2, 234–237.

Conn, H. O. (1983). *Hepatology (N.Y.)* **3,** 121–123.

Conrad, M. E., Schwartz, F. D., and Young, A. A. (1964). *Am. J. Med.* **37,** 789–801.

Cosgriff, T. M., and Arnold, W. J. (1976). *JAMA, J. Am. Med. Assoc.* **235,** 1362–1363.

Creutzfeldt, W., Severidt, H. J., Schmitt, H., Gallasch, E., Arndt, H. J., Brachmann, M., Schmidt, G., and Tschaepe, O. (1966). *Dtsch. Med. Wochenschr.* **91,** 1813–1820.

Damodaran, K., and Hartfall, S. J. (1944). *Br. Med. J.* **2,** 587–590.

Davison, A. M., Williams, I. R., Mawdsley, C., and Robson, J. S. (1972). *Br. Med. J.* **1,** 409–411.

Degos, F., Degott, C., Bedrossian, J., Camilieri, J. P., Barbanel, C., Duboust, A., Rueff, B., Benhamon, J. P., and Kreis, H. (1980). *Transplantation* **29,** 100–102.

Deutsch, E. (1965). *Prog. Liver Dis.* **2,** 69–83.

Dische, E. F., and Golding, J. R. (1957). *Br. Med. J.* **2,** 738–740.

Drüeke, T., Barbanel, C., Jungers, P., Digeon, M., Poisson, M., Brivet, F., Trecon, C., Feldmann, G., Crosnier, J., and Bach, J. F. (1980). *Am. J. Med.* **68,** 86–90.

Duffy, J., Lidsky, M. D., Sharp, J. T., Davis, J. S., Person, D. A., Hollinger, F. B., and Min, K. W. (1976). *Medicine (Baltimore)* **55,** 19–37.

Dusheiko, G., Song, E., Bowyer, S., Whitcutt, M., Maier, G., Meyers, A., and Kew, M. C. (1983). *Hepatology (N.Y.)* **3,** 330–336.

Eisenburg, J., Meister, P., Holl, J., and Grunst, J. (1975). *Fortschr. Med.* **93,** 1085–1092.

Elling, H., Skinhoj, P., and Elling, P. (1980). *Ann. Rheum. Dis.* **39,** 511–513.

Ellis-Pegler, R., Sutherland, D. C., Douglas, R., Woodfield, D. G., and Wilson, J. D. (1977). *Clin. Exp. Immunol.* **36,** 221–226.

Enk, B., and Friss, T. (1971). *Nord. Med., NM* **86,** 1148–1150.

Gahl, G. M., Hess, G., Arnold, W., and Grams, G. (1979). *Nephron* **24,** 58–63.

Galambos, J. F. (1963). *Gastroenterology* **44,** 267–274.

Galbraith, R. M., El Sheikh, N., Portmann, B., Eddleston, A. L. W., Williams, R., Parsons, V., Bewick, M., and Ogg, C. S. (1976). *Br. Med. J.* **1,** 1495–1497.

Galli, M., and Invernizzi, F. (1981). *Ann. Intern. Med.* **95,** 522.

Garibaldi, R. A., Forrest, J. N., Bryan, J. A., Hanson, B. F., and Dismukes, E. E. (1973). *JAMA, J. Am. Med. Assoc.* **225,** 384–389.

Gardner, H. T., Rovelstad, R. A., Moore, D. J., Streitfield, F. A., and Knowlton, M. (1949). *Ann. Intern. Med.* **30,** 1009–1019.

Gellis, S. S. (1945). *JAMA, J. Am. Med. Assoc.* **128,** 1158–1159.

Gelpi, A. P. (1970). *Am. J. Gastroenterol.* **53,** 41–44.

Gerety, R. J., and Schweitzer, I. L. (1977). *J. Pediatr. (St. Louis)* **90,** 368–374.

Gianotti, F. (1973). *Arch. Dis. Child.* **48,** 794–799.

Gianotti, F. (1978). *N. Engl. J. Med.* **298,** 460.

Gillespie, W. J. (1973). *J. R. Coll. Surg. Edinburgh* **18,** 120–122.

Gimson, A. E. S., White, Y. S., Eddleston, A. L. W. F., and Williams, R. (1983). *Gut* **24,** 1194–1198.

Gione, E., Blomhoff, J. P., and Wienecke, J. (1971). *Scand, J. Gastroenterol.* **6,** 161–168.

Giraud, P., Dronet, J., and Dupay, J. M. (1975). *Lancet* 2, 1088–1089.

Gocke, D. J., Hsu, K., Morgan, C., Bombardieri, S., Lockshin, M., and Christian, C. L. (1970). *Lancet* 2, 1149–1153.

Gocke, J. S. (1975). *Am. J. Med. Sci.* **270**, 49–52.

Govindarajan, S., Chin, K. P., Redeker, A. G., and Peters, R. L. (1984). *Gastroenterology* **86**, 1417–1420.

Greenberg, H. B., Robinson, W. S., Knauer, C. M., and Gregory, P. B. (1981). *Hepatology (N.Y.)* **1**, 54–57.

Gregory, P. B., Knauer, C. M., and Kempson, R. L. (1976). *N. Engl. J. Med.* **294**, 681–687.

Gross, P. A., and Gerding, D. N. (1971). *Gastroenterology* **60**, 898–902.

Hagler, L., Pastore, R. A., and Bergin, J. J. (1975). *Medicine (Baltimore)* **54**, 139–164.

Halpern, M. S., England, J. M., Deery, D. T., Petcu, D. J., Mason, W. S., and Molnar-Kimber, K. L. (1983). *Proc. Natl. Acad. Sci. U.S.A.* **80**, 4865–4869.

Hampers, C. L., Prager, D., and Senior, J. R. (1964). *N. Engl. J. Med.* **271**, 749–754.

Harrison, T. J., Tsiquaye, K., and Zuckerman, A. J. (1983). *J. Virol. Methods* **6**, 295–302.

Havens, W. P., and Marck, R. E. (1946). *Am. J. Med. Sci.* **212**, 129–138.

Henkin, R. I., and Smith, F. R. (1971). *Lancet* **1**, 823–826.

Hirsch, H. Z., Ainsworth, S. K., De Beukelaer, M., Brissie, R. M., and Hennigar, G. R. (1981). *Am. J. Clin. Pathol.* **75**, 597–602.

Hoefs, J. C., Renner, I. G., Ashcavai, M., and Redeker, A. G. (1980). *Gastroenterology* **79**, 191–194.

Hoofnagle, J. H., Dusheiko, G. M., and Shafer, D. F. (1982). *Ann. Intern. Med.* **96**, 447–449.

Horak, W. (1983). *In* "Viral Hepatitis: Laboratory and Clinical Science" (F. Deinhardt and J. Deinhardt, eds.), pp. 295–316. Dekker, New York.

Ishimaru, Y., Ishimaru, H., Toda, G., Baba, K., and Mayumi, M. (1976). *Lancet* **1**, 707–709.

Jilg, W., Delhoune, C., Deinhardt, F., Roumeliotou-Karayannis, A. J., Papaevangelou, G. J., Mushawar, I. K., and Overby, L. R. (1984). *J. Med. Virol.* **13**, 171–178.

Jones, D. P. (1979). *In* "Problems in Liver Diseases" (C. S. Davidson, ed.), pp. 255–260. Thieme, Stuttgart.

Jones, G. P., and Evans, E. G. (1951). *Br. Med. J.* **2**, 451–452.

Kaboth, U., Schober, A., Klinge, O., Lowitz, H. D., Quellhorst, E., Scheler, F., and Creutzfeld, W. (1971). *Dtsch. Med. Wochenschr.* **96**, 1235–1242.

Kam, W., Rall, L. B., Smuckler, E. A., Schmid, R., and Rutter, W. J. (1982). *Proc. Natl. Acad. Sci. U.S.A.* **79**, 7522–7526.

Kew, M. C., Purves, L. R., and Bersohn, J. (1973). *Gut* **14**, 939–942.

Kirel, R. M. (1961). *Am. J. Dig. Dis.* **6**, 1017–1031.

Kleinknecht, C., Levy, M., Peix, A., Broyer, M., and Courtecuisse, V. (1979). *J. Pediatr. (St. Louis)* **95**, 946–952.

Koff, R. S. (1978). "Viral Hepatitis." Wiley, New York.

Koff, R. S., and Galambos, J. (1982). *In* "Diseases of the Liver" (L. Schiff and E. R. Schiff, eds.), 5th ed., pp. 461–610. Lippincott, Philadelphia, Pennsylvania.

Koff, R. S., Grady, G. F., and Chalmers, T. C. (1967). *N. Engl. J. Med.* **276**, 703–710.

Kosmidis, J. C., and Leader-Williams, L. K. (1972). *Clin. Exp. Immunol.* **11**, 31–35.

Krugman, S., and Gocke, D. J. (1978). "Viral Hepatitis." Saunders, Philadelphia, Pennsylvania.

Krugman, S., Overby, R. L., Mushahwar, I., Ling, C. M., Frösner, G., and Deinhardt, F. (1979). *N. Engl. J. Med.* **300**, 101–196.

Kudzma, D. J., Peterson, E. W., and Knudsen, K. B. (1969). *Arch. Intern. Med.* **124**, 322–325.

Laverdant, C., Molinie, C., Essioux, H., and Daly, J. P. (1978). *Gastroenterol. Clin. Biol.* **2**, 652–653.

Lechner, K., Niessner, H., and Thaler, E. (1977). *Semin. Thromb. Hemostasis* **4**, 40–56.

Lee, A. K. Y., Ip, H. M. H., and Wong, V. C. W. (1978). *J. Infect. Dis.* **138**, 668–671.

Leone, M. C., Ratner, F., Diefenbach, W. C. L., Eads, M. G., Lieberman, J. E., and Murray, R. I. (1954). *Ann. N.Y. Acad. Sci.* **57,** 948–961.

Levin, S., and Hahn, T. (1982). *Lancet 1,* 592–594.

Levo, Y., Gorevic, R. D., Kassab, H. J., Zucker-Franklin, D., and Franklin, E. C. (1977). *N. Engl. J. Med.* **296,** 1501–1504.

Lieberman, H. M., LaBrecque, D. R., Kew, M. C., Hadziyannis, S. J., and Shafritz, D. A. (1983). *Hepatology (N.Y.)* **3,** 285–291.

Lucke, B., and Mallory T. (1946). *Am. J. Pathol.* **22,** 867–945.

Lynne-Davis, P., and Sproule, B. J. (1967). *J. Can. Med. Assoc.* **96,** 1110–1112.

McCarthy, D. J., and Ormiste, V. (1973). *Arch. Intern. Med.* **132,** 264–268.

McIntyre, N. (1978). *Gut* **19,** 526–530.

Mandal, B. K., and Allbeson, M. (1972). *Lancet 2,* 1322.

Maretic, Z., and Kuze-Capar (1970). *Z. Kreislauf forsch.* **59,** 1116–1124.

Matern, S., and Gerok, W. (1979). *Acta Hepato-Gastroenterol.* **26,** 185–189.

Mathiesen, L. R., Skinhoj, P., Nielsen, J. O., Purcell, R. H., Wong, D., and Ranek, L. (1980). *Gut* **21,** 72–77.

Modai, M., and Theodor, E. (1970). *Gastroenterology* **58,** 379–387.

Molnar, J. G., and Gitnick, G. L. (1977). *Gastroenterology* **72,** 1103.

Nagaratnam, N., De Silva, D. P. K. M., and Gunawardene, K. R. W. (1971). *Postgrad. Med. J.* **47,** 785–788.

Nagington, J., Cossart, Y. E., and Cohen, B. J. (1977). *Lancet 1,* 558–560.

Overby, L. R. (1983). *In* "Viral Hepatitis: Laboratory and Clinical Science" (F. Deinhardt and J. Deinhardt, eds.), pp. 159–198. Dekker, New York.

Palmer, E. D. (1951). *Am. J. Dig. Dis.* **18,** 323–325.

Par, A., Berna, K., Hollos, J., Kovacs, M., Miszlai, Z., Patakfalvi, A., and Javor, T. (1977). *Lancet 1,* 702.

Piazza, M., Guadignino, W., and Picciotto, L. (1983). *Hepatology (N.Y.)* **3,** 45–49.

Poller, L. (1978). *In* "Recent Advances in Blood Coagulation" (L. Poller, ed.), pp. 267–292. Churchill-Livingstone, Edinburgh and London.

Public Health Laboratory Service Survey (1976). *Br. Med. J.* **1,** 1579–1581.

Randomized Trial of Steroid Therapy in Acute Liver Failure (1979). *Gut* **20,** 620–623.

Rashid, H., Morley, A. R., Ward, M. K. Kerr, D. N. S., and Codd, A. A. (1981). *Br. Med. J.* **2,** 948–949.

Redeker, A. G., Schweitzer, J. L., and Yamahiro, H. S. (1976). *N. Engl. J. Med.* **294,** 728–729.

Repsher, L. H., and Freebern, R. K. (1969). *N. Engl. J. Med.* **281,** 1393–1396.

Rizzetto, M. (1983). *Hepatology (N.Y.)* **3,** 729–737.

Robinson, W. S. (1983). *In* "Viral Hepatitis: Laboratory and Clinical Science" (F. Deinhardt and J. Deinhardt, eds.), pp. 57–116. Dekker, New York.

Roggendorf, M., Deinhardt, F., Frösner, G. G., Scheid, R., Bayerl, B., and Zachoval, R. (1981). *J. Clin. Microbiol.* **13,** 618–626.

Saunders, S. J., Dowdle, E. B., and Fiskerstrand, C. (1978). *Gut* **19,** 930–934.

Schimmelpfennig, W. (1981). *Dtsch. Gesundheitswes.* **36,** 1321–1324.

Schmidt, E., and Schmidt, F. W. (1983). *In* "Viral Hepatitis: Laboratory and Clinical Science" (F. Deinhardt and J. Deinhardt, eds.), pp. 411–487. Dekker, New York.

Schmidt, E., and Schmidt, F. W. (1984). *Dtsch. Med. Wochenschr.* **109,** 139–144.

Schomerus, H., Wiedmann, K. H., and Dölle, W. (1984). *Hepatology (N.Y.)* **4,** 331–335.

Schweitzer, I. L. (1973). *Am. J. Med.* **55,** 762–771.

Schweitzer, I. L., Weiner, J. M., McPeak, C. M., and Thursby, M. W. (1975). *JAMA, J. Am. Med. Assoc.* **233,** 979–980.

Sears, D. A., George, J. N., and Gold, M. S. (1975). *Arch. Intern. Med.* **135**, 1585–1589.
Seeff, L. B., Zimmermann, H. J., Wright, E. C., and the V. A. Cooperative Study Group (1977). *Gastroenterology* **72**, 111–121.
Sergent, J. S., Lockshin, M. D., Christian, C. L., and Gocke, D. J. (1976). *Medicine (Baltimore)* **55**, 1–18.
Sheehy, T. W., Artenstein, M. S., and Green, R. W. (1964). *JAMA, J. Am. Med. Assoc.* **190**, 1023–1028.
Shimizu, M., Ohyama, M., Takahashi, Y., Udo, K., Kojima, M., Kametani, M., Tsuda, F., Takai, E., Miyakawa, Y., and Mayumi, M. (1983). *Gastroenterology* **84**, 604–610.
Shimizu, Y., and Kitamoto, O. (1963). *Gastroenterology* **44**, 740–744.
Siegel, M. (1966). *N. Engl. J. Med.* **274**, 768–771.
Siegel, M. (1973). *JAMA, J. Am. Med. Assoc.* **226**, 1521–1524.
Siegert, W., Grunst, J., Wilmanns, W., Frösner, G. G., and Deinhardt, F. (1979). *Infection* **7**, 220–222.
Slusarczyk, J., Michalak, T., Mazarewicz-de Mezer, T., Krawczynski, K., and Nowoslawski, A. (1980). *Am. J. Pathol.* **98**, 29–43.
Smedile, A., Farci, P., and Verme, G. (1982). *Lancet* **2**, 945–947.
Smith, C. J., and Merigan, T. C. (1983). *In* "Viral Hepatitis: Laboratory and Clinical Science" (F. Deinhardt and J. Deinhardt, eds.), pp. 491–512. Dekker, New York.
Stevens, C. E., and Szmuness W. (1980). *In* "Virus and the Liver" (L. Bianchi, W. Gerok, K. Sickinger, and G. A. Stalder, eds.), pp. 285–291. MTP Press Ltd., Lancaster.
Stevens, C. E., Beasley, R. P., Tsui, J., and Lee, W. C. (1975). *N. Engl. J. Med.* **292**, 771–774.
Stewart, J. S., Farrow, L. J., Clifford, R. E., Lamb, S. G. S., Coghill, N. F., Lindon, R. L., Sanderson, J. M., Dodd, P. A., Smith, H. G., Preece, J. W., and Zuckerman, A. J. (1978). *Q. J. Med.* **187**, 365–384.
Stutz, R., Blum, A. L., Haemmerli, U. P., Schmid, P., and Schmid, M. (1969). *Am. J. Med.* **47**, 93–100.
Szmuness, W., Prince, A. M., Grady, G. F., Mann, M. K., Levine, R. M., Giedman, E. A., Jacobs, M. J., Josephson, A., Ribot, S., Shapiro, F. L., Stenzel, K. H., Suki, W. N., and Vyas, G. (1974). *JAMA, J. Am. Med. Assoc.* **227**, 901–906.
Szmuness, W., Stevens, C. E., Harley, E. J., Zang, E. A., Oleszko, R., William, D. C., Sadovsky, R., Morrison, J. M., and Kellner, A. (1980). *N. Engl. J. Med.* **303**, 833–841.
Tabor, E., Gerety, R. J., Hoofnagle, J. H., and Barker, L. F. (1976). *Gastroenterology* **71**, 635–640.
Tabor, E., Gerety, R. J., Barker, L. F., Howard, C. R., and Zuckerman, A. J. (1978). *J. Med. Virol.* **2**, 295–303.
Tabor, E., Krugman, S., Weiss, E. C., and Gerety, R. J. (1981). *J. Med. Virol.* **8**, 277–282.
Takekoshi, Y., Tanaka, M., Shida, N., Satake, Y., Saheki, Y., and Matsumoto, S. (1978). *Lancet* **2**, 1065–1068.
Takekoshi, Y., Tanaka, M., Miyakawa, Y., Yoshizawa, H., Takahashi, K., and Mayumi, M. (1979). *N. Engl. J. Med.* **300**, 814–819.
Trepo, C. G., Robert, D., Mutin, J., Trepo, D., Sepetjern, M., and Prince, A. M. (1976). *Gut* **17**, 10–13.
Vahrman, J. (1971). *Br. Med. J.* **2**, 466–467.
Verme, G., Bonino, F., and Rizzetto, M., eds. (1983). "Viral Hepatitis and Delta Infection," Prog. Clin. Biol. Res., Vol. 143. Alan R. Liss, Inc., New York.
Villa, E., Theodossi, A., Portmann, B., Eddleston, A. L. W., and Williams, R. (1981). *Gastroenterology* **80**, 1048–1053.
Villa, E., Bardir, T., Grisendi, A., Bellenzani, S., Rubbiani, L., Ferretti, J., De Palma, M., and Manenti, F. (1982). *Lancet* **2**, 1243–1244.

Viola, C., Vineta, L., Bosch, J., and Rodes, J. (1983). *Hepatology (N.Y.)* **3**, 1013–1015.
Ware, A. J., Jones, R. E., and Shorey, J. W. (1974). *Am. J. Gastroenterol.* **62**, 130–133.
Ware, A. J., Cuthbert, J. A., Shorey, J., Gurian, L. E., Eigenbrodt, E. H., and Combes, B. (1981). *Gastroenterology* **80**, 219–224.
Weiss, T. D., Cheng, C. J., Baldessare, A. C., and Zuckner, J. (1978). *Am. J. Med.* **64**, 269–273.
Weston, M. J. C., Talbot, C., Howorth, P. J. N., Mant, A. K., Capildeo, R., and Williams, R. (1976). *Br. Heart J.* **38**, 1179–1188.
Wicks, R. C. (1975). *Am. J. Dig. Dis.* **20**, 518–522.
Wolf, J. E., Perkins, H. A., Schreeder, M. T., and Vincenti, F. (1979). *Ann. Intern, Med.* **91**, 412–413.

Chapter 7

Chronic Hepatitis B

STEN A. IWARSON
Department of Infectious Diseases
University of Göteborg
Östra Hospital
Göteborg, Sweden

I. The Carrier State of HBV

A. The Asymptomatic Carrier

Individuals with chronic HBV infection can be divided into two groups, those with chronic hepatitis B and those who are asymptomatic, "healthy" carriers of HBV (Table I, Fig. 1). The patients with chronic hepatitis B usually have elevated serum aminotransferase activities. Liver biopsies of these patients reveal chronic inflammatory changes as well as liver cell necrosis. They may or may not be symptomatic, but most are seropositive for HBeAg, DNA polymerase, and HBV DNA.

The so-called "healthy" carrier state of HBV is usually associated with normal liver function, no detectable markers of HBV replication, and no detectable circulating virions. The HBV genome seems to be expressed mainly by production of HBsAg-bearing particles in individuals who are usually seronegative for HBeAg, HBV DNA, and DNA polymerase.

HEPATITIS B   119   Copyright © 1985 by Academic Press, Inc.
All rights of reproduction in any form reserved.
ISBN 0-12-280672-7

TABLE I
Chronic Sequelae of HBV Infection
and Classification

The asymptomatic carrier state
Chronic hepatitis B
    Chronic persistent hepatitis (CPH)
    Chronic active hepatitis (CAH)
    Chronic lobular hepatitis (CLH)
Liver cirrhosis
Hepatocellular carcinoma

During recent years it has become clear that chronic hepatitis B and the asymptomatic carrier state are not so much two separate forms of disease as they are two stages of the same chronic viral infection. Thus, when patients with chronic hepatitis B are followed prospectively, a certain percentage enter a spontaneous and often permanent remission of disease activity with serum enzymes falling to normal. This remission that seems to occur in 10 to 20% of such patients each year is almost invariably accompanied by loss of serum HBeAg and seroconversion to anti-HBe (Realdi *et al.*, 1980; Hoofnagle *et al.*, 1981; Norkrans *et al.*, 1982; Liaw *et al.*, 1982).

Seroconversion from HBeAg to anti-HBe denotes a transition from an active phase of disease to an asymptomatic carrier state. This transition is important in our understanding of the natural history of chronic HBV infections.

A late result of chronic HBV infection appears to be hepatocellular cancer (Table I). The distribution of this type of cancer parallels that of chronic HBV infection; it is especially prevalent in certain regions of Asia and Africa (see Chapter 12).

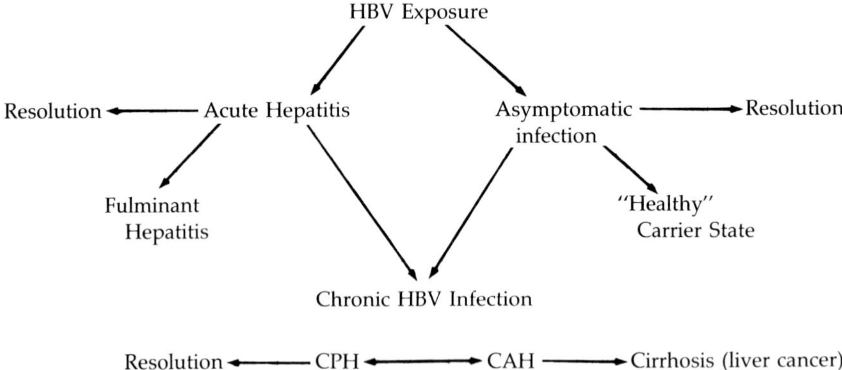

Figure 1. The main chronic sequelae of HBV infection (schematic description).

The prevalence of HBV carriers in the general population varies considerably, being rather low (0.1–0.5%) in Western Europe and the United States, but high in certain regions of Africa and Asia, where up to 20% are carriers. The prevalence of the carrier state is influenced by several factors including sex, age at exposure, and geographical region. In high prevalence areas like Southeast Asia and China many children are infected perinatally by their virus-carrier mothers. This type of vertical transmission of HBV was followed by chronic HBV infection in ~90% of children in an Asian population (Beasley *et al.*, 1983).

The high frequency of vertical HBV transmission in certain Asian populations may be explained by the fact that mothers in these areas are virus carriers, while HBsAg-positive Caucasian mothers more often are carriers of an integrated nonreplicative form of HBV (Derso *et al.*, 1978).

In population studies within Europe and the United States, HBsAg has been detected significantly more frequently in males. Male/female ratios as high as 2.7 have been reported (Szmuness *et al.*, 1978). The excess incidence in males seems to be confined to young adults; in children and adults over 40 years of age, the HBsAg rates are similar in the two sexes. Young males may have an enhanced HBV exposure because of drug addiction or homosexuality, but males also seem to retain HBV to a greater extent.

In areas where HBV infection is relatively uncommon, the highest prevalence of HBsAg is found in the 20 to 40-year age group, while the prevalence of anti-HBs continues to increase with age. The decline in rates of HBsAg positives in ages over 40 indicates that the carrier state is not lifelong.

In countries with low HBsAg carrier rates, most carriers are of the "healthy" type with a nonreplicative form of HBV. In areas with high rates, most carriers have a chronic HBV infection with circulating virions. However, the transition from one stage to the other, from active viral replication to genome-integrated HBsAg production may result in misinterpretations.

Recently Brechot *et al.* (1981) were able, using a hybridization technique, to clearly distinguish between the chronic carrier of HBV and the healthy carrier of HBsAg. The former condition was characterized by free viral DNA in the liver and viral DNA as well as HBeAg in the serum, while healthy HBsAg carriers are distinguished by the presence of integrated HBV DNA sequences in the liver cell without presence of viral DNA or HBeAg in serum.

Other studies using molecular hybridization techniques have shown that the HBV genome can exist in the liver in two forms, either as free, episomal, or extrachromosomal DNA or as integrated or chromosomal DNA (Shafitz *et al.*, 1981; Chen *et al.*, 1981).

Chronic HBV infection can thus be considered as having an early "replicative" phase during which chronic hepatitis B disease activity is present and a later "nonreplicative" phase when the necroinflammatory activity ceases. During the later phase, HBsAg may persist even though replicative forms of HBV may not be detectable in liver or serum, suggesting that HBsAg but not intact HBV can be synthesized by the hepatocytes containing integrated forms of HBV DNA only.

Certain distinguishing characteristics between HBsAg-positive healthy "nonreplicative" HBV carriers and individuals with chronic hepatitis B have been put forward. First, there seem to be differences in the distribution of HBcAg and HBsAg within the liver cell. Intranuclear HBcAg is found in many hepatocytes from patients with chronic hepatitis B but in few liver cells from healthy HBsAg carriers. On the other hand, the cytoplasmic HBsAg is present in few hepatocytes of patients with chronic liver disease, while in "healthy" carriers up to 50% of the liver cells may contain HBsAg (Woolf, 1974). Other investigators have found a focal cytoplasmic distribution of HBsAg in patients with HBV-associated liver damage and a more diffuse distribution in healthy carriers of HBsAg (Tapp and Jones, 1977; see also Chapters 11 and 13).

The "e" antigen–antibody system has long been considered a reliable marker separating most healthy HBsAg carriers from patients with HBV-associated chronic liver disease, since HBeAg is associated with active viral replication and is not found in the serum of healthy carriers who in many cases already have anti-HBe (Magnius *et al.*, 1975) (see also Chapter 4).

It has also been suggested that testing for IgM anti-HBc may help in differentiating healthy carriers of HBsAg from patients with HBsAg-positive acute or chronic hepatitis (Feinman *et al.*, 1982). However, Lemon and Hoofnagle (1982), who also studied chronic HBsAg carriers for the presence of IgM anti-HBc found 22 of 23 DNA polymerase-positive carriers but also 6 of 9 DNA polymerase-negative carriers positive for IgM anti-HBc by a solid-phase radioimmunoassay (RIA). These findings led the authors to conclude that even if IgM anti-HBc is present in most HBsAg carriers with markers of active HBV replication, the finding of IgM anti-HBc also in many anti-HBe-positive, DNA polymerase-negative carriers makes it a serologic marker of dubious value for predicting viral replication or infectivity. Obviously, more data are needed to understand the mechanism of transition from IgM to IgG anti-HBc response.

An interesting approach to studying the carrier state was taken by Kato *et al.* (1982), who analyzed the production of interferon by lymphocytes in HBsAg carriers with normal liver function and normal liver histology compared with carriers with chronic liver disease. The interferon production was found to be normal in healthy carriers, whereas it was significantly decreased in HBsAg-positive patients with chronic active hepatitis and cirrhosis. These authors suggest that an impaired interferon response may be causally related to the development of chronic liver disease in hepatitis B infections. This is of a special interest since interferon has been used as a therapeutic agent in chronic hepatitis B infection.

B. Liver Disease in the Asymptomatic Carrier

Even if a healthy carrier of HBV has been defined as someone who is asymptomatic and has no biochemical or histological evidence of liver disease, most studies of chronic carriers have included asymptomatic carriers as well as those with chronic hepatitis B.

As was pointed out in the early 1970s, HBsAg carriers with normal serum aminotransferase levels in most cases also had normal liver histology. However, racial factors also seem to play an important role in this context. For example, in Germany and Sweden ~90% of diagnosed asymptomatic native carriers have normal aminotransferases and no sign of chronic hepatitis histologically, while in other study populations ~50% or more of diagnosed asymptomatic carriers had evidence of chronic persistent hepatitis in spite of normal aminotransferase levels (Table II).

More reproduceable results are found when asymptomatic carriers with raised aminotransferases are studied. In the series presented in

TABLE II

Liver Histology in 220 Asymptomatic HBsAg-Positive Individuals with Normal Serum Aminotransferase Levels

		Liver histology			
Reference	Number of patients	Normal	Minor alterations	CPH[a]	CAH
Klinge and Bannash (1971)	21	14	3	4 (19)	0
Iwarson *et al.* (1973)	19	10	5	4 (21)	0
Woolf (1974)	16	3	3	10 (56)	0
Anderson *et al.* (1974)	31	13	0	18 (58)	0
Shrago *et al.* (1977)	26	8	3	15 (58)	0
Velasco *et al.* (1978)	19	6	1	12 (63)	0
Deurmeyer *et al.* (1982)	88	63	15	6 (7)	4

[a]Percentages in parentheses.

TABLE III
Liver Histology in 91 Asymptomatic HBsAg-Positive Individuals with Elevated Serum
Aminotransferase Levels

| | | Histological findings in liver biopsies | | | |
Reference	Number of patients	Normal	CPH	CAH and/or cirrhosis	Other reaction
Velasco *et al.* (1978)	19	4	9	3	3
Woolf (1974)	18	0	14	4	0
Feinman *et al.* (1975)	11	0	9	1	1
Anderson *et al.* (1974)	13	0	11	2	0
Vittal *et al.* (1974)	30	2	28	0	0

Table III, a normal liver histology was present (on an average) in only 10% of carriers, while as many as 20% had histological evidence of chronic active hepatitis and/or cirrhosis.

Recently, Deurmeyer *et al.* (1982) in a prospective study attempted to evaluate the prognosis in 88 asymptomatic HBsAg carriers found among blood donors. An initial liver biopsy was followed by a repeat biopsy ~4 years later. As many as 78 carriers had normal liver histology or minor alterations both initially and during follow-up. All these individuals were lacking detectable markers of HBV replication such as intrahepatic HBcAg and serum HBeAg. One of 6 carriers with chronic persistent hepatitis (CPH) on initial biopsy had progressed to chronic active hepatitis (CAH) after 4 years, while among 4 carriers with CAH at diagnosis, 1 showed only minimal alterations when rebiopsied. Obviously an asymptomatic carrier of HBsAg with normal liver histology at diagnosis usually remains normal.

The delta (δ) agent, which was first described in 1977 by Rizzetto, may be of importance for "healthy" carriers of HBsAg since superinfection of carriers by δ may occur. (Rizzetto *et al.*, 1977). This agent has been seen mainly in the Mediterranean area and in drug addicts from western Europe and the United States, but the distribution of the δ agent seems to be worldwide (Rizzetto *et al.*, 1983). HBV acts as a helper for the replication of the δ agent, and δ infection can take place only in association with concomitant HBV infection.

Delta infection may be transmitted by inocula containing both δ and HBV, or by superinfection of an HBsAg carrier with the δ agent. If simultaneous infection occurs and HBV replication is transient, the δ agent does not outlive HBV, and the harm done by this agent is very limited. In the event of superinfection of an HBV carrier, the continued HBV replication provides conditions appropriate for the full expression of the δ agent in terms of liver damage.

In HBsAg carriers with anti-HBe in serum, the chronic HBV infection is often asymptomatic (Magnius *et al.*, 1975), but if δ superinfection occurs, progressive liver disease may develop (Rizzetto *et al.*, 1983).

C. Alcohol and the Asymptomatic HBsAg Carrier State

An interesting approach to chronic liver disease in asymptomatic HBsAg carriers was taken by Villa *et al.* (1982). This Italian group studied the susceptibility of HBsAg carriers to the hepatotoxic effect of ethanol in 296 carriers who were followed for up to $3\frac{1}{2}$ years with repeated biochemical and clinical examinations. A control group of HBsAg-negative blood donors matched by age, sex, occupation, and duration and type of ethanol intake was studied in the same way. A significantly higher proportion of HBsAg-positive subjects had hepatic abnormalities when the daily ethanol consumption exceeded 60 g. Overall, HBsAg carriers seemed to be at risk of hepatic abnormalities when drinking an amount of ethanol that was harmless for HBsAg-negative subjects. The authors concluded that it is advisable to suggest complete abstinence from ethanol for HBsAg carriers.

Vargas *et al.* (1982) studied the percentage of patients with active HBV infection among 60 alcoholic cirrhotics who had consumed >80 g of alcohol daily for >10 years. These authors found that one-third of the alcoholics had signs of active HBV infection, a significantly higher prevalence than in their controls. However, in a Scandinavian study Orrholm *et al.* (1981) retrospectively found an increased prevalence of current or past HBV infection in all types of alcohol-related liver injury, progressive or nonprogressive, and concluded that coincident HBV infection probably plays a minor role in the rate of progression of alcohol-related liver disease.

Recently Bassendine *et al.* (1983) reported that in 56 Caucasian patients with biopsy-proven alcoholic liver disease, no increased prevalence of any serum marker of HBV was found when compared with a control population without liver disease. Thus, even if the association of HBV infection with the different alcohol-related liver lesions is not fully clarified, these British data suggest that HBV infection has no major role in determining the rate of progression of alcohol-induced liver disease. Another British study (Saunders *et al.*, 1982) reached the same conclusion, but pointed out that even if hepatitis B infection does not enhance the development of chronic liver disease in heavy drinkers, an exception has to be made for those who remain positive for HBsAg.

Bassendine and her colleagues (1983) also reported that the incidence of antibody to HBsAg and HBcAg was significantly increased in patients with cryptogenic CAH. The British group also found the incidence of HBsAg and anti-HBc to be significantly higher in patients with hepatocellular cancer than in the control population. These observations suggest that HBV may be giving rise to both cryptogenic CAH and liver cell cancer in the population concerned, and that the two diseases could represent two stages of chronic HBV infection. These findings are interesting, and if confirmed, may shed new light on the pathogenesis of cryptogenic CAH.

II. Chronic Hepatitis B

A. Predicting Chronicity

The progression of acute hepatitis B to chronic liver disease may be influenced by a variety of factors, including the immune status of the patients, underlying diseases, corticosteroid treatment, etc. Tests for serum aminotransferases are unreliable for predicting chronicity, and the appearance of a liver biopsy specimen should not be regarded as prognostic until at least 6 months or even 1 year from onset of jaundice.

After clinically apparent hepatitis B, complete recovery with clearance of HBV occurs in 90 to 95% of the cases within 6 months. On the other hand, this means that up to 10% of patients with acute clinical hepatitis B may become persistently infected with the hepatitis B virus. Unfortunately, HBV persistence is associated with the development of chronic liver disease in the majority of patients (Nielsen *et al.*, 1971; Redeker, 1975; Norkrans *et al.*, 1976).

Chronic HBV infection may also present insidiously with a mild acute attack more likely to proceed to chronicity (Nielsen *et al.*, 1974; Sherlock, 1976). For this reason, hospitalized patients may not be the ideal group for studying progression to chronicity. An experimental study using the inoculation of contagious material into volunteers showed that among 12 individuals who became HBsAg carriers, only 2 had experienced acute icteric disease, whereas among 103 subjects who cleared the antigen, 75% had had icteric disease (Barker and Murray, 1971). Furthermore, a severe or fulminant acute attack of hepatitis B rarely is followed by persistent infection or chronicity in survivors (Karvountsis *et al.*, 1974).

Perinatal exposure to HBV is followed by chronic infection with a very high frequency. Beasley and his colleagues (1983) in Taiwan found that >90% of children perinatally exposed to HBV became chronically infected, while this outcome occurred in <5% of infected adolescents.

Several reports have appeared on the predictive value of different alterations in liver histology during and following an acute attack of hepatitis B. In 1970, Boyer and Klatskin suggested the prognostic value of confluent necrosis with bridging between vascular structures. Patients with bridging necrosis were more likely to develop cirrhosis, while patients with the usual "spotty" necrosis seemed to have a more benign course. In a well-defined Danish series of patients with biopsy-verified acute hepatitis B, morphological features such as piecemeal necrosis, destruction of the limiting plates of the portal tracts, and portal infiltration by plasma cells proved most useful in predicting a chronic outcome (Dietrichson *et al.*, 1975). In a study by Vanstapel *et al.* (1983), the predictive value of piecemeal necrosis in acute hepatitis B was investigated, and follow-up revealed an evolution to chronicity in a very high percentage of cases with piecemeal necrosis in the original liver biopsy.

Quantitative determination of HBsAg in serum has also been suggested to be of value in predicting the prognosis of an acute attack of hepatitis B (Frösner *et al.*, 1982). These authors determined HBsAg quantitatively in patients with acute hepatitis B, and found that patients with clearance of HBsAg from the circulation within 6 months showed at least a 50% reduction in antigen concentration within 20 days after onset of jaundice. No such decrease in HBsAg titer was found in patients who became chronic HBV carriers.

In Italy, Careboda *et al.* (1982) found persistence of circulating HBsAg–IgM complexes in acute hepatitis B to be a possible marker of chronic evolution. Serial serum samples from 110 patients with acute hepatitis B were tested for HBsAg/IgM complexes by a solid-phase radioimmunoassay. In 102 patients the infection resolved; in these patients, HBsAg–IgM complexes were either absent or disappeared from the serum within 4 weeks of admission. This occurred long before HBsAg had been cleared and ALT levels had returned to normal. Eight patients developed chronic HBV infection and progressive liver disease. In these patients, HBsAg–IgM complexes were detectable in the serum on admission and never disappeared.

The prognostic meaning of the e system in acute hepatitis B was partly clarified in the mid-1970s using the immunodiffusion method to detect HBeAg (Nielsen *et al.*, 1974; Norkrans *et al.*, 1976; Tabor *et al.*, 1977). Later studies using more sensitive techniques have shown that clearing of HBeAg within 10 weeks after onset of jaundice during an acute attack of hepatitis B regularly indicates clearing of HBV also within a short time with a favorable prognosis in most cases. In contrast, hepatitis B patients carrying HBeAg for >10 weeks after onset of jaundice seem to be at greater risk of developing chronic HBV infections (Norkrans *et al.*, 1979; Aldershvile *et al.*, 1980; Tabor *et al.*, 1980).

B. The HBeAg System in Chronic Hepatitis B

Realdi and his co-workers (1980) studied the behavior of the e system in 50 patients with chronic hepatitis B, and observed that of 29 cases initially HBeAg positive, 13 lost this antigen and 10 seroconverted to anti-HBe during a follow-up period of 2 to 7 years. Seroconversion to anti-HBe was associated with a reduction in the activity of virus replication that prevailed in patients who progressed to liver cirrhosis. Improvement in serum aminotransferase levels occurred in cases who seroconverted to anti-HBe, independently of the histologic evolution in liver; immunosuppressive therapy seemed to delay seroconversion but did not affect its incidence. These results suggest that in chronic hepatitis B, HBeAg in serum identifies an early, although prolonged, course of active viral replication that is frequently followed by the disappearance of virus particles from serum and the appearance of anti-HBe. This latter event, however, does not always seem to indicate a favorable prognosis.

In a study by Hoofnagle *et al.* (1981), the natural history of chronic hepatitis B was studied during a follow-up period of up to 6 years in a population that included 20 CAH and 5 CPH patients. Initially, all were positive for HBsAg and had serum aminotransferase elevations. Only 1 patient lost HBsAg reactivity during follow-up, but in 13 (52%), seroconversion from HBeAg to anti-HBe occurred. These patients became negative for serum DNA polymerase, and their elevated serum aminotransferase levels fell to normal and remained so. In contrast, 12 patients who remained HBeAg positive continued to have elevated serum aminotransferase levels.

These data also indicate that many patients with chronic hepatitis B may have a spontaneous remission of active disease accompanied by the disappearance of HBeAg and DNA polymerase. However, this study also showed that seroconversion to anti-HBe did not prevent progressive liver disease, since 11 of 13 patients had developed CAH or cirrhosis on liver biopsy at the end of follow-up. In several patients, cirrhosis seemed to develop before there was a spontaneous resolution in disease activity and seroconversion to anti-HBe. Such patients appeared to have inactive or "burnt-out" cirrhosis.

Andres *et al.* 1981 studied the prognostic indications of DNA polymerase and HBeAg in HBV-associated chronic liver disease. Fifty patients with HBsAg as well as DNA polymerase and HBeAg in their serum were contrasted with 46 HBsAg-positive patients who had neither DNA polymerase nor HBeAg in serum. Progressive liver disease (cirrhosis included) was more common in DNA polymerase and HBeAg-negative patients than in those who were positive. Similar findings were recently reported by Norkrans *et al.* (1982). Among 5 patients who were still

HBsAg-positive 1 year after the acute attack and had developed anti-HBe at that point, 4 developed CAH and/or cirrhosis during a 5-year period of follow-up.

Liaw *et al.* (1982) found that a majority of their patients who seroconverted from HBeAg to anti-HBe had an exacerbation of their chronic liver disease. Hoofnagle (1983) has interpreted this as "immune clearance" of hepatocytes containing replicative forms of HBV genome. If so, this may indicate that the "terminating" immune attack in hepatitis B is directed against liver cells producing intact HBV.

HBeAg occurs both free and in association with IgG in the circulation of individuals infected with HBV. Based on the observation that free HBeAg migrates faster than IgG-bound HBeAg on electrophoresis in polycylamide gel, Takahashi *et al.* (1979) determined free and IgG-bound forms of HBeAg. They found a gradual decrease of free HBeAg and a shift to IgG-bound forms of HBeAg in six patients with resolving acute hepatitis B. The same events took place in one experimentally inoculated chimpanzee in which IgG-bound HBeAg eventually disappeared and anti-HBe developed in serum.

More recently, Sagnelli *et al.* (1982) described the separation of free and IgG-bound HBeAg by protein A-bearing *Staphlococcus aureus*. High values of IgG-bound HBeAg were frequently observed in patients with CAH. It is possible that the determination of free and IgG-bound forms of HBeAg may provide a new means to predict the outcome of acute HBV infections.

Some years ago, Cochrane *et al.* (1976) suggested that in addition to the known immunological reactions against viral antigens that occur during the acute phase of viral hepatitis, autoimmune reactivity directed against a liver-specific protein may be initiated; if this reactivity persists, chronic hepatitis may develop. This suggestion was based on studies of lymphocyte cytotoxicity for isolated hepatocytes, which frequently was found to be significantly increased in HBsAg-positive patients who exhibited the features of chronic aggressive hepatitis in follow-up liver biopsies.

C. The Delta Agent in Chronic Hepatitis B

The HBsAg-associated δ antigen appears to be a defective hepatotropic agent that requires obligatory helper functions of the hepatitis B virus for its replication. The δ agent may be associated with acute as well as with chronic hepatitis B. The different expressions of δ-associated hepatitis B infection may be explained by the defective nature of this agent. Because of the dependence on concomitant HBV replication, infection with the δ agent can take place only in association with ongoing HBV infection (Rizzetto *et al.*, 1977, 1983).

In δ-associated chronic hepatitis, the δ agent may be demonstrated in the liver and/or its antibody (anti-δ) may be found in the blood. As a rule, anti-δ persists in high titer in chronic δ-associated HBV infections. An analysis of 131 Italian HBV carriers with intrahepatic δ antigen showed that δ-associated liver disease was chronic active hepatitis in 70% of the patients. Liver cirrhosis was found in 20% of these patients, while persistent or lobular hepatitis was diagnosed in very few (Rizzetto *et al.*, 1979).

After an observation period of 2 to 6 years, chronic δ-associated hepatitis had progressed to cirrhosis in ~40% of these Italian patients who had no nodular transformation in the initial biopsy. Cirrhosis developed whether or not the initial histological diagnosis was chronic persistent or chronic lobular hepatitis B.

Obviously the δ agent may be associated with the type of chronic progressive liver disease that is unresponsive to immunosuppressive treatment. Therefore, δ-positive HBV carriers with morphological changes of chronic persistent or chronic lobular hepatitis must be interpreted with caution because of their tendency to progress to chronicity.

In the sera of patients from southern Italy, anti-δ was found in 65–80% of patients with hepatitis B progressing to chronicity. At clinical presentation, many of them had anti-HBe in serum and lacked IgM anti-HBc. These patients thus probably represent so-called healthy carriers of HBsAg who have become superinfected with the δ agent. An interesting aspect of δ infection in chronic carriers is its association with a depression in HBsAg titer, which may temporarily make it difficult to detect this antigen.

Delta infection in a chronic HBV carrier may sometimes be associated with termination of the carrier state. In a Swedish series of 191 HBsAg carriers, 10% lost HBsAg over a 12-year period (Moestrup *et al.*, 1983). Fourteen of these patients were drug addicts, of whom 9 had markers of δ infection. In three cases, HBV clearance and seroconversion to anti-HBs coincided with an acute attack of δ hepatitis, which suggests a possible relationship between δ infection and HBsAg clearance in these cases. The impact of δ infection on chronic hepatitis B outside Italy is little known; δ infection has a worldwide distribution, yet is predominant in the Mediterranean area. In Europe and the United States, δ infection has mainly been found in drug addicts and occasionally in hemophiliacs (Hansson *et al.*, 1982; Tedder *et al.*, 1983; Raimondo *et al.*, 1982).

TABLE IV
Association of Clinical Presentation and Histological Outcome in 16 Patients with HBV-Associated Chronic Persistent Hepatitis B[a,b]

Liver histology at the end of follow-up	Presentation at diagnosis		
	Acute	Insidious	Asymptomatic
Healed	0	0	1
CPH	5	2	1
CAH (mild)	1	6	0

[a]Mean follow-up period, 5.6 years.
[b]From Chadwick *et al.* (1979).

D. Chronic Persistent Hepatitis B

1. Clinical Course and Diagnosis. Chronic persistent hepatitis (CPH) may follow an acute attack of clinically recognized hepatitis B, but may also present insidiously (Table IV). Symptoms are usually mild and may include periods of fatigue and discomfort over the liver region. A slightly enlarged liver may be found at examination, but serum aminotransferases (ALT, AST) seldom exceed five times the upper normal limit. Serum gamma globulin levels, as well as coagulation tests, are normal, and autoantibodies are not found (or if so, occur in very low titers). Most patients with HBV-associated chronic persistent hepatitis B are young or middle-aged males.

DeGroote *et al.* (1968) defined the histological signs of CPH as "Chronic inflammatory infiltration, mostly portal, with preserved lobular architecture, and little or no fibrosis as well as piecemeal necrosis." In CPH the architecture of the liver parenchyma is preserved, and the main alteration is portal inflammation. The histological appearances of chronic persistent hepatitis are not specific; clinical as well as laboratory data must be considered in reaching a correct diagnosis. A majority of diagnosed cases of CPH seem to be caused by HBV (Chadwick *et al.*, 1979; Aldershvile *et al.*, 1982).

Chronic active hepatitis is distinguished from CPH by the characteristic disturbances of the lobular architecture with severe periportal lesions and piecemeal as well as bridging necrosis. The morphological lesions of chronic persistent hepatitis may also be observed in patients with inflammatory bowel disease, in certain collagen disorders, and in association with other systemic diseases. Alcoholic liver disease may at times be difficult to distinguish morphologically from CPH.

TABLE V

Seroconversion Rate (HBeAg to anti-HBe) in 39 Patients with HBsAg- and HBeAg-Positive
Chronic Persistent Hepatitis

			Findings at latest follow-up	
References	Number of CPH patients	Follow-up period (years)	Still HBeAg positive (number)	Seroconversion to anti-HBe (number)
Realdi *et al.* (1980)	7	2–7	6 ⎫	1 ⎫
Norkrans *et al.* (1980)	5	2–7	3 ⎬ 74%	2 ⎬ 26%
Hoofnagle *et al.* (1981)	5	1–6	3 ⎪	2 ⎪
Aldershvile *et al.* (1982)	14	1–5	11 ⎭	3 ⎭

Most patients developing chronic persistent hepatitis after an acute
attack of hepatitis B have continued replication of HBV with HBsAg as
well as HBeAg in serum. Subsequently, seroconversion from HBeAg to
anti-HBe may occur. Norkrans *et al.* (1982) prospectively followed 17
patients who had been HBsAg- and HBeAg positive for at least 1 year
after the acute attack of hepatitis B. The follow-up continued for up to 8
years. Eight of these patients remained persistently HBsAg- and HBeAg
positive during the follow-up period, and 7 had CAH on liver biopsy at
the end of follow-up.

Nine patients (53%) cleared HBeAg (all within 2 years of onset) but
remained HBsAg positive during follow-up. Seven of them had histological signs of CPH in the latest liver biopsy. These findings suggest
that prolonged detection of HBeAg (for several years) is unusual in a
case of CPH and should indicate repeated liver biopsies to reevaluate the
diagnosis.

2. Prognosis and Treatment. In general, chronic persistent hepatitis B
can be considered a relatively benign condition. Patients developing
chronic disease after a clinical attack of hepatitis B in most cases show a
picture of CPH (Redeker, 1975; Norkrans *et al.*, 1976a). These studies
presented rather short follow-up periods. The incidence of CAH may
increase somewhat with time, particularly among male homosexuals. In
a Danish study of well-defined CPH cases of HBV origin, 6 of 23 Caucasian patients who were followed for an average of 3 years developed
mild chronic active hepatitis (25%). Five of these 6 patients were persistently HBeAg positive; the majority were male homosexuals (Aldershvile *et al.*, 1982).

In a British study, Chadwick *et al.* (1979) found development of mild
CAH in 7 of 16 patients with CPH of HBV origin after an average follow-

up of 5 years. The progression to CAH was not associated with any change in symptoms or biochemical test results (Table IV).

Dudley and co-workers (1971) showed that the serum concentration of HBsAg tended to be higher in patients with CPH than in those with histological signs of chronic active hepatitis of cirrhosis. This finding was later confirmed in another British study that also found a possible relationship between CPH patients with a low serum concentration of HBsAg and progression to CAH (Chadwick *et al.*, 1979).

The prognostic implications of the e system in patients with HBV-associated chronic persistent hepatitis was studied in 14 Danish patients (10 male homosexuals). They were followed for an average of 3 years; 11 of the 14 patients were persistently HBeAg positive. Of these HBeAg-positive patients, 5 developed chronic active hepatitis (CAH) or cirrhosis. A further 9 patients were HBsAg positive, but were HBeAg negative at the time of CPH diagnosis. Only 1 developed CAH during follow-up (Aldershvile *et al.*, 1982) (Table V).

However, even if seroconversion from HBeAg to anti-HBe may be a good sign in many patients, this is not always the case. First, long-term HBsAg carriers are at risk for developing hepatocellular carcinoma, and second, superinfection with the δ agent may occur. Also, reactivation of the disease may occur, for instance if immunosuppressive treatment is initiated. This latter occurrence indicates an incomplete eradication of replicative forms of HBV in anti-HBe-positive individuals. Finally, the liver cell of the anti-HBe positive HBsAg carrier may be damaged by other hepatotropic viruses as well as by alcohol or drugs.

Immunosuppressive treatment with corticosteroids or azathioprine should not be given to patients with chronic persistent hepatitis B. Such therapy may favor viral replication, lengthen the course of the disease, and cause undesirable side effects (Alberti *et al.*, 1981; Sagnelli *et al.*, 1980) (see also Chapter 10).

No dietary regimen is indicated in CPH, but some patients complain of food intolerance and may prefer to avoid certain foods. Additional vitamins are often given but hardly required in most cases.

3. Varieties of Chronic Persistent Hepatitis.

a. Chronic lobular hepatitis. Sometimes the histological features of acute hepatitis B persist for >4–6 months indicating unresolved acute hepatitis. Prolonged histological abnormalities may be accompanied by impaired liver function. This condition, known as chronic lobular hepatitis (CLH), often has clinical and laboratory features similar to those of convalescent hepatitis B.

Histologically, the liver lesions of chronic lobular hepatitis resemble those of acute viral hepatitis with hepatocellular necrosis, focal regeneration, and inflammation. The enlarged portal tracts are inflamed and only occasionally does fibrosis progress to scarring (Popper *et al.*, 1982).

According to a recent study in Taiwan (Liaw *et al.*, 1982) CLH occurs mainly in young males and may be indistinguishable from slow-resolving acute hepatitis B. Chronic lobular hepatitis may extend for several years with remissions and relapses. No evidence of progression to cirrhosis was found in the Taiwan study, however, during an average of nearly 5 years of follow-up. It seems that this uncommon variety of hepatitis B in general has a favorable prognosis and does not require specific treatment.

b. Nonspecific reactive hepatitis. This is a mild form of chronic hepatitis that may be seen in patients who show malaise and/or hepatomegaly for a rather long period (often years) after an acute attack of hepatitis B. Sometimes these patients have a history of drug addiction. The main finding is elevated or fluctuating serum aminotransferase levels; the term "transaminitis" has been proposed for this condition. The prognosis seems to be good, with complete histological resolution except for minor scars or pigmented macrophages in the liver of some patients (Popper and Schaffner, 1976).

E. Chronic Active Hepatitis B

Chronic active hepatitis B is a chronic inflammatory liver lesion with disarrangement of the architecture of the liver lobules and with liver cirrhosis as a possible final development. It may develop after an acute attack of hepatitis B, but may also present silently. CAH may be of varied etiology, and HBV contributes to a minority of diagnosed cases, at least in Caucasian populations (Lindberg *et al.*, 1978a; Hodges *et al.*, 1982; Holdstock *et al.*, 1983). Other forms of the disease include drug-induced and autoimmune CAH. Non-A, non-B hepatitis also carries the risk of progression to CAH (Table VI).

1. Clinical Course and Diagnosis. The clinical picture of HBsAg positive CAH may be variable, but persistent elevation of serum aminotransferases is a common finding. Symptoms may include fatigue and anorexia, but some patients are asymptomatic until late stages and may present with portal hypertension. In HBsAg-positive chronic active hepatitis, autoantibodies such as antinuclear factor and smooth muscle antibody are absent or present in low titers, and γ globulin levels are normal or

TABLE VI
Percentage of HBsAg-Positive Cases of Histologically Verified CAH in Different Countries

Country	Number of patients	HBsAg (%)	References
England	31	6	Holdstock *et al.* (1983)
England	61	20	Hodges *et al.* (1982)
Sweden	66	20	Lindberg *et al.* (1978)
Belgium	34	50	DeGroote *et al.* (1978)
Iraq	83	91	Holdstock *et al.* (1983)

[a]Third-generation tests for HBsAg.

only moderately increased. A great majority of the patients are young or middle-aged males; as a rule the development of HBV-associated CAH is a gradual and silent process (Table VII).

According to DeGroote *et al.* (1968), CAH is histologically characterized by "piecemeal necrosis, new fiber formation and lymphocytic infiltration of portal tracts and lobules. Features of acute hepatitis may be superimposed and connective tissue septa may be present. Signs of liver-cell regeneration are usually seen and the borderline between CAH and cirrhosis is not sharp." A main difference between fully developed cirrhosis and CAH is that in liver cirrhosis nodular regeneration has led to a complete and irreversible loss of the normal hepatic architecture. The lesions of chronic active hepatitis may be reversible. The severity of the liver lesion may vary in different parts of the liver and histological signs of cirrhosis and CAH may coexist.

Piecemeal necrosis, a key sign in CAH, may be defined as "a destruction of liver cells at an interface between parenchyma and connective tissue." This process is regularly accompanied by lymphocyte or plasma

TABLE VII
Different Characteristics of Autoimmune and HBV-Associated Chronic Active Hepatitis

	Autoimmune type	HBV-Associated type
Predominant sex	Female	Male
Serum HBsAg	Negative	Positive
Serum anti-HBc	Negative	Positive
Serum gamma globulin	Markedly increased	Normal
Smooth muscle antibody	High serum titers	Absent or low titers
Response to immunosuppresive therapy	Usually good	None

cell infiltrates. The inflammatory reaction extends beyond the portal areas into the liver lobule, eroding the limiting plate. HBV-associated chronic persistent hepatitis may at times be difficult to distinguish from chronic active hepatitis, as borderline cases are common. In CPH, however, the lobular architecture is intact. No piecemeal necrosis, bridging necrosis, or rosette formation is seen.

2. Immunosuppressive Treatment. There is no convincing evidence that corticosteroids or other immunosuppresive agents are beneficial in the treatment of HBV-associated CAH. Corticosteroids can lead to temporary improvement in serum aminotransferases (Dudley *et al.*, 1971), but are ineffective in extending life expectancy (Schalm *et al.*, 1976).

Alberti *et al.* (1981) studied the levels of hepatitis B virus DNA polymerase over variable periods of time in 16 HBV carriers, and found that carriers receiving immunosuppressive drugs showed a progressive increase in DNA polymerase during therapy, but returned to pretreatment levels after therapy was withdrawn. Similar findings have been reported by Sagnelli *et al.* (1980), who found that long-term prednisone and/or azathioprine treatment seem to favor the replication of HBV in patients with chronic active hepatitis B.

In a Hong Kong study, Lam *et al.* (1981) found that corticosteroids may induce biochemical relapses and increase the frequency of complications in HBsAg-positive CAH. Fifty-one patients were pair randomized to receive either placebo or prednisolone. After initial remission, the dosage of prednisolone was decreased from 15–20 to 10 mg/day; this dosage was continued for up to $3\frac{1}{2}$ years. Prednisolone-treated individuals experienced a lower remission rate, a higher relapse rate, and a decreased survival rate than did placebo-treated individuals. This study has been criticized for its definite conclusions, and some of its statistical analyses are open to question. Recently Wu *et al.* (1982) presented histological confirmation of the failure of steroid therapy in HBsAg-positive patients with CAH.

A randomized multicenter clinical trial in Europe, which included 89 patients with HBV-associated CAH, was recently reported (E. Juhl and N. Tygstrup, personal communication). The treatment was either placebo or 10 mg/day of prednisolone, which was initiated when serum ALT levels reached more than twofold the upper limit of normal. The code was broken when it was found that nine deaths had occurred in one group versus only two in the other group. The high death rate occurred in the prednisolone-treated group, and all deaths were either the result of hematemesis or hepatic failure. In the placebo group there was one suicide and one case of septicemia. The survival rate was significantly different according to log rank analysis ($p = .025$) in the two groups, which otherwise had similar clinical and laboratory variables. Consequently, the authors conclude that corticosteroid treatment can reduce survival in HBsAg-positive CAH.

The statement some years ago by Wright *et al.* (1977) that the only patient with CAH who may benefit to a degree that outweights toxicity from therapy are symptomatic, HBsAg-negative patients with severe histological abnormalities seems more and more valid.

Some authors recommend a therapeutic trial of steroids during 3 to 6 months in cases of progressive HBsAg-positive liver disease (Boyer and Miller, 1982). After this period, the treatment should be terminated if symptoms are not alleviated, or if biochemical improvement does not occur, or if side effects develop. Otherwise, steroid therapy should continue at low dosage. Against the background of a prolonged period of HBsAg positivity, an increasing titer of HBV markers, and a reduced survival rate following immunosuppressive therapy, therapeutic steroid trials seem doubtful.

A possible explanation for the different effects of steroids in HBV-associated CAH and autoimmune CAH was given by Nouri-Aria *et al.* (1982), who found a defect in Con-A-induced suppressor-cell activity in 22 patients with autoimmune CAH and in 26 patients with HBsAg-positive CAH as compared with controls. Normal values were, however, observed in patients with autoimmune hepatitis in whom a remission had been induced and maintained by treatment with prednisolone. The loss of suppressor-cell activity in chronic active hepatitis B may allow liver damage to continue, and the reversal of the defect in autoimmune forms of CAH by administration of prednisolone provides a plausible explanation for the efficacy of this treatment. The contrasting responses to prednisolone in autoimmune and HBsAg-positive chronic active hepatitis suggest that the nature of this suppressor-cell defect may be different in these two forms of CAH.

Antiviral therapy, which is probably a better therapeutic approach in chronic active hepatitis B than are immunosuppressive agents, are covered in Chapter 10.

3. Prognosis. Prognostic studies in HBV-associated CAH have shown variable results; some studies have suggested a better outcome than in a patient with the classical autoimmune type of CAH (Dudley *et al.*, 1971; Czaja *et al.*, 1981; Lindberg *et al.*, 1978b), while others have found a worse prognosis in HBV-associated CAH (Schalm *et al.*, 1976; DeGroote *et al.*, 1978). The long-term follow-up of 17 HBV-associated CAH cases by de Groote *et al.* showed a transition to cirrhosis in 70% between the second and the fifth year of their disease. All these patients had received immunosuppressive treatment, however.

HBsAg-positive chronic active hepatitis with HBeAg in the serum has often been regarded as a progressive disorder with a poor prognosis. These conclusions have at least in part been based on cross-sectional studies of patients with active disease (Elefthériou *et al.*, 1975; Sagnelli *et al.*, 1978) and may not give a true picture of the natural history of HBV-associated CAH.

Realdi *et al.* (1980) followed 50 HBsAg-associated cases of CAH for 2 to 7 years, and found that seroconversion from HBeAg to anti-HBe occurred in ~30% of cases and was associated with a striking reduction in the activity of virus replication and transaminase levels independently of the histologic evolution. These results as well as those of Hoofnagle *et al.* (1981) suggested that in HBsAg-positive chronic active hepatitis, HBeAg in serum identifies a prolonged phase of active virus replication that is frequently followed by the disappearance of virus particles from serum and the appearance of anti-HBe as a sign of the integration of viral DNA in liver cell DNA. This event does not necessarily imply a good prognosis, as it seems to occur mainly in those who develop cirrhosis (Hoofnagle, 1983; Liaw, 1982).

Apparently HBV-associated CAH may proceed slowly to cirrhosis in certain cases, while in other patients the disease progresses very little over the years. The impact of superinfection with the δ agent has been little studied outside Italy, and remains one possibility which must be pursued. Racial factors must be considered as well, since striking geographical differences appear in the reported prevalence of HBV-associated CAH (Table VI). Finally, the use of corticosteroids for several years in many cases may have affected the outcome.

The course of HBsAg-positive CAH in an Asian population was studied by Lo *et al.* (1982) in Taiwan. They followed 76 HBsAg-positive CAH-patients for an average of ~4 years. At the time of the last follow-up, about half either had evidence of progressive liver disease or had died. Of 15 deaths, 9 were due to complications of chronic liver disease and 6 to hepatocellular carcinoma. Obviously the course of HBsAg-positive CAH was much more progressive in this predominantly male Chinese population as compared with, for example, caucasian populations.

Even if the prognosis in HBsAg-positive chronic active hepatitis is variable, the mode of presentation provides some information to the clinician. Those cases presenting with complications of CAH or cirrhosis (such as ascites) clearly have a poor prognosis. In those patients who have been discovered incidentally or who have been followed since their acute hepatitis, the prognosis is uncertain but may well be good since the latent period for development of clinically overt cirrhosis is often long. Further longitudinal studies of HBV-associated CAH patients who received no immunosuppressive treatment are needed to clarify the natural history of HBV-associated CAH.

A potential sequel of chronic hepatitis B is the development of hepatocellular carcinoma, which is common in those areas of the world where chronic HBV infection is common, namely in parts of Africa and Asia. Patients with hepatocellular carcinoma in these regions are much more frequently HBsAg positive than are controls from the same geographical area, suggesting an etiological role of HBV in hepatic cell oncogenesis (see Chapter 12).

F. Chronic HBV-Associated Liver Disease in Special Groups of Patients

1. Homosexual Men. Of homosexual males attending veneral disease clinics, up to 5% may be symptomless carriers of HBsAg, while ~50% may have anti-HBs (Jeffries *et al.*, 1973; Szmuness *et al.*, 1975; Coleman *et al.*, 1977; Iwarson *et al.*, 1980). Ellis *et al.* (1979) studied the prevalence of chronic liver disease in a population of male homosexuals attending veneral disease clinics in London. Over 2600 homosexual males were surveyed; 129 (5%) were found to carry HBsAg. Forty-three of 65 (66%) of these carriers had abnormal liver function tests. Among those with abnormal serum aminotransferases, 9 had asymptomatic acute hepatitis with liver function tests returning to normal with time. Of the remaining HBsAg carriers, 25 accepted a liver biopsy; 23 (92%) had signs of chronic liver disease. The histological appearance was that of chronic active hepatitis in 10 cases, active cirrhosis in 4, chronic persistent hepatitis in 9, and only minimal changes in 2. HBeAg was demonstrable in the serum of 12 of 14 patients with CAH, and in 6 of 9 with CPH.

In another British study, Viola *et al.* (1981) studied 100 consecutive HBsAg carriers seen at a teaching hospital in London. Ninety-four were males, of which 82% were homosexuals, demonstrating the epidemiological impact of male homosexuals in the spread of hepatitis B. These authors considered liver biopsy as the only reliable means of diagnosing the type and severity of liver disease in these male homosexuals. The seroconversion rate of HBeAg to anti-HBe was low (9.7%) during nearly 4 years of follow-up, and very few patients had developed signs of advanced liver disease. This very informative study clearly shows the high risk of hepatitis B exposure in male homosexuals, the apparent tendency to persistent HBV infection, and the development of chronic liver disease.

In a recent Danish study on patients with chronic persistent hepatitis, 10 of 14 males with a histological diagnosis of CPH were homosexuals. All were HBsAg positive and remained so during the period of follow-up (1–7 years). Among 11 of 14 patients who remained HBeAg positive during the period of study, 5 progressed to CAH or cirrhosis, again suggesting a worse prognosis of HBV-associated chronic liver disease in male homosexuals as compared with nonhomosexuals. In the Danish study, only 2 of 28 nonhomosexuals with CPH (7%) progressed to CAH or cirrhosis during the period of follow-up (Aldershvile *et al.*, 1982).

Recent studies of the immune response in male homosexuals have revealed severe impairment in a large percentage. This may be one explanation for the high frequency of chronic HBV infection in male homosexuals (Gottlieb *et al.*, 1981; Masur *et al.*, 1981; Centers for Disease Control, 1982). Schreeder *et al.* (1982) found that seropositivity for HBV markers was significantly related to the duration of regular homosexual activity and to the number of nonsteady male sexual contacts. Genital–anal and oral–anal intercourse also were significantly related to evidence of HBV infection. Other investigators have pointed out that the highest frequency of HBV markers as well as of opportunistic infections are found in sexually active male homosexuals that have many partners.

2. Hemophiliacs. Serologic evidence of past or present hepatitis B infection was found in 90% of 136 hemophiliacs in a study by Gerety *et al.* (1980). Of 34 patients 10 years of age or younger, 85% already had serologic evidence of prior or ongoing hepatitis B infection. Similar findings have been reported by Scaroni *et al.* (1980). Although the great majority of hemophiliacs have hepatitis B markers in serum, prospective studies have shown that <10% of patients with persistently elevated aminotransferases are chronically infected with HBV. In addition, only 20% of those with chronic hepatitis have persistent HBV infection (Mannucci *et al.*, 1975; Hoofnagle and Seeff, 1976; White *et al.*, 1982).

Yannitsiotis *et al.* (1977) found chronic liver disease in 47 of 101 Greek hemophiliacs. The prevalence of chronic liver disease was, however, not higher in HBsAg-positive than HBsAg-negative hemophiliacs. In an American study, White *et al.* (1982) tried to determine the severity of liver disease in multiply transfused hemophiliacs with aminotransferase (ALT) abnormalities. Of 15 patients with persistently elevated ALT levels, 13 had serologic evidence of prior exposure to HBV, but none had clinical evidence of liver disease. Liver biopsies revealed CPH or other mild forms of liver disease in 14 of the 15 patients. Patients with CPH tended to have higher ALT elevations than patients with histologically milder forms of hepatic inflammation, but there was no correlation between liver histology and hepatitis B serology.

Kim *et al.* (1980) studied 103 patients treated with factor VIII and factor IX concentrates for 6 to 36 months; 51% showed elevated ALT levels for >6 months. Only 8 patients were HBsAg positive for >6 months, but overall 77% had anti-HBs in serum. Six acute episodes of hepatitis were attributed to HBV and another six to non-A, non-B agents. Obviously chronic HBV-associated liver disease is a problem in hemophiliacs with persistent HBV replication.

Hasiba *et al.* (1980) studied liver enzymes (ALT and AST) and HBV serological markers in >500 American hemophiliacs receiving blood products, and found persistence of HBsAg for >12 months in 6% of the patients. Anti-HBs was detected in 90% of patients treated with factor VIII or factor IX concentrates but in only 49% of patients treated with fresh frozen plasma or cyroprecipitate.

In a study by Rizzetto *et al.* (1979), sera from chronic HBsAg carriers among former blood donors and hemophiliacs in Maryland were tested by RIA for antibodies to the δ antigen (anti-δ). Anti-δ was not detected in any of 81 sera from HBsAg-positive former blood donors. In contrast, 45% of HBsAg-positive hemophiliacs had detectable anti-δ. As part of the same study, 22 AHF or factor IX concentrates were tested and found negative for the δ antigen.

It has been assumed that persistently raised aminotransferase levels in hemophiliacs mainly are due to chronic non-A, non-B hepatitis infection (Gerety *et al.*, 1980), but other hypotheses have also been put forward. Myers *et al.* (1980) suggested hypersensitivity reactions as a possible explanation. Some kind of autoimmune reaction has also been proposed as an explanation, since autoantibodies are often found in hemophiliacs with chronic liver disease. It may, however, be concluded that the natural history of chronic liver disease in hemophiliacs is not well defined, even if the exclusion of other possible etiologies leaves non-A, non-B hepatitis as a possible explanation both for the elevated aminotransferase levels and the liver abnormalities seen in many hemophiliacs. Apparently chronic HBV infection does not play a major role in the high frequency of chronic liver dysfunction found in hemophiliacs. The possibility of vaccinating the newly diagnosed hemophiliac against hepatitis B should further reduce the impact of HBV infection in hemophiliacs.

3. Hemodialysis and Renal Transplant Patients. There appears to be a high risk for development of chronic liver disease in hemodialysis as well as in renal transplant patients who become chronically infected

TABLE VIII
Chronic HBV-Associated Liver Disease among Dialysis and Renal Transplant Patients

		Histological findings in liver biopsies		
References	Number of patients	Normal picture or minor histological lesions	CPH	CAH/cirrhosis number (%)[a]
Coughlin *et al.* (1980)	21	14	2	5 (24)
Galbraith *et al.* (1979)	15	6	4	5 (33)
Miller *et al.* (1978)	23	—	11	12 (52)
Nordenfelt *et al.* (1975), Löfgren *et al.* (1982)	29	9	16	4 (14)

[a] Percentages in parentheses.

with HBV. Most of these patients have no clinical symptoms but show mild increases in serum aminotransferase levels. Examination of liver biopsies may, however, reveal a severe chronic hepatitis. In an Australian study by Coughlin *et al.* (1980), 7 of 21 patients who were HBsAg positive for at least 6 months developed chronic liver disease during a 5-year follow-up period; 5 progressed to CAH or cirrhosis. The livers of the remaining 14 HBV carriers did not show any evidence of progression to chronicity (Table VIII). In all, the incidence of HBsAg in 141 patients who received renal transplants in this center during 1972–1977 was 16%, while in 181 patients on maintenance hemodialysis the incidence of HBsAg was 6%.

Another study concerning the outcome of HBV-associated liver disease in transplant patients was reported by Degos *et al.* (1980). Serial liver biopsies were performed on the day of transplantation and at 1 and 3 years later. Almost all patients (97%) who later developed chronic hepatitis already had abnormal liver histology prior to transplantation. Most HBsAg-positive patients with mild chronic hepatitis before transplantation developed chronic aggressive hepatitis after transplantation. The relative risk of contracting chronic hepatitis was 30-fold greater for HBsAg-positive recipients of renal transplants than for HBsAg-negative recipients.

In a large center in the United States, a study of 162 renal transplant recipients revealed only six acute episodes of liver disease attributable to hepatitis B virus. Four of these progressed to chronic liver disease (Ware *et al.*, 1979). In another study conducted in the United States by La-Quaglia *et al.* (1981), chronic liver disease developed in 35 of 405 renal transplant patients; very few of these chronic cases were HBV associated. Apparently HBV-related chronic liver disease does not play a major role in renal transplant patients even if a certain number of patients do have a chronic asymptomatic HBV infection, especially when the patients are on immunosuppressive treatment.

In a series presented by Galbraith *et al.* (1979), development of chronic liver disease occurred in 9 of 15 HBsAg-positive patients with chronic renal disease. In a similar study by Miller *et al.* (1978) that included 23 HBsAg-positive dialysis patients who were followed for an average of 9 months, 12 patients (52%) had a histological picture of CAH on liver biopsy with erosion of the limiting plate and bridging necrosis. The remaining 11 had features of unresolved hepatitis (Table VIII). Four of the CAH patients had progressed to chronicity quite silently, which seems to be common in hemodialysis patients.

Among 27 Swedish patients who died during regular dialysis treatment, 17 were HBsAg positive at death. Twelve had signs of CPH or CAH when autopsied. The duration of hemodialysis treatment and time of HBsAg carriership showed the same variation among patients with or without signs of chronic hepatitis (Nordenfelt *et al.*, 1975).

In a later study in the same center (Löfgren *et al.*, 1982) a serological follow-up of 50 HBsAg-positive hemodialysis patients showed that only 10 (20%) seroconverted to anti-HBs during the period of follow-up (from 6 months to several years). These Scandinavian dialysis patients as a rule had a clinically mild liver disease with slight or moderate elevations in serum aminotransferase levels. Twelve HBsAg-positive patients died. Histological changes consistent with CAH were observed in two patients, CPH in six, and normal findings in four.

The prognosis of the liver disease among HBsAg-positive dialysis or renal transplant patients with chronic persistent hepatitis histologically is usually good, and therapeutic intervention appears not to be necessary. It is not quite clear whether the natural history of CAH is different in these patients, but Strom and Merrill (1977) have suggested that renal transplant patients with liver failure may benefit from a discontinuation of azathioprine. Since patients with chronic active hepatitis rarely have serious rejection episodes, there may be little advantage to and potential harm in continuing azathioprine therapy.

In general chronic HBV infection does not seem to influence significantly the clinical condition or the long-term prognosis in hemodialysis or renal transplant patients even if histological studies in certain cases show rather severe liver lesions.

4. Drug Addicts. Hepatitis B infection is a major problem in drug addicts, and development of chronic HBV-associated liver disease seems to occur more often in them than in nonaddicts. In a study including >350 acute hepatitis B cases in patients aged 15–45 years, progression to chronicity was documented in 14.4% of drug addicts compared with 5.3% of nonaddicts ($p < .01$) (Norkrans *et al.*, 1976a). The chronic liver disease was associated with continued replication of HBV in about one-half of the addicts but in 80% of nonaddicts, possibly indicating that factors other than persistent HBV replication alone were active.

The observation that severe chronic liver disease may develop following an acute attack of hepatitis B in spite of a rapid clearance of HBsAg and normalization of serum aminotransferase levels was reported in the early 1970s (Cherubin *et al.*, 1972). In a later study by Arnold (1982), histological signs of CAH appeared in 21 of 48 addicts studied (43%); 10 were HBsAg negative. In many cases, progression to CAH took place in spite of almost normal levels of serum aminotransferases (Table IX). Similar findings have been reported by Seeff *et al.* (1975). In this study, 25% of drug addicts biopsied because of persistently abnormal serum transaminase levels revealed histological characteristics of CAH or cirrhosis. This led the authors to suggest that every drug addict with persistently abnormal aminotransferases (>3 months), particularly when accompanied by a positive test for HBsAg, should have a liver biopsy performed.

Addicts may also show an intense portal and intralobular inflammation with eosinophilic leukocytes and macrophages present. This type of inflammation may proceed to granuloma formation, and is believed to result from intravenously injected contaminants such as talc, baking soda, etc. (Min *et al.*, 1974).

Multiple attacks of jaundice are much more common among drug addicts than in nonaddicts. The different icteric episodes may result from single attacks of hepatitis A, hepatitis B, and non-A, non-B hepati-

TABLE IX

Histological Studies of Liver Biopsies in Drug Addicts Correlated with Their ALT Levels[a]

	Number	ALT < 50 U/liter	ALT > 50 U/liter	HBsAg-positive, number (%)[b]
CPH	16	5	11	8 (50)
CAH	21	5	16	11 (55)
Nonspecific reaction	6	2	4	0
Normal histology	5	4	1	0

[a]From studies of Cherubin *et al.* (1972) and Arnold (1982).
[b]Percentages in parentheses.

tis. Certain icteric attacks seem to be associated with a histological picture of nonspecific or unresolved hepatitis on liver biopsy, and may possibly be explained as toxic reactions (Iwarson *et al.*, 1973a). However, to distinguish between individual bouts of acute hepatitis and exacerbations of the original illness or fluctuations during the course of a chronic disease is difficult. In one study of 33 addicts who had experienced at least 2 attacks of jaundice, 23 episodes (32%) were explained as hepatitis A and 30 as hepatitis B (42%). Finally, 18 episodes (25%) were caused by neither of these viruses (Norkrans *et al.*, 1980a). In spite of their recurrent attacks of jaundice, the liver disease in these Scandinavian addicts seemed to have a rather benign course.

In addicts with chronic HBV infection, concurrent infection with the δ agent is common, as shown by the presence of anti-δ in 27% of symptomless Italian addicts with HBsAg, and the finding of δ markers in 64% of addicts with HBsAg-positive hepatitis in different parts of Europe (Raimondo *et al.*, 1982).

The presence of δ markers in addicts, with acute disease and two bouts of aminotransferase elevations a few weeks apart, suggests that this biphasic hepatitis may result from double infection with HBV and δ, with sequential expression of the two agents. This was verified in two chimpanzees experimentally infected with separate inocula containing HBV and δ. Each animal had two separate hepatitis episodes, one of which was accompanied by the presence of intrahepatic HBcAg and the other by intrahepatic δ (Rizzetto *et al.*, 1982).

The clinical features of δ infection were analyzed in a large Swedish study including 191 HBsAg carriers and nearly 600 cases of acute hepatitis B (Moestrup *et al.*, 1983). Delta infection proved to occur almost exclusively in drug addicts. In chronic HBsAg carriers, the most common clinical manifestation of δ infection was an episode of acute δ-positive hepatitis. During the period of δ infection, the HBsAg titer decreased, and in 3 of 26 cases seroconversion from HBsAg to anti-HBs occurred. In addicts with acute hepatitis B the clinical picture did not distinguish between those with and without simultaneous δ infection. The progression to HBV carrier state was similar whether or not the patient was infected simultaneously with the δ agent.

In addition to chronic liver disease, drug addicts also develop other types of HBsAg-related complications, presumably as a result of immune complex formation. Renal disease like membranoproliferative or focal glomerulonephritis, which manifest as the nephrotic syndrome, has been reported (Kilcoyne *et al.*, 1972; Knieser *et al.*, 1974). Polyarteritis and necrotizing angiitis have also been described in addicts, primarily among amphetamine users (Gocke *et al.*, 1970; Citron *et al.*, 1970).

G. Chronic HBV-Associated Liver Disease in Childhood

Perinatal transmission of HBV from mother to child may occur when the mother either develops acute hepatitis B late in pregnancy or is a chronic carrier of HBV with circulating virions. In hyperendemic areas such as parts of Asia where the rate of chronic HBV carriers is high, transmission from carrier mothers is the predominant mode of spread of hepatitis B infection (Stevens *et al.*, 1975; Okada *et al.*, 1975).

Babies usually become infected with HBV at birth and most often develop a chronic carrier state that is associated with biochemical and histological signs of chronic persistent hepatitis (Schweitzer, 1975). In rare instances, CAH or cirrhosis may develop. The development of acute icteric hepatitis B with subsequent clearing of HBsAg may occur as well. Occasional cases of acute fulminant hepatitis B have also been described (Wright *et al.*, 1970; Fawaz *et al.*, 1975; Shiraki *et al.*, 1980, Tong *et al.*, 1981).

Most studies on the transmission of HBV from mother to infant indicate that the transmission occurs mainly in mothers with serological markers of circulating HBV such as HBeAg and DNA polymerase at the time of delivery. In contrast, infants born to HBsAg-positive mothers who have anti-HBe in their serum have been reported to escape chronic infection more often (Okada *et al.*, 1976; Gerety and Schweitzer, 1977).

In a study by Stevens *et al.* (1979), 45 of 47 Chinese infants born to HBeAg-positive mothers had evidence of HBV infection, and 40 became chronic HBsAg carriers. On the other hand, none of 14 infants born to anti-HBe positive mothers became chronically HBsAg positive, although 3 of them had serological evidence of transient HBV infection.

Tong *et al.* (1981) found three mothers with both HBeAg and anti-HBe in their serum. All three transmitted HBV to their infants, while two carrier mothers with only anti-HBe did not transmit HBV to their babies. These findings are similar to those reported by Stevens *et al.* (1979). More recently two reports have documented a total of five cases of acute hepatitis B in infants born to anti-HBe positive carrier mothers (Shiraki *et al.*, 1980; Sinatra *et al.*, 1982). Four of these five children were of Asian origin. The mother of the fifth child was a carrier found to be anti-HBe positive 3 months after delivery. These reports as well as those of others (Papaevangelou and Hoofnagle, 1979) indicate that infants born to asymptomatic anti-HBe positive HBsAg-carrier mothers may become infected with HBV and may display clinical responses ranging from asymptomatic transient viremia with development of anti-HBs to mild clinical disease, but do not become chronic carriers of HBV.

The transmission of HBV from an anti-HBe-positive mother to her offspring may be due to continued viral replication with circulating virions in spite of seroconversion to anti-HBe. One possible explanation for this is that termination of the HBV infection occurs gradually and was not complete at the time of delivery.

The follow-up period in some of the chronically HBV-infected infants reported by Tong *et al.* (1981) is now >10 years. All have remained HBsAg positive, and some continue to show periodic increases in their serum ALT levels. Among eight children with an initial histological diagnosis of chronic persistent hepatitis, three developed spider angiomas, three showed hepatomegaly, and another two had both angiomas and hepatomegaly. Thus, although children with chronic persistent hepatitis usually remain clinically stable there is a possibility that a more serious type of liver disease may eventually develop, at least in an Asian population (Table X).

In a study from Vienna, Sacher *et al.* (1979) followed six HBsAg-positive children who were admitted because of suspected liver disease. These children (aged 3 months to 14 years) were followed for ~3 years, and elimination of HBsAg was noted in only one. Three children showed mild CPH, and one had histological evidence of CAH. In 26 German children (aged 7 months to 14 years) with chronic hepatitis B infection, CPH was histologically diagnosed in 15 while CAH was seen in 9. Two of these children had only minimal abnormalities in liver histology, and 8 had additional diseases including hemophilia and heart disease (Bosch *et al.*, 1980).

One of the most extensive long-term follow-ups of chronic hepatitis B

TABLE X

Histological Findings in Liver Biopsies of Children with HBsAg-Positive Chronic Liver Disease

Reference	Number of patients	"Minimal changes"	CPH	CAH
Sacher *et al.* (1979)	5	2	2	1
Bosch *et al.* (1980)	26	2	15	9
Bortolotti *et al.* (1981)	35	1	18	16[a]
Total	66	5 (7%)	35 (53%)	26 (40%)

[a]Cirrhosis in two patients

in children was reported by Bortolotti *et al.* (1981), who studied 35 children 1–11 years of age known to be HBsAg carriers for at least 6 months prior to the study. Ten had had an acute icteric hepatitis, while the rest had not. Although approximately three-fourths of the children were asymptomatic, only one was a healthy carrier of HBsAg. Eighteen children presented a histological picture of CAH, and 16 had histological evidence of CPH (Table VII). A high percentage also had markers of circulating virions. During a follow-up period of an average of 3 years, serum aminotransferase levels became normal in 5 CPH patients, and liver histology normalized in 3. Two of 5 untreated children with CAH showed complete remission, while this was observed in only 1 of 11 CAH patients who had received immunosuppressive treatment. These results indicate the possibility of spontaneous remission of HBsAg-positive CAH and CPH in children. The study raises obvious doubts about the usefulness of immunosuppressive therapy in children with chronic hepatitis B.

Extrahepatic manifestations of HBV infection have been found in children as well as in adults. In 1974, Brzosko *et al.* described glomerulonephritis associated with hepatitis B. More recently, membraneous glomerulonephritis in HBsAg-positive children was reported (Takekoshi *et al.* 1979; Ito *et al.*, 1981). HBeAg was found in serum as well as in the kidneys of these children. In two children, seroconversion from HBeAg to anti-HBe was associated with improvement in renal histology. It is supposed that the kidney damage was caused by HBeAg–anti-HBe complexes in these Japanese infants.

References

Alberti, A., Pontisso, P., and Realdi, G. (1981). *J. Med. Virol.* **8,** 223–229.

Aldershvile, J., Frösner, G. G., Nielsen, J. O., Hardt, F., Deinhardt, F., and Skinhøj, P. (1980). *J. Infect. Dis.* **141,** 293–298.

Aldershvile, J., Dietrichson, O., Skinhøj, P., Kryger, P., Mathiesen, L. R., Christoffersen, P., Nielsen, J. O., and the Copenhagen Hepatitis Acuta Programme (1982). *Hepatology (N.Y.)* **2,** 243–246.

Anderson, K. E., Sun, S. C., Berg, H. S., and Chang, N. K. (1974). *Am. J. Dig. Dis.* **19,** 693–703.

Andres, L., Sawhney, V. K., Scullard, G. H., Smith, J. L., Merigan, T. C., Robinson, W. S., and Gregory, P. B. (1981). *Hepatology (N.Y.)* **1,** 583–585.

Arnold, W. (1982). *In* "The European Meeting on Vaccination against Hepatitis b2 (MSD)."

Barker, L. F., and Murray, R. (1971). *JAMA, J. Am. Med. Assoc.* **216,** 1970.

Bassendine, M. F., Della Seta, L., Salmeron, J., Thomas, H. C., and Sherlock, S. (1983). *Liver* **3,** 65–70.

Beasley, R. P., Hwang, L. Y., Stevens, C. E., Lin, C. C., Hsieh, F. J., Wang, K. Y., Sun, T. S., and Szmuness, W. (1983). *Hepatology (N.Y.)* **3**, 135–141.

Bortolotti, F., Cadrobbi, P., Crivellaro, C., Bertaggia, A., Alberti, A., and Realdi, G. (1981). *Gut* **22**, 499–504.

Bosch, C., Becker, M., Rotthauwe, H. W., and Födisch, H. J. (1980). *Eur. J. Pediatr.* **135**, 169–173.

Boyer, J. L., and Klatskin, G. (1970). *N. Engl. J. Med.* **283**, 1063.

Boyer, J. L., and Miller, D. J. (1982). *In* "Diseases of the Liver" (L. Schiff and E. R. Schiff, eds.), 5th ed., pp. 799–800. Lippincott, Philadelphia, Pennsylvania.

Brechot, C., Scotto, J., Charnay, P., Hadchouel, M., Degos, F., Trepo, C., and Tiollais, P. (1981). *Lancet* **2**, 765–768.

Brzosko, W. J., Nazarewicz, T., Krawczynski, K., Morzycka, M., and Nowoslawski, A. (1974). *Lancet* **2**, 477–479.

Careboda, F., de Franchis, R., D'Arminio Monforte, A., Vecchi, M., Rossi, E., Primignani, M., Palla, M., and Dioguardi, N. (1982). *Lancet* **2**, 355–360.

Centers for Disease Control (1982). *N. Engl. J. Med.* **306**, 248–252.

Chadwick, R. G., Galizzi, J., Jr., Heathcote, J., Lyssiotis, T., Cohen, B. J., Scheur, P. J., and Sherlock, S. (1979). *Gut* **20**, 372–377.

Chen, D. S., Sung, J. L., and Lai, M. Y. (1981). *Gastroenterology* **80**, 880–881.

Cherubin, C. E. *et al.* (1972). *Ann. Intern. Med.* **76**, 385–389.

Citron, R. H., Halpern, M., and Mowann, M. (1970). *N. Engl. J. Med.* **283**, 1005–1011.

Cochrane, A. M. G., Moussouros, A., Smith, A., Thomson, A. D., Eddleston, A. L. W. F., and Williams, R. (1976). *Gut* **17**, 714–718.

Coleman, J. C., Waugh, M., and Dayton, R. (1977). *Br. J. Vener. Dis.* **53**, 132.

Coughlin, G. P., van Deth, A. G., Disney, A. P. S., Hay, J., and Wangel, A. G. (1980). *Gut* **21**, 118–122.

Czaja, A. L., Ludwig, J., Baggenstoss, A. H., and Wolf, A. (1981). *N. Engl. J. Med.* **304**, 5–9.

Degos, F., Degott, C., Bedrossian, J., Camilieri, J. P., Barbanel, C., Duboust, A., Rueff, B., Benhamou, J. P., and Kreis, H. (1980). *Transplanation* **29**, 100–102.

DeGroote, J., Desmet, V. J., Gedigk, P., Korb, G., Popper, H., Poulsen, H., Scheuer, P. J., Schmid, M., Thaler, H., Uehlinger, E., and Wepler, W. (1968). *Lancet* **2**, 626.

DeGroote, J., Fevery, J., and Lepoutre, L. (1978). *Gut* **19**, 510–513.

Derso, A., Boxall, E. H., Tarlow, M. J., and Flewett, T. H. (1978). *Br. Med. J.* **1**, 949–952.

Deurmeyer, H. H., Arnold, W., Klinge, O., Schönborn, H., Hess, G., and Meyer zum Büschenfelde, K. H. (1982). *In* "Viral Hepatitis" (W. Szmuness, H. J. Alter, and J. E. Maynard, eds.), pp. 681–682. Franklin Inst. Press, Philadelphia, Pennsylvania.

Dietrichson, O., Juhl, E., Christoffersen, P., Elling, P., Feber, V., Iversen, K., Nielsen, J. O., Petersen, P., and Poulsen, H. (1975). *Acta Pathol. Microbiol. Scand., Sect. A* **83A**, 183–188.

Dudley, F., Fox, R., and Sherlock, S. (1971). Lancet 2, 1–3.

Eleftheriou, N., Thomas, H. C., Heathcote, J., and Sherlock, S. (1975). *Lancet* **2**, 1171–1173.

Ellis, W. R., Coleman, J. C., Fluker, J. L., Keeling, P. W. N., Banatuala, J. E., Murray-Lyon, I. M., Evans, B. A., Bull, J., Simmons, P. D., Willcox, J. R., and Thompson, R. P. H. (1979). *Lancet* **1**, 903–904.

Fawaz, K. A., Grady, G. F., Kaplan, M. M., and Gellis, S. S. (1975). *N. Engl. J. Med.* **293**, 1357.

Feinman, S., Cooler, N., Sinclair, J. C., Wrobel, D., and Berris, B. (1975). *Lancet* **2**, 609.

Feinman, S. V., Overby, L. R., Berris, B., Chau, K., Schable, C. A., and Maynard, J. E. (1982). *Hepatology (N.Y.)* **2**, 795–799.

Frösner, G. G., Schomerus, H., Wiedmann, K. H., Zachoval, R., Bayerl, B., Bäcker, U., Gathof, G. A., and Sugg, U. (1982). *Eur. J. Clin. Microbiol.* **1,** 52–58.

Galbraith, R. M., El Sheikh, N., and Portmann, B. (1979). *Br. Med. J.* **1,** 1495–1597.

Gerety, R. J., and Schweitzer, I. L. (1977). *J. Pediatr. (St. Louis)* **90,** 368.

Gerety, R. J., Eyster, M. E., Tabor, E., Drucker, J. A., Lusch, C. J., Prager, D., Rice, S. A., and Bowman, H. S. (1980). *J. Med. Virol.* **6,** 111–118.

Gocke, D. J., Hsu, K., Morgan, C., Bombardieri, S., Lockshin, M., and Christian, C. L. (1970). *Lancet 2,* 1149–1153.

Gottlieb, M. S., Schroff, R., Schanker, H. M., Weisman, J. D., Fan, T. P., Wolf, R. A., and Saxon, A. (1981). *N. Engl. J. Med.* **305,** 1425–1431.

Hansson, B., Moestrup, T., Widell, A., and Nordenfelt, E. (1982). *J. Infect. Dis.* **146,** 472–478.

Hasiba, U., Eyster, M. E., Gill, F. M., Kajanu, M., Lewis, J. H., Lusch, C. J., Prager, D., Rice, S. A., and Shapiro, S. S. (1980). *Dig. Dis. Sci.* **25,** 776–782.

Hodges, J. R., Millward-Sadler, G. H., and Wright, R. (1982). *Lancet 1,* 550–552.

Holdstock, G., Rassam, S., Millward-Sadler, G. H., and Wright, R. (1983). *Liver* **3,** 2–7.

Hoofnagle, J. H. (1983). *Gastroenterology* **84,** 422–424.

Hoofnagle, J. H., and Seeff, L. B. (1976). *In* Natl. Inst. Health Rep. 77-1089, pp. 55–66. U.S. Department of Health, Education and Welfare, Washington, D.C.

Hoofnagle, J. H., Dusheiko, G. M., Seeff, L. B., Jones, E. A., Waggoner, J. G., and Bales, Z. B. (1981). *Ann. Intern. Med.* **94,** 744–748.

Ito, H., Hattori, S., Matusda, I., Amamiya, S., Hajikano, H., Yoshizawa, H., Miyakawa, Y., and Mayumi, M. (1981). *Lab. Invest.* **44,** 214–220.

Iwarson, S., Lundin, P., Holmgren, J., and Hermodsson, S. (1973a). *J. Infect. Dis.* **127,** 544–550.

Iwarson, S., Magnius, L., Lindholm, A., and Lundin, P. (1973b). *Br. Med. J.* **1,** 84–87.

Iwarson, S., Johannison, G., Löwhagen, G.-B., and Emilsson, A.-C. (1980). *Infection* **8,** 223–225.

Jeffries, D. J., James, W. H., Jerferiss, F. J. G., MacLeod, K. G., and Willcox, R. R. (1973). *Br. Med. J.* **2,** 455–456.

Karvountsis, G. G., Redeker, A. G., and Peters, R. L. (1974). *Gastroenterology* **67,** 870–877.

Kato, Y., Nakagawa, H., Kobayashi, K., Hattori, N., and Hatano, K. (1982). *Hepatology (N.Y.)* **2,** 789–790.

Kilcoyne, M. M., Daly, J. D., Gocke, J. D., Thomson, G. E., Meltzer, J. I., Hsu, K. C., and Tannenbaum, M. (1972). *Lancet 1,* 17–20.

Kim, H., Saidi, P., Ackley, A., Bringelsen, K., and Goche, D. (1980). *Gastroenterology* **79,** 1159.

Klinge, O., and Bannash, P. (1971). *Verh. Dtsch. Ges. Pathol.* **52,** 568–573.

Knieser, M. R., Jenis, E. H., and Lowenthal, D. T. (1974). *Arch. Pathol.* **97,** 193–200.

Lam, K. C., Lai, C. L., Ng, R. P., Trepo, C., and Wu, P. C. (1981). *N. Engl. J. Med.* **304,** 380–386.

LaQuaglia, M. P., Tolkoff-Rubin, N. E., and Dienstag, J. L. (1981). *Transplantation* **32,** 504–506.

Lemon, S., and Hoofnagle, J. (1982). *In* "Viral Hepatitis" (W. Szmuness, H. J. Alter, and J. E. Maynard, eds.), pp. 723–724. Franklin Inst. Press, Philadelphia, Pennsylvania.

Liaw, Y. F., Chu, C. M., Chen, T. J., Lin, D. Y., Chang-Chien, C. S., and Wu, C. S. (1982). *Hepatology (N.Y.)* **2,** 258–262.

Lindberg, J., Lindholm, A., and Iwarson, S. (1978a). *J. Infect. Dis.* **137,** 189–193.

Lindberg, J., Frösner, G., Hansson, B. G., Hermodsson, S., and Iwarson, S. (1978b). *Scand. J. Gastroenterol.* **13,** 525–527.

Lo, K. J., Tong, M. J., Chien, M.-C., Tsai, Y.-T., Liaw, Y. F., Yang, K.-C., Chian, H., Liu, H.-C., and Lee, S.-D. (1982). *J. Infect. Dis.* **146**, 205–210.

Löfgren, B., Nordenfelt, E., Lindholm, T., and Lindergård, B. (1982). *Scand. J. Infect. Dis.* **14**, 165–169.

Magnius, L. O., Lindholm, A., Lundin, P., and Iwarson, S. (1975). *JAMA, J. Am. Med. Assoc.* **231**, 356.

Mannucci, P. M., Capitanio, A., Del Ninno, E., Colombo, M., Pareti, F., and Ruggeri, Z. M. (1975). *J. Clin. Pathol.* **28**, 620–624.

Masur, H., Michelis, M. A., Greene, J. B. *et al.* (1981). *N. Engl. J. Med.* **305**, 1431–1438.

Miller, D. J., Williams, A. E., Le Bouvier, G. L., Dwyer, J. M., Grant, J., and Klatskin, G. (1978). *Gastroenterology* **74**, 1208–1213.

Min, K. W., Gyorkey, F., and Cain, D. (1974). *Arch. Pathol.* **98**, 331–335.

Moestrup, T., Hansson, B.-G., Widell, A., and Nordenfelt, E. (1983). *Br. Med. J.* **286**, 87–90.

Myers, T. J., Trembevilla-Zubiri, C. L., Klatsky, A. U., and Rickles, F. R. (1980). *Blood* **55**, 748–751.

Nielsen, J. O., Dietrichson, O., Elling, P., and Christoffersen, P. (1971). *N. Engl. J. Med.* **285**, 1157–1160.

Nielsen, J. O., Dietrichson, O., and Juhl, E. (1974). *Lancet* 2, 913.

Nordenfelt, E., Lindholm, T., and Henriksson, H. (1975). *Scand. J. Urol. Nephrol.* **9**, 277–281.

Norkrans, G., Hermodsson, S., Lundin, P., and Iwarson, S. (1976a). *Infection* **4**, 70–72.

Norkrans, G., Magnius, L., and Iwarson, S. (1976b). *Br. Med. J.* **1**, 740–742.

Norkrans, G., Frösner, G., and Iwarson, S. (1980a). *JAMA, J. Am. Med. Assoc.* **234**, 1056–1058.

Norkrans, G., Nordenfelt, E., Hermodsson, S., and Iwarson, S. (1980b). *Scand. J. Infect. Dis.* **12**, 159–160.

Norkrans, G., Lindberg, J., Frösner, G., Hermodsson, S., Lundin, P., and Iwarson, S. (1982). *Scand. J. Gastroenterol.* **17**, 383–387.

Nouri-Aria, K. T., Hegarty, J. E., Graeme, J. M., Alexander, M. B., Eddleston, A. L. W. F., and Williams, R. (1982). *N. Engl. J. Med.* **306**, 1301–1304.

Okada, K., Yamada, T., and Miyakawa, Y. (1975). *J. Pediatr. (St. Louis)* **87**, 360.

Okada, K., Kamiyama, I., Inomata, M., Imai, M., Miyakawa, Y., and Mayumi, M. (1976). *N. Engl. J. Med.* **294**, 746.

Orrholm, M., Aldersvhile, J., and Tage-Jensen, U. (1981). *J. Clin. Pathol.* **34**, 1378–1380.

Papaevangelou, G., and Hoofnagle, J. H. (1979). *Pediatrics* **63**, 602–605.

Popper, H., and Schaffner, F. (1976). *Prog. Liver Dis.* **5**, 531–558.

Popper, H., Thung, S. N., and Gerber, M. A. (1982). *In* "Viral Hepatitis" (W. Szmuness, H. Alter, and J. Maynard, eds.). Franklin Inst. Press, Philadelphia, Pennsylvania.

Raimondo, G., Smedile, A., Gallow, L., Balbo, A., Ponzetto, A., and Rizzetto, M. (1982). *Lancet* 1, 249–251.

Realdi, G., Alberti, A., Rugge, M., Bortolotti, F., Rigoli, A. M., Tremolada, F., and Ruol, A. (1980). *Gastroenterology* **79**, 195–199.

Redeker, A. G. (1975). *Med. Clin. North Am.* **59**, 1168.

Rizzetto, M., Canese, M. G., Arico, S., Crivelli, O., Trepo, C., Bonino, F., and Verme, G. (1977). *Gut* **18**, 997.

Rizzetto, M., Shih, J. W. K., Gocke, D. J., Purcell, R. H., Verme, G., and Gerin, J. L. (1979). *Lancet* 2, 986.

Rizzetto, M., Smedile, A., and Farci, P. (1982). *Scand. J. Infect. Dis., Suppl.* **36**, 74–75.

Rizzetto, M., Verme, G., Recchia, S., Bonino, F., Farci, P., Arico, S., Calzia, R., Picciotto, A., Colombo, M., and Popper, H. (1983). *Ann. Intern. Med.* **98**, 437–441.

Sacher, M., Eder, G., Bianchi, L., Gudat, F., and Thaler, H. (1979). *Wien. Klin. Wochenschr.* **91**, 722–726.

Sagnelli, E., Vernace, S. J., and Paronetto, F. (1978). *Gastroenterology* **75**, 864–868.

Sagnelli, E., Maio, G., Felaco, F. M., Crescenzo, M. I., Manzillo, G., Pasquale, G., Filippini, P., and Piccinino, F. (1980). *Lancet 2*, 395–397.

Sagnelli, E., Triolo, G., Vernace, S., and Paronetto, F. (1982). *In* "Viral Hepatitis" (W. Szmuness, H. J. Alter, and J. E. Maynard, eds.). Franklin Inst. Press, Philadelphia, Pennsylvania.

Saunders, J., Haines, A., Postman, B., Wodali, A., Powell-Hackson, P., Davis, M., and Williams, R. (1982). *Lancet 1*, 1381.

Scaroni, C., Cancellieri, V., Carnelli, V., Moroni, G. A., and Angeli, M. (1980). *Lancet 2*, 537–538.

Schalm, S. W., Summerskill, W. H. J., Gitnick, G. L., and Elveback, L. R. (1976). *Gut* **17**, 781–786.

Schreeder, M. T., Thompson, S. E., Hadler, S. C., Bergquist, K. R., Zaidi, A., Maynard, J. E., Ostrow, D., Judson, F. N., Braff, E. H., Nylund, T., Moore J. N., Jr., Gardner, P., Doto, I. L., and Reynolds, G. (1982). *J. Infect. Dis.* **146**, 7–15.

Schweitzer, I. L. (1975). *Prog. Med. Virol.* **20**, 27.

Seeff, L. B., Zimmerman, H. J., Wright, E. C. *et al.* (1975). *Am. J. Med. Sci.* **270**, 41–47.

Shafitz, D. A., and Key, M. C. (1981). *Hepatology (N.Y.)* **1**, 1–18.

Sherlock, S. (1976). *Lancet 2*, 354–356.

Shiraki, K., Yoshihara, N., Sakurai, M., Eto, T., and Kawana, T. (1980). *J. Pediatr.* **97**, 768.

Shrago, S. S., Auslander, M. O., and Gitnick, G. L. (1977). *Lab. Med.* **101**, 648–651.

Sinatra, F. R., Shah, P., Weissman, J. Y., Thomas, D. W., Merritt, R. J., and Tong, M. J. (1982). *Pediatrics* **70**, 557–559.

Stevens, C. E., Beasley, R. P., Tsui, J., and Lee, W.-C. (1975). *N. Engl. J. Med.* **292**, 771.

Stevens, C. E., Neurath, R. A., Beasley, R. P., and Szmuness, W. (1979). *J. Med. Virol.* **3**, 237–241.

Strom, T. B., and Merrill, J. P. (1977). *N. Engl. J. Med.* **296**, 225–226.

Szmuness, W., Much, M. I., Prince, A. M., Hoofnagle, J. H., Cherubin, C. E., Harley, E. J., and Block, G. H. (1975). *Ann. Intern. Med.* **83**, 489–495.

Szmuness, W., Harley, E., Ikram, H., and Stevens, C. (1978). *In* "Viral Hepatitis" (G. N. Vyas, S. N. Cohen, and R. Schmid, eds.), pp. 297–320. Franklin Inst. Press, Philadelphia, Pennsylvania.

Tabor, E., Gerety, R. J., and Barker, L. F. (1977). *J. Infect. Dis.* **136**, 541–547.

Tabor, E., Frösner, G., Deinhardt, F., and Gerety, R. J. (1980). *J. Med. Virol.* **6**, 91–99.

Takahashi, M., Miyakawa, Y., Gotanda, T., Mishiro, S., Imai, M., and Mayumi, M. (1979). *N. Engl. J. Med.* **300**, 814–819.

Takehoshi, Y., Tanaka, M., and Miyakawa, Y. (1979). *N. Engl. J. Med.* **300**, 814.

Tapp, E., and Jones, D. M. (1977). *J. Clin. Pathol.* **30**, 671–674.

Tedder, R., Briggs, M., and Howell, D. (1983). *Lancet 1*, 764–765.

Tong, M. J., Thursby, M. W., Lin, J. H., Hejssman, J. Y., and McPeak, C. M. (1981). *Prog. Med. Virol.* **27**, 137–147.

Vanstapel, M. J., van Steenbergen, W., de Wolf-Peeters, C., Desmyter, J., Fevery, J., DeGroote, J., and Desmet, V. J. (1983). *Liver* **3**, 46–57.

Vargas, V., Pedreira, J. D., Esteban, R., Hernández-Sanchez, J. M., Guardia, J., and Bacardi, R. (1982). *In* "Viral Hepatitis" (W. Szmuness, H. J. Alter, and J. E. Maynard, eds.). Franklin Inst. Press, Philadelphia, Pennsylvania.

Velasco, M., Gonzales-Ceron, M., de la Fuente, C., Ruiz, A., Dorso, S., and Katz, R. (1978). *Gut* **19**, 569–571.

Villa, E., Barchi, T., Grisendi, A., Bellentani, S., Rubbiani, L., Ferretti, I., de Palma, M., and Manenti, F. (1982). *Lancet* 2, 1243–1244.

Viola, L. A., Coleman, J. C., Fluker, J. L., Murray-Lyon, I. M., Barrison, I. G., Paradinas, J. F., and Evans, B.-A. (1981). *Lancet* 2, 1156–1159.

Vittal, S. B. V., Dourdourekas, D., and Shobassay, N. (1974). *Am. J. Clin. Pathol.* **62**, 649–654.

Ware, A. J., Luby, J. P., Hollinger, B., Eigenbrodt, E. H., Cuthbert, J. A., Atking, C. R., Shorey, J., Huk, A. R., and Combes, B. (1979). *Ann. Intern. Med.* **91**, 364–371.

White, G. C., Zeitler, K. D., Lesesne, H. R., McMillan, C. W., Warren, M. S., Roberts, H. R., and Blatt, P. M. (1982). *Blood* **60**, 1259–1262.

Woolf, I. L. (1974). *In* "Symposium on the Carrier State." Br. Soc. Gastroenterol., Aviemore.

Wright, E. C., Seeff, L. B., Berk, P. D., Jones, E. A., and Plotz, P. H. (1977). *Gastroenterology* **73**, 1422–1430.

Wright, R., Perkins, J. R., and Bower, B. D. (1970). *Br. Med. J.* **4**, 719.

Wu, P. C., Lai, C. L., Lam, K. C., and Ho, J. (1982). *Hepatology (N.Y.)* **2**, 777–783.

Yannitsiotis, A., Bossinakiou, I., Louisou, K., Panayotopolou, C., and Mandalaki, T. (1977). *Scand. J. Haematol.* **30**, 11–15.

Chapter 8

Follow-Up and Management of Hepatitis B Carriers

RICHARD E. SAMPLINER
Gastroenterology Section
Veterans Administration Medical Center
and University of Arizona Health Sciences Center
Tucson, Arizona

I. Definition of the Chronic Carrier of HBsAg

The chronic carrier of hepatitis B is an individual with hepatitis B surface antigen (HBsAg) detectable in the serum for 6 months or longer. The hepatocytes of the carrier are chronically infected with the hepatitis B virus (HBV), and are directed by the viral genome to produce excess HBsAg. As a result of this chronic infection, the carrier circulates HBsAg and may manifest a variety of serological markers reflecting the presence of the virus—the hepatitis B e antigen (HBeAg), the enzyme DNA polymerase—or the host's reaction to the virus—the antibody to hepatitis B core antigen (anti-HBc), and the antibody to e antigen (anti-HBe). The frequency and significance of these hepatitis B serological markers in carriers will be discussed below.

The term "carrier" in general medical usage indicates an infected individual who can transmit an etiological agent, but who lacks manifestations of the disease caused by the agent. Because of the complex-

155

Copyright © 1985 by Academic Press, Inc.
All rights of reproduction in any form reserved.
ISBN 0-12-280672-7

ities of the agent–host interaction in the case of HBV and the difficulty of noninvasive hepatic evaluation, an operational definition of the chronic carrier of HBsAg is the persistence of HBsAg over a period of time independent of the health of the carrier. The wide spectrum of hepatic manifestations of HBV infection ranging from a normal liver to severe chronic active hepatitis and primary hepatocellular carcinoma (PHC) will be discussed in the evaluation of the liver disease of the carrier. On a population scale, it is not feasible to define the status of the liver in each carrier, although at a clinical level such definition may be desirable. Our operational definition of the carrier state will include all individuals with chronic HBV infection, whatever the liver manifestations.

The minimum duration of the carrier state is based upon the clearance of HBsAg by 6 months in 90 to 95% of patients with acute hepatitis B (Nielsen *et al.*, 1971; Redeker, 1975; Hoofnagle, 1978). The remaining 5–10% of patients become carriers and circulate HBsAg for a prolonged interval.

II. The Magnitude of the Problem of the Carrier

The carrier can be identified in many settings—population screening programs, blood donor screening, and evaluation of patients with suspected or known liver disease. Based upon the prevalence of HBsAg in volunteer blood donors, it has been estimated that there are 1 million carriers in the United States (Szmuness, 1975). From population surveys, the worldwide estimate for carriers exceeds 170 million (Szmuness, 1978), but numbers alone do not define the magnitude of the health problem. The frequency of chronic liver disease in carriers and the risk of carriers developing PHC highlight the direct health impact. The reservoir for transmission of HBV provided by carriers emphasizes the public health problem.

III. The Implications of Being a Carrier

The major impact of the carrier state is on both the individual and the public health. The assessment of the health of the carrier and the risk of transmission of hepatitis B by the carrier will determine the appropriate follow-up and management.

A. Evaluation of the Carrier

The focus of a primary care physician is on the health of the individual patient. This focus is appropriate for the chronic carrier of HBsAg. With a spectrum of liver involvement ranging from none that is apparent to potentially lethal chronic active hepatitis with cirrhosis, evaluation of the liver is the key for determining the prognosis of an individual carrier. Medical history is of little help in evaluating the carrier. The majority do not have a history of viral hepatitis, and presumably have had a subclinical infection. Symptoms short of jaundice are notoriously nonspecific and insensitive in relation to liver disease. The first step in the laboratory evaluation of the carrier is the determination of serum alanine aminotransferase (ALT) and aspartate aminotransferse (AST) activity (Fig. 1). If the aminotransferase activity is normal, the likelihood of liver involvement affecting survival is remote and further evaluation at that point in time is unnecessary. In reviewing series of 15 or more carriers with normal aminotransferases, only 1.7% (9 of 513) had chronic active hepatitis and/or cirrhosis (Reinicke *et al.*, 1972; Iwarson *et al.*, 1972; Anderson *et al.*, 1974; Woolf *et al.*, 1974; Schaefer *et al.*, 1974; Feinman *et al.*, 1975; Holtermuller *et al.*, 1975; Villeneuve *et al.*, 1976; Koretz *et al.*, 1978; Velasco *et al.*, 1978; Sampliner *et al.*, 1979; Liaw and Sung, 1979; De-Franchis *et al.*, 1980; Gonzalez-Molina *et al.*, 1980; Dormeyer *et al.*, 1981). Once chronic active hepatitis has been histologically excluded, the prognosis of the carrier is excellent. Of 104 chronic carriers with serial liver

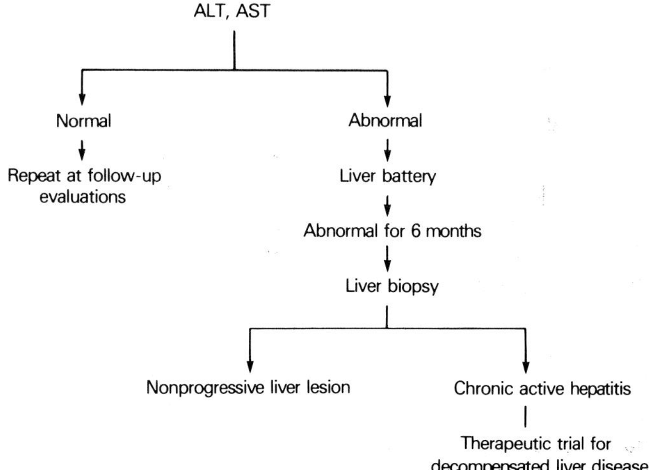

Figure 1. Evaluation of chronic carriers of HBsAg.

biopsies, only 2 progressed to chronic active hepatitis during an interval of 1.5 to 4 years (Dormeyer *et al.*, 1981; Sun *et al.*, 1976). These two patients may represent an unusual evolution of chronic persistent hepatitis, or the sampling of liver by the original needle biopsy may have inadequately represented their liver pathology (Soloway *et al.*, 1971).

If the serum AST and/or ALT activity of a carrier are abnormal, then a complete battery of liver tests is indicated, including alkaline phosphatase, albumin, globulin, bilirubin, and prothrombin time. Even though abnormalities other than serum aminotransferase activity are unusual in asymptomatic carriers, establishing a baseline liver profile is important. The finding of abnormal aminotransferases should be confirmed by repeat testing at 3- to 6-month intervals. If the aminotransferase levels remain elevated for 6 months or longer, a liver biopsy is indicated. The current state of the art for diagnosing liver disease does not offer a reliable noninvasive method to recognize chronic active hepatitis. Preliminary data do suggest that tests measuring specific liver functions (the aminopyrine breath test and serum bile acid concentrations) correlate with histologic severity of chronic hepatitis (Monroe *et al.*, 1982). If further studies support these data, true liver function tests may be of value in selecting patients for liver biopsy. Currently the carrier's prognosis can be best established by defining liver histology. Further developments in hepatology may yield sensitive functional tests that will obviate the need to obtain tissue.

In reviewing the larger series of carriers with abnormal aminotransferase activity at the time of liver biopsy, 19% (37 of 199) had chronic active hepatitis and/or cirrhosis (Singleton *et al.*, 1971; Bolin *et al.*, 1973; Simon and Patel, 1974; Vittal *et al.*, 1974; Anderson *et al.*, 1974; Woolf *et al.*, 1974; Feinman *et al.*, 1975; Villeneuve *et al.*, 1976; Velasco *et al.*, 1978; Liaw and Sung, 1979; Sampliner *et al.*, 1979; Gonzales-Molina *et al.*, 1980; Reesink *et al.*, 1980). The magnitude of the elevation of aminotransferase activity seems less important than the persistence of an elevation, for chronic active hepatitis can be found histologically when the serum aminotransferase elevation is twofold or less above normal values. In the 10–15% of carriers with persistent aminotransferase elevations, at least half have chronic active hepatitis (Reesink *et al.*, 1980; Sampliner *et al.*, 1982).

The underlying assumption of the above discussion relating serum aminotransferase elevation to chronic active hepatitis is that liver histology is the best available prognostic indicator for liver disease. Chronic active hepatitis is a liver disease that frequently progresses to cirrhosis and that shortens survival (Boyer, 1976). The finding of chronic persistent hepatitis has not been discussed because of the self-limited nature and benign prognosis of this liver disease.

The last issue for the carrier's personal health is PHC. The relative risk of PHC in a carrier is the highest documented for any neoplasm independent of a genetic syndrome, 224 for male carriers in Taiwan compared to an HBsAg-negative control group (Beasley, 1982). The carrier's risk for PHC may not be as high in the United States as in Taiwan, but a preliminary retrospective study suggests that it is significantly greater than that of the general population (Prince and Alcabes, 1982). Not only are there epidemiologic data supporting the role of HBV in oncogenicity, but integration of HBV DNA into the host genome has been documented in carriers with PHC (Brechot *et al.*, 1980; Shafritz and Kew, 1981). Whether integration of viral DNA with the host genome is sufficient or whether a co-carcinogen is necessary for the production of PHC is not yet clear. PHC may develop in a carrier with or without underlying cirrhosis of the liver. Early recognition of PHC for effective therapeutic intervention is difficult. Although α-fetoprotein can be markedly elevated at the time of detection of PHC, the tumor may already be unresectable (Kubo *et al.*, 1978). In addition, α-fetoprotein may not become elevated with the development of PHC. In spite of these shortcomings, the serum α-fetoprotein remains the best available test for early recognition of PHC.

B. The Carrier and the Public Health

The chronic carrier of HBsAg serves as a reservoir of hepatitis B infection. Among the best-documented examples of the carrier as a source of transmission are the blood donor, the new mother, and the health care worker who has violated medical technique. With the screening of volunteer blood donors for HBsAg, the asymptomatic carrier has been nearly eliminated from the blood donor pool. Hepatitis B now accounts for <10% of posttransfusion hepatitis (Alter *et al.*, 1975a). On a global basis, the carrier mother may well be the most important source of HBV transmission. Although less of a problem in the United States (Schweitzer, 1975), a high frequency of transmission from the carrier mother to her infant has been well documented in Taiwan (Stevens *et al.*, 1975). Such perinatal transmission has been estimated to account for 40% of the carriers in the general population of Taiwan.

A small number of health care worker carriers have been identified as sources of infection for their patients (Levin *et al.*, 1974; Grob and Moeschlin, 1975; Goodwin *et al.*, 1976; Rimland *et al.*, 1977; Collaborative

Study, 1980). Although not all health care worker carriers transmit hepatitis B (Alter *et al.*, 1975b; Williams *et al.*, 1975; Gerber *et al.*, 1977; LaBrecque and Dhand, 1981), the risk has created a major controversy as to the need for occupational restriction. Careful evaluation of each transmission episode reveals a break in accepted technique that has resulted in patient exposure. The commonality of these examples of carriers as a source of transmission is an infectious carrier, an exposure, and a susceptible host; each of these three elements is necessary for transmission.

A great effort has been made to identify the subgroup of carriers who are infectious, those at greatest risk of transmitting hepatitis B. HBeAg has been documented to be a marker of infectivity (Alter *et al.*, 1976; U.S. National Heart and Lung Institute, 1976; Okada *et al.*, 1976). DNA polymerase, an enzyme associated with the core of the HBV, is also an indicator of relative infectivity (Alter *et al.*, 1976). Other markers of active viral replication (high-titer anti-HBc, HBV DNA; Bonino *et al.*, 1981) or of intense viral infection [high-titer HBsAg, Dane particles in the serum, hepatitis B core antigen (HBcAg) in hepatocytes] also presumably correlate with infectivity (Table I). There are many interrelationships among the above HBV markers. Unfortunately, no single study evaluates all of the markers in one group of patients. There is a high correlation between the presence of HBeAg and hepatitis B-specific DNA polymerase (Alter *et al.*, 1976; Imai *et al.*, 1976). Furthermore, HBeAg correlates with high-titer HBsAg (Trepo *et al.*, 1976; Stevens *et al.*, 1978), the finding of Dane particles in the serum (Takahashi *et al.*, 1976; Tong *et al.*, 1977), and of HBcAg in the hepatocyte (Hess *et al.*, 1977). Although HBcAg is not found free in the serum, it can be detected in Dane particle preparations, and correlates with the finding of HBcAg in the liver (Rizzetto *et al.*, 1981). HBeAg connotes relative risk of infectivity, but it does not define other factors important for transmission, the size of the inoculum, the mode of exposure, and the susceptibility of the exposed host. Carriers with anti-HBe have also been documented to transmit hepatitis B (Ste-

TABLE I
Correlates of HBV Replication and Infectivity

HBeAg
DNA polymerase
High-titer HBsAg
Dane particles by electronmicroscopy
HBV DNA
HBcAg in hepatocytes
High-titer anti-HBc
Anti-HBc IgM

vens *et al.*, 1978; Werner and Grady, 1982). HBV DNA may well be the most specific indicator of HBV infection and may better define individuals with a high risk of transmission (Lieberman *et al.*, 1983).

An understanding of the nature of the exposure necessary for transmission is crucial for the development of effective interventions. Although HBsAg has been detected in many body fluids, blood is clearly the most important source of infection. Blood has a higher titer of HBsAg and presumably a higher concentration of complete hepatitis B virions than either semen or saliva (Heathcote *et al.*, 1974). The skin is such an effective barrier against viral penetration that percutaneous or permucosal exposure to blood is necessary for transmission Outside of the medical environment and the setting of intravenous drug abuse, percutaneous exposure is unusual. Sexual intercourse provides permucosal exposure and therefore is a likely route of transmission. Recent evidence in homosexual men demonstrates that what appears to be permucosal transmission may in fact be percutaneous because of the high frequency of bleeding rectal mucosal lesions (Reiner *et al.*, 1982). Permucosal salivary exposure is insufficient for transmission in an animal model (Bancroft *et al.*, 1977), and saliva does not seem to be an important naturally occurring mode of transmission.

Finally, the susceptible host lacks prior experience with hepatitis B, that is, antibody to HBsAg (anti-HBs). With rare exceptions (Koziol *et al.*, 1976), only a massive exposure to HBV will result in hepatitis B in an individual with high titer anti-HBs (Trepo and Prince, 1976). The new inactivated hepatitis B vaccine (Szmuness *et al.*, 1980), which induces anti-HBs in the recipient, offers the opportunity to eliminate susceptible hosts in high-risk populations.

IV. Epidemiology and Serology

The epidemiological characteristics of the carrier in the United States have been most extensively evaluated in potential volunteer blood donors found to have HBsAg. Such carriers can be characterized as low-income males, nonwhites, or (if white) young, single, poorly educated males of foreign origin (Szmuness *et al.*, 1978). Caucasian carriers are more frequently male, live in the inner city, and are foreign born; if U.S. born, they have foreign-born fathers, are non–Jewish, single, live in crowded conditions, have a relatively poor education and low family income, more frequently have been tattooed, and have a history of viral hepatitis. In contrast, nonwhite carriers differ from controls only with respect to being more frequently male and having a low family income. The large number of risk factors for whites may reflect the acquisition of HBsAg as an adult in contrast to acquisition in childhood by the nonwhite.

The above characteristics of the carrier result from the combination of the likelihood of HBV exposure and the likelihood of HBsAg persistence. With the major routes of transmission being percutaneous, permucosal, and perinatal, exposure results from intravenous drug abuse, occupational activity, sexual practices, and family contact. Given effective exposure to HBV, factors associated with persistence include race, immune status, age, and sex. The high frequency of HBsAg persistence in Chinese–Americans (14.2 versus 5.5% in Caucasian volunteer blood donors in New York) is evidence for a racial effect (Szmuness *et al.*, 1978). Association of HBsAg with Down's syndrome, lymphocytic leukemia, Hodgkin's disease, lepromatous leprosy, and maintenance hemodialysis therapy supports a role for host immune status. Infections in childhood (Gerety *et al.*, 1974) and in males (Blumberg *et al.*, 1972) increase the likelihood of becoming a carrier in the range of 8- and 1.6-fold, respectively. Patients with mild or subclinical hepatitis B infections seem more likely to become carriers (Barker and Murray, 1971).

The vast majority of individuals infected with HBV clear HBsAg and resolve the HBV infection as heralded by the development of anti-HBs. Why carriers fail to clear HBsAg and usually fail to develop anti-HBs is not understood. No specific immune defect has been reproducibly documented in carriers. Recently a failure of carrier lymphocytes to produce anti-HBs has been reported (Dusheiko *et al.*, 1981). Yet, carriers are able to respond to HBV infection with the production of anti-HBc and anti-HBe. A carrier can even produce anti-HBs directed to heterotypic HBsAg determinants (Tabor *et al.*, 1977).

Having considered the epidemiology of the carrier, we now turn to the serological characteristics. The serology of the carrier is a manifestation of HBV infection of the liver. The HBV genome directs the carrier's hepatocytes to produce HBV, including a massive excess of HBsAg. Figure 2 demonstrates the serological events in the development of the carrier state after acute clinical hepatitis B. The depicted serological sequence of infection is the same in the absence of a clinical illness. Virtually all carriers have anti-HBc (Hoofnagle *et al.*, 1973), reflecting ongoing HBV infection. Anti-HBc can be the only marker of HBV infection and as such, when present in high titer, can indicate a "low-level carrier" (Kojima *et al.*, 1977). Because the infectious dose of HBV can be associated with a level of HBsAg undetectable by radioimmunoassay, a

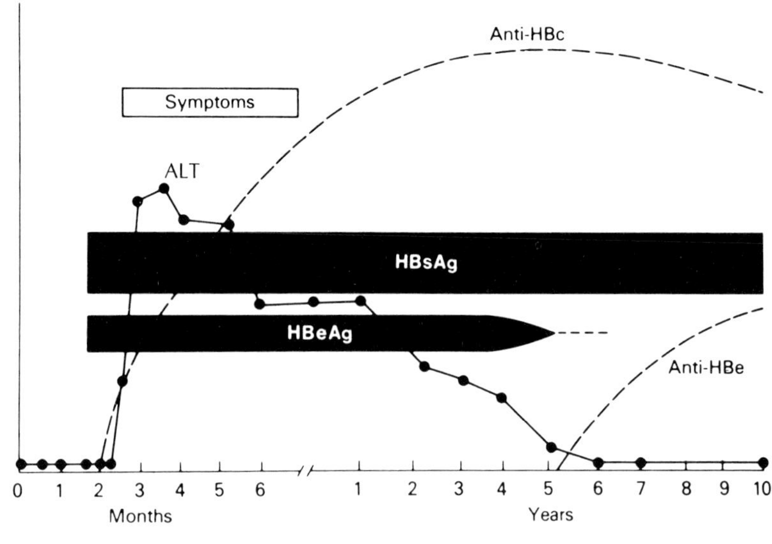

Figure 2. The serological events associated with development of the carrier after acute hepatitis B.

carrier with anti-HBc alone can serve as a source of HBV infection. Such "low-level" carriers have been implicated in the transmission of HBV in the posttransfusion setting (Hoofnagle *et al.*, 1974).

Anti-HBc IgM, another indicator of active HBV replication, has been detected in 35 to 83% of carriers (Roggendorf *et al.*, 1981; Gerlich *et al.*, 1980; Dormeyer *et al.*, 1981). Like HBeAg (see below), anti-HBc IgM may prove a means of placing an individual in the time course of infection. With appropriate dilution of sera and selection of a cut-off value, anti-HBc IgM can discriminate current from remote infections (Chau *et al.*, 1983; Chapter 3). Anti-HBs is infrequently detected in carriers, and is usually of low titer and directed at an HBsAg determinant different from that of the circulating HBsAg (Le Bouvier *et al.*, 1976; Tabor *et al.*, 1977). The frequency of HBeAg in carriers is a function of the specific population, ranging from 4% in volunteer blood donors to 64% in dialysis patients (Szmuness, 1978). The frequency of HBeAg may be related to the time course of the hepatitis B infection; more recently infected carriers are more likely to have HBeAg, and therefore more likely to be infectious. The δ agent is a defective virus requiring HBV for its synthesis. It was originally observed in Italy and is most commonly found in intravenous drug abusers (Rizzetto *et al.*, 1981). The detection of anti-δ in a carrier indicates infection with the δ agent and may result in superimposed fulminant hepatitis (Hadler *et al.*, 1984) or may herald progression to chronic liver disease (Smedile *et al.*, 1981).

The family of the carrier is of special interest as a microcosm displaying the results of HBV exposures and HBsAg persistence. Although retrospective studies of families cannot elucidate the time sequence of cases, information can be gained on the role of genetics, age of exposure, route of exposure, and resulting serological markers. Household contacts of carriers have an HBsAg prevalence seven- to eightfold, and anti-HBs prevalence threefold, that of contacts of HBsAg negative controls (Szmuness *et al.*, 1975; Bernier *et al.*, 1982). This high prevalence supports person-to-person transmission as an important mode within the household. Infection with HBV under the age of 10 years is associated with a higher frequency of HBsAg persistence (Skinhoj, 1979). Family studies have highlighted the importance of mother-to-child transmission, even in the United States (Sampliner *et al.*, 1981; Bernier *et al.*, 1982). Recognition of this mode is possible in the high-risk environment of the family of a carrier. HBeAg and elevated DNA polymerase activity have been associated with a higher frequency of serological evidence of hepatitis B infection in spouses and sexual partners (Perrillo *et al.*, 1979).

V. The Duration of the Carrier State

Once established, the duration of the carrier state is prolonged. However, there are a number of lines of evidence suggesting that the carrier state can spontaneously terminate. The prevalence of HBsAg in populations decreases with advanced age. This decrease could result from clearance of HBsAg by carriers, or alternatively, be accounted for by increased mortality of carriers. In two populations who presumably become infected in childhood, Chinese–Americans and mentally handicapped, HBsAg titers decrease significantly with age (Szmuness *et al.*, 1978). Projecting from these data, if followed long enough a carrier's HBsAg titer may become undetectable. The most direct evidence for the self-limited nature of the carrier state comes from a number of large groups of carriers detected as volunteer blood donors who have been followed prospectively. In one group followed for 4 to 20 months, 13 of 210 (6.2%) cleared HBsAg (Szmuness *et al.*, 1973). In a group followed for 2 to 42 months (an average of 15 months), 4 of 414 (1.0%) carriers cleared HBsAg (Helske, 1974). (These studies were reported before the consensus definition of 6 months duration of the carrier state.) In the last-mentioned study, HBsAg clearance occurred at 4, 4, 6, and 6 months, respectively. The 4- to 6-month time of clearance in this study highlights the importance of the six-month criterion for the carrier state. In a group of carriers followed for 6 to 76 months (a mean of 44 months), 1 of 227 (0.4%) cleared HBsAg (Sampliner *et al.*, 1982). This individual remained anti-HBc positive and failed to develop anti-HBs. With the presence of HBsAg documented for 6 months, clearance of HBsAg would appear to be an unusual event.

Spontaneous clearance of HBsAg may be even more uncommon in carriers with underlying chronic hepatitis. Seven carriers (six with chronic persistent hepatitis) followed subsequent to episodes of acute hepatitis B were documented to clear HBsAg and develop anti-HBs after 13 to 98 months (Lindsay *et al.*, 1981). Unfortunately, the denominator population was not determinable in this study.

Spontaneous or therapeutic clearance of HBV serological markers other than HBsAg is more common. Thirteen of 29 patients with chronic hepatitis B and HBeAg by immunodiffusion who were followed for 2 to 7 years cleared HBeAg, 10 seroconverting to anti-HBe (Realdi *et al.*, 1980). All who cleared HBeAg also cleared HBV-specific DNA polymerase. Six of the 13 patients had been treated with corticosteroids and/or azathioprine. Seroconversion from HBeAg to anti-HBe was associated with progressive reduction in serum aminotransferase levels, but with histological progression to cirrhosis in 6 of 8 patients with chronic active hepatitis on initial biopsy. In another series, 13 of 25 patients with chronic hepatitis B and HBeAg by radioimmunoassay spontaneously seroconverted to anti-HBe over 1–6 years (Hoofnagle *et al.*, 1981). The seroconverters all became negative for DNA polymerase, and most exhibited a decrease in HBsAg titer, 1 clearing HBsAg completely. The seroconverters also had a spontaneous fall of serum aminotransferase levels into the normal range. These studies suggest that HBeAg and DNA polymerase are markers of an early period in the time course of chronic HBV infection. Although "early," this period may have a duration of years.

VI. Follow-up and Management of the Carrier

A. The Carrier and Liver Disease

Periodic determination of HBsAg and serum aminotransferase activity is necessary in order to make clinical decisions concerning an individual carrier. HBsAg persistence must be documented, and clearance, although unusual, needs to be recognized because of its importance. Clearance of HBsAg implies resolution of underlying liver disease, elimination of the risk for transmission of hepatitis B to others, and possibly elimination of the risk for PHC. Persistently elevated serum aminotransferase activity indicates the need for liver biopsy to diagnose chronic active hepatitis, a potentially progressive liver disease. Normal serum aminotransferase levels indicate that any liver disease is likely to be nonprogressive.

The role of corticosteroid therapy for chronic hepatitis B disease is controversial. Corticosteroids favor HBV replication (Sagnelli *et al.*, 1980), and may even have a deletorious effect on the course of the liver disease (Lam *et al.*, 1981). However, at a clinical level, therapeutic options are extremely limited. A trial of corticosteroid therapy is appropriate for a patient with decompensated liver disease (major interference with performance status, jaundice, and/or ascites) and chronic active hepatitis with bridging necrosis by liver biopsy. At an experimental level, antiviral therapy consisting of interferon and adenine arabinoside is available. Antiviral therapy has cleared HBsAg from only 3 of 32 carriers with chronic hepatitis B (Scullard *et al.*, 1981a). The effect of antiviral therapy on other HBV markers has been greater. HBeAg and DNA polymerase activity cleared in 12 of 32 patients, implying a diminution of infectivity that has been documented in chimpanzee studies (Scullard *et al.*, 1982). The impact of antiviral therapy on the underlying liver disease has been disappointing. Chronic active hepatitis regressed to chronic persistent hepatitis in 6 of 18 patients, 5 of the 6 having had a "successful" serological response (Scullard *et al.*, 1981b).

Determination of HBeAg is helpful in relation to infectivity and liver disease activity. A carrier with HBeAg should have his or her e antigen status periodically determined. Seroconversion from HBeAg to anti-HBe may signal resolution of inflammatory activity in the liver and indicate a lessened risk of transmission if an exposure occurs. Any clinical problem in a carrier that could be related to liver disease should be thoroughly evaluated. This evaluation may need to include liver biopsy to assess the current activity of the liver disease. The ideal frequency of periodic evaluations is not clear. After initial detection of HBsAg, a minimum of 6-month testing for 1 year is appropriate. Subsequent follow-up at yearly intervals is preferable. Until a better screening test is defined, an elevated serum α fetoprotein level should precipitate a workup for PHC.

B. The Carrier and the Public Health

A major aspect of the management of a carrier is informing the individual of the risk of transmission to others and educating him/her as to reasonable measures to avoid transmission. Yet, our knowledge of the precise modes and the exact risks of transmission is incomplete, and the education of the carrier is, therefore, a delicate process. Our goal is an informed carrier who will behave socially and occupationally in a manner unlikely to transmit hepatitis B. There can be a fine line between responsible behavior, to avoid transmission, and social and occupational paralysis. The carrier should not—and need not—be the twentieth-century leper (Mosley, 1975). The physician's knowledge of the individual carrier will make possible personally directed information sessions. Availability to answer the carrier's questions will provide support and help ensure appropriate adjustment (Kiernan and Powers, 1979).

A general list of do's and don'ts can be formulated for the carrier (Table II). The carrier should not share articles that could penetrate his/her skin or be contaminated with blood, such as razor blades, nail files and clippers, scissors, toothbrushes, and douche and enema equipment. A carrier should take care of his/her own abrasions and lacerations or seek medical attention. Blood contamination should be promptly cleaned, and soiled items disposed of or laundered. Skin breaks should be covered. The carrier must inform medical personnel of his/her status, and he/she must not donate blood. A balanced view needs to be maintained so that unnecessary barriers are not erected in the carrier's life. The data from family studies do not suggest the need for eliminating normal family contact (Perillo *et al.*, 1979; Bernier *et al.*, 1982). However, the carrier does have the responsibility of informing sexual partners of the risk of transmission of hepatitis B. Partners may agree on the use of a condom or may choose to have the nonimmune partner vaccinated with the hepatitis B vaccine.

Avoidance of transmission by the carrier health worker rests on application of accepted techniques of medical practice. Measures for medical environmental control have been carefully defined and applied (Bond *et al.*, 1977; Public Health Laboratory Service, 1974). The carrier health worker has a special responsibility to prevent transmission.

TABLE II
Advice for Hepatitis B Carriers

DO	Inform health care personnel that you are a carrier
	Inform sexual partner of risk of transmission
	Cover skin breaks
	Clean any blood spill
	Seek medical care for unexplained illness
DO NOT	Donate blood
	Share items that can penetrate skin or contact mucosal surfaces

VII. Unresolved Issues

A. Detection of Liver Disease

How can we better detect and evaluate the liver disease of the carrier? Currently the best screen for progressive liver disease is serum aminotransferase activity. Yet, sampling of liver histology is still necessary to achieve adequate clinical specificity. A more sensitive and specific noninvasive test for the detection of chronic active hepatitis is needed. A functional test of the liver such as the aminopyrine breath test may be of value in selecting patients for liver biopsy. HBeAg was initially touted as an indicator of severe liver disease. With the availability of more sensitive assays for HBeAg and the evaluation of more extensive patient populations, it has become clear that HBeAg indicates an active viral replication stage rather than a stage of histological severity of liver disease (Andres *et al.*, 1981).

What is effective therapy for chronic hepatitis B liver disease? The ineffectiveness of corticosteroids and the unimpressive preliminary results of antiviral therapy have been discussed. Effective therapy will require a breakthrough in the understanding of the pathogenesis of the liver disease or in the development of new therapeutic modalities.

How can we better detect and more effectively treat PHC in the carrier? Once again, our current best screening test, α-fetoprotein, is inadequate. Progress will depend upon the development of new serological techniques and/or more effective surgical or chemotherapeutic intervention.

B. Prevention of Transmission and Eradication of the Carrier State

What are the precise modes of transmission of the carrier other than blood contact? Do some carriers need to be excluded from some occupations? Specific restrictions of carrier activity can be justified only on the basis of data demonstrating the mode and risk of spread. The impact of the unresolved issues of transmission will be blunted by the availability of the hepatitis B vaccine. The vaccine can interrupt the chain of transmission, but it is expensive and on a global basis will be in limited supply for years. Future vaccines containing specific hepatitis B antigenic determinants produced by genetic technology may be amenable to more rapid and greater volume production. On a global basis, only extensive vaccination of infants will reduce the population of carriers.

The final unresolved issue is the eradication of the carrier state. Current antiviral therapy is more effective in reducing infectivity than in eliminating HBsAg. New agents or new combinations of existing agents will be needed to eradicate the carrier state. Unraveling the biology of the HBV has led to many scientific advances. Only further advances will provide solutions to the unresolved issues of the carrier.

References

Alter, H. J., Holland, P. V., Morrow, A. G., Purcell, R. H., Feinstone, S. M., and Moritsugu, Y. (1975a). *Lancet 2*, 838–841.

Alter, H. J., Chalmers, T. C., Freeman, B. M., Lunceford, J. L.,Lewis, L. L., Holland, P. V., Pizzo, P. A., Plotz, P. H., and Meyer, W. J. (1975b). *N. Engl. J. Med.* **292**, 454–457.

Alter, H. J., Seeff, L. B., Kaplan, P. M., McAuliffe, V. J., Wright, E. C., Gerin J. L., Purcell, R. H., Holland, P. V., and Zimmerman, H. J. (1976). *N. Engl. J. Med.* **295**, 909–913.

Anderson, K. E., Sun, S.-C., Berg, H. S., and Chang, N.-K. (1974). *Dig. Dis. Sci.* **19**, 693–703.

Andres, L. L., Sawhney, V. K., Scullard, G. H., Smith, J. L., Merigan, T. C., Robinson, W. S., and Gregory, P. B. (1981). *Hepatology (N.Y.)* **1**, 583–585.

Bancroft, W. H., Snitbhan, R., Scott, R. M., Jingpalapong, M., Watson, W. T., Tanticharoenyos, P., Karwacki, J. J., and Srimarnt, S. (1977). *J. Infect. Dis.* **135**, 79–85.

Barker, L. F., and Murray, R. (1971). *JAMA, J. Am. Med. Assoc.* **216**, 1970–1976.

Beasley, R. P. (1982). *Hepatology (N.Y.)* **2**, 215–265.

Bernier, R. H., Sampliner, R., Gerety, R., Tabor, E., Hamilton, F., and Nathanson, N. (1982). *Am. J. Epidemiol.* **116**, 199–211.

Blumberg, R. S., Sutnick, A. I., London, W. T., and Melartin, L. (1972). *Arch. Intern. Med.* **130**, 227–231.

Bolin, T. D., Davis, A. E., and Liddelow, A. G. (1973). *Gut* **14**, 365–368.

Bond, W. W., Peterson, N. J., and Favero, M. S. (1977). *Health Lab. Sci.* **14**, 235–252.

Bonino, F., Hoyer, R., Nelson, J., Engle, R., Verme, G., and Gerin, J. (1981). *Hepatology (N.Y.)* **1**, 386–391.

Boyer, J. L. (1976). *Gastroenterology* **70**, 1161–1171.

Brechot, L., Pourcel, C., Louise, A., Rain, B., and Tiollais, P. (1980). *Nature (London)* **286**, 533–535.

Chau, K. H., Hargie, M. P., Decker, R. H., Mushahwar, I. K., and Overby, L. R. (1983). *Hepatology* **3**, 142–149.

Collaborative Study by Central Public Health Laboratories (1980). *Lancet 1*, 1–6.

DeFranchis, R., D'Arminio, A., Vecchi, M., Ronchi, G., DelNinno, E., Parravicini, A., Ferroni, P., and Zanetti, A. R. (1980). *Gastroenterology* **79**, 521–527.

Dormeyer, H. H., Arnold, W., Schonborn, H., Braun, B., Klinge, O., Pfeifer, U., Knolle, J., Hess, G., Kryger, P., Nielsen, J. O., and Meyer Zum Buschenfelde, K.-H. (1981). *J. Infect. Dis.* **144**, 33–37.

Dusheiko, G. M., Hoofnagle, J. H., Cooksley, W. G., Minuk, G. Y., and Jones, E. A. (1981). *Hepatology (N.Y.)* **1**, 507.

Feinman, S. V., Cooter, N., Sinclair, J. C., Wrobel, D. M., and Berris, B. (1975). *Gastroentrology* **68**, 113–120.

Gerber, M. A., Lewin, E. B., and Gerety, R. J. (1977). *J. Pediatr. (St. Louis)* **91**, 120–122.

Gerety, R. J., Hoofnagle, J. H., Markenson, J. A., and Barker, L. F. (1974). *J. Pediatr. (St. Louis)* **84**, 661–665.

Gerlich, W. H., Luer, W., Thomssen, R., Study Group for Viral Hepatitis of Deutsche Forschungsgemeinschaft (1980). *J. Infect. Dis.* **142,** 95–101.

Gonzalez-Molina, A., Sarrion, J. V., Rayon, M., Rodrigo-Moreno, M., Primo, J., Berengner, J., Marty, M. L., Serra, M., Baguera, J., and Sanchez-Cuenca, J. M. (1980). *Gastroenterology* **78,** 1652–1653.

Goodwin, D. J., Fannin, S. L., Roberts, R. R., Edwards, V. M., and Mosley, J. W. (1976). *Gastroenterology* **71,** 408.

Grob, P. J., and Moeschlin, P. (1975). *N. Engl. J. Med.* **293,** 197.

Hadler, S. C., Monzon, M. D., Ponzetto, A., Anzola, E., Rivero, D., Mondolfi, A., Bracho, A., Francis, D. P., Gerber, M. A., Thung, S., Gerin, J., Maynard, J. E., Popper, H., and Purcell, R. H. (1984). *Ann. Intern. Med.* **100,** 339–344.

Heathcoat, J., Cameron, C., and Dane, D. (1974). *Lancet 1,* 71–73.

Helske, T. (1974). *Scand. J. Haematol., Suppl.* **22,** 1–54.

Hess, G., Arnold, W., Shih, F. W.-K., Kaplan, P. M., Purcell, R. H., Gerin, J. L., and Meyer Zum Buschenfelde, K. H. (1977). *Infect. Immunol.* **17,** 550–554.

Holtermuller, K. H., Baumeister, H. G., Schafer, A., Eckardt, V., Arndt-Hauser, A., Ewe, K., Waudel, E., Baas, N., and Overby, L. R. (1975). *Gastroenterology* **69,** 830.

Hoofnagle, J. H. (1978). *In* "Viral Hepatitis." (G. N. Vyas, S. N. Cohen, and R. Schmid, eds.), pp. 219–242. Franklin Inst. Press, Philadelphia, Pennsylvania.

Hoofnagle, J. H., Gerety, R. J., and Barker, L. F. (1973). *Lancet 2,* 869–873.

Hoofnagle, J. H., Gerety, R. J., Ni, L. Y., and Barker, L. F. (1974). *N. Engl. J. Med.* **290,** 1336–1340.

Hoofnagle, J. H., Dusheiko, G. M., Seeff, L. B., Jones, E. A., Waggoner, J. G., and Bales, Z. B. (1981). *Ann. Intern. Med.* **94,** 744–748.

Imai, M., Tachibana, F. L., Moritsugu, Y., Miyakawa, Y., and Mayumi, M. (1976). *Infect. Immun.* **14,** 631–635.

Iwarson, S., Lindholm, A., and Lundin, P. (1972). *Vox Sang.* **22,** 501–509.

Kiernan, T. W., and Powers, R. J. (1979). *JAMA, J. Am. Med. Assoc.* **241,** 585–587.

Kojima, M., Udo, K., Takahashi, Y., Yoshizawa, G., Usuda, F., Itoh, Y., Miyakawa, K., and Mayumi, M. (1977). *Gastroenterology* **73,** 664–667.

Koretz, R. L., Lewin, K. J., Reghun, D. J., and Gitnick, G. L. (1978). *Gastroenterology* **69,** 830.

Koziol, D. E., Alter, H. J., Kirchner, J. P., and Holland, P. V. (1976). *J. Immunol.* **117,** 2260–2262.

Kubo, V., Okuda, K., Musha, H., and Nakashima, T. (1978). *Gastroenterology* **74,** 578–582.

LaBrecque, D. R., and Dhand, A. K. (1981). *Hepatology (N.Y.)* **1,** 398–400.

Lam, K. C., Lai, C. L., Trepo, C., and Wu, P. C. (1981). *N. Engl. J. Med.* **304,** 380–386.

Le Bouvier, G. L., Capper, R. A., Williams, A. E., Pelletier, M., and Katz, A. J. (1976). *J. Immunol.* **117,** 2262–2264.

Levin, M. L., Maddrey, W. C., Wands, J. R., and Mendeloff, A. I. (1974). *JAMA, J. Am. Med. Assoc.* **228,** 1139–1140.

Liaw, Y.-F., and Sung, J.-L. (1979). *Gastroenterology* **76,** 1084.

Lieberman, H. M., LaBrecque, D. R., Kew, M. C., Hadziyannis, S. J., and Shafritz, D. A. (1983). *Hepatology* **3,** 285–291.

Lindsay, K. L., Redeker, A. G., and Ashcavi, M. (1981). *Hepatology (N.Y.)* **1,** 586–589.

Monroe, P. S., Baker, A. L., Schneider, J. F., Kragor, P. S., Klein, P. D., and Schoeller, N. (1982). *Hepatology (N.Y.)* **2,** 317–322.

Mosley, J. W. (1975). *N. Engl. J. Med.* **292,** 477–478.

Nielson, J. O., Dietrichson, O., Elling, P., and Christoffersen, P. (1971). *N. Engl. J. Med.* **285,** 1157–1160.

Okada, K., Kamiyama, I., Inomata, M., Imai, M., Miyakawa, Y., and Mayumi, M. (1976). *N. Engl. J. Med.* **294**, 746–749.

Perrillo, R. P., Gelb, L., Campbell, C., Wellinghoff, W., Ellis, F. R., Overby, L., and Aach, R. D. (1979). *Gastroenterology* **76**, 1319–1325.

Prince, A. M., and Alcabes, P. (1982). *Hepatology (N.Y.)* **2**, 155–205.

Public Health Laboratory Service (1974). *Br. Med. J.* **4**, 751–754.

Realdi, G., Alberti, A., Rugge, M., Bortolotti, F., Rigoli, A. M., Tremolada, F., and Ruol, A. (1980). *Gastroenterology* **79**, 195–199.

Redeker, A. G. (1975). *Am. J. Med. Sci.* **270**, 9–16.

Reesink, H. W., Wesdorp, I. C. E., Grijm, R., Hengeveld, P., Jobsis, A. C., Aay, C., and Reerink-Brongers, E. E. (1980). *Vox Sang.* **38**, 138–146.

Reiner, N. E., Judson, F. N., Bond, W. W., Francis, D. R., and Peterson, N. J. (1982). *Ann. Intern. Med.* **96**, 170–173.

Reinicke, V., Dybkjaer, E., Poulsen, H., Banke, D., Lylloff, K., and Nordenfelt, E. (1972). *N. Engl. J. Med.* **286**, 867–870.

Rimland, D., Parkin, W. E., Miller, G. B., and Schrack, W. D. (1977). *N. Engl. J. Med.* **296**, 953–958.

Rizzetto, M., Shih, J., W.-K., Verme, G., and Gerin, J. L. (1981). *Gastroenterology* **80**, 1420–1429.

Roggendorf, M., Deinhardt, F., Frosner, G. G., Scheid, R., Bayerl, B., and Zachoval, R. (1981). *J. Clin. Microbiol.* **13**, 618–626.

Sagnelli, E., Maio, G., Felaco, F. M., Izzo, C. M., Manzillo, G., Pasquale, G., Filippini, P., and Piccinino, F. (1980). *Lancet* **2**, 395–397.

Sampliner, R. E., Hamilton, F. A., Iseri, O. A., Tabor, E., and Boitnott, J. (1979). *Am. J. Med. Sci.* **277**, 17–22.

Sampliner, R. E., Loevinger, B. L., Tabor, E., and Gerety, R. J. (1981). *Am. J. Epidemiol.* **113**, 50–54.

Sampliner, R., Carney, E., Tabor, E., and Gerety, R. (1982). *In* "Viral Hepatitis" (W. Szmuness, H. J. Alter, and J. E. Maynard, eds.), pp. 722–723. Franklin Inst. Press, Philadelphia, Pennsylvania.

Schaefer, R. A., Finlayson, N. D. C., and Prince, A. M. (1974). *J. Clin. Invest.* **53**, 71.

Schweitzer, I. L. (1975). *Am. J. Med. Sci.* **270**, 287–291.

Scullard, G. H., Pollard, R. B., Smith, J. L., Sacks, S. L., Gregory, P. B., Robinson, W. S., and Merigan, T. C. (1981a). *J. Infect. Dis.* **143**, 772–783.

Scullard, G. H., Andres, L. L., Greenberg, H. B., Smith, J. L., Sawhney, V. K., Neal, E. A., Mahal, A. S., Popper, H. Merigan, T. C., Robinson, W. S., and Gregory, P. B. (1981b). *Hepatology (N.Y.)* **1**, 228–232.

Scullard, G. H., Greenberg, H. B., Smith, J. L., Gregory, P. B., Merigan, T. C., and Robinson, W. S. (1982). *Hepatology (N.Y.)* **2**, 39–49.

Shafritz, D. A., and Kew, M. C. (1981). *Hepatology (N.Y.)* **1**, 1–8.

Simon, J. P., and Patel, S. K. (1974). *Gastroenterology* **66**, 1020–1028.

Singleton, J. N., Merrill, D. A., Fitch, R. A., Kohler, P. F., and Rettberg, W. A. H. (1971). *Lancet* **2**, 785–787.

Skinhoj, P. (1979). *Trans. R. Soc. Trop. Med. Hyg.* **73**, 549–552.

Smedile, A., Dentico, P., Zanetti, A., Sagnelli, E., Nordenfelt, E., Actis, G. L., and Rizzetto, M. (1981). *Gastroenterology* **81**, 992–997.

Soloway, R. D., Baggenstoss, A. H., Schonfield, L. J., and Summerskill, W. M. (1971). *Am. J. Dig. Dis.* **16**, 1082–1086.

Stevens, C. E., Beasley, R. P., Tsui, J., and Lee, W.-C. (1975). *N. Engl. J. Med.* **292**, 771–774.

Stevens, C. E., Neurath, A. R., Szmuness, W., Beasley, R. P., and Ikram, H. (1978). *In* "Viral Hepatitis" (G. N. Vyas, S. N. Cohen, and R. Schmid, eds.), pp. 211–215. Franklin Inst. Press, Philadelphia, Pennsylvania.

Sun, S., Beasley, R. P., Anderson, K. E., Berg, H. S., Hsu, C.-P., and Lee, W.-C. (1976). *Am. J. Dig. Dis.* **21,** 366–369.

Szmuness, W. (1975). *Am. J. Pathol.* **81,** 629–649.

Szmuness, W. (1978). *Prog. Med. Virol.* **24,** 40–69.

Szmuness, W., Prince, A. M., Brotman, B., and Hirsch, R. L. (1973). *J. Infect. Dis.* **127,** 17–25.

Szmuness, W., Harley, E. J., and Prince, A. M. (1975). *Am. J. Med. Sci.* **270,** 293–304.

Szmuness, W., Harley, E. J., Ikram, H., and Stevens, C. E. (1978). *In* "Viral Hepatitis" (G. N. Vyas, S. N. Cohen, and R. Schmid, eds.), pp. 297–320. Franklin Inst. Press, Philadelphia, Pennsylvania.

Szmuness, W., William, D. C., Sadovsky, R., Morrison, J. M., and Kellner, A. (1980). *N. Engl. J. Med.* **303,** 833–841.

Tabor, E., Gerety, R. J., Smallwood, L. A., and Barker, L. F. (1977). *J. Immunol.* **118,** 369–370.

Takahashi, K., Imai, M., Tsuda, F., Takahashi, T., Miyakawa, Y., and Mayumi, M. (1976). *Gastroenterology* **117,** 102–105.

Tong, M. J., Stevenson, D., and Gordon, I. (1977). *J. Infect. Dis.* **135,** 980–984.

Trepo, C. G., and Prince, A. M. (1976). *Ann. Intern. Med.* **85,** 429–430.

Trepo, C. G., Magnius, L. O., Schaefer, R. A., and Prince, A. M. (1976). *Gastroenterology* **71,** 804–808.

U.S. National Heart and Lung Institute Collaborative Study Group and Pheonix Laboratories Division (1976). *Lancet 2,* 492–494.

Velasco, M., González-Cerón, M., de la Fuente, C., Ruiz, A., Donoso, S., and Katz, R. (1978). *Gut* **19,** 569–571.

Villeneuve, J. P., Richer, G., Cote, J., Guevin, R., Marleau, D., Joly, J. G., and Viallet, A. (1976). *Dig. Dis. Sci.* **21,** 18–25.

Vittal, S. B. V., Dourdourekas, D., Shobassy, N., Gerber, M., Telischi, M., Szanto, P. B., Steicmann, F., and Clowdus, B. V. (1974). *Am. J. Clin. Pathol.* **62,** 649–654.

Werner, B. G., and Grady, G. F. (1982). *Ann. Intern. Med.* **97,** 367–369.

Williams, S. V., Pattison, C. P., and Berquist, K. R. (1975). *JAMA, J. Am. Med. Assoc.* **232,** 1231–1233.

Woolf, I. L., Boyes, B. E., Jones, D. M., Whittaker, J. S., Tapp, E., MacSween, R. N. M., Renton, P. H., Stratton, F., and Dymock, I. W. (1974). *J. Clin. Pathol.* **27,** 348–352.

Chapter 9

Therapy of Chronic Hepatitis B

JAY H. HOOFNAGLE
Liver Diseases Section
Digestive Diseases Branch
National Institute of Arthritis, Diabetes and Digestive and Kidney Diseases
National Institutes of Health
Bethesda, Maryland

I. Chronic Hepatitis B

A. Introduction

Chronic hepatitis B is perhaps the major single cause of liver disease in the world today. This disease affects at least 5% of the world's population and is an important cause of both cirrhosis and hepatocellular car-

Copyright © 1985 by Academic Press, Inc.
All rights of reproduction in any form reserved.
ISBN 0-12-280672-7

cinoma (Szmuness, 1975; Beasley *et al.*, 1981; Hoofnagle and Alter, 1984). Unfortunately, there is at present no specific therapy for this disease. No manipulations of diet, no recommendations regarding exercise, and no biological or pharmacological agents have been shown to beneficially affect the natural history of this disease.

B. Experimental Therapies

In recent years, several forms of experimental therapy have been attempted in patients with chronic hepatitis B (Table I). Basically, these experimental agents fall into two categories; first, agents that inhibit viral replication, and second, therapies that modulate the immune response to the viral infection. In the first category, the most promising agents have been human leukocyte interferon and adenine arabinoside (Smith and Merigan, 1982). In the second category, the most promising therapies have been transfer factor, immune RNA, and short courses of immunosuppression. Studies on the pathogenesis of chronic hepatitis B suggest that this disease is due to a deficient or abnormal host immune response that permits infection with the hepatitis B virus (HBV) to persist (Dienstag, 1984). Thus, therapy of this disease might be directed at either the viral replication or the abnormality of immune responsiveness.

TABLE I
Therapies for Chronic Hepatitis B

Antiviral agents
    Human leukocyte (α) interferon
    Human fibroblast (β) interferon
    Human immune (γ) interferon
    Adenine arabinoside (Ara-A)
    Adenine arabinoside monosphosphate (Ara-AMP)
    Acyclovir
    Ribavirin
    Phosphonoformic acid (PFA)
    Intercalating agents (quinacrine)
Immunomodulating therapies
    Plasmapheresis
    Hepatitis B immune globulin
    Hepatitis B vaccine
    Transfer factor
    Immune RNA
    Levamisole
    Bacillus Calmette–Guérin
    Immunosuppression

Complicating this schema are recent data suggesting that drugs which inhibit HBV replication may also cause some degree of immunosuppression (Scullard *et al.*, 1979), and agents used to modulate the immune system may promote HBV replication (Scullard *et al.*, 1981c). The beneficial effect of an antiviral agent may, thus, be offset by its concurrent immunosuppressive effects. Design of therapies might best be aimed at both components of this illness: the viral replication and the host immunological response.

C. Goals of Therapy

Design of therapies for chronic hepatitis B should also begin with a full understanding of the goals of therapy. The primary goal is, of course, a complete cure of the infection (Table II). Thus, one would hope that treatment would lead to eradication of the virus and resolution of the liver disease. Evidence of such an outcome would be the disappearance of HBsAg and viral markers including HBeAg, DNA polymerase, and HBV DNA, as well as return of serum alanine and aspartate aminotransferase activities (ALT and AST) to the normal range. Such an outcome, while very desirable, may not be practical.

Another goal of therapy, which is perhaps less ambitious but nonetheless important, is amelioration of the chronic liver disease. Evidence for this outcome would be the disappearance of clinical symptoms of hepatitis, normalization of the serum ALT and AST activities, improvement in other liver function tests (such as serum albumin levels, prothrombin time, and bile acid levels), and improvement in the liver biopsy histology.

A final goal of therapy is a reduction in infectivity or in the level of viral replication. Evidence of this outcome would be the disappearance of serum HBeAg, DNA polymerase, and HBV DNA (Scullard *et al.*, 1981b). These latter two goals of therapy may be practical using some of the recent experimental approaches to treatment. Furthermore, loss of serum markers of HBV such as HBeAg and DNA polymerase is frequently accompanied by an amelioration of the liver disease despite the persistence of HBsAg (Scullard *et al.*, 1981a; Hoofnagle *et al.*, 1981).

D. Natural History

The natural history of chronic hepatitis B is discussed in detail in Chapter 8 and will only be summarized here. Shown in Fig. 1 is the usual course of chronic infection with HBV. This course can be separated into three stages (Hoofnagle and Seeff, 1982): a period of acute or

TABLE II
Goals of Therapy for Chronic Hepatitis B

Outcome	End point in serum test results			
	HBsAg	HBeAg	HBV DNA and DNA polymerase	Serum aminotransferase
Cure of infection	Negative	Negative	Negative	Normal
Amelioration of disease	Positive	Positive or Negative	Positive or Negative	Normal
Decrease in infectivity	Positive	Negative	Negative	Abnormal or Normal

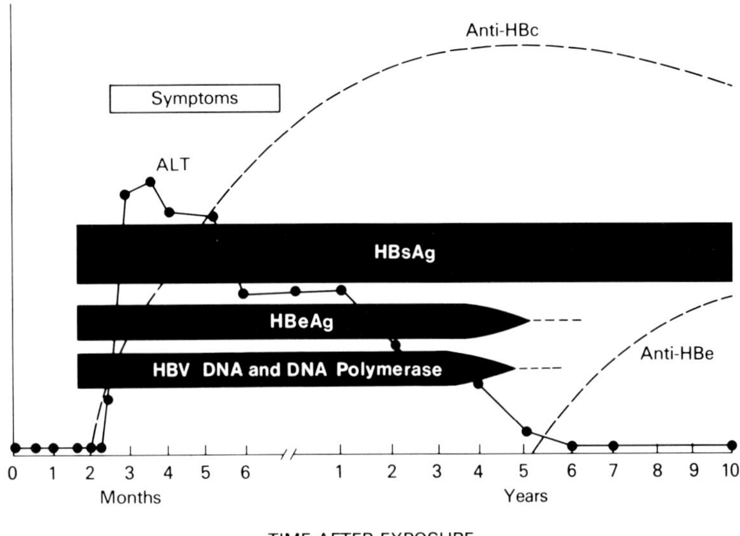

Figure 1. Typical course of chronic hepatitis B. Abbreviations: HBsAg, hepatitis B surface antigen; HBeAg, Hepatitis B e antigen; anti-HBc, antibody to hepatitis B core antigen; anti-HBe, antibody to hepatitis B e antigen; ALT, alanine aminotransferase (SGPT).

subacute hepatitis, a period of chronic hepatitis, and finally a period that is usually referred to as the asymptomatic "healthy" carrier state.

At the onset of infection, serum levels of HBV (as reflected by serum HBV DNA, DNA polymerase, and HBeAg) rise to high levels and persist (Kaplan *et al.*, 1973; Krugman *et al.*, 1974; Krugman *et al.*, 1979; Bonino *et al.*, 1981). During this early phase, serum aminotransferase activities (ALT and AST) are increased, but are usually not as high as in acute viral hepatitis. Serum bilirubin levels are rarely elevated, and symptoms are mild, if present at all. Indeed, a large percentage of patients with chronic hepatitis B cannot date the onset of their disease and deny a previous history of acute hepatitis or jaundice. Nevertheless, an "acute" or "subacute" phase of illness usually occurs and lasts for 2 to 6 months.

After the initial few months of infection, serum aminotransferase activities usually fall to a lower level, but remain elevated (in the range of 2 to 10 times the upper limit of normal). This second period can be considered a stage of chronic hepatitis. Symptoms are mild, if present at all, and consist largely of fatigability and loss of usual stamina (Hoofnagle and Alter, 1984). The serum markers of HBeAg, HBV DNA, and DNA polymerase persist, but often will slowly decline in titer with time. This chronic hepatitis phase lasts for as short a period as 1 year to as long as several decades. The chronic hepatitis can be severe leading ultimately to cirrhosis and hepatocellular failure, or it can be mild and asymptomatic and not associated with any serious permanent liver damage.

The third stage of chronic HBV infection begins when serum aminotransferase activities fall into the normal or near-normal range, and serum markers of virus (HBeAg, HBV DNA, and DNA polymerase) disappear. Generally, HBsAg persists at moderate or low titers. The best single serological marker of the transition of the second to the third stage is the seroconversion from HBeAg to anti-HBe (Realdi *et al.*, 1980; Hoofnagle *et al.*, 1981). The transition that accompanies the loss of serum HBV markers indicates the end of the chronic hepatitis disease activity and a decrease in infectivity. Patients during this last stage of HBV infection usually have normal serum aminotransferase activities and inactive liver disease. It has been referred to as the "healthy" or asymptomatic chronic HBsAg carrier state.

This transition from chronic hepatitis to an inactive liver disease and seroconversion from HBeAg to anti-HBe actually indicates a decrease or perhaps even a termination of viral replication. Even though HBsAg persists in the serum, markers of the intact virus are no longer present. This suggests that the viral infection has become latent. Molecular hybridization studies suggest that this transition from HBeAg to anti-HBe seropositivity is also accompanied by a change in the state of the HBV genome in the liver; a disappearance of replicative forms of HBV DNA (free or episomal DNA) in the hepatocyte and the persistence of only nonreplicative forms of the viral genome (integrated or chromosomal HBV DNA) (Tiollais *et al.*, 1981; Brechot *et al.*, 1981). For this reason, the three stages of chronic HBV infection might best be referred to as either "replicative" (the acute and chronic hepatitis stages) or "nonreplicative" (the asymptomatic HBsAg carrier state) (Hoofnagle and Alter, 1984) (Table III).

Most patients who are HBeAg positive are in an active, replicative phase, and those without HBeAg who have anti-HBe are usually in a latent, nonreplicative phase of illness. There are, however, important and striking exceptions to this simple categorization of patients on the basis of HBeAg positivity. Testing for HBeAg in serum is not a perfect means of discriminating between these two states of the HBV genome. Some patients with anti-HBe have significant ongoing liver disease with elevated serum aminotransferase activities and active HBV replication (Hadziyannis *et al.*, 1983). Some of these patients are suffering from a reactivation of HBV infection so that even though they are negative for HBeAg, they have episodic bouts of HBV replication with return of HBV

TABLE III

Stages of Chronic Hepatitis B[a]

Stage (State of virus)	Timing	ALT/AST	HBsAg	HbeAg/ anti-HBe	Serum HBV DNA	Liver HBV DNA
Acute Hepatitis (replicative)	Early (1–6 months)	>10 ×	+++	HBeAg	++	Free
Chronic Hepatitis (replicative)	Early (1–20 years)	2–20 ×	++	HBeAg	++	Free (± integrated)
Healthy Carrier (nonreplicative)	Late (decades)	<2 ×	+	Anti-HBe	−	Integrated
Reactivation (low level replicative)	Late	2–20 ×	+	Anti-HBe	+	Free and integrated

[a]ALT, Alanine aminotransferase; AST, aspartate aminotransferase; HBsAg, hepatitis B surface antigen; HBeAg, hepatitis B e antigen; anti-HBe, antibody to HBeAg; HBV, hepatitis B virus.

DNA and DNA polymerase activity and elevations in serum aminotransferase activities (Davis *et al.*, 1984a). Other patients with anti-HBe appear to have persisting low levels of viral replication with an accompanying chronic hepatitis and detectable levels of HBV DNA and DNA polymerase activity in serum (Bonino *et al.*, 1984). Because the viral replication is low grade, HBeAg is not present in serum and HBV DNA may be difficult to detect or present intermittently. Other means of detecting low levels of ongoing HBV replication include assaying for IgM anti-HBc in serum (Sjogren *et al.*, 1984), staining for HBcAg in liver tissue (Hadziyannis, 1983; Bonino *et al.*, 1984), and assaying for the presence of episomal forms of HBV DNA in liver (Brechot *et al.*, 1981). Patients with low levels of HBV replication and episodic reactivation are especially prone to developing cirrhosis (Hoofnagle and Alter, 1984).

Antiviral therapy for chronic hepatitis B has been largely and correctly directed towards patients in the "replicative" phases of illness and especially those patients who are seropositive for HBeAg and DNA polymerase (Smith and Merigan, 1982). Treatment of HBsAg positive patients with anti-HBe is usually without demonstrable effect (Bassendine *et al.*, 1981). However, further studies are needed to document whether patients with low levels of viral replication and patients suffering from reactivation of chronic disease are helped by antiviral therapy.

The aim of therapy has been to terminate and eradicate viral replication, which should lead to a permanent loss of serum HBeAg, HBV DNA, and DNA polymerase in the serum as well as HBcAg and episomal forms of HBV DNA in liver. The majority of such patients will then enter a clinical remission with disappearance of symptoms and normalization of serum aminotransferase activities. In a small number of patients, the loss of replicative forms of HBV will also result in the disappearance of serum HBsAg and even in the development of anti-HBs. However, many patients with chronic hepatitis B already have integrated forms of HBV DNA in liver that are probably capable of independently directing the synthesis of HBsAg. For this reason, patients may continue to have HBsAg in serum despite the loss of all evidence of active viral replication (Tiollais *et al.*, 1981). Merigan (1982) has classified responses to antiviral therapy into three types: type I, in which all serological markers (DNA polymerase, HBeAg, and HBsAg) are permanently lost; type II, in which the HBV markers of active viral replication (DNA polymerase and HBeAg) are permanently lost but HBsAg persists; and type III, in which DNA polymerase transiently falls to negative but returns when therapy is discontinued.

II. Antiviral Agents

The major approach to treatment of chronic hepatitis B has been to attempt to inhibit or terminate the persistent viral replication. Antiviral agents hold great promise for the therapy of this disease. However, at present the development of antiviral drugs is still in its infancy; there are few agents that are effective, safe, and easy to administer. Most antivirals act by blocking viral RNA or DNA polymerases and by causing termination of the growing nucleic acid. Antiviral agents typically inhibit viral polymerases more potently than host cellular polymerases. Agents that have been used in the treatment of chronic hepatitis B include the interferons, adenine arabinoside, ribavirin, acyclovir, phosphonoformic acid, and the intercalating agents.

A. The Interferons

The interferons are a family of proteins synthesized and secreted by cells in response to viral and other forms of stimuli. The interferons are defined by their characteristic biological activities which include antiviral, antiproliferative, and immunomodulatory effects (Friedman, 1981; Kirchner, 1984). Many mammalian cells produce interferon in response to viral infections. The interferon produced then acts on other cells by binding to cell surface membranes, activating cellular enzymes, leading to the synthesis of mRNA and proteins which in turn interfere in growth of viruses and synthesis of viral proteins. Interferon thus acts by inducing an antiviral state. Its specific site of action in the inhibition of viral replication is not known and may differ with each different virus.

Interferon is actually a heterogeneous group of proteins. Unlike other hormone-like factors such as insulin or glucagon, interferons have a high degree of cell and species specificity. Interferons produced in non-human species are generally not active in man. In addition, different human cells produce different forms of interferon that have different activities. The three major forms of human interferon are the following: α or leucocyte interferon, which is produced by leukocytes; β or fibroblast interferon, which is synthesized by fibroblasts; and γ or type II ("immune") interferon, which is produced by lymphocytes in response to some nonspecific mitogens (Stewart, 1979; Stiehm *et al.*, 1982). These three forms of human interferon have different potencies and different effects.

The mode of action of interferon has led to the suggestion that it is important in recovery from viral infections. Thus, patients with persistent infections such as chronic hepatitis B may have deficient interferon production and administration of interferon may help to eliminate the viral infection. Indeed, at least one study has shown that patients with acute viral hepatitis usually have high levels of serum interferon and their peripheral blood leukocytes are in an "antiviral" state (Levin and Hahn, 1982). In contrast, patients with chronic hepatitis B do not have detectable levels of serum interferon, and their cells are not in an antiviral state (Ponzetto *et al.*, 1979). Furthermore, peripheral blood mononuclear cells from patients with chronic viral hepatitis produce only low amounts of alpha interferon after viral challenge (Kato *et al.*, 1982; Davis *et al.*, 1984b).

In 1976, Greenberg and co-workers from Stanford University first reported on the effect of human leukocyte (α) interferon on chronic hepatitis B. They treated four patients with doses of 1 to 10 million units (mu) per day for periods ranging from 1 week to several months. Treatment led to an immediate decrease in serum levels of HBV DNA and DNA polymerase. Short courses were followed by a rapid return of HBV markers to previous levels. However, in two patients treated for prolonged periods, HBV DNA and DNA polymerase remained undetectable even after therapy was stopped (Fig. 2). These patients eventually became HBeAg negative and underwent a clinical remission in disease activity. One patient later became HBsAg negative (Scullard *et al.*, 1982).

Later studies of α interferon by this same group, however, did not yield similarly promising results (Table IV). Scullard *et al.* (1981a,b,c, 1982) have summarized the total experience of the Stanford group with anti-

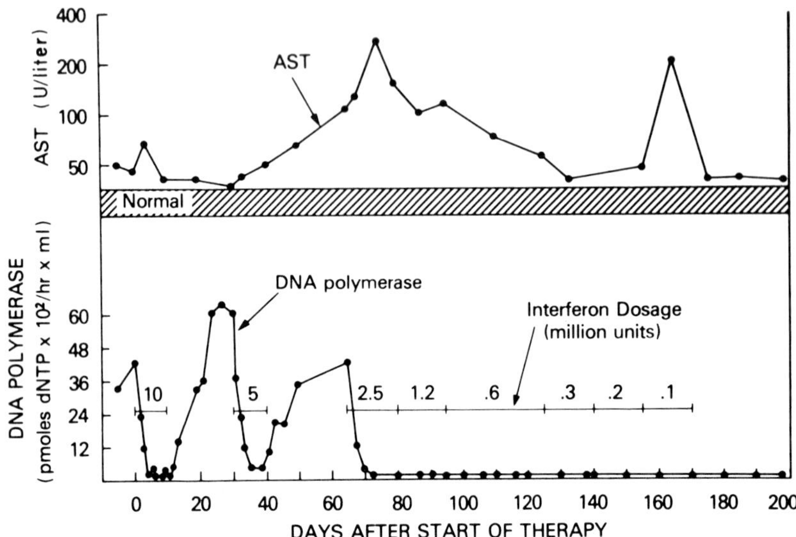

Figure 2. Course of a patient with chronic hepatitis B who was treated with human alpha interferon. Abbreviations: AST, aspartate aminotransferase; U, international units; dNTP, deoxy nucleotide triphosphate. Adapted from Scullard *et al.* (1981a).

viral agents in chronic hepatitis B. A total of 16 patients were treated using interferon alone, in doses ranging from 2 to 20 mu per day, given either in multiple 10- to 14-day courses or continuously for 5 to 6 months. The total dosage per patient ranged from 400 to 900 mu. All 16 patients demonstrated a dramatic decline in serum HBV DNA and DNA polymerase during treatment; but in the majority, these markers returned to pretreatment levels when the interferon injections were stopped. In only 4 of 16 patients (25%) did serum HBV DNA and DNA polymerase remain undetectable once interferon was discontinued. These 4 patients subsequently lost HBeAg reactivity and demonstrated an improvement in their clinical disease.

Early reports from other groups on the effect of human leukocyte interferon on chronic hepatitis B have not been as encouraging as initial reports. Investigators from King's College Hospital, London (Scullard *et al.*, 1979) reported using human leukocyte interferon in dosages of 1 to 3 mu per day for 5 weeks in seven patients and for 5 months in one patient with chronic hepatitis B. Clear-cut and reproducible inhibition of serum levels of HBV DNA polymerase and Dane particles occurred in only one patient. These authors noted that interferon had immunosuppressive effects and postulated that these might offset its antiviral effects.

TABLE IV
Summary of Studies on Interferon Therapy of Chronic Hepatitis B

Reference	Type (and total dose) of interferon[a]	Permanent response
Scullard et al. (1979)	α (35–350 mu)	17% (1/8)
Weimar et al. (1980)	α (165 mu)	20% (2/10)
Scullard et al. (1981b)	α (400–900 mu)	25% (4/16)
Lok et al. (1983)	α (~500 mu)	46% (5/11)
Dooley et al. (1983)	α* (54–1035 mu)	22% (2/9)
Smith et al. (1983)	α* (9–1552 mu)	0% (0/9)
Omata et al. (1984)	α* (1000–2800 mu)	0% (0/15)
Dusheiko et al. (1984)	α* (342–1500 mu)	40% (4/10
Kingham et al. (1978)	β (140 mu)	0% (0/2)
Weimar et al. (1977)	β (18–42 mu)	0% (0/5)
Muller et al. (1982b)	β (332–800)	12% (1/8)
Scullard et al. (1981b)	α** (400–900 mu)	43% (7/16)
Smith et al. (1982a)	α** (420–560 mu)	10% (1/10)

[a]mu, Million units; *, recombinant interferon; **, interferon in combination with adenine arabinoside or adenine arabinoside monophosphate.

Weimar and associates (1980) from Erasmus University, Rotterdam, the Netherlands conducted a randomized double-blind, placebo-controlled study on human leukocyte interferon. Ten patients received daily injections of interferon for 6 weeks. The dosage was initially 12 mu daily and was decreased by one-half each week so that the average total dosage was 165 mu per patient. Only transient and partial inhibition of serum DNA polymerase activity was noted. Among 10 treated patients, none became DNA polymerase negative during therapy. In follow up only 2 patients (20%) had a permanent disappearance of serum DNA polymerase activity, subsequently seroconverted from HBeAg to anti-HBe, and had an improvement in clinical status (Schalm and Heijtink, 1982). Among the 10 placebo-treated controls, 4 (40%) eventually lost HBeAg reactivity along with serum DNA polymerase and had a remission in hepatitis disease activity. Thus, leukocyte interferon given in this dosage–schedule did not appear to result in an increased rate of permanent serological or clinical remissions.

All of the early studies of α interferon employed human leukocyte interferon prepared by Cantell and associates at the State Serum Institute in Helsinki, Finland, from buffy-coat preparations from human blood donors (Cantell and Hirvonen, 1978). Only small amounts of impure interferon (less than 2% pure) were available. Thus, lack of a high rate of response in these studies may have been due to the low dosages given and the short courses of therapy. The major hindrance to clinical studies on interferon was the lack of inexpensive and highly purified preparations. This hindrance has been overcome through advances in molecular biology. Recombinant DNA human α, β, and γ interferons have been developed and produced in large quantities (Goeddel *et al.*, 1980). These newer interferons are highly purified (greater than 95% pure) and have similar potencies, pharmacokinetics, and side effects as the leukocyte-derived interferons (Gutterman *et al.*, 1982). Furthermore, interferon derived from a lymphoblastoid cell line has been isolated, characterized, and purified in large amounts. Preliminary trials indicate that this lymphoblastoid interferon has potencies similar to leukocyte-derived and recombinant interferons (Weller *et al.*, 1982d). These new interferons will allow for definitive large-scale, controlled trials of therapy for this disease.

Investigators at the Royal Free Hospital, London have employed lymphoblastoid interferon in patients with chronic hepatitis B (Weller *et al.*, 1982d; Lok *et al.*, 1983, 1984). They treated 11 patients with lymphoblastoid interferon intramuscularly at a dosage of 10 mu/m^2 daily for 5 days and then 3 times weekly for 8 weeks. The thrice-weekly injections were as effective as daily injections in lowering serum hepatitis B virus levels. HBV DNA and DNA polymerase decreased in all 11 patients and became negative in five. Four patients subsequently lost HBeAg and two also became HBsAg negative. The high response rate (45%) and loss of HBsAg in some patients after prolonged interferon therapy was encouraging and has led to an ongoing randomized controlled trial of interferon by this group.

Four groups of investigators have reported preliminary results using high doses of recombinant human α interferon (Omata *et al.*, 1983, 1984; Dooley *et al.*, 1983, 1984; Smith *et al.*, 1983; Dusheiko *et al.*, 1984). In these studies, gradually increasing doses (from 1 to 100 mu) of interferon were administered on a twice-daily, daily, or three-times-a-week schedule. The duration of treatment varied from 12 to 90 days. These studies demonstrated that doses of interferon above 9 to 18 mu are poorly tolerated and are not associated with an increased degree of inhibition of serum levels of HBV DNA or DNA polymerase. Dooley *et al.* (1983) from the National Institutes of Health treated 9 patients with multiple 2-week courses of interferon at dosages of 18 to 68 mu three times a week. Two of the nine patients (22%) had a permanent loss of HBV DNA and HBeAg with treatment and one of these patients later became HBsAg negative. Both had a clinical remission in their disease. Dusheiko *et al.* (1984) from Johannesburg, South Africa, treated 10 patients with recombinant α interferon at dosages of 18 to 50 mu three times a week for 4 to 8 weeks. Permanent loss of HBV DNA, DNA polymerase, and HBeAg occurred in four patients (40%), three of whom later became HBsAg negative. In contrast, Omata *et al.* (1984) from Japan treated 15 patients and Smith *et al.* (1983) from Stanford University treated 10 patients with multiple 2-week courses of recombinant α interferon without a permanent response to therapy in any patient. These pilot studies have yielded important information of the pharmacokinetics and tolerance of high doses of interferon in patients with chronic hepatitis B. The long-term beneficial effects of prolonged interferon therapy in preliminary studies have been sufficiently encouraging to lead to large scale controlled trials which are now underway in both the United States and Europe.

Reports on the use of fibroblast interferon in chronic hepatitis B have been less promising than those using leukocyte interferon. In an early study, Desmyter and co-workers (1976) from Leuven, Belgium, treated one human patient and two chronic HBsAg carrier chimpanzees with 10 mu of fibroblast interferon every other day for 2 weeks. Serum HBsAg and aminotransferase activities did not change, but there was a marked decrease in the amount of HBcAg present in liver biopsy tissue taken during treatment. These changes returned to pretreatment levels when interferon injections were stopped. Results of testing for serum HBV DNA and DNA polymerase were not reported.

Subsequently, two European groups have reported on the effects of fibroblast interferon in series of patients with chronic hepatitis B. Kingham and co-workers (1978) from Southhampton, England, treated two patients with 10 mu daily for 2 weeks. They noted no effect on aminotransferase activities, HBsAg titer, HBeAg or Dane particles. An unexpected finding was a marked decrease in serum anti-HBc titers. Weimar and associates (1977) from the Netherlands treated two patients twice weekly and three patients daily with 2 to 8 mu of fibroblast interferon. No effect was noted on serum levels of DNA polymerase, HBeAg, or HBsAg, and serum aminotransferase activities did not change. Subsequently, Weimar and associates (1979) compared the effects of fibroblast and leukocyte interferon (both at doses of 3 mu daily for 2 weeks) and found decreases in serum DNA polymerase only with the leukocyte form of interferon.

Müller and associates (1982a) from Hannover and Munich, West Germany conducted a randomized, controlled trial of fibroblast interferon. Eight patients received 332 to 800 mu of interferon in varying dosage schedules over a 6-month period. In all eight patients serum levels of DNA polymerase fell, and in six, it became undetectable. However, in the majority of patients this effect was transient, and DNA polymerase activity returned to pretreatment levels even while therapy was continued. Only one of the eight patients demonstrated a permanent loss of DNA polymerase and subsequently lost both serum HBeAg and HBsAg and had a concurrent remission in disease activity. None of the controls had a similar decrease in serum hepatitis B virus markers. Thus, despite early promising results, fibroblast interferon has not been shown to be effective in inducing a long-term improvement in chronic hepatitis B.

Recombinant β and γ interferon have recently been prepared in sufficient quantities and with suitable purity to begin human studies. There have been no reports on the use of these recombinant interferons in chronic hepatitis B.

Another approach to interferon therapy in chronic hepatitis B was reported by Purcell and associates (1976) from the National Institutes of Health, who used interferon inducers. They treated two chronic HBsAg carrier chimpanzees with polyriboinosinic–polyribocytidylic acid poly-*l*-lysine carboxymethyl cellulose complex (PICLC) for 2 weeks during a preliminary study and for 7 weeks in a subsequent trial. PICLC led to the appearance of detectable serum interferon in both animals and subsequently to a decrease in serum DNA polymerase and HBeAg. However, these viral markers returned to pretreatment values when PICLC was discontinued. This approach to treatment of chronic hepatitis B has not been studied further, largely because of the toxicities of most efficient interferon inducers.

The disparate results using interferon require explanation. One reason for the differing results is the possibility of variation in the potencies of the interferon preparations used. Thus, fibroblast interferon may not be as potent an inhibitor of hepatitis B virus replication as leukocyte interferon (Weimar *et al.*, 1979). Furthermore, different lots of interferon and different cloned molecules of these lymphokines may vary in potency, in metabolic distribution, and in clearance rate.

Another reason for the differences in results among different groups of investigators is the dosage of interferon used and the duration of therapy. Merigan and co-workers (1980) have claimed that permanent responses to therapy require treatment with more than 400 mu given over 5 to 6 months. Administration of these dosages is now practical using the lymphoblastoid and recombinant interferons. The maximum dosage of interferon that can be tolerated for a prolonged period of time is probably in the range of 2 to 10 mu daily. Administration of interferon every other day or three times weekly may be as effective as daily inter-

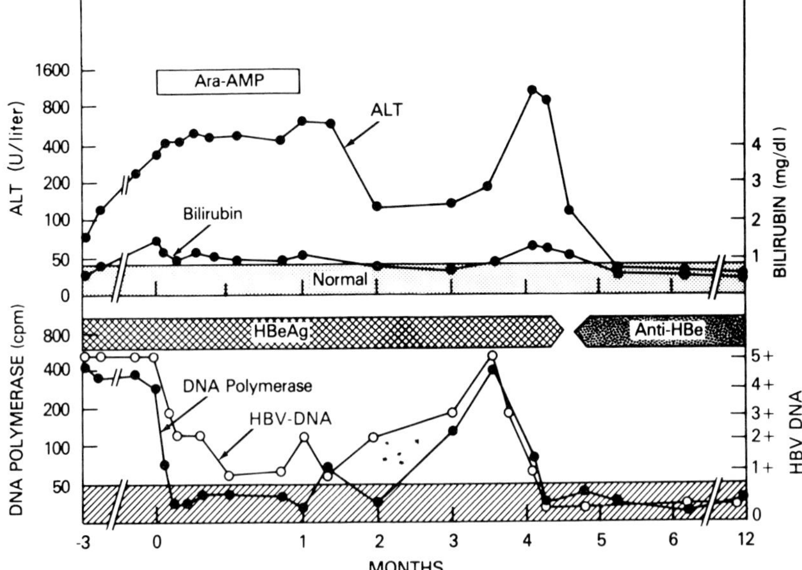

Figure 4. Course of a patient with chronic hepatitis B who was treated with adenine arabinoside monophosphate (Ara-AMP) for four weeks (Hoofnagle et al., 1982b). Abbreviations: see legend to Fig. 1.

levels of hepatitis B virus returned to pretreatment values soon after discontinuation of the drug. The course of a patient demonstrating a permanent response to therapy is shown in Fig. 4.

Controlled trials of Ara-AMP treatment of chronic hepatitis B using more prolonged periods of treatment or multiple courses of therapy have now been conducted both in Europe and the United States (Table

TABLE VI

Summary of Four Prospective Randomized Controlled Trials of Ara-AMP

	Long-term beneficial responses	
Reference	Ara-AMP[a] group	Control group
Hoofnagle et al. (1984b)	20% (2/10)	20% (2/10)
Perrillo et al. (1985)	5% (1/18)	5% (1/17)
Thomas and Lok (1983)	26% (4/15)	0% (0/14)
Trepo et al. (1984)	55% (10/18)	26% (5/9)

[a]Ara-AMP, Adenine arabinoside monophosphate.

VI). Hoofnagle *et al.* (1984a) from the National Institutes of Health performed a randomized, controlled trial of a 28-day course of Ara-AMP in 20 patients. Patients received 10 mg/kg/day iv for the first 5 days in hospital and were then followed as outpatients on 5 mg/kg/day im for 23 days. This therapy resulted in a prompt decrease in DNA polymerase levels in all patients. This decrease was sustained for the 28 days of outpatient therapy. One year after starting therapy, four treated patients had lost HBV DNA and HBeAg and had entered a clinical remission in disease. Interestingly, the disappearance of HBV DNA and DNA polymerase actually occurred after therapy was discontinued. In addition, two of the four responders subsequently suffered a relapse in disease with return of HBeAg, DNA polymerase, and HBV DNA. At the conclusion of the trial, 20% of both the treated and untreated patient groups had become HBeAg negative and had a sustained improvement in their liver disease. Subsequently, these investigators treated ten more patients with three, 10-day courses of Ara-AMP (10 mg/kg/day) (Hoofnagle *et al.*, 1985). Only one patient (10%) had a serological response to therapy. In follow up this patient also suffered a relapse in disease with reactivation of the underlying chronic hepatitis B virus infection (Davis *et al.*, 1984a).

Perrillo *et al.* (1985) from Washington University, St. Louis, entered 35 patients with chronic hepatitis B into clinical trials using either one or two 28-day courses of Ara-AMP (10 mg/kg/day for 5 days, followed by 5 mg/kg/day for 23 days). One of the 18 treated patients as well as one of the 17 control patients had a sustained loss of DNA polymerase activity and HBeAg during the course of follow-up evaluation. These two trials from the United States suggested that 28-day courses of Ara-AMP were not effective in inducing a sustained serological and clinical improvement in chronic hepatitis B.

Trials of Ara-AMP therapy in the United Kingdom and France have yielded different results. Investigators at the Royal Free Hospital, London (Thomas and Lok, 1983), entered a total of 29 patients into a randomized controlled trial of Ara-AMP given im for 28 days. Four of 15 treated patients, but none of 14 controls had a sustained serological response. Trepo *et al.* (1984) from Lyons, France, entered 37 patients into a randomized controlled trial of Ara-AMP (10 mg/kg/day for 5 days followed by 5 mg/kg/day for 23 days). Ten of 18 treated (55%) as opposed to 5 of 19 (26%) untreated patients had a sustained response to therapy as defined by a loss of HBeAg or DNA polymerase or both.

The widely different results between studies conducted in the United States and those conducted in Europe have invited analyses of the characteristics of patients who responded to Ara-AMP therapy. Investigators from the Royal Free Hospital (Novick *et al.*, 1984) suggested that male homosexual patients are less likely to respond to Ara-AMP therapy than heterosexual patients. In their combined experience, none of 13 homosexual patients but 8 of 16 heterosexual patients responded to Ara-AMP therapy. The trial conducted in France did not include any male homosexuals and reported the highest response rate to this drug. In contrast, 40–65% of patients entered into studies in the United States were male homosexuals and both studies reported low rates of response. Since male homosexual patients frequently have underlying immunodeficiencies, their lack of response to Ara-AMP therapy may have been due to their relative immune hyporesponsiveness. This was an atrractive hypothesis to explain the differences between trials conducted in Europe and those conducted in the United States. However, analysis of the studies from the United States does not support the role of homosexuality in the poor outcome of those trials. In the combined results on 26 patients treated at the National Institutes of Health, 2 of 17 male homosexual patients exhibited a sustained serological and clinical response to therapy, whereas none of 9 heterosexuals responded. Furthermore, studies from Japan (Omata *et al.*, 1984) and later studies from the United Kingdom (Lok *et al.*, 1983) have found a low rate of permanent responses to Ara-AMP therapy. The small numbers of responders in all of these studies interferes with a meaningful analysis of the factors that determined outcome of therapy. While much attention is paid to the identification of the type of patient who responds best to antiviral chemotherapy, it is obvious that what is most needed is therapy that would be beneficial for all patients with chronic hepatitis B.

Ara-A and Ara-AMP have significant toxic effects. Prolonged or high-dose therapy commonly causes anorexia, nausea, and fatigue; vomiting and diarrhea can also occur. Both drugs cause mild but reversible bone marrow suppression; the platelet count is usually affected most and may decrease by half. The most troublesome side effects, however, have been the neuromuscular toxicities of Ara-A and Ara-AMP. With dosages in excess of 10 mg/kg/day, headaches, lethargy, stupor, and tremors may develop. These symptoms can last several weeks and may be associated with EEG changes. Sacks and co-workers (1979) from Stanford University reported one patient who developed progressive stupor, followed by seizures, coma, and respiratory arrest during combined interferon and Ara-AMP therapy. Recovery was slow but eventually complete. Several fatalities due to Ara-A neurotoxicity have been reported in patients treated for other conditions (Sacks *et al.*, 1979; VanEtta *et al.*, 1981). In addition, Ara-A and Ara-AMP given in lower doses for prolonged periods frequently lead to a peculiar neuromuscular pain syndrome (Preiksaitis *et al.*, 1981: Hoofnagle *et al.*, 1982b). Patients describe muscle cramps, especially in large muscle groups, which are worse with rest and are improved with exercise or massage. This toxicity can be severe and disabling, and can persist for as long as 2 months after therapy is discontinued. Neuromuscular toxicity occurs in as many as 50% of patients treated with Ara-AMP for 28 days. The cause of this pain syndrome is unknown; it occurs rarely in patients treated with Ara-A for viral infections other than hepatitis. The troublesome side effects and lack of high rate of response have led to a discontinuation of trials of Ara-AMP in chronic hepatitis B.

C. Acyclovir

Acyclovir [9-(2-hydroxyethoxymethyl)guanine] is a new nucleoside analog with potent and unique antiviral activities against many herpes viruses (Schaeffer *et al.*, 1978; Elion, 1982). Acyclovir is so named because it has an acyclic side chain substituted for the usual cyclic carbohydrate moiety in guanosine (Fig. 5). Acyclovir is relatively nontoxic, and its antiviral activities are mainly against the herpes group of viruses, especially herpes simplex types 1 and 2. Acyclovir must first be activated to its monophosphate form, a reaction catalyzed by the herpes virus-specific thymidine kinases but not by cellular thymidine kinases. Furthermore, the triphosphate form of acyclovir is selectively more potent against viral DNA polymerases than against host cellular DNA polymerases. For these reasons, acyclovir is potentially an ideal agent for herpes virus infections, and numerous studies have revealed that it is effective therapy for both systemic and local herpes virus infections (Straus *et al.*, 1982).

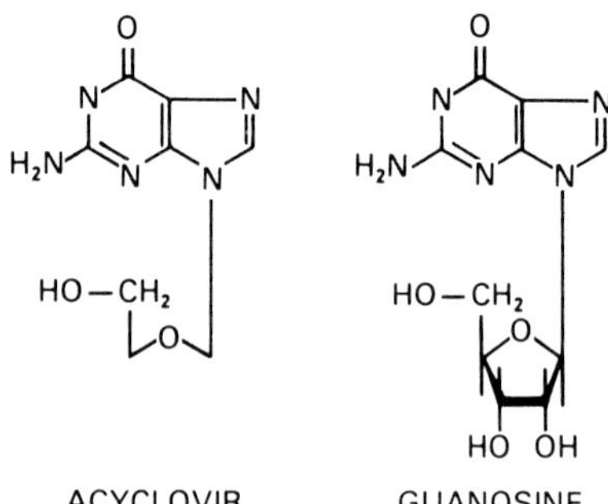

Figure 5. Structures of acyclovir and guanosine.

The hepatitis B virus has not been shown to possess an endogenous thymidine kinase, and infection with this virus is not known to induce such an enzyme in cells. Nevertheless, several groups of investigators have reported successful results of treating small numbers of patients with chronic hepatitis B using acyclovir. Smith and co-workers (1982b) from Stanford University treated three patients with 10 separate 7- to 14-day courses of acyclovir in doses ranging from 15 to 45 mg/kg/day iv. Each course was associated with a decrease in serum levels of DNA polymerase activity. However, inhibition of serum hepatitis B virus was usually partial and DNA polymerase returned to pretreatment levels as soon as acyclovir was discontinued. One of the three patients, nevertheless, remained DNA polymerase negative after a fourth course of therapy. These investigators concluded that acyclovir had some activity against hepatitis B virus but was inadequate as a single agent. Weller and associates (1982b) from the Royal Free Hospital, London, treated four patients with chronic hepatitis B using iv acyclovir at a dosage of 5 to 15 mg/kg/day for 5 to 7 days. A decrease in serum levels of HBV DNA and DNA polymerase occurred with doses of 10 to 15 mg/kg/day; however, in no case was this inhibition complete or permanent.

Alexander *et al.* (1984) from King's College Hospital, London, have recently conducted a controlled trial of acyclovir in chronic hepatitis B. They entered 30 patients into this trial, 15 of whom received 45 mg/kg/day of acyclovir by continuous iv infusion for 28 days. Serum levels of DNA polymerase fell only slightly during acyclovir treatment. One year after entering the study, 4 treated and 2 untreated patients had lost DNA polymerase and HBeAg.

Acyclovir can be administered by the oral route, but plasma drug levels are not as high as with iv therapy (Van Dyke *et al.*, 1982). Acyclovir is relatively nontoxic. Unlike other nucleoside analogs such as Ara-A or Ara-AMP, acyclovir produces little or no bone marrow suppression. Known side effects of acyclovir include transient minor increases in serum ALT levels and mild degrees of renal toxicity. Animal studies suggest that acyclovir can lead to crystal deposition in renal tubules, and rapid, iv administration of acyclovir in man has led to transient increases in serum creatinine levels (Brigden *et al.*, 1982). However, when administered by slow iv infusion to a well-hydrated patient who is without kidney disease, renal toxicity is rare.

Thus, acyclovir is a promising antiviral agent that may be valuable in combination with other agents as therapy of chronic hepatitis B. The recent development of an analog of acyclovir (6-deoxyacyclovir: procyclovir) that is well absorbed by the oral route promises to provide a practical form of this drug to evaluate in long-term therapeutic trials.

D. Ribavirin

Ribavirin (1-β-D-ribofuranosyl-1,2,4-triazole-3-carboxamide) is a nucleoside analog that is active *in vitro* against a wide range of both RNA and DNA viruses (Fig. 6) (Sidwell *et al.*, 1972). Sidwell and associates (1977) demonstrated that ribavirin has a marked effect in preventing death in mice infected with murine hepatitis virus (an RNA coronavirus). Ribavirin is concentrated in the liver, and acts to inhibit the enzymes involved in guanosine monophosphate synthesis.

Ayrosa-Galvao and co-workers (Ayroso-Galvao and Castro, 1977) from Brazil reported favorable results using ribavirin in a large number of patients with acute hepatitis. Results of testing for hepatitis B virus markers were not described. Denes *et al.* (1976) from the Center for Disease Control, Phoenix, Arizona, treated two chronically HBsAg-positive chimpanzees with ribavirin and noted no significant change in serum HBsAg or serum aminotransferase activities. A similar lack of effect on HBsAg and aminotransferase activities was noted by Kew and Seftel (1977) from Johannesburg, South Africa, in a study of 13 patients with chronic hepatitis B who were treated with 800 to 1200 mg of ribavirin daily for 10 to 28 days. Finally, Jain and co-workers (1978) from the Royal Free Hospital, London, conducted a double-blind, placebo-controlled trial of ribavirin (200 mg orally four times daily) in six patients with chronic HBsAg positive hepatitis. Patients were treated with either ribavirin or placebo for 4 weeks and were then changed over to the other therapy. There were no consistent changes in either aminotransferase activities, HBsAg concentrations, or DNA polymerase activity in serum. Thus, data in both chimpanzee and human studies suggest that ribavirin has no inhibitory effect on hepatitis B virus replication and does not beneficially alter the course of chronic hepatitis B.

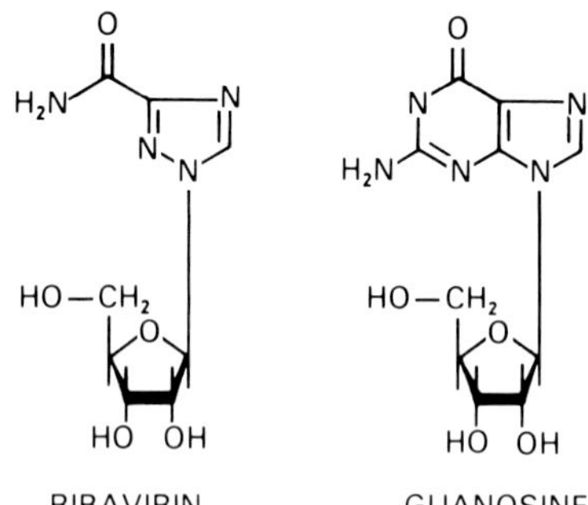

Figure 6. Structures of ribavirin and guanosine.

E. Phosphonoformic Acid

Trisodium phosphonoformic acid (PFA) and phosphonoacetic acid (PAA) are pyrophosphate analogs (Fig. 7) that interfere with the attachment of polymerases to triphosphate nucleotides during RNA and DNA synthesis (Helgstrand *et al.*, 1978). The trisodium salts of PFA and PAA inhibit *viral* polymerase activity at concentrations far below those that block *host, cellular* polymerase activity and are thus potentially useful antiviral compounds. Nordenfelt and co-workers (1979) from Lund, Sweden, demonstrated that PFA is a potent in vitro inhibitor of hepatitis B virus DNA polymerase activity. Concentrations required to inhibit this DNA polymerase were not toxic to mammalian cellular DNA synthesis and can be achieved *in vivo.* PAA, which is a potent inhibitor of herpes virus replication, was not effective against hepatitis B virus DNA polymerase. These results were confirmed and extended by Hess and co-workers (1980) from Berlin, West Germany, who demonstrated that PFA was a noncompetitive inhibitor of hepatitis B virus DNA polymerase that appears to interact with the pyrophosphate binding site of the elongating DNA molecule.

PFA in a topical formulation is currently undergoing evaluation in man as treatment for cutaneous herpes simplex. A parenteral form of the drug was evaluated in two chronic HBsAg carrier chimpanzees (R. Johnson and R. H. Purcell, personal communication.) Administration of the drug led to an inhibition of serum levels of DNA polymerase and a decrease in liver cell HBcAg reactivity, as assessed by immunofluorescence microscopy of liver biopsy tissue. Further evaluation in chimpanzees was made difficult by the necessity of administering PFA by slow iv infusions several times daily. Reports on the use of parenteral PFA for chronic hepatitis B in man have not appeared. Unfortunately, the phosphate moiety of PFA becomes incorporated into bone where further metabolic turnover is slow, being measured in years. Concerns over possible long-term toxicity of PFA retained in bone tissue have stood in the way of further studies of this drug in man.

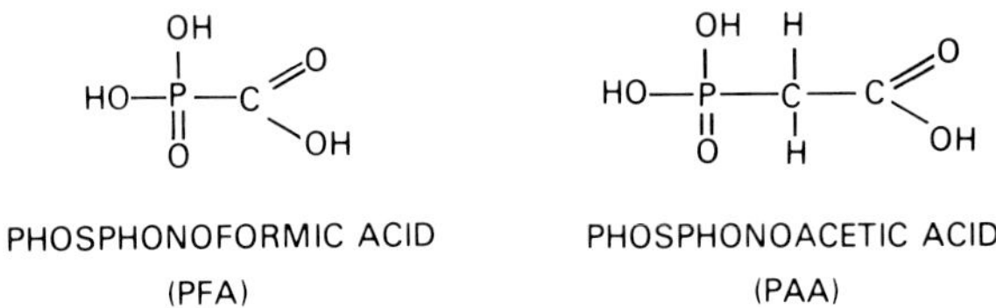

Figure 7. Structures of phosphonoformic acid (PFA) and phosphonoacetic acid (PAA).

F. Intercalating Agents

The intercalating agents interfere with DNA polymerase reactions *in vitro* and have been proposed as modes of therapy for chronic hepatitis B (Hirschman and Garfinkel, 1978). Examples of intercalating agents that are relatively nontoxic include quinacrine, chloroquine, chlorpromazine, and primaquine. Uncontrolled studies conducted at the Royal Free Hospital, London (Thomas and Lok, 1983), suggested that they were not active *in vivo* in lowering hepatitis B virus levels in serum. Bodenheimer *et al.* (1983) conducted a randomized controlled trial of quinacrine using a maintenance dosage of 100 mg/day for months in 22 patients with chronic hepatitis B. There was no evidence of inhibition of DNA polymerase levels or of a sustained clinical improvement in liver disease in any of the ten quinacrine-treated patients. These results indicate that intercalating agents are unlikely to exert a sufficiently antiviral effect to be useful agents in the treatment of chronic hepatitis B.

G. Combination Therapy

The somewhat discouraging results obtained with the use of interferon and Ara-AMP alone led Merigan and co-workers to attempt chemotherapy using a combination of these agents (Merigan, 1982). They used a variety of dosages and drug regimens, including therapy with both agents concurrently as well as alternating cycles of each. Among 16 patients treated with combinations of Ara-A and interferon, permanent inhibition of serum DNA polymerase was found in 7 (43%) and complete clearance of serological markers including HBsAg occurred in 2 (12%) (Scullard *et al.*, 1981b). Patients who responded with clearance of DNA polymerase usually experienced a subsequent clinical remission in symptoms and disease activity. Furthermore, such patients could be shown to have a marked decrease (if not complete clearance) of serum infectivity (Scullard *et al.*, 1982). This rate of response was higher than with interferon alone (25%) or Ara-A alone (16%) (Table IV). In a later report from Stanford University, Smith *et al.* (1982a) described results of combined chemotherapy with interferon and Ara-AMP using various dosage regimens. Permanent inhibition of DNA polymerase with eventual loss of HBeAg was noted in only 1 of 10 (10%) patients.

These early results of combination chemotherapy were promising but suffered from the same shortcomings as other studies of antiviral therapy of this disease: they lacked suitable randomized, concurrently followed, untreated control patients. Since the spontaneous rate of improvement in chronic hepatitis B can be as high as 30% per year, it is difficult to say that the results obtained in these studies were greater than would have occurred by chance. For this reason, Merigan and co-workers at Stanford University embarked upon a large, randomized, placebo-controlled, double-blind study of antiviral therapy using a combination of human leukocyte interferon (buffy-coat derived) and Ara-AMP (Merigan, 1982). After preliminary evaluation, all patients were started on a 6-month course of therapy with twice daily im injections. The patients were randomized into three groups: Group 1 to receive 1 month of interferon alternating with 1 month of Ara-AMP for 6 months; Group 2 to receive 1 month of Ara-AMP alternating with 1 month of placebo for 6 months; and Group 3 to receive 6 months of placebo injections. Unfortunately, the combined chemotherapy was found to be too toxic; the majority of patients receiving both interferon and Ara-AMP developed the neuromuscular pain syndrome. The combined arm (Group 1) of this controlled trial was discontinued, but results of the treatment with monthly courses of Ara-AMP have yet to be reported.

A similar high rate of toxicity with the combination of interferon and Ara-AMP was found by Müller *et al.* (1984) from West Germany. It is probable that interferon alters the metabolism of other drugs including Ara-AMP. This finding reinforces the fact that combinations of medications may not result in additive beneficial effects but almost always result in additive adverse side effects.

Nevertheless, combined antiviral chemotherapy still holds the most promise for therapy of chronic hepatitis B. Studies to date indicate that interferon, Ara-AMP and acyclovir all have some effect of hepatitis B virus replication and that long-term therapy will induce remissions in disease in a small percentage of patients. It is hoped that a combination of these drugs might yield a higher rate of response. Future trials of antiviral therapy in chronic hepatitis B will probably focus on combinations of α interferon, acyclovir, procyclovir, and possibly γ interferon.

III. Agents That Affect the Immune System

Considerable evidence indicates that the host immune response plays a major role in the development, course, and outcome of chronic hepatitis B (Levy and Chisari, 1981; Dienstag, 1984). Another approach to therapy of this disease is the use of treatments or agents that modulate, enhance, or suppress the immune system. Two major difficulties have hindered studies using this approach to therapy. First, the nature of the underlying immunological deficiency in chronic hepatitis B remains unclear. It has been suggested that patients with this disease have an abnormality in T-lymphocyte function. However, most studies of specific and nonspecific T-cell function in this disease have revealed minimal if any abnormalities in the majority of patients (Dienstag, 1984). A second difficulty with immunomodulation as an approach to therapy is that there are few agents that are safe and that lead to an effective enhancement or modulation of the immune response. If the development of antiviral agents is in its infancy, the development of immunomodulating agents is in its perinatal period.

A. Plasmapheresis

Plasmapheresis has been proposed as a means of therapy for several diseases with suspected immunological etiologies. Plasmapheresis may play a special role in those diseases in which circulating immune complexes are present. Because high levels of HBsAg and HBV can be present in plasma, and because circulating immune complexes are detectable in some forms of chronic hepatitis B, plasmapheresis has been attempted as a means of therapy for this disease. Case reports of beneficial responses to plasmapheresis have been published (Chalopin *et al.*, 1980), but there have not been any sizeable prospective or randomized trials of this therapy. Shown in Fig. 8 are results of serum testing for HBsAg, HBeAg, and DNA polymerase in a patient who underwent extensive plasmapheresis for suspected polyarteritis nodosa due to chronic HBV infection (J. H. Hoofnagle, J. L. Gerin, and A. S. Fauci, unpublished observations). Each 2-liter plasmapheresis led to an abrupt decrease in levels of HBsAg, HBeAg, and DNA polymerase. However, these viral markers returned to pretreatment levels within hours to days. A 4-week course of plasmapheresis performed three times each week led to a 50% decrease in HBsAg titer but to no change in serum HBeAg or DNA polymerase. The amount of HBsAg present in serum in chronic hepatitis B is so great (in the range of 1 to 500 mcg/ml) that even extensive plasmapheresis will not reduce this to undetectable levels (below 500 pcg/ml).

Actually, plasmapheresis is used extensively in patients with chronic hepatitis B in order to provide source plasma for the hepatitis B virus vaccine (Szmuness *et al.*, 1980). Plasmapheresis donors for the vaccine must have high levels of serum HBsAg and are commonly seropositive for HBeAg. Two-unit plasmaphereses are performed on each donor once a week. There have been no reports of either beneficial or harmful long-term effects of such plasmaphereses. We have followed three patients with mild chronic hepatitis B who have undergone regular plas-

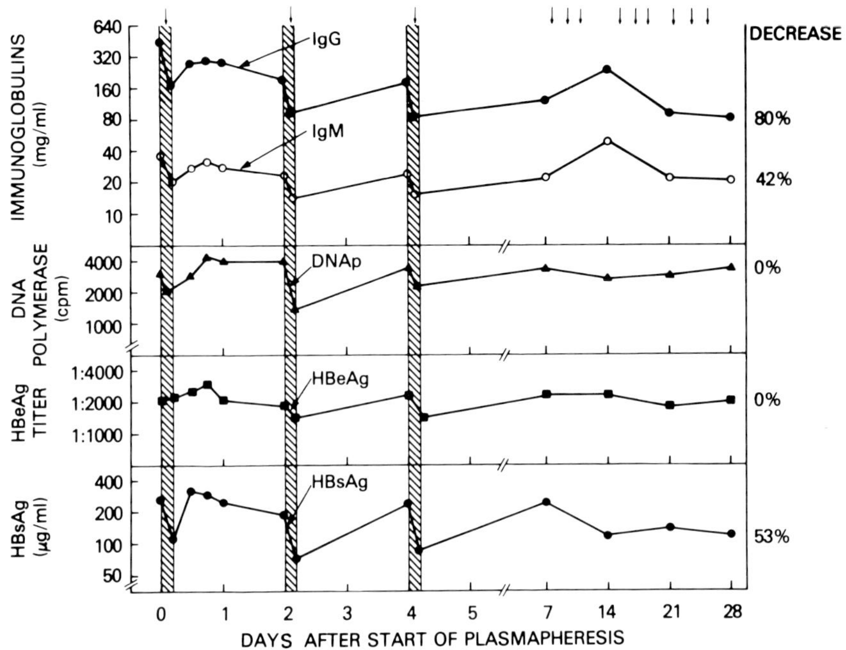

Figure 8. Course of a patient with chronic hepatitis B who was treated with intensive plasmaphereses (↓) for 4 weeks. The total percent decrease of each marker is shown on the right of the figure. Abbreviations: see legend to Fig. 1.

mapheresis once weekly for the past 2 years without change in serum HBsAg, HBeAg, or DNA polymerase. Thus, plasmapheresis has not been shown to be beneficial for patients with chronic hepatitis B.

B. Immunoglobulin Therapy

From 30 to 40% of patients with chronic hepatitis B have both HBsAg as well as antibody to HBsAg (anti-HBs) in serum (Hoofnagle and Alter, 1984). The anti-HBs, however, is heterotypic, meaning that it is directed against a subdeterminant of HBsAg that is not present in the serum. Chronic HBsAg carriers do not have homotypic anti-HBs; they appear not to make antibody to the large amounts of HBsAg that circulate in the serum. It has been suggested that the lack of HBsAg clearance in patients with this disease may be due to an inadequate production of homotypic anti-HBs. One approach to therapy is, therefore, the infusion of serum or globulin preparations with high titers of this antibody.

Reed and co-workers (1973) from King's College Hospital, London, treated five patients with chronic hepatitis B with an immune globulin preparation containing high titers of anti-HBs (hepatitis B immune globulin, HBIG). Patients were given 300–400 ml by slow iv infusion over an 8-hr period. The infusions were well tolerated; no patient developed evidence of immune complex disease. A transient decrease in HBsAg titers was noted in the three patients with the lowest initial levels of HBsAg. However, this effect was not sustained and no consistent permanent effect on HBsAg titers or disease activity was found. It should be noted that all patients were concurrently receiving immunosuppressive therapy and that the period of follow-up evaluation was brief.

HBIG or plasma containing high titers of anti-HBs has also been used to treat acute fulminant hepatitis. Three uncontrolled studies suggested a beneficial effect (Gocke, 1971; Dupuy *et al.*, 1975; Gateau *et al.*, 1976), but a multicenter randomized, placebo-controlled study conducted by the Acute Hepatic Failure Study Group (1977) failed to show any benefit from therapy with HBIG. Unfortunately, the amount of anti-HBs containing HBIG used in the controlled study was not equal to that used in previously published reports.

Thus, passive infusion of anti-HBs-rich plasma or globulin preparations can temporarily reduce HBsAg titers, but has not been reported to induce a permanent beneficial effect on this disease. The expense of HBIG and the potential for inducing immune complex-related complications in nonimmunosuppressed individuals make passive immunotherapy an unlikely mode of treatment for chronic hepatitis B.

C. Vaccination

The recent development of a hepatitis B vaccine promises to provide a safe and effective means of preventing this liver disease (Szmuness *et al.*, 1980). The vaccine induces anti-HBs in >90% of normal recipients. The fact that chronic HBsAg carriers lack homotypic anti-HBs and appear to have immunological tolerance to HBsAg has led to the suggestion that vaccination with HBsAg might have a beneficial effect in this condition.

Tabor and co-workers (1976) at the Office of Biologics, Bethesda, Maryland, immunized a chronic HBsAg carrier (subtype **adw**) chimpanzee with purified HBsAg of the opposite subtype (**ayw**). The chimpanzee developed antibody to the ''y'' subdeterminant but did not become HBsAg negative.

Dienstag and colleagues (1982) from Boston, Massachusetts, treated

16 chronic HBsAg carriers with hepatitis B virus vaccine (40 μg of HBsAg/**adw**) im each month for 6 months. The study was discontinued early when two recipients developed marked increases in serum aminotransferase activities after the second and fourth injections. None of the 16 patients subsequently cleared HBsAg. One of the 10 HBeAg-positive recipients lost this reactivity, and serum aminotransferase activities improved in several other treated patients. However, the authors concluded that these changes were not related to vaccination. This study was not controlled, and results of testing for HBsAg and HBeAg titers and serum HBV DNA and DNA polymerase were not reported.

Schalm and co-workers (1982) from the Netherlands recently summarized an ongoing double-blind randomized trial of hepatitis B virus vaccine treatment of patients with chronic hepatitis B. Forty-nine individuals were randomized to receive either 3 μg of vaccine (both **adw** and **ayw** subtypes) or placebo at monthly intervals for 3 months. Changes in HBsAg or HBeAg and serum aminotransferase activities occurred among the 29 vaccine recipients at a frequency similar to that among the 20 placebo recipients.

Thus, vaccination with hepatitis B virus vaccine has not been shown to have any therapeutic benefit in this disease. More in-depth analysis of the published reports on vaccination is warranted.

D. Transfer Factor

Transfer factor is a soluble protein of low molecular weight (<10,000) that is produced by T lymphocytes and that is capable of transferring or augmenting cell-mediated immunity to specific antigens (Lawrence, 1969). Transfer factor has been successfully used to treat immune deficiency syndromes (Levin *et al.*, 1973) and to provide specific cell-mediated immunity to viral infections (Drew *et al.*, 1973). Several groups of investigators have employed transfer factor in the treatment of chronic hepatitis B (Table VII).

Kohler and associates (1974) from Denver, Colorado, treated an HBsAg-positive infant on two occasions with lymphocyte transfer factor from the child's mother (who had recovered from hepatitis B). Serum aminotransferase activities increased shortly after both injections but eventually fell into the normal range 6 months later. There was a concurrent decrease in HBsAg titer. In a second patient, transfer factor therapy had no effect on serum enzymes or HBsAg titer. Grob and co-workers (1975) in Switzerland treated a single patient with HBsAg-positive polyarteritis nodosa and a child with chronic hepatitis with transfer factor.

TABLE VII
Summary of Studies on Transfer Factor Therapy of
Chronic Hepatitis B

Reference	Number treated	Beneficial response[a]
Kohler *et al.* (1974)	2	50%
Grob *et al.* (1975)	1	0%
Jain *et al.* (1977)	6	0%
Sano *et al.* (1977)	5	0%
Pizza *et al.* (1979)	9	55%
Shulman *et al.* (1976)	6	83%

[a]Definition of beneficial response varies with each study.

There was a transient increase in HBsAg titers after treatment, but no beneficial effect on the disease was noted.

Jain and associates (1977) from the Royal Free Hospital, London, treated six patients, first with "nonspecific" transfer factor (from donors without anti-HBs) followed by "specific" transfer factor (from donors recently recovered from hepatitis B). Transient increases in serum aminotransferase activities were seen in three of the six patients after specific transfer factor treatment but in none of those treated with the nonspecific material. At follow-up, no beneficial therapeutic effect of the treatment was noted.

Two other negative studies have been reported. Tong and associates (1976) from Los Angeles treated a single patient and Sano and associates (1977) from Kyoto, Japan, five patients with multiple doses of transfer factor. Both groups demonstrated the transfer of cell-mediated immunity to HBsAg (as monitored by *in vitro* assays), but in neither study did the patients demonstrate any permanent improvement in clinical, biochemical, or serological indices of disease.

Two groups of investigators have reported positive results using transfer factor. Pizza and co-workers (1979) from Bologna, Italy, treated nine patients with a transfer factor prepared from a lymphoblastoid cell line. An increase in serum aminotransferase activities occurred in all but one patient after the initial dose of transfer factor. On follow-up, one patient became HBsAg-negative and five demonstrated improvements in serum aminotransferase activities. Finally, Shulman *et al.* (1975, 1976) from Gainesville, Florida, have conducted a randomized, double-blind, controlled trial of transfer factor. At least moderate improvements in clinical, histological, and biochemical indices of disease were noted in five of six transfer-factor-treated patients but in only two of six placebo-treated recipients. In neither of these reports were results of hepatitis B virus levels reported, and follow-up was brief.

Thus, transfer factor prepared from lymphocytes of patients recovering from acute hepatitis B can transfer immune reactivity to HBsAg as assessed by *in vitro* assays and it may cause transient changes in serum HBsAg titers and aminotransferase activities. However, permanent beneficial effects on disease activity or serological markers of infection have not been consistently demonstrated. More thorough evaluation of the effects of transfer factor therapy on hepatitis B virus markers is warranted. The lack of standardization and assays for stability and potency of transfer factor make any studies of this material difficult.

E. Immune RNA

RNA extracted from lymphocytes of lymph nodes or spleens can transfer specific immunity to nonimmune animals (Fishman and Adler, 1976). This "immune RNA" is similar to transfer factor in action, but consists of a nondialyzable, high molecular weight nucleic acid rather than a dialyzable, low molecular weight protein.

Vyas and colleagues (1974) from the University of California, San Francisco, demonstrated that delayed hypersensitivity to HBsAg (as assayed by skin testing and migration inhibition of peritoneal exudate cells) could be transferred to nonimmune guinea pigs using an RNA extract from hyperimmunized guinea pig spleen cells. These authors suggested that such a restoration of T-lymphocyte immune responsiveness to HBsAg might benefit patients with chronic hepatitis B.

Liu *et al.* (1982) from Peking University, People's Republic of China, prepared immune RNA from extracts of lymph nodes and spleens of horses that had been hyperimmunized with HBsAg. This hepatitis B immune RNA was administered 1 to 2 times per week for 6 months to 50 patients with chronic hepatitis B. A majority of treated patients (80%) subsequently demonstrated a decrease in HBsAg titer, and 20% cleared HBsAg. Serum aminotransferase activities decreased in 64% of treated patients and became normal in 44%. In a control group of 21 patients, only 3 (14%) showed a decrease in HBsAg titer and none became HBsAg negative. Furthermore, only 2 (10%) of the controls had a decrease in serum aminotransferase activities. Side effects were said not to occur. These authors did not report results of testing for other HBV markers, and it is not clear whether the study was truly randomized. This very promising report has not been followed by further controlled studies of immune RNA therapy.

F. Bacillus Calmette–Guérin

Vaccination with Bacillus Calmette–Guérin (BCG) can lead to enhancement of cell-mediated immune responses and has been proposed as a means of restoring immune responsiveness.

Brzosko *et al.* (1978) from Warsaw, Poland, treated 20 children with chronic hepatitis B with weekly vaccinations of BCG. A total of 5.4 ml of BCG was administered over a 4 to 6-month period. On follow up 1 year later, all of the children were clinically improved. Serum aminotransferase activities were normal in all 20 children, and 8 had become HBsAg negative. A control group was not studied, and serum HBeAg and DNA polymerase levels were not reported.

Bassendine *et al.* (1980) from the Royal Free Hospital, London, treated nine patients with a total dose of 0.3 mg of BCG over a 10- to 20-week period. Two of five patients with HBeAg and DNA polymerase reactivity in serum had a disappearance of these viral markers with therapy. One of four patients with anti-HBe who were nonreactive for DNA polymerase lost HBsAg with treatment. Side effects were few. While these reports were encouraging, further studies on BCG immunotherapy of chronic hepatitis B have not appeared. Some of the apparent responses to BCG noted in this study may have been due to previous withdrawal of immunosuppressive therapy (Weller *et al.*, 1982c).

G. Levamisole

Levamisole (tetramisole) is an antihelminthic agent that has been extensively used in veterinary medicine (Fig. 9) (Thienpoint *et al.*, 1966). Studies have shown that levamisole is capable of enhancing both humoral and cellular immune responses (Renoux and Renoux, 1972). Levamisole has been proposed as an immunomodulating agent that might play an ancillary role in the chemotherapy of viral infections and cancer (Hadden *et al.*, 1977; Tripodi *et al.*, 1973).

Par and co-workers (1977) from Hungary conducted a placebo-controlled trial of levamisole (150 mg/day for 2 weeks) in 50 patients with acute viral hepatitis. Among the 25 patients with hepatitis B, serum

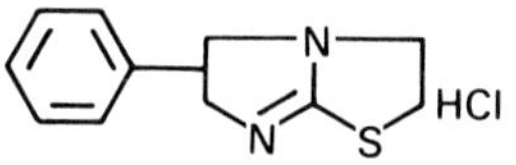

Figure 9. Structure of levamisole.

aminotransferase activities and HBsAg titers fell more quickly in the levamisole-treated than in the placebo-treated patients. After 3 months, evidence for chronic hepatitis was present in only 4% (1 of 23) levamisole-treated but in 30% (8 of 27) placebo-treated patients. Results of testing for other hepatitis B virus markers were not given. Furthermore, more in-depth analyses of this study have not been published.

DeCree and associates (1974) from Belgium treated 18 patients with chronic hepatitis B with oral levamisole. The initially depressed levels of serum complement improved on therapy while HBsAg titers decreased. Evidence for a long-lasting beneficial response was not reported. Masi *et al.* (1978) from Bologna, Italy treated 5 children with chronic hepatitis B using levamisole at a dosage of 2 mg/kg/day for 3 days a week for 4 weeks. They noted marked changes in numbers of peripheral blood B and T lymphocytes and in surface markers during treatment. Serum aminotransferase activities also increased. After 5 months of follow-up, no consistent improvements in disease activity or HBsAg titers were noted.

Fattovich *et al.* (1982) from Padua, Italy, treated eight children with chronic hepatitis B with 2.5 mg/kg levamisole twice a week for 6 to 18 months. Six of the eight children became HBeAg negative on therapy and one also lost HBsAg. These six children showed marked improvements in serum aminotransferase activities and liver biopsy histopathology. These uncontrolled results prompted this group of investigators to begin a long-term, randomized, placebo-controlled trial of levamisole therapy that is still ongoing.

Chadwick and co-workers (1980) from the Royal Free Hospital, London, treated eight patients with chronic hepatitis B with levamisole at a dosage of 150 mg daily for 6 to 8 weeks. Treatment led to an increase towards normal of circulating E-receptor-bearing T lymphocytes and a restoration of cellular immune responsiveness to HBsAg in three of eight patients. These three patients concurrently demonstrated rises in serum aminotransferase activities. However, serum DNA polymerase and HBeAg remained unchanged, and follow-up demonstrated no permanent improvement in indices of disease activity or liver biopsy histopathology.

Thus, levamisole can improve some of the abnormalities of cellular immune function that have been noted in chronic hepatitis B (Verhaegen *et al.*, 1977). However, the drug has not been definitely shown to lower serum hepatitis B virus markers or to have a long-lasting effect on the course of this infection. Results of a controlled trial of levamisole from Italy are still awaited. A possible ancillary role for levamisole in combination with other antiviral agents deserves further study.

H. Immunosuppression

Corticosteroids with or without other immunosuppressive agents have been used as the standard therapy of chronic hepatitis for the past 20 years. However, the role of these agents in the treatment of patients with chronic hepatitis B remains controversial (Hoofnagle, 1982; Davis and Czaja, 1981). Three randomized trials conducted in the late 1960s and early 1970s demonstrated that corticosteroids prolonged survival and decreased mortality of chronic active hepatitis (Cook *et al.*, 1971; Murray-Lyon *et al.*, 1973; Summerskill *et al.*, 1975). These studies were performed before HBsAg testing was available and before the significance of this viral marker was known. Subsequent analyses indicated that the majority of the patients in those studies were HBsAg negative and probably were suffering from chronic autoimmune hepatitis (Wright *et al.*, 1977).

Reanalysis of the Mayo Clinic trials of corticosteroid treatment for chronic active hepatitis by Schalm and associates (1976) demonstrated that HBsAg-positive individuals responded less well to this immunosuppressive regimen than HBsAg-negative individuals. Unfortunately, there were too few HBsAg-positive patients in the control group to assess whether corticosteroid treatment was more beneficial than no treatment at all. These data supported the clinical experience of investigators who suggested that corticosteroids were not particularly beneficial in this disease (Reynolds, 1980).

Lam and associates (1981) from the University of Hong Kong reported results of a randomized, single-blind, controlled trial of prednisolone in patients with chronic hepatitis B. In this study, 51 patients were pair randomized to receive either placebo or 15 to 20 mg of prednisolone daily. After initial remission, the dose of prednisolone was decreased to 10 mg/day, and was continued for as long as $3\frac{1}{2}$ years. Actuarial analysis revealed that prednisolone-treated patients experienced a lower remission rate, a higher relapse rate, and a lower survival rate than did placebo-treated patients. This study was flawed by serious errors in the statistical analyses. Furthermore, results of testing for the viral markers HBeAg, HBV DNA, and DNA polymerase were not reported. Nevertheless, these findings suggested that corticosteroids are not beneficial and may be deleterious in chronic hepatitis B.

Recently, the European Association for the Study of the Liver (1984) presented data from a multicenter trial of corticosteroid therapy of chronic hepatitis B. Ninety-four patients were treated with either prednisolone (10 mg/day) or placebo. After 5 years, analysis revealed a significantly higher mortality rate among the corticosteroid treated group and the trial was discontinued. These studies indicate that long-term prednisolone therapy is probably detrimental in patients with chronic hepatitis B.

The reason for the poor response of this disease to corticosteroid therapy has been suggested by studies on the effects of immunosuppression on serum levels of hepatitis B virus and its associated markers. Scullard *et al.* (1981c) from Stanford University measured serum levels of HBsAg and DNA polymerase in 21 patients withdrawn from immunosuppressive therapy of prednisolone with or without azathioprine (Table VIII). DNA polymerase fell in all 21 patients, becoming undetectable in 8 (38%). HBsAg titers decreased in 17 patients, but none became seronegative. The authors also reported results of serum hepatitis B virus markers in 3 patients that were given a 12-week course of prednisolone (30 mg/day for 4 weeks, 20 mg/day for 4 weeks, and a tapering dosage for the remaining 4 weeks) (Fig. 10). Serum DNA polymerase activity and HBsAg titers increased during therapy in all 3 patients. These authors concluded that immunosuppressive therapy enhances hepatitis B virus replication. Thus, therapy with corticosteroids may be deleterious in chronic hepatitis B because they increase viral synthesis and block the natural loss of hepatitis B virus markers that occurs spontaneously in 10 to 30% of patients each year (Realdi *et al.*, 1980; Hoofnagle *et al.*, 1981). Similar results of immunosuppression on hepatitis B virus markers (DNA polymerase and serum HBcAg) have been reported by others (Sagnelli *et al.*, 1980; Weller *et al.*, 1982a).

While long-term therapy with corticosteroids is probably deleterious, short-term treatment with immunosuppressive agents may yet have a role in the therapy of chronic hepatitis B. Several groups of investigators have noted that a high proportion of patients withdrawn from cor-

TABLE VIII

Retrospective Studies on Effect of Withdrawal of Corticosteroids on Serum DNA Polymerase and Hepatitis B e Antigen (HBeAg)

Reference	Number of patients withdrawn	Percentage with loss of	
		DNA Polymerase	HBeAg
Scullard *et al.* (1981c)	21	38%	NR[a]
Hoofnagle (1982)	15	47%	47%
Müller *et al.* (1981)	11	NR	46%
Weller *et al.* (1982a)	9	89%	44%
Total	56	51%	46%

[a]NR, Not reported.

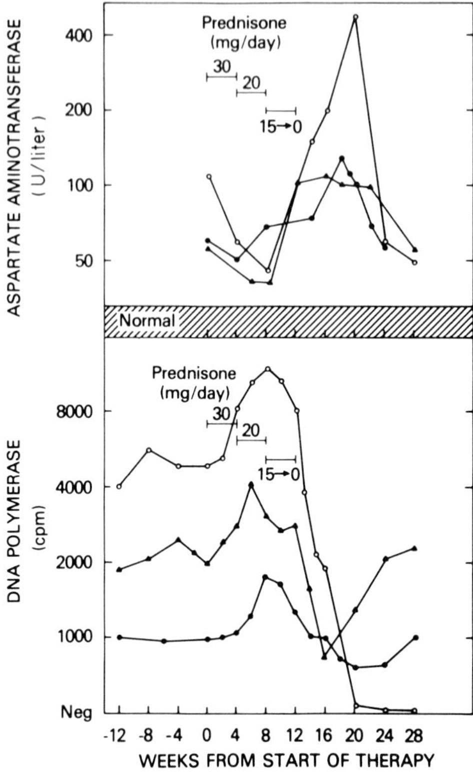

Figure 10. Course of three patients with chronic hepatitis B who were treated with a 12-week course of prednisone in gradually decreasing dosages. Adapted from Scullard *et al.* (1981c).

ticosteroids subsequently undergo a seroconversion from HBeAg to anti-HBe and an improvement in serum aminotransferase activities (Scullard *et al.*, 1981c; Hoofnagle, 1982; Müller *et al.*, 1982a; Weller *et al.*, 1982a) (Table VIII). The frequency of this response to withdrawal of immunosuppression was ~50%, which is far higher than might be expected to occur by chance during the 6-month period of observation in these studies. This increased frequency of seroconversion from HBeAg to anti-HBe after withdrawal of corticosteroids can be explained in several ways.

First, immunosuppressive therapy may retard the occurrence of a spontaneous seroconversion from HBeAg to anti-HBe. When corticosteroids are then discontinued, the excess number of seroconversions represent cases that would have undergone this seroconversion had corticosteroids not been given (a "catch-up" phenomenon). This possibility is supported by the absence of seroconversions that occur in patients while on immunosuppressive therapy.

Second, patients who are chosen to receive immunosuppressive therapy may be those who are most likely to undergo a spontaneous seroconversion from HBeAg to anti-HBe. A period of transient worsening of chronic hepatitis often immediately precedes the seroconversion from HBeAg to anti-HBe (Liaw *et al.*, 1983). For this reason, patients in the process of undergoing a seroconversion from HBeAg to anti-HBe may be placed on corticosteroids in an attempt to treat the sudden worsening of the chronic hepatitis.

Third, the administration and subsequent abrupt withdrawal of immunosuppressive therapy may *induce* seroconversion from HBeAg to anti-HBe. As shown in Fig. 10, the administration of corticosteroids usually causes a decrease in serum aminotransferase activities. Sudden withdrawal of therapy leads to an excacerbation of chronic hepatitis, typically occurring 1 to 2 months afterwards. During this exacerbation, serum levels of HBV DNA and DNA polymerase decrease, sometimes falling into the negative range and remaining negative. This can be followed by a seroconversion from HBeAg to anti-HBe and a clinical remission. These possibilities have led to the suggestion that a short, high-dose course of immunosuppressive therapy might be beneficial for patients with chronic hepatitis B (Hoofnagle, 1982; Chiaramonte *et al.*, 1982). The rationale for this is that abrupt discontinuation of immunosuppressive therapy might lead to an exacerbation of disease (converting the chronic to an acute hepatitis) that would cause an immune clearance of virus and permanent loss of serum hepatitis B virus markers. Indeed, just such an exacerbation followed by remission has been reported to occur in chronic HBsAg carriers treated with intensive chemotherapy for carcinoma or lymphoma (Lightdale *et al.*, 1980; Hoofnagle *et al.*, 1982a). Disturbing, however, are the reports of severe exacerbations and even fulminant hepatitis occurring after discontinuation of immunosuppressive therapy (Galbraith *et al.*, 1975; Hoofnagle *et al.*, 1982a).

These considerations led to the initiation of a randomized, double-blind, placebo-controlled trial of a short, high-dose course of prednisolone in patients with chronic hepatitis B (Hoofnagle *et al.*, 1984a). Fifteen patients were entered into this trial; 10 received prednisolone (60 mg/day for 2 weeks followed by 30 mg/day for 2 weeks followed by abrupt withdrawal) and 5 received placebo tablets. Serum aminotransferase activities decreased in all 10 patients during therapy with prednisolone and then 4 to 10 weeks afterwards rebounded to levels higher than pretreatment values. None of the treated or control patients lost HBV DNA, DNA polymerase, or HBeAg during the subsequent year of follow-up evaluation, and three treated patients suffered a severe and prolonged exacerbation of disease during the rebound period after pred-

TABLE IX
Prospective Studies on the Effect of Short Courses of Corticosteroids on the Course of Chronic Hepatitis B

Reference	Peak dosage of corticosteroid	Duration of treatment	Permanent responses
Scullard *et al.* (1982c)	30 mg Prednisone	12 weeks	0% (0/3)
Rakela *et al.* (1983)	60 mg Prednisolone	6 weeks	0% (0/6)
Hoofnagle *et al.* (1984a)	60 mg Prednisolone	4 weeks	0% (0/10)
Omata *et al.* (1984)	40 mg Prednisolone	8 weeks	20% (2/10)

nisolone withdrawal. Liver biopsy histology revealed worsening of the chronic hepatitis in over half of the treated patients but in none of the controls. A similar lack of permanent seroconversion and remission in disease following purposeful, short-term ("pulse") prednisolone therapy has been reported by others (Table IX) (Nair *et al.*, 1983).

These findings suggest that both long-term and short-term corticosteroid therapy is contraindicated in cases of chronic hepatitis B. However, two groups of investigators have employed a short-course of prednisolone immediately before treatment with antiviral agents (Table X). Perrillo *et al.* (1985) treated patients who had previously not responded to courses of Ara-AMP alone with a 1-month course of prednisolone followed (4 weeks later) with a 1-month course of Ara-AMP. Five of the 11 patients had a permanent loss of serum DNA polymerase activity and HBeAg. Similarly, Omata and co-workers (1984) from Chiba, Japan, treated patients with a variety of schedules including recombinant α interferon, Ara-AMP, prednisolone, and a short course of prednisolone followed by either Ara-AMP or interferon. Permanent loss of hepatitis B virus markers occurred in 6 of 9 (67%) patients treated with prednisolone followed by Ara-AMP and in 3 of 5 (60%) treated with prednisolone followed by interferon. In contrast, none of 15 patients

TABLE X
Short Course of Prednisolone Followed by Antiviral Therapy of Chronic Hepatitis B

Reference	Antiviral agent[a]	Permanent responses
Omata *et al.* (1984)	Ara-AMP	67% (6/9)
Omata *et al.* (1984)	α Interferon	60% (3/5)
Perrillo *et al.* (1985)	Ara-AMP	45% (5/11)

[a]Ara-AMP, Adenine arabinoside monphosphate.

responded to interferon alone; 1 of 10 responded to Ara-AMP alone and 2 of 10 to prednisolone alone. These results suggest that the response rate to antiviral therapy can be increased by inducing an exacerbation of the underlying disease using abrupt withdrawal of immunosuppressive therapy. This intriguing approach to antiviral therapy needs to be evaluated in careful prospective studies.

IV. Conclusions

The therapy of chronic hepatitis B remains controversial and unsatisfactory. In the last several years, advances in understanding the hepatitis B virus and the diseases that it causes have allowed for better and more rational approaches to therapy of this disease. Promising beneficial results have been obtained with a variety of agents including human leukocyte interferon, adenine arabinoside monosphosphate, acyclovir, transfer factor, and immune RNA. Combinations of these agents or use of antiviral chemotherapy after a short course of immunosuppression have become the focus of major attention. Other approaches to therapy that have not been adequately evaluated and have not been discussed in this review include the flavinoid cyanidanol (Conn, 1983), the antiviral agent insoprine (Hadden *et al.*, 1977), and other, less well-studied immunomodulating agents such as thymosin (Goldstein *et al.*, 1981), penicillamine (Stern *et al.*, 1977), Freund's adjuvant (Brozosko *et al.*, 1978), and *Corynebacterium parvum*.

In addition, modifications of currently employed agents may provide more satisfactory and less toxic approaches to treatment, such as the targeting of antiviral agents to the liver by the use of monoclonal antibodies (Shouval *et al.*, 1981) or modified asialoglycoproteins (Ashwell and Steer, 1981). Presently the only satisfactory approach to the control of chronic hepatitis B is its prevention. It is hoped that the hepatitis B vaccine will eventually lead to a decrease in the prevalence of this disease. Until that occurs, the problems of chronic hepatitis B and its long-term consequences are such that major efforts need to continue in developing therapies for this chronic liver disease.

References

Acute Hepatic Failure Study Group (1977). *Ann. Intern. Med.* **86,** 272–277.
Alexander, G. J. M., Hegarty, J. E., Fagan, E., Guarascio, P., Eddleston, A. L. W. F., and Williams, R. (1984). *J. Hepatology* **1,** S3.

Ashwell, G., and Steer, C. J. (1981). *JAMA, J. Am. Med. Assoc.* **246,** 2358–2364.

Ayrosa-Galvao, P.A., and Castro, I. O. (1977). *Ann. N.Y. Acad. Sci.* **284,** 278–283.

Bassendine, M. F., Weller, I. V. D., Murray, A., Summers, J., Thomas, H. C., and Sherlock, S. (1980). *Gut* **21,** A915.

Bassendine, M. F., Chadwick, R. G., Salmerson, J., Shipton, U., Thomas, H. C., and Sherlock, S. (1981). *Gastroenterology* **80,** 1016–1022.

Beasley, R. P., Hwang, L. Y., Lin, C. C., and Chin, C. S. (1981). *Lancet* **2,** 1129–1133.

Bodenheimer, H. C., Schaffner, F., Vernace, S., Hirschman, S. Z., Goldberg, J. D., and Chalmers, T. (1983). *Hepatology* **3,** 936–938.

Bonino, F., Hoyer, B., Nelson, J., Engle, R., Verme, G., and Gerin, J. (1981). *Hepatology* **1,** 386–391.

Bonino, F., Negro, F., Chiaberge, E., and Crivelli, O. (1984). *In* "Viral Hepatitis and Delta Infection" (G. Verme, F. Bonino, and M. Rizzetto, eds.), pp. 337–344. Liss, New York.

Brechot, C., Hadchouel, M., Scotto, J., Degos, F., Charnay, P., Trepo, C., and Tiollais, P. (1981). *Lancet* **2,** 765–768.

Brigden, D., Rosling, A. E., and Woods, N. C. (1982). *Am. J. Med.* "Acyclovir Symposium", pp. 182–185.

Brozosko, W. J., Debski, R., and Derecka, K. (1978). *Lancet* **2,** 311.

Cantell, K., and Hirvonen, S. (1978). *J. Gen. Virol.* **39,** 541–543.

Chadwick, R. G., Bassendine, M. F., Crawford, E. M., Thomas, H. C., and Sherlock, S. (1978). *Br. Med. J.* **2,** 531–533.

Chadwick, R. G., Jain, S., Cohen, B. J., Scott, G. M., Thomas, H. C., and Sherlock, S. (1980). *Scand. J. Gastroenterol.* **15,** 973–978.

Chalopin, J. M., Rifle, G., Turc, J. M., Cortet, P., and Severac, M. (1980). *Br. Med. J.* **1,** 368.

Chiaramonte, M., Floreani, A., Martinez, D. DeLazzari, F., and Naccarato, R. (1982). *Ann. Intern. Med.* **97,** 451–452.

Conn, H. O. (1983). *Hepatology* **3,** 121–123.

Cook, G. C., Mulligan, R., and Sherlock, S. (1971). *Q. J. Med.* **40,** 159–185.

Davis, G. L., and Czaja, A. J. (1981). *J. Clin. Gastroenterol.* **3,** 381–388.

Davis, G. L., Hoofnagle, J. H., and Waggoner, J. G. (1984a). *Gastroenterology* **86,** 230–235.

Davis, G. L., Jicha, J. L., and Hoofnagle, J. H. (1984b). *Gastroenterology* **86,** 1315.

DeCree, J., Verhaegen, H., Decock, W., and Brugmans, J. (1974). *Digestion* **10,** 306.

Denes, A. E., Ebert, J. W., Berquist, K. R., Murphy, B. L., and Maynard, J. E. (1976). *Antimicrob. Agents Chemother.* **10,** 571–572.

Desmyter, J., Ray, M. B., DeGroote, J., Bradburne, A. F., Desmet, V. J., Edy, V. G., Biuiau, A., DeSomer, P., and Mortelmans, J. (1976). *Lancet* **2,** 645–647.

Dienstag, J. L. (1984). *In* "Viral Hepatitis and Liver Diseases" (G. N. Vyas, J. L. Dienstag, and J. H. Hoofnagle, eds.), pp. 135–166. Grune & Stratton, New York.

Dienstag J. L., Stevens, C. E., Bhan, A. K., and Szmuness, W. (1982). *Ann. Intern. Med.* **96,** 575–579.

Dolen, J. G., Carter, W. A., Horoszewicz, J. S., Vladutin, A. L., Leigowitz, A. I., and Nolan, J. P. (1979). *Am. J. Med.* **67,** 127–131.

Dooley, J. S., Davis, G. L., Waggoner, J. G., and Hoofnagle, J. H. (1983). *Hepatology* **3,** 853.

Dooley, J. S., Peters, M., Davis, G. L., and Hoofnagle, J. H. (1984). *In* "Viral Hepatitis and Liver Disease" (G. N. Vyas, J. L. Dienstag, and J. H. Hoofnagle, eds.), p. 662. Grune & Stratton, New York.

Drew, W. L., Blume, M. R., Minter, R., Silverberg, I., and Rosenbaum, E. H. (1973). *Ann. Intern. Med.* **79,** 747–748.

Dupuy, J. M., Frommel, D., and Alagille, D. (1975). *Lancet* **1,** 191–194.

Dusheiko, G. M., DiBisceglie, A., Bowyer, S., Sacks, E., Kew, M. C. (1984). *J. Hepatol.* **1,** 789.

Elion, G. B. (1982). *Am. J. Med.* "Acyclovir Symposium," pp. 7–13.

European Association for the Study of the Liver. (1984). *Gastroenterology* **86**, 1317.

Fattovich, G., Cadrobbi, P., Crivellaro, C., Pornaro, E., Alberti, A., and Realdi, G. (1982). *Digestion* **25**, 131–137.

Fishman, M., and Adler, F. L. (1976). *In* "Immune RNA in Neoplasia" (M. A. Fink, ed.), pp. 53–59. Academic Press, New York.

Friedman, R. M. (1981). "Interferons: A Primer." Academic Press, New York.

Galbraith, R. M., Eddleston, A. L. W. F., Williams, R., Zuckerman, A. J., and Bagshawe, K. D. (1975). *Lancet* 2, 528–530.

Gateau, P., Opolon, P., Nusinovici, V., Ropars, C., and Caroli, J. (1976). *Digestion* **14**, 304–310.

Gocke, D. J. (1971). *N. Engl. J. Med.* **284**, 919–922.

Goeddel, D. V., Yelverton, E., Ullrich, A., Heyneker, H. L., Miozzari, G., Holmes, W., Seeburg, P. H., Dull, T., May, L., Stebbing, N., Crea, R., Maeda, S., McCandliss, R., Sloma, A., Tabor, J. M., Gross, M., Familletti, P. C., and Pestka, S. (1980). *Nature (London)* **287**, 411–416.

Goldstein, A. L., Low, T. L. K., Thurman, G. B., Zata, M. M., Hall, N., Chen, J., Hu, S.-K., Naylor, P. B., and McClure, J. E. (1981). *Recent Progr. Horm. Res.* **37**, 369–415.

Greenberg, H. B., Pollard, R. B., Lutwick, L. I., Gregroy, P. B., Robinson, W. S., and Merigan, T. C. (1976). *N. Engl. J. Med.* **295**, 517–522.

Grob, P. J., Franke, C., Reymond, J. F., and Frei-Wettstein, M. (1975). *Eur. J. Clin. Invest.* **5**, 33–43.

Gutterman, J. U., Fine, S., Quesada, J., Horning, S. J., Levine, J. F., Alexanien, R., Bernhardt, L., Kramer, M., Spiegel, H., Colburn, W., Trown, P., Merigan, T., and Dziewanowski, Z. (1982). *Ann. Intern. Med.* **96**, 549–556.

Hadden, J. W., Lopez, C., O'Reilly, R. J., and Hadden, E. M. (1977). *Ann. N.Y. Acad. Sci.* **284**, 139–152.

Hadziyannis, S. J., Lieberman, H. M., Karvountzis, G. G., and Shafritz, D. A. (1983) *Hepatology* **3**, 656–663.

Helgstrand, E., Eriksson, B., Johnansson, N. G., Lannero, B., Larsson, A., Misiorny, A., Noren, J. O., Sjoberg, B., Stenberg, K., Stening, G., Stridh, S., Oberg, B., Alenius, S., and Philipson, L. (1978). *Science* **201**, 819–821.

Hess, G., Arnold, W., and Meyer zum Büschenfelde, K.-H. (1980). *J. Med. Virol.* **5**, 309–316.

Hirschman, S. Z., and Garfinkel, E. (1978). *Nature (London)* **271**, 681–683.

Hoofnagle, J. H. (1982). *In* "Viral Hepatitis" (W. Szmuness, H. J. Alter, and J. E. Maynard, eds.), pp. 573–583. Franklin Inst. Press, Philadelphia, Pennsylvannia.

Hoofnagle, J. H., and Alter, H. J. (1984). *In* "Viral Hepatitis and Liver Disease" (G. N. Vyas, J. L. Dienstag, and J. H. Hoofnagle, eds.), pp. 97–113. Grune & Stratton, New York.

Hoofnagle, J. H., and Seeff, L. B. (1982). *Progr. Liver Dis.* **7**, 469–479.

Hoofnagle, J. H., Dusheiko, G. M., Seeff, L. B., Jones, E. A., Waggoner, J. G., and Bales, Z. B. (1981). *Ann. Intern. Med.* **94**, 744–748.

Hoofnagle, J. H., Dusheiko, G. M., Schafer, D. F., Jones, E. A., Micetich, K. C., Young, R. C., and Costa, J. (1982a). *Ann. Intern. Med.* **96**, 447–449.

Hoofnagle, J. H., Minuk, G. Y., Dusheiko, G. M., Schafer, D. F., Johnson R., Straus, S. E., Jones, E. A., Gerin, J. L., and Ishak, K. (1982b). *Hepatology* **2**, 784–788.

Hoofnagle, J. H., Davis, G. L., Hanson, R. G., Avigan, M., Peters, M. G., Pappas, S. C., Seeff, L. B., and Jones, E. A. (1984a). *Gastroenterology* **86**, 1324.

Hoofnagle, J. H., Hanson, R. G., Minuk, G. Y., Pappas, S. C., Schafer, D. F., Dusheiko, G. M., Straus, S. E., Popper, H., and Jones, E. A. (1984b). *Gastroenterology* **86**, 150–157.

Hoofnagle, J. H., Davis, G. L., Hanson, R. G., Pappas, S. C., Peters, M. G., Avigan, M. I., Waggoner, J. G., Howard, R., Jones, E. A., and Straus, S. E. (1985). *J. Med. Virol.* **15,** 121–128.

Jain, S., Thomas, H. C., and Sherlock, S. (1977). *Clin. Exp. Immunol.* **30,** 10–15.

Jain, S., Thomas, H. C., Oxford, J. S., and Sherlock, S. (1978). *J. Antimicrob. Chemother.* **4,** 367–373.

Kaplan, P. M., Greenman, R. L., Gerin, J. L., Purcell, R. H., and Robinson, W. S. (1973). *J. Virol.* **12,** 995–1005.

Kato, Y., Nakagawa, H., Kobayashi, K., Hattori, N., and Hatano, K. (1982). *Hepatology* **2,** 789–790.

Kew, M. C., and Seftel, H. C. (1977). *Br. Med. J.* **1,** 904.

Kingham, J. G. C., Ganguly, N. K., Shaari, Z. D., Mendelson, R., McGuire, M. J., Holgate, S. J., Cartwright, T., Scott, G. M., Richards, B. M., and Wright, R. (1978). *Gut* **19,** 91–94.

Kirchner, H. (1984). *Springer Semin. Immunopathol.* **7,** 347–374.

Kohler, P. F., Trembath, J., Merrill, D. A., Singleton, J. W., and Dubois, R. S. (1974). *Clin. Immunol. Immunopathol.* **2,** 465–471.

Krugman, S., Hoofnagle, J. H., Gerety, R. J., Kaplan, P. M., and Gerin, J. L. (1974). *N. Engl. J. Med.* **290,** 1331–1335.

Krugman, S., Overby, L. R., Mushahwar, I. K., Ling, C.-M., Frosner, G. G., and Deinhardt, F. (1979). *N. Engl. J. Med.* **300,** 101–107.

Lam, K. C., Lai, C. L., Ng, R. P., Trepo, C., and Wu, P. C. (1981). *N. Engl. J. Med.* **304,** 380–386.

Lawrence, H. S. (1969). *Adv. Immunol.* **11,** 195–266.

Levin, A. S., and Hahn, T. (1982). *Lancet* **1,** 592–594.

Levin, A. S., Spitter, L. E., and Fudenberg, H. H. (1973). *Annu. Rev. Med.* **24,** 175–208.

Levy, G. A., and Chisari, F. V. (1981). *Springer Semin. Immunopathol.* **3,** 439–459.

Liaw, Y.-F., Chu, C.-M., Huang, J.-J., Lin, D.-Y., and Chang-Chien, C.-S. (1983). *Gastroenterology* **84,** 216–219.

Lightdale, C. J., Idram, H., and Pinsky, C. (1980). *Cancer* **46,** 1117–1122.

Liu, S.-S., Lian, C.-F., Hao, F.-Y., and Zheng, C.-X. (1982). *Lancet* **1,** 197–198.

Lok, A. S. F., Karayiannis, P., Brown, D., Fowler, M. J. F., Monjardino, J., Thomas, H. C., and Sherlock, S. (1983). *Hepatology* **3,** 865.

Lok, A. S. F., Weller, I. V. D., Karayiannis, P., Brown, D., Fowler, J. F., Monjardino, J., Thomas, H. C., and Sherlock, S. (1984). *Liver* **4,** 45–49.

Masi, M., Paolucci, P., Timoncini, C., Iantini, M. P., Leggieri, G., Chiodo, F., and Franceschi, C. (1978). *Arch. Dis. Child.* **53,** 764–765.

Merigan, T. C. (1982). *In* "Viral Hepatitis" (W. Szmuness, H. J. Alter, and J. E. Maynard, eds.), pp. 537–540. Franklin Inst. Press, Philadelphia, Pennsylvania.

Merigan, T. C., Robinson, W. S., and Gregory, P. B. (1980). *Lancet* **1,** 422–423.

Müller, R., Vido, I., and Schmidt, F. W. (1981). *Lancet* **1,** 1323–1324.

Müller, R., Deinhardt, F., Hofschneider, H. P., Schmidt, F. W., Siegert, W., and Vido, I. (1982a). *In* "Viral Hepatitis" (W. Szmuness, H. J. Alter, and J. E. Maynard, eds.), pp. 648–649. Franklin Inst. Press, Philadelphia, Pennsylvania.

Müller, R., Vido, I., and Schmidt, F. W. (1982b). *In* "Viral Hepatitis" (W. Szmuness, H. J. Alter, and J. E. Maynard, eds.), p. 647. Franklin Inst. Press, Philadelphia, Pennsylvania.

Müller, A., Vido, I., and Schmidt, F. W. (1984). *In* "Viral Hepatitis and Liver Disease" (G. N. Vyas, J. L. Dienstag, and J. H. Hoofnagle, eds.), pp. 669–670. Grune & Stratton, New York.

Murray-Lyon, I. M., Stern, R. B., and Williams, R. (1973). *Lancet* **1,** 735–737.

Nair, P., Tong, M. J., Stevenson, D., Roskamp, D., and Boone, C. (1983). *Hepatology* **3**, 877.

Nordenfelt, E., Helgstrand, E., and Öberg, B. (1979). *Acta Pathol. Microbiol. Scand., Sect. B* **87**, 75–76.

Novick, D. M., Lok, A. S. F., and Thomas, H. C. (1984). *J. Hepatol.* **1**, 29–35.

Omata, M., Imazeki, F., Yokosuka, O. , Uchiumi, K. , Mori, J., and Okuda, K. (1983). *Gastroenterology* **84**, 1264.

Omata, M., Yokosuka, O., Imazeki, F., and Okuda, K. (1984). *In* "Viral Hepatitis and Liver Disease" (G. N. Vyas, J. L. Dienstag, and J. H. Hoofnagle, eds.), p. 670. Grune & Stratton, New York.

Par, A., Barna, K., Hollos, I., Kovacs, M., Miszlai, Z. S., Patakjalvi, A., and Javor, T. (1977). *Lancet 1*, 702.

Perrillo, R., Regenstein, F., Bodicky, C., Campbell, C., Sanders, G., and Sunwoo, Y. C. (1985). *Gastroenterology* **88**, 780–786.

Pizza, G., Viza, D., Roda, A., Aldini, R., Roda, E., and Barbara, L. (1979). *N. Engl. J. Med.* **300**, 1332.

Pollard, R. B., Smith, J. L., Neal, A., Gregory, P. B., Merigan, T. C., and Robinson, W. S. (1978). *JAMA, J. Am. Med. Assoc.* **239**, 1648–1650.

Ponzetto, A., Zucca, M., Marcucci, F., Rizzetto, M., Actis, G. C., Bonino, F., and Gioannini, P. (1979). *J. Med. Virol.* **4**, 43–50.

Preiksaitis, J. K., Lank, B., Ng, P. K., Brox, L., LePage, G. S., and Tyrrell, D. L. J. (1981). *J. Infect. Dis.* **144**, 358–364.

Purcell, R. H., Gerin, J. L., London, W. T., Wagner, J., McAuliffe, V. J., Popper, H., Palmer, A. E., Lvorsky, E., Kaplan, P. M., Wong, D. C., and Levy, H. B. (1976). *Lancet* **2**, 757–761.

Rakela, J., Redeker, A. G., and Weliky, B. (1983). *Gastroenterology* **84**, 956–960.

Realdi, E., Alberti, A., Rugge, M., Bortolotti, F., Rigoli, A. M., Tremolada, F., and Ruol, A. (1980). *Gastroenterology* **79**, 195–199.

Reed, W. D., Eddleston, A. L. W. F., Cullens, H., Williams, R., Zuckerman, A. J., Peters, D. K., Williams, D. G., and Maycock, W. D. A. (1973). *Lancet 2*, 1347–1351.

Renoux, G., and Renoux, M. (1972). *J. Immunol.* **109**, 761–765.

Reynolds, T. B. (1980). *Am. J. Med.* **69**, 485–487.

Sacks, S. L., Smith, J. L., Pollard, R. B., Sawhney, V., Mahol, A. S., Gregory, P., Merigan, T. C., and Robinson, W. S. (1979). *JAMA, J. Am. Med. Assoc.* **241**, 28.

Sagnelli, E., Manzillo, G., Maio, G., Pasquale, G., Felaco, F. M., Filippini, P., Izzo, C. M., and Piccinino, F. (1980). *Lancet 2*, 395–397.

Sano, M., Takeuchi, T., Adachi, M., and Ito, K. (1977). *N. Engl. J. Med.* **296**, 53.

Schaeffer, H. J., Beauchamp, L., deMiranda, P., Elion, G. B., Bauer, D. J., and Collins, P. (1978). *Nature (London)* **272**, 583–585.

Schalm, S. W., and Heijtink, R. A. (1982). *Hepatology* **2**, 791–794.

Schalm, S. W., Summerskill, W. H. J., Gitnick, G. L., and Elveback, L. R. (1976). *Gut* **17**, 781–786.

Schalm, S. W., Heijtink, R. A., vanBlankenstein, M., and Vreugdehil, A. (1982). *Hepatology* **2**, 750.

Scullard, G. H., Alberti, A., Wansbrough-Jones, M. H., Howard, C. R., Eddleston, A. L. W. F., Zuckerman, A. J., Cantell, K., and Williams, R. (1979). *J. Clin. Lab. Immunol.* **1**, 277–282.

Scullard, G. H., Andres, L. L., Greenberg, H. B., Smith, J. L., Sawhney, W. K., Neal, E. A., Mahal, A. S., Popper, H., Merigan, T. C., Robinson, W. S., and Gregory, P. B. (1981a). *Hepatology* **1**, 228–232.

Scullard, G. H., Pollard, R. B., Smith, J. L., Sacks, S. L., Gregory, P. B., Robinson, W. S., and Merigan, T. C. (1981b). *J. Infect. Dis.* **143,** 772–783.

Scullard, G. H., Smith, C. I., Merigan, T. C., Robinson, W. X., Gregory, P. B. (1981c). *Gastroenterology* **81,** 987–991.

Scullard, G. H., Greenberg, H. B., Smith, J. L., Gregory, P. B., Merigan, T. C., and Robinson, W. S. (1982). *Hepatology* **2,** 39–49.

Shouval, D., Wands, J. R., Zurawski, V. R., and Shafritz, D. A. (1981). *Hepatology* **1,** 547 (57A).

Shulman, S. T., Howlett, S. A., Hutto, J. H., Ayoub, E. M., and McGuigan, J. E. (1975). *Clin. Res.* **23,** 257A.

Shulman, S. T., Hutto, J. H., Ayoub, E. M., and McGuigan, J. E. (1976). *N. Engl. J. Med.* **195,** 898.

Sidwell, R. W., Huffman, J. H., Khare, C. P., Allen, L. B., Witkowski, J. T., and Robins, R. K. (1972). *Science* **177,** 705–706.

Sidwell, R. W., Huffman, J. H., Campbell, N., and Allen, L. B. (1977). *Ann. N.Y. Acad. Sci.* **284,** 239–246.

Sjogren, M. H., Hoofnagle, J. H., and Gerin, J. L. (1984). *Gastroenterology* **86,** 1341.

Smedley, H., Katrak, M., Sikora, K., and Wheeler, T. (1983). *Br. Med. J.* **286,** 262–264.

Smith, C. I., and Merigan, T. C. (1982). *Prog. Liver Dis.* **7,** 481–494.

Smith, C. I., Kitchen, L. W., Scullard, G. H., Robinson, W. S., Gregory, P. B., and Merigan, T. C. (1982a). *JAMA, J. Am. Med. Assoc.* 247, 2261–2265.

Smith, C. I., Scullard, G. H., Gregory, P. B., Robinson, W. S., and Merigan, T. C. (1982b). *Am. J. Med.* "Acyclovir Symposium," pp. 267–270.

Smith, C. I., Weissberg, J., Bernhardt, L., Merigan, T. C., and Robinson, W. S. (1983). *J. Infect. Dis.* **148,** 907–913.

Stern, R. B., Wilkinson, S. P., Howorth, P. J. N., and Williams, R. (1977). *Gut* **18,** 19–22.

Stewart, W. E., II (1979). "The Interferon System." Springer-Verlag, Berlin.

Stiehm, E. R., Kronenberg, L. H., Rosenblatt, H. M., Bryson, Y., and Merigan, T. C. (1982). *Ann. Intern. Med.* **96,** 80–93.

Straus, S. E., Smith, H. A., Brickman, C., deMiranda, P., McLaren, C., and Keeney, R. E. (1982). *Ann. Intern. Med.* **96,** 265–269.

Summerskill, W. H. J., Korman, M. G., Ammon, H. V., and Baggenstoss, A. H. (1975). *Gut* **16,** 876–883.

Szmuness, W. (1975). *Am. J. Pathol.* **81,** 629–649.

Szmuness, W., Stevens, C. E., Harley, E. J., Zang, E. A., Oleszka, W. R., William, D. C., Sadovsky, R., Morrison, J. M., and Kellner, A. (1980). *N. Engl. J. Med.* **303,** 833–841.

Tabor, E., Gerety, R. J., Smallwood, L. A., and Barker, L. F. (1976). *J. Immunol.* **117,** 2038–2040.

Thienpont, D., Vanparijs, O. F. J., Raeymaekers, A. H. M., Vandenberk, J., Demoen, P. J. A., Allewijn, F. T. N., Marsboom, R. P. H., Niemegeers, C. J. E., Schellekens, K. H. L., and Janssen, P. A. J. (1966). *Nature (London)* **20,** 1084–1086.

Thomas, H. C., and Lok, A. S. F. (1983). *In* "Viral Hepatitis and Delta Infection" (G. Verme, F. Bonino, and M. Rizzetto, eds.), pp. 379–393. Liss, New York.

Tiollais, P., Charnay, P., and Vyas, G. N. (1981). *Science* **213,** 406–411.

Tong, M. J., Nystrom, J. S., Redeker, A. G., and Marshall, G. J. (1976). *N. Engl. J. Med.* **295,** 209–211.

Trepo, C., Hantz, O., Ouzan, D. Chossegros, P., Chevallier, P., Berthillon, P., and Brette, R. (1984). *Hepatology* **4,** 1055.

Tripodi, D., Parks, L. C., and Brugmans, J. (1973). *N. Engl. J. Med.* **289,** 354–357.

Trown, P. W., Kramer, M. J., Dennin, R. A., Jr., Connell, E. V., Palleroni, A. V., Quesada, J., Gutterman, J. U. (1983). *Lancet 1*, 81–84.

Van Dyke, R. B., Conner, J. D., Wyborny, C., Hintz, M., and Keeney, R. E. (1982). *Am. J. Med.* "Acyclovir Symposium," pp. 172–175.

VanEtta, L., Brown, J., Mastri, A., and Wilson, T. (1981). *JAMA, J. Am. Med. Assoc.* **246**, 1703–1705.

Verhaegen, H., DeCree, J., DeCock, W., and Vergruggen, F. (1977). *Clin. Exp. Immunol.* **27**, 313–318.

Vyas, G. N., Ibrahim, A. B., Rao, K. R., and Likhite, V. (1974). *Nature (London)* **247**, 377–378.

Weimar, W., Heijtink, R. A., Schalm, S. W., van Blankentstein, M., Schellekens, H., Masurel, N., Edy, V. G., Billiau, A., and DeSomer, P. (1977). *Lancet 2*, 1282.

Weimar, W., Heijtink, R. A., Schalm, S. W., and Schellekens, H. (1979). *Eur. J. Clin. Invest.* **9**, 151–154.

Weimar, W., Heijtink, R. A., TenKate, F. J. P., Schalm, S. W., Masurel, N., and Schellekens, H. (1980). *Lancet 1*, 336–338.

Weller, I. V. D., Bassendine, M. R., Murray, A. K., Summers, J., Thomas, H. C., and Sherlock, S. (1980). *Gastroenterology* **79**, 1129.

Weller, I. V. D., Bassendine, M. F., Craxi, A., Fowler, M. J. F., Monjardino, J., Thomas, H. C., and Sherlock, S. (1982a). *Gut* **23**, 717–723.

Weller, I. V. D., Bassendine, M. F., Murray, A. K., Thomas, H. C., and Sherlock, S. (1982b). *Gut* **23**, 650–655.

Weller, I. V. D., Carreno, V., Fowler, M. J. F., Monjardino, J., Makinen, D., Thomas, H. C., and Sherlock, S. (1982c). *Lancet 1*, 273.

Weller, I. V. D., Fowler, M. J. F., Monjardino, J., Carreno, V., Thomas, H. C., and Sherlock, S. (1982d). *Philos. Trans. R. Soc. London, Ser. B.* **299**, 125–144.

Whitley, R. J., Soong, S.-J., Dolin, R., Galasso, G. J., Ch'ien, L. T., Alford, C. A., and the Collaborative Study Group (1977). *N. Engl. J. Med.* **297**, 289–294.

Wright, E. C., Seeff, L. B., Berk, P. D., Jones, E. A., and Plotz, P. H. (1977). *Gastroenterology* **73**, 1422–1430.

Chapter 10

Immunopathogenesis of Acute and Chronic Hepatitis B

R. JAMES KLINGENSTEIN* AND JULES L. DIENSTAG

Gastroenterology Unit (Medical Services)
Massachusetts General Hospital
and the Department of Medicine
Harvard Medical School
Boston, Massachusetts

I. Introduction

In most clinically apparent cases of hepatitis B virus (HBV) infection, hepatocellular necrosis is followed by virus elimination and complete recovery. A small proportion of infected persons fail to clear the virus from their hepatocytes, however, permitting continued viral replication. These patients exhibit a spectrum of chronic liver diseases ranging from chronic active hepatitis (CAH) with severe liver inflammation to asymptomatic chronic hepatitis B infection with normal or near-normal hepatic morphology. The existence of the asymptomatic chronic carrier state suggests that HBV is not a directly cytopathic agent; rather, liver cell necrosis may be due to an attack by the host's immune system on virally altered hepatocytes (Edgington and Chisari, 1975), a notion fostered by the close proximity of lymphoid cells to necrotic hepatocytes in acute

*Present address: Newton Wellesley Hospital, Newton, Massachusetts.

Copyright © 1985 by Academic Press, Inc.
All rights of reproduction in any form reserved.
ISBN 0-12-280672-7

and chronic hepatitis B. This hypothesis has immense appeal, and has generated many investigations designed to prove its validity. Although much has been learned, it has been difficult to verify the hypothesis. Nevertheless, available evidence provides substantial support for a contribution by the host immune system to the varied outcomes of acute HBV infection.

II. Liver Membrane Antigens

Necrosis of liver cells, regardless of the initiating process, is effected by disruption of the cell plasma membrane. Because of this fact, there has been increasing emphasis on the role of alterations of cell-surface membranes in hepatocellular disease, and especially on characterization of liver cell-surface antigens. Attention has thus been focused on localization of these antigens in hepatocytes during HBV infections. Hepatitis B surface antigen (HBsAg) has received the most attention, because development of antibody (anti-HBs) to it during acute infection coincides with resolution of disease. Hepatitis B surface antigen can be demonstrated most easily on hepatocytes from immunosuppressed patients with hepatitis B, presumably because of restricted elimination of these infected hepatocytes (Ray et al., 1976; Gudat and Bianchi, 1977). During ongoing necrosis of infected hepatocytes, virus antigen localization on cells is less clear. In acute hepatitis B, expression of HBsAg on the hepatocyte surface has been found in single cell suspensions (Alberti et al., 1976) but not in frozen sections (Ray et al., 1976). Conversely, in HBV-induced CAH, HBsAg has been demonstrated on the surface of biopsy-derived hepatocytes in frozen sections (Ray et al., 1976) but not in single cell suspensions (Alberti et al., 1976). There is general agreement, however, that HBsAg can be expressed on the liver cell surface, at least under some conditions, and that it potentially might serve as a target for immunological attack.

In contrast, intracytoplasmic HBsAg is not thought to play a pathogenetic role in hepatic injury, because the amounts found are inversely proportional to the degree of liver damage (Ray et al., 1976; Nowoslawski et al., 1975). Hepatitis B core antigen (HBcAg), although usually detected primarily in liver cell nuclei, has also been proposed as a target antigen (Edgington and Chisari, 1975) and has been seen in close proximity to (Ray et al., 1976) and on the hepatocyte membrane. The importance of HBcAg as a liver cell target antigen seemed improbable because development of antibody to HBcAg (anti-HBc) appears to serve only as a marker of HBV infection and to provide no detectable antiviral function. In addition, electron microscopic studies have localized HBcAg to the sub-membranous region of hepatocytic cytoplasm rather than to the surface membrane (Gudat and Bianchi, 1977). Newer information, however, suggested that HBcAg is expressed on the surface of the hepatocyte but is obscured by IgG (Trevisan *et al.*, 1982), and may be the target antigen against which immunological attack occurs.

Among the various and conflicting schemes of tissue localization of HBV antigens in hepatocytes, unanimity does exist for the observation that chronic active hepatitis is associated with nuclear localization of HBcAg in the hepatocyte (Ray *et al.*, 1976; Alberti *et al.*, 1976; Bianchi and Gudat, 1979; Trevisan *et al.*, 1979; Realdi *et al.*, 1979). Alberti *et al.* (1976) detected membrane-bound IgG on liver cells in such cases of chronic active hepatitis; in subsequent studies they found that anti-HBc could be eluted from the hepatocyte membrane and that surface membrane expression of HBcAg increased after removal of surface-bound IgG by elution (Trevisan *et al.*, 1982). These findings suggest that surface membrane IgG is directed against HBcAg on the membrane surface.

Furthermore, Eddleston and his colleagues (Eddleston *et al.*, 1982; Mieli-Vergani *et al.*, 1982; Mondelli *et al.*, 1982; Naumov *et al.*, 1984) published a series of papers in which peripheral blood lymphocyte cytotoxicity in patients with chronic HBV infection was measured against their autologous hepatocytes isolated from biopsy specimens. They found that in chronic hepatitis B, cytotoxicity was increased and confined primarily to the purified T cell-enriched fractions; that T-cell cytotoxicity was restricted to HBeAg-positive patients, that is, those with viral replication; that cytotoxicity could be blocked by the addition of anti-HBc, but not HBsAg, anti-HBs, liver-specific protein (LSP), or aggregated IgG; that T-cell cytotoxicity in this sytem occurred in patients with HBcAg detectable in liver cells, and that cytotoxicity was accompanied by a reduction in HBcAg-expressing but not HBsAg-expressing hepatocytes. As control targets, these investigators used autologous fibroblasts, against which they found only low-level T-cell cytotoxicity that was not blocked by addition of exogenous anti-HBc (Mondelli *et al.*, 1982). These findings suggested that cytolytic T cells from patients with HBsAg-positive chronic active hepatitis are directed against HBcAg on the membrane surface. These observations led to the hypothesis that in hepatocytes with nuclear expression of HBcAg and active virus replication, HBcAg is also expressed at the cell membrane. In this scheme, liver cells with nuclear HBcAg from patients with chronic active hepatitis would also be the ones likely to have membrane HBcAg and to be susceptible to attack by cytolytic T cells. Thus, competition between anti-HBc and cytolytic T cells at the cell-surface membrane could determine the extent of hepatocytolysis, and further that anti-HBc bound to hepatocytes via membrane HBcAg could actually modulate the expression by the cell of cytolytic cell-inviting HBcAg. Such modulation of target cell membrane antigen expression by antibody has been described in other viral infections in which persistent infection occurs despite an immune response to viral antigens.

Binding of IgG anti-HBc to hepatocyte membranes, however, is insufficient to explain the pathogenesis of liver injury in HBV-induced liver disease, because such binding, which reflects virus replication, can be detected even in patients with minimal or no histological liver damage. Similarly, T-cell cytotoxicity for autologous hepatocytes was observed not only in patients with chronic active hepatitis B but also in patients with chronic persistent hepatitis B and in those with near-normal liver morphology. No increased cytotoxicity was found in 50% of patients with HBsAg-positive chronic active hepatitis with cirrhosis (Mondelli *et al.*, 1982). Moreover, the presence of anti-HBc in high titer is universal in acute and chronic HBV infection, and the concept of modulation of hepatocytolysis by anti-HBc would require a qualitative or quantitative distinction in anti-HBc between cases with minimal and substantial liver injury. No such distinction has ever been supported by laboratory observation. The importance of deposition of IgG in chronic active hepatitis B is also rendered questionable by recent reports that fail to uphold the specificity of the association between surface IgG and chronic active hepatitis B (Realdi *et al.*, 1979; Meliconi *et al.*, 1983).

The evidence for virus-specific T-cell cytotoxicity directed against HBcAg expressed on the hepatocyte membrane is not conclusive; there are both clinical and laboratory observations that this hypothesis cannot accommodate, and the supporting *in vitro* cytotoxicity studies, all originating from a single laboratory, have not been confirmed. On the other hand, this hypothesis merits serious consideration. If indeed HBcAg is the target for cytolytic T cells, other factors, such as target cell properties and immunoregulatory function, may explain differences in outcomes among those infected with HBV.

Endogenous liver antigens may also serve as targets of immunologic attack. Meyer zum Buschenfelde and Miescher (1972) described two antigens obtained from supernatants of human liver homogenates fractionated by column chromatography. One protein, designated LP-1, was shown to be a low-density macromolecular lipoprotein on the hepatocyte membrane, whereas LP-2 was derived from the cytoplasm. Studies suggested that these proteins were organ specific but not species specific, that is, human liver-specific protein (LSP, which, through common usage, usually refers to LP-1) demonstrated partial antigenic cross-reactivity with LSP prepared from other mammalian species (Hopf *et al.*,

1974). Studies have shown that LSP preparations are far more complex than originally suspected. They consist of phospholipids, triglycerides, and multiple protein-containing components (McFarlane *et al.*, 1977), and include at least two liver-specific determinants, one of which is species cross-reactive and the other human specific (Hutteroth and Meyer zum Buschenfelde, 1978). In addition, another liver membrane antigen (LMAg) has been identified that is also species nonspecific but distinct from LSP.

Immunologically mediated attack against self-antigens on hepatocytes is an inviting explanation for liver diseases such as "lupoid hepatitis" that are thought to be caused by autoimmune reactions. Potentially, however, attack against these antigens may result from infection with hepatitis B virus. Eddleston and Williams (1974) postulated that T cells recognizing viral determinants activate B cells whose progeny synthesize anti-LSP, leading to a state of continuous autoimmunity when a defect in anti-HBs production allows persistent viral replication. While there is little evidence to support this concept, the possibility that the immune response to liver cell membrane antigens plays a role in liver injury was explored by Meyer zum Buschenfelde and associates (1972), who injected rabbits repeatedly over many months with LSP in complete Freund's adjuvant. Eventually, a liver lesion characterized by portal tract infiltration and piecemeal necrosis developed in many of the animals, and the appearance of this histological alteration appeared to correlate with delayed hypersensitivity to LSP (Meyer zum Buschenfelde and Hopf, 1974). All the rabbits produced antibodies to LP-2 (not to LP-1), and those in which CAH-like lesions developed, were shown to have antibodies coating their hepatocytes. Mononuclear infiltrations of kidneys and lungs, however, also developed in the rabbits, and these findings suggested, as do more recent studies (Behrens and Paronetto, 1979; Behrens *et al.*, 1979), that LSP is not truly specific for liver. Nevertheless, these findings do suggest that sensitization to hepatocyte membrane antigens may produce hepatic damage. Additional studies are required to characterize truly liver-specific membrane proteins and to evaluate their role in liver injury.

III. Humoral Immunity

Initial attempts to detect antibodies against liver-specific antigens in sera from patients with hepatitis proved difficult. Antibodies to LP-2 were detected by passive hemagglutination in a few cases, but only in low titers (Meyer zum Buschenfelde, 1968). Then, Hopf *et al.* (1975) examined suspensions of viable human hepatocytes by direct immunofluorescence for the presence of surface-bound IgG, and found positive hepatocyte membrane staining in 5 of 6 untreated patients with chronic hepatitis and in 2 of 27 others on immunosuppressive therapy. Similar results were obtained in HBsAg-positive and HBsAg-negative patients. Patients with acute hepatitis A, chronic persistent hepatitis, and other liver diseases did not have detectable antibodies to hepatocyte membranes, and thus served as negative controls. In addition, the pattern of fluorescence staining on hepatocyte surface membranes was linear in HBsAg-negative patients but granular [this is the antibody reported subsequently to be anti-HBc (Trevisan *et al.*, 1982), as discussed above] in HBsAg-positive cases (Hopf *et al.*, 1976a).

This called to mind a similar dichotomy of patterns seen in glomerulonephritis, in which linear staining is thought to represent an autoantibody against glomerular basement membrane and granular-staining immune complex deposition. By analogy to glomerulonephritis, therefore, an autoantibody might be present in lupoid hepatitis, while immune complexes might produce the granular pattern in HBsAg-positive CAH. These findings were not confirmed by Alberti *et al.* (1976), who found granular IgG deposits on the hepatocellular surface of both HBsAg-positive and -negative CAH patients. Moreover, whether the granular patterns observed in these studies were actually due to deposition of immune complexes was not determined. Alternatively, granular fluorescence patterns might have been produced by redistribution of cell membrane proteins subsequent to cross-linking by antibody (patching). Another possibility, that fluoresceinated IgG might have bound to hepatocyte Fc receptors (Hopf *et al.*, 1976b) in a nonspecific fashion, was not excluded by the use of $F(ab')_2$ reagents in these studies. Moreover, even if immune complexes do bind to hepatocytes in CAH, their pathogenetic importance is questionable. Liver cell membrane-bound immune complexes have been demonstrated as well in rheumatoid arthritis, systemic lupus erythematosus, mixed cryoglobulinemia, and Sjogren's syndrome in the absence of liver damage (Realdi *et al.*, 1979).

Hopf *et al.* (1976a) also detected an antibody in the serum of patients with HBsAg-negative chronic hepatitis that bound in a linear pattern to membranes of isolated rabbit hepatocytes. This putative liver membrane autoantibody (LMA), directed against LMAg, could be adsorbed from serum by preparations of LSP but not by homogenates of human nonhepatic tissues (Hopf *et al.*, 1976a; Tage-Jensen *et al.*, 1977), and appeared to be absent in HBsAg-positive CAH. The two distinct immunofluorescence patterns on hepatocytes and the presence of LMA only in HBsAg-negative chronic hepatitis suggested an immunological distinction between HBsAg-negative and -positive cases. That hepatocyte-bound immunoglobulins are actually important in producing cell damage, although suggested in the case of HBV-induced disease (see above), has never been shown definitively.

With the subsequent development of a sensitive radioimmunoassay for anti-LSP, investigators found that unlike LMA, anti-LSP was detected in almost all patients with acute hepatitis and untreated CAH (both HBsAg-positive and HBsAg-negative) and also in patients with chronic persistent hepatitis (CPH) but at lower levels (Jensen *et al.*, 1978; Kakumu *et al.*, 1979). Jensen *et al.* (1978) postulated that anti-LSP might participate in the final common pathway of liver cell damage in both HBsAg-negative and HBsAg-positive liver injury. Alternatively, however, these observations might represent a humoral immune response to antigens liberated by hepatocyte necrosis that played no pathogenetic role in liver injury (Dienstag and Isselbacher, 1978).

Evidence suggesting that LSP and LMAg are distinct (Meyer zum Buschenfelde *et al.*, 1979) and that anti-LSP develops in both HBsAg-positive and -negative CAH is increasing, while LMA occurs mainly in patients with HBsAg-negative CAH. Still, the significance of these two liver antigens and the concept of liver-specific antigens remain controversial. Although LSP is purported to be liver specific, it is labile and therefore prepared under conditions that leave it contaminated with other large and/or hydrophobic hepatocellular molecules. In addition, Behrens and Paronetto (1979), comparing LSP and LP-2 with similarly prepared kidney tissue analogs KSP and KP-2, found the characteristics of the liver and kidney preparations to be virtually identical. Furthermore, when they examined sera from patients with CAH for the presence of antibodies to these antigens, they found that sera were able to induce antibody-dependent cellular cytotoxicity (ADCC) against erythrocytes coated with one of the kidney antigens as well as those coated with either LSP or LP-2 (Behrens *et al.*, 1979). They concluded that LSP and LP-2 are not liver specific, and that antibodies in sera of patients with CAH detect liver cell membrane antigens sharing common determinants with kidney cells. Clarification of the liver specificity of so-called liver-specific membrane proteins and their role in the pathogenesis of liver cell injury will require additional purification and characterization of liver membrane components.

Potential Immunopathological Role for Humoral Immunity

There are several possible mechanisms whereby humoral immunity to viral and cell surface antigens might damage hepatocytes during hepatitis B virus infections. One is by initiating complement-mediated cytolysis. This possibility is supported by the finding that fractional catabolic rates of C1q (Potter *et al.*, 1980) and C3 (Thomas *et al.*, 1979) are elevated in HBsAg-positive CAH but not in HBsAg-negative cases. However, Paronetto *et al.* (1973) studied 13 patients with CAH, both HBsAg-positive and -negative, and found that their sera could not mediate cytotoxicity when mixed with autologous hepatocytes and complement, despite the fact that the patients' sera, but not normal sera, bound to hepatocytes derived from patients with CAH. Therefore, the increase in complement turnover in HBsAg-positive CAH seemed most consistent with complement activation by circulating immune complexes rather than by liver-bound antibody. Further evidence against a cytotoxic role for antibodies recognizing liver cell surface antigens derives from clinical observations. There are reports of both HBsAg-positive and -negative hepatitis occurring in patients with hypogammaglobulinemia (Tong *et al.*, 1977; Solley *et al.*, 1979). Furthermore, the administration of anti-HBs to patients with HBsAg-positive CAH has not resulted in increased hepatocellular necrosis (Kohler *et al.*, 1974; Reed *et al.*, 1973).

Tissue deposition of immune complexes is a second potential mechanism whereby a product of humoral immunity could mediate hepatic damage during HBV infections. Circulating immune complexes can be detected with several different assays in a large proportion of patients with both HBsAg-positive and HBsAg-negative hepatitis (Thomas *et al.*, 1978). In HBsAg-positive acute and chronic hepatitis, serum has been shown to contain cryoprecipitable material that includes immunoglobulin, HBsAg, and complement components (Wands *et al.*, 1975a; McIntosh *et al.*, 1976). In some patients these complexes deposit in extrahepatic tissues and cause a variety of immune complex-mediated syndromes (Dienstag, 1981). Almeida and Waterson (1969) noted differences in HBsAg–anti-HBs complexes detected by electron microscopy in liver biopsy homogenates from patients with different clinical expressions of HBV infection. Fulminant hepatitis was reported to be associated with complexes in antibody excess, chronic active hepatitis with complexes in antigen excess, and asymptomatic chronic HBV carriage with HBsAg in the absence of antibody. Based on a correlation between degree of liver injury and quantity of immune complexes in serum, they proposed that the pathogenesis of hepatocellular necrosis in patients with HBV infection was similar to the vascular injury mediated by immune complex deposition in serum sickness. Similarly, Nowoslawski *et al.* (1975) reported a correlation between the intensity of liver cell necrosis and the quantity of intrahepatic HBsAg-containing immune complexes, and suggested a role for these complexes in the pathogenesis of hepatitis B-induced liver damage.

Abundant evidence, however, challenges the concept of a pathogenetic role for circulating immune complexes in liver injury, whether or not associated with HBV infection. In experimental models of acute and chronic immune complex disease, liver disease is distinctly absent as a component of the systemic illness. Furthermore, even when antigen–antibody complexes are injected directly into the portal vein of experimental animals, the hepatic lesion that results is one of ischemic hepatocellular necrosis (Sabesin, 1963), unrelated to the histologic lesion of acute or chronic hepatitis. Moreover, circulating immune complexes can be detected in most diseases of the liver (Thomas *et al.*, 1978) and probably *result from* rather than *cause* liver disease. Thus if the normal phagocytic capacity of Kupffer cells is impaired or overwhelmed, gut-derived immune complexes that should have been cleared in the liver could gain access to the systemic circulation. The findings of Almeida and Waterson (1969) and Nowoslawski *et al.* (1975) notwithstanding, other studies have shown no correlation between the presence or quantity of circulating immune complexes and the presence or severity of liver disease in patients with HBV infection (Prince and Trepo, 1971). In this regard, asymptomatic HBsAg carriers with normal liver morphology have been shown to harbor circulating immune complexes. Therefore, hepatocyte-bound immune complexes appear merely to reflect binding of IgG to Fc receptors on the hepatocyte surface.

Others have suggested that *intracellular,* rather than circulating, immune complexes may participate in the pathogenesis of hepatitis B-induced liver injury. Gerber *et al.* (1976) found that in CAH, but not in acute hepatitis, those nuclei that contained HBcAg also contained IgG. That these nuclei could also fix complement *in vitro* reinforced the authors' contention that the intranuclear IgG was complexed to antigen. These findings, however, defy simple interpretation, because circulating IgG would not be expected to penetrate intact hepatocyte membranes. Conceivably, circulating anti-HBc might enter membranes rendered penetrable by primary hepatocytolytic mechanisms, and thus gain entry to the nucleus where HBcAg resides. Alternatively, there is evidence that IgG can penetrate viable human peripheral blood mononuclear cells via Fc receptors, and perhaps damage the cells (Alarcon-Segovia *et al.*, 1978, 1979). Theoretically, IgG molecules could penetrate viable hepatocytes in the same way via Fc receptors on the hepatocyte membrane (Hopf *et al.*, 1976a). Still another possibility is that hepatocytes might take up circulating intact immune complexes (Hopf *et al.*, 1981), in which case the intranuclear IgG might have been bound to antigens other than HBcAg; however, the intranuclear rather than intracytoplasmic location of the complexes is inconsistent with this possibility. On balance, it seems doubtful that intranuclear HBcAg–anti-HBc complexes in HBsAg-positive CAH are of primary importance in cell injury.

A third mechanism whereby humoral immunity could contribute to hepatocyte injury in HBV infection is by priming target cells for attack by antibody-dependent cellular cytotoxicity (ADCC), mediated by Fc receptor-bearing lymphocytes lacking T- and B-cell markers and known as killer or K cells (but also by polymorphonuclear leukocytes, monocytes, and perhaps some T cells). This cytotoxic effector mechanism will be discussed in the following section (Section IV).

IV. Cellular Immunity

A. Lymphocyte Sensitization

The leukocyte migration test was used early in the search for evidence of cell-mediated immunity to hepatocellular membrane antigens in hepatitis. In this test, peripheral blood lymphocytes are mixed with an antigen and assayed for release of leukocyte migration inhibitory factor (LIF), a lymphokine released preferentially by those T cells that presumably have been presensitized to the antigen *in vivo*. Initially, a crude extract of homogenized normal human liver was used as the test antigen, and conflicting findings emerged; both inhibition and stimulation of migration were detected in leukocytes from patients with CAH compared to normal controls (Bacon *et al.*, 1972; Smith *et al.*, 1972). Because stimulation may have resulted from suboptimal antigen preparation or concentration, Miller *et al.* (1972) prepared LP-1 for further experiments by the method of Meyer zum Buschenfelde. Lymphocytes from 11 of 16 patients with CAH inhibited leukocyte migration after exposure to LP-1, while only 1 showed stimulation; however, one-half of the patients were receiving prednisone, which was subsequently shown to diminish migration inhibition (Lee *et al.*, 1975). This confusion carried over into studies of lymphokine elaboration in the presence of LSP when testing for HBsAg became available, and the behavior of antigen-positive and -negative cases was found to be similar (Lee *et al.*, 1975).

Testing for cellular immunity to HBsAg in a variety of HBsAg-positive patients demonstrated release of macrophage migration inhibitory factor (Howlett and McGuigan, 1975), but conflicting results appeared and were interpreted as evidence for and against a role for antiviral cellular immunity in HBV infection (Dudley *et al.*, 1972b; deMoura *et al.*, 1975; Ito *et al.*, 1972). Admittedly, however, the antigen preparations used in these studies were poorly characterized. Other groups addressed the same issue by attempting to measure liver or virus antigen-specific transformation of lymphocytes from patients with hepatitis B. Ortona *et al.* (1979) demonstrated blastogenesis in 8 of 10 HBsAg-positive and in 12 of 15 HBsAg-negative CAH patients when their lymphocytes were exposed to rabbit LSP. Tong *et al.* (1975) studied lymphocyte proliferation to purified HBsAg in HBsAg-positive patients, and found that proliferative responses were lower in CAH than in acute disease but greater than in patients with CPH or chronic carriage of HBsAg; another group agreed that in patients recovering from acute hepatitis B, lymphocyte proliferation to HBsAg developed (Yeung-Laiwah *et al.*, 1973). These studies suggested lymphocyte sensitization to hepatocyte and viral antigens in patients with HBV infection; however, the assays used relied on indirect indicators of cell-mediated immunity, namely detection of lymphokine release or lymphocyte stimulation. Furthermore, these results have been difficult to reproduce.

B. Lymphocyte Effector Function

This uncertainty and the imprecision of these methods fostered interest in measuring *in vitro* cellular cytotoxicity by peripheral blood lymphocytes as a more meaningful reflection of interactions between effector lymphocytes and target hepatocytes. A variety of target cells has been used, because of the limited availability and viability of autologous human hepatocytes. The first target cells used in these studies were rabbit hepatocytes. Thomson *et al.* (1974) found that lymphocytes from 20 of 22 patients with CAH were significantly more cytotoxic for isolated rabbit hepatocytes than those from healthy controls or patients with other chronic liver diseases. Eighteen of the patients were receiving immunosuppressive agents, and the 2 without enhanced killing were from this group. The HBsAg status of the patients was not determined. When blocking studies were performed to determine the specificity of this reaction, both human and rabbit LSP preparations were shown to inhibit cytotoxicity markedly. In contrast, a human kidney protein fraction prepared in a manner identical to that for LSP failed to inhibit cytotoxicity, suggesting that LSP was the specific target of the cytotoxic cells. Moreover, antibodies to LSP elicited in guinea pigs also blocked the reaction. These antibodies were shown by direct immunofluorescence to bind to the target cells, but an important immunofluorescence control, normal guinea pig serum, was not used to rule out nonspecific blocking by cross-reacting antibodies. These observations are consistent with antibody-independent cell-mediated killing, with LSP producing blockade by binding to lymphocyte surface receptors for antigen, and with anti-LSP covering antigenic sites on the target cell surfaces to prevent interaction with lymphocytes.

In a subsequent report from the same group, Cochrane *et al.* (1976) measured cytotoxicity of lymphocyte subpopulations. Cells from 12 of 17 patients with CAH (4 were HBsAg positive) were cytotoxic for rabbit hepatocytes; preparations enriched for non-T cells were cytotoxic in all 12 cases, whereas preparations enriched for T cells were cytotoxic in only 1 case. HBsAg-positive and HBsAg-negative cases reacted similarly. In 6 patients, the addition of aggregated IgG significantly reduced cytotoxicity, presumably by blocking Fc receptors on K cells. Thus, the authors concluded that the effector cell was a K cell mediating an ADCC reaction directed against antibody-coated liver-specific membrane lipoprotein on the target cell surface. The methods these investigators used to isolate lymphocyte populations are controversial, however, and there is no evidence to support their supposition that antibody might have been secreted by B lymphocytes or that immune complexes passively transferred on Fc receptor-positive cells might have dissociated and bound to the target cells. Moreover, had the potential for ADCC been present, the added anti-LSP would have been expected to enhance rather than inhibit cytotoxicity. And the ability of lymphocyte-inhibiting factors that may be liberated from the liver during homogenization (Schumacher *et al.*, 1974) to modulate cellular immune reactions in a nonspecific manner might explain the successful "blocking" by LSP of rabbit hepatocyte injury by effector cells.

Wands *et al.* (1975b) used Chang cells, a purported liver cell line derived from normal human liver (Chang, 1954), as target cells in studies of spontaneous and mitogen-induced cell-mediated cytotoxicity. Increased cytotoxicity was found in patients with acute and chronic active, but not chronic persistent, hepatitis. Most of the patients were positive for HBsAg, although asymptomatic chronic carriers of HBsAg were not examined. In similar studies, Kakumu *et al.* (1978b) also found enhanced cell-mediated cytotoxicity by lymphocytes from patients with CAH for Chang cell targets, and undertook studies in which the responsible effector cell was characterized as nonmonocyte, non-T, and complement receptor-positive; again, cytotoxicity was diminished by addition of LSP or complexed IgG (Kakumu *et al.*, 1978a). While these workers also concluded they were observing ADCC, questions raised by the absence of antibodies to target cells and the ability of LSP to inhibit cytotoxicity were not answered. The latter point is particularly important, because most Chang cells available today lack LSP on their surface membrane (Mutchnik *et al.*, 1978). Moreover, currently available Chang cells have chromosomal and isoenzyme features not of liver cells but of HeLa cells (Nelson-Rees and Flandermeyer, 1976; Lavappa *et al.*, 1976), and Vierling *et al.* (1977) demonstrated that cytotoxicity by lymphocytes from patients with chronic liver disease for Chang cells was paralleled by that for EL-4 mouse sarcoma cells. Anti–Chang cell cytotoxicity thus appears not to have been directed against liver antigens but rather to reflect spontaneous cell-mediated cytotoxicity (SCMC), that is, nonspecific cytolysis directed against tumor and other antigen-modified cells that can be mediated by macrophages, granulocytes, and natural killer (NK) lymphocytes.

The demonstration by Hopf *et al.* (1975, 1976b) of IgG bound to the surface membrane of hepatocytes from patients with CAH suggests that ADCC might mediate hepatic injury in this disease. This concept was reinforced by Kawanishi and MacDermott (1979), who found that sera from patients with HBsAg-positive and -negative CAH, but not CPH or normals, could support ADCC by normal human lymphocytes against rabbit hepatocytes. Another group suggested that the monocyte/macrophage might mediate hepatic injury. Using avian erythrocytes coated with LSP as target cells, Vogten *et al.* (1978) found that 50% of the patients studied with CAH had cytotoxic lymphocytes, compared to 5% of healthy controls. Cytotoxicity was abolished by depletion of monocytes, conflicting with the finding of Kakumu *et al.* (1978b) that depletion of monocytes did not diminish cytotoxicity. As in previous studies, cytotoxicity was diminished by LSP, anti-LSP, and aggregated IgG, which again made identification of the mechanism of cytotoxicity difficult to discern. Recruited and activated macrophages may release proteolytic enzymes that can damage hepatic parenchymal cells, which might account for the findings in this study. Alternatively, these findings may represent another demonstration of enhanced SCMC.

Other groups prepared target cells by coupling HBsAg to their surfaces. Alberti *et al.* (1977) studied cell-mediated cytotoxicity against HBsAg-coated chicken red blood cells. They found increased killing by lymphocytes from patients with acute and chronic active hepatitis B, relative to that by cells from normals and chronic carriers of HBsAg. Lysis could be inhibited by addition of HBsAg or uncoated target cells. Similar studies with similar results were obtained with HBsAg-coated Chang cells (El Sheikh *et al.*, 1978) and rabbit red blood cells (Warnatz *et al.*, 1979) as targets. In each of these studies, lymphocyte depletion experiments suggested that cytotoxicity was mediated by T cells, supporting the hypothesis of Dudley *et al.* (1972a) that hepatocyte injury in hepatitis B is mediated by classical cytolytic T cells. In light of modern understanding of cytotoxic T-cell function, however, these results are difficult to interpret. T-Cell cytolysis requires simultaneous recognition by the effector cell of self-histocompatibility antigen and target antigen expressed on, rather than bound artificially to, the cell membrane of the target cell (Zinkernagel and Doherty, 1979). Therefore, to demonstrate T-cell cytolysis, these studies would have been required to use human target cells HLA matched with effector lymphocytes.

A critical flaw in most of these studies was failure to include patients with asymptomatic chronic carriage of HBsAg. One might predict low cytotoxicity in these patients because their immune systems presumably are not inducing liver injury. This issue was addressed by Dienstag and Bhan (1980), who used the PLC/PRF/5 hepatocellular carcinoma cell line as a target cell for studies of *in vitro* cytotoxicity. This cell line, derived from an HBsAg-positive patient (Macnab *et al.*, 1976), provides target cells with both HBsAg and "LSP" expressed naturally on their surface membranes (Alexander *et al.*, 1978). They found that lymphocytes from chronically HBsAg-positive patients had significantly greater cytotox-icity for PLC/PRF/5 cells than did those from patients with acute or resolved HBV infection, acute or chronic viral and nonviral liver diseases unassociated with HBV, and normals. However, not only patients with CAH, but also chronic HBsAg carriers, who have little or no liver damage associated with their HBV infection, and patients with CPH, demonstrated increased killing. In addition, similarly enhanced cytotox-icity was detected when other liver-derived and nonliver-derived cell lines, which did not express HBsAg or LSP, were used as targets, and cytotoxicity for PLC/PRF/5 cells could be blocked by these nonliver/non-virus antigen-bearing cells. The effector cells appeared to be non-phagocytic, nonadherent lymphocytes that bore IgG Fc receptors, did not rosette with sheep erythrocytes, and whose cytotoxic potential was enhanced by interferon (Dienstag *et al.*, 1982). Thus, enhanced *in vitro* cytotoxicity in chronically HBsAg-positive patients appeared to repre-sent enhanced NK activity, and did not account for the clinical dif-ferences among patients with chronic carriage of HBsAg, CPH, and CAH. Kawanishi *et al.* (1980) confirmed these results in HBsAg-positive CAH, although not in asymptomatic carriers, and also showed that SCMC was enhanced by interferon, a characteristic of NK activity. In contrast, Chisari *et al.* (1981b) were not able to confirm enhanced cyto-toxicity against PLC/PRF/5 cells in HBsAg-positive CAH. Nevertheless, these several studies taken together emphasize the need to view crit-ically investigations designed to evaluate antigen-specific cellular cytolysis. In the absence of human, antigen-bearing, HLA-matched tar-get cells, classic T-cell cytolysis probably does not occur; cytotoxicity observed under these nonantigen-specific circumstances, including that described in many of the previously published studies of cellular cyto-toxicity, probably represents SCMC.

Given the limitations of using tumor and animal cells as target cells in assays of cell-mediated cytotoxicity, several groups have sought evidence for cytotoxicity against autologous hepatocytes isolated from liver biopsy specimens. Wands and Isselbacher (1975) reported enhanced killing of both autologous hepatocytes and Chang cells by peripheral lymphocytes from patients with CAH, relative to that seen in CPH and healthy controls. Six of the 9 patients were HBsAg positive, but chronic HBsAg carriers were not examined. Paronetto and Vernace (1975) reported similar findings using early subcultures of autologous liver cells, although in their assay, cells from CPH patients also demonstrated enhanced killing. Thus, patients with CAH have circulating lymphocytes that are capable of destroying their own liver cells *in vitro*. Geubel *et al.* (1976) found significantly greater hepatocyte killing by autologous lymphocytes than by normal allogeneic lymphocytes, but only in one-half of both HBsAg-positive and -negative CAH patients studied; one-third of patients actually showed less killing than normals. In addition, these investigators and others (Dienstag and Bhan, 1980) found that cytotoxicity was markedly decreased in patients being treated with immunosuppressive agents such as prednisone, regardless of whether therapy was effective in controlling disease. Therefore, rather than reflecting a beneficial pharmacological modulation of the hepatocytolytic pathogenic process *in vivo*, the effect of prednisone therapy on cytotoxicity most likely represents the inhibitory activity of corticosteroids on cytolytic effector lymphocytes *in vitro* (Parillo and Fauci, 1978).

Examining patients with chronic hepatitis B, Eddleston *et al.* (1982) found the greatest cytotoxicity for autologous hepatocytes in CAH and the least in patients with near-normal liver histology. The surprise finding in these studies was that anti-HBc but not anti-HBs could block cytotoxicity. As discussed above, a series of investigations by Eddleston and colleagues and Alberti and colleagues suggested that T cell cytotoxicity directed against membrane HBcAg may play a central role in the immunopathogenesis of liver injury associated with HBV.

V. Immunoregulatory Serum Factors

Endogenous factors suppressing cellular immunity have also attracted increasing interest. Serum from patients with acute and chronic, viral and nonviral hepatitis has been found to contain a factor(s) that inhibits *in vitro* cytotoxicity by autologous or allogeneic lymphocytes (Wands *et al.*, 1975b; Kakumu *et al.*, 1978a; Paronetto and Vernace, 1975). Some of these factors have been characterized as lipoproteins and have been shown to inhibit T-cell erythrocyte rosetting (Chisari *et al.*, 1976) and lymphocyte mitogenesis (Geubel *et al.*, 1976; Brattig and Berg, 1976). One group noted a similar phenomenon in patients with cholestatic liver disease (Tavassolie and Kawanishi, 1978), and demonstrated a correlation between the presence of serum inhibitory factors and increased levels of circulating bile acids (Kawanishi *et al.*, 1980). It has been proposed that during hepatitis, factors are released from infected liver that suppress the immune response and limit the degree of hepatic injury (Brattig and Berg, 1983). What role these factors may play in the development of chronic hepatitis, and whether they play any particular role in liver injury associated with HBV infection, remains unknown.

VI. Cellular Immune Regulation

Immune suppression may also be mediated by cellular mechanisms. A reasonable hypothesis worth considering is that lack of normal suppressor cell function might allow a limited or persistent cellular immune response directed against hepatocyte antigens in acute or chronic hepatitis. Hodgson *et al.* (1978) studied concanavalin A-induced suppressor cell activity in 14 patients with CAH, 3 of whom were HBsAg positive. They found defective mitogen-stimulated suppressor cell function in the majority of CAH patients, but normal suppressor cell function in patients with acute hepatitis or other inflammatory diseases. These findings were confirmed in HBsAg-negative CAH by de Galocsy *et al.* (1981) and Tremolada *et al.* (1980), although in the latter study suppressor cell activity was normal in HBsAg-positive cases. Using a different assay system, Kakumu *et al.* (1980) measured the ability of fractionated T cells to suppress pokeweed mitogen-induced blastogenesis and found decreased suppressor T-cell activity in 50% of both HBsAg-positive and HBsAg-negative CAH. Finally, Chisari *et al.* (1981a) identified a defect in HBsAg-positive acute and chronic active hepatitis of an adherent, radio-resistant cell (presumably a monocyte) normally capable of suppressing mixed lymphocyte reactions. These observations raise the possibility that defective immune regulation might provide a permissive environment for harmful, unchecked cellular and humoral immune reactivity. The suppressor cell defects observed in acute and chronic hepatitis, however, do not necessarily contribute to the development of liver injury but alternatively may result from the liver disease. The same phenomenon can be demonstrated in alcoholic hepatitis (Kawanishi *et al.*, 1981), a liver disease that does not resemble CAH or viral liver injury clinically or pathologically, although it is associated with immunological abnormalities.

VII. Lymphocyte Subpopulations

Lymphocyte subpopulations in patients with acute and chronic hepatitis have been studied in an attempt to gain insight into the regulatory and effector lymphocytes that effect hepatic injury. Early studies concentrated on determinations of percentages of circulating B and T lymphocytes, and yielded conflicting findings from which no conclusions could be drawn. The development of monoclonal antibodies to helper–inducer (T4) and cytotoxic–suppressor (T8) T-cell subsets permitted further analysis of T-cell populations. In acute hepatitis B, the ratio of T4/T8 positive cells was found to be minimally (Klingenstein *et al.*, 1981) or significantly (Thomas *et al.*, 1982) reduced, while in chronic active hepatitis B the ratio was heterogeneous (Klingenstein *et al.*, 1981) or low (Thomas *et al.*, 1982). The decreased ratio in acute hepatitis B returns to normal upon recovery, paralleling changes seen in other viral infections including those caused by Epstein–Barr virus (Waele *et al.*, 1981) and cytomegalovirus (Rubin *et al.*, 1981). Of paramount importance, however, was the fact that the ratios in asymptomatic chronic HBsAg carriers were consistently reduced (Klingenstein *et al.*, 1981), perhaps reflecting an increase in suppressive immunoregulatory forces limiting immunological attack on infected hepatocytes.

Because changes in peripheral lymphocytes might not necessarily reflect the characteristics of the cells found at the site of tissue injury, other investigators examined liver-derived lymphocytes. Miller *et al.* (1977) isolated lymphocytes from liver biopsy specimens obtained from patients with chronic hepatitis, enumerated T and B lymphocytes, and found a predominance of T cells in the hepatic infiltrates of all patients. This pattern was not unique to chronic hepatitis; Husby *et al.* (1975) reported similar results in intact histological sections of liver from patients with alcoholic liver disease. Miller *et al.* (1977), however, found that the ratio of T cells to B cells was much lower in HBsAg-negative than in HBsAg-positive CAH (2:1 compared to 20:1), a dichotomy that the authors suggested was further evidence that HBsAg-positive and -negative CAH resulted from different pathogenetic processes. In a subsequent study, Miller *et al.* (1978) could isolate large numbers of Fc receptor-positive "null" lymphocytes from the livers of HBsAg-negative patients but not HBsAg-positive patients with CAH. Although these findings supported the postulated role of K cell-mediated ADCC in HBsAg-negative CAH, they challenged the hypothetical contribution of ADCC to HBsAg-positive CAH.

Using monoclonal antibodies, Pape *et al.* (1983) showed that the T cells infiltrating the liver in chronic hepatitis B were of the cytotoxic–suppressor (T8) subset. Others found a lower percentage of this subset in the inflammatory hepatic infiltrates of patients with HBeAg-positive chronic hepatitis B than in anti-HBe-positive cases or in lupoid CAH (Montano *et al.*, 1983). The infiltrating T cells tend to bear Ia markers, the hallmark of "activated" T cells (Colucci *et al.*, 1983). Taken together, studies of lymphocyte phenotype markers in blood and liver support the notion that the immune system causes the liver injury seen in hepatitis B infection. They suggest that cytotoxic effector cells make up a large proportion of lymphocytes infiltrating the liver in chronic hepatitis B, and support an increase in suppressor influences as a factor responsible for the minimal hepatic inflammation seen in the chronic HBsAg carrier state.

VIII. Discussion

A plethora of data suggests that the immune system plays a causative role in the production of liver injury in hepatitis B. This follows directly from the supposition that HBV is a noncytopathic virus, and that the mononuclear cells adjacent to dying hepatocytes in hepatic infiltrates are responsible for the death of those cells.

It is clear that humoral and cellular immune responses to viral antigens develop following acute HBV infection. This is easiest to document in terms of humoral immunity, with development of antibodies to HBsAg, HBcAg, and HBeAg during or after infection. Whether anti-HBs plays a role in the destruction of virally infected hepatocytes is more difficult to determine. As reviewed above, it is difficult to demonstrate HBsAg on the surface of hepatocytes during acute hepatitis B. It is thought that this results from rapid elimination of infected hepatocytes; alternatively, surface membrane expression of HBsAg may be obscured the coating of infected hepatocytes by IgG. Recent data, however, show that this IgG binds to HBcAg rather than to HBsAg.

Cell-mediated immunity seems more likely to play the major role in production of liver injury in hepatitis B infections. This notion derives from several clinical observations. First, in persons with alleged defects in cellular immunity, such as patients with Down's syndrome, lepromatous leprosy, and chronic renal failure, asymptomatic HBsAg carriage is more likely than is chronic hepatitis to develop after acute HBV infection (Blumberg *et al.*, 1970).

Second, when chemotherapy is discontinued in an immunosuppressed HBsAg-positive person, such as a patient with malignancy, fulminant hepatocellular necrosis may occur, presumably as a result of the return of cellular immune responsiveness (Galbraith *et al.*, 1975). Third, in patients with HBsAg-positive CAH, elevations of serum aminotransferase activity develop following treatment with levamisole (Thomas *et al.*, 1977) and transfer factor (Kohler *et al.*, 1974), agents thought to stimulate cellular immunity, but not following "humoral reconstitution" by infusion of anti-HBs (Reed *et al.*, 1973).

As we have reviewed, there is a wealth of data showing that patients with chronic hepatitis B have circulating lymphocytes that are cytotoxic for autologous and nonautologous hepatocytes. Many of these cellular phenomena can be found in forms of liver damage that are thought less likely to be immunologically mediated, however. Such phenomena may be secondary to liver injury. In this regard, Smith *et al.* (1980a) demonstrated a specific cellular immune response to liver cell antigens (but not to kidney or spleen cell antigens) in mice with nonimmunologic liver injury induced by carbon tetrachloride. Sensitized lymphocytes from affected mice, however, did not cause hepatocellular necrosis when administered to syngeneic mice. Furthermore, mice depleted of their T lymphocytes by perinatal thymectomy did not mount a cellular immune response to liver antigens, but toxic hepatitis developed nevertheless (Smith *et al.*, 1980b). Therefore, despite the apparent liver specificity of cellular immune responses demonstrated by Smith *et al.* (1980a,b) *in vitro*, these responses appear to have *resulted from* the liver injury and not to have participated in its pathogenesis. Thus, even the best *in vitro* assay of cellular immunity cannot distinguish primary pathological events from epiphenomena.

Problems of data interpretation are further compounded by the absence of suitable target cells for cytotoxicity assays. The most meaningful target cells are those syngeneic to the lymphocyte donor, such as autologous hepatocytes. While autologous hepatocytes are theoretically preferable to tumor cells and rabbit hepatocytes as target cells, however, self- or viral antigens might be removed from, or neoantigens exposed on, target cells during preparation. Furthermore, even when autologous hepatocytes are used as targets, these target cells are not autologous to lymphocytes from normal controls. Therefore, these experiments cannot include all the proper controls.

The type(s) of effector mechanisms involved in destruction of infected hepatocytes are also not certain. We presume that NK cells, which will frequently attack virally infected targets, are probably not the effector cells, because asymptomatic HBsAg carriers have high NK activity but near-normal livers. Histologic analysis suggests that T8-positive T cells might be the effectors, and these presumably would be antigen specific. Which antigens they recognize are unknown. Despite early advocacy for autoimmunity induced by HBV, it seems unlikely that LSP is the target antigen. One might have presumed that the target was HBsAg; however, Eddleston *et al.* (1982) found cytotoxicity by lymphocytes from patients with chronic hepatitis for autologous hepatocytes to be blocked by exogenous anti-HBc, not by HBsAg or anti-HBs. This suggests again the novel concept that HBcAg might be a target antigen.

All of the clever *in vitro* manipulations designed thus far have not explained why chronic hepatitis B develops in some patients and what determines where in the clinical spectrum a patient will fall. While the pathogenesis of liver injury associated with HBV infection has been attributed to impaired T-cell recognition and cytolysis, ADCC, defective suppressor cell function, immune inhibitory factors in serum and liver, specific patterns of intrahepatocytic virus antigen expression, and sensitization to liver cell membrane antigens, *in vitro* studies have not substantiated any of these hypotheses definitively. Moreover, the glib dismissal of humoral immune mechanisms in the pathogenesis of liver injury may warrant reconsideration; a defective humoral immune response could be contributory. In this regard, chronic HBsAg carriers appear to have a specific B-cell defect in anti-HBs production as determined in B- and T-cell co-culture experiments (Duscheiko *et al.*, 1983). Theoretically, an inadequate B-cell response or elaboration of nonneutralizing antibody might allow unchecked virus antigen and infectious particles to flood the circulation, continuously infecting new hepatocytes and perpetuating the disease despite the presence of intact cellular immune recognition and effector mechanisms. Even the observed B-cell defect, however, may result from rather than contribute to chronic infection.

In simple terms, our understanding of the immunopathogenesis of hepatitis B remains elementary at best. Despite the many *in vitro* immunological investigations and hypotheses, a direct immunological role in the pathogenesis of liver disease has not been proven. Many aspects of the immune response remain to be elucidated. Chief among these is the specificity of immunological attack on the liver. Studies of potential liver cell target antigens have not established the existence or specificity of a unique liver membrane antigen, and the viral target antigen involved is not certain. In addition, genetic influences over immune responsiveness, established in mouse cytolytic T-cell responses, have not been addressed in considerations of the immunopathogenesis of human hepatitis B. Moreover, besides host immune factors, virus factors that we may only now be on the threshold of discovering may play a role in determining the outcome of HBV infection. There has always been disagreement as to whether the immune responses studied *in vitro* play a primary causal role in hepatitis or are secondary phenomena, such as those which result from portasystemic shunting (Webb *et al.*, 1980) or those seen in hepatotoxic liver injury (Smith *et al.*, 1980a,b). This debate will continue until better *in vitro* models are developed that more closely approximate *in vivo* conditions or until animal models amenable to laboratory investigation become available. Productive research in the future is likely to derive from experimental models that evaluate effector cytotoxicity and immune regulation with specificity for virus and host antigens.

References

Alarcon-Segovia, D., Ruiz-Arguelles, A., and Fishbein, E. (1978). *Nature (London)* **271**, 67–69.

Alarcon-Segovia, D., Ruiz-Arguelles, A., and Llorente, L. (1979). *J. Immunol.* **122**, 1855–1862.

Alberti, A., Realdi, G., Tremolada, F., and Spina, G. P. (1976). *Clin. Exp. Immunol.* **25**, 396–402.

Alberti, A., Realdi, G., Bortolotti, F., and Rigoli, A. M. (1977). *Gut* **18**, 1004–1009.

Alexander, J., Macnab, G., and Saunders, R. (1978). *Perspect. Virol.* **10**, 103–110.

Almeida, J. D., and Waterson, A. P. (1969). *Lancet 2*, 983–986.

Bacon, P. A., Berry, H., and Brown, R. (1972). *Gut* **13**, 427–429.

Behrens, U. J., and Paronetto, F. (1979). *Gastroenterology* **77**, 1045–1052.

Behrens, U. J., Vernace, S., and Paronetto, F. (1979). *Gastroenterology* **77**, 1053–1061.

Bianchi, L., and Gudat, F. (1979). *Prog. Liver Dis.* **6**, 371–392.

Blumberg, B. S., Sutnick, A. I., and London, W. T. (1970). *Am. J. Med.* **48**, 1–8.

Brattig, N. W., and Berg, P. A. (1976). *Clin. Exp. Immunol.* **25**, 40–49.

Brattig, N. W., and Berg, P. A. (1983). *Hepatology 3*, 639–646.

Chang, R. S. (1954). *Proc. Soc. Exp. Biol. Med.* **87**, 440–443.

Chisari, F. V., Routenberg, J. A., and Edgington, T. S. (1976). *J. Clin. Invest.* **57**, 1227–1238.

Chisari, F. V., Castle, K. L., Xavier, C., and Anderson, D. S. (1981a). *J. Immunol.* **126**, 38–44.

Chisari, F. V., Bieber, M. S., Josepho, C. A., Xavier, C., and Anderson, D. S. (1981b). *J. Immunol.* **126**, 45–49.

Cochrane, A. M. G., Moussouros, A., Thomson, A. D., Eddleston, A. L. W. F., and Williams, R. (1976). *Lancet 1*, 441–444.

Colucci, G., Colombo, M., Del Nino, E., and Paronetto, F. (1983). *Gastroenterology* **85**, 1138–1145.

de Galocsy, C., Jenkins, P. J., Mieli-Vergani, G., Eddleston, A. L. W. F., and Williams, R. (1981). *Clin. Exp. Immunol.* **43,** 486–490.

deMoura, M. C., Vernace, S. J., and Paronetto, E. (1975). *Gastroenterology* **69,** 310–317.

Dienstag, J. L. (1981). *Semin. Liver Dis.* **1,** 45–57.

Dienstag, J. L., and Bhan, A. K. (1980). *J. Immunol.* **125,** 2269–2276.

Dienstag, J. L., and Isselbacher, K. J. (1978). *N. Engl. J. Med.* **299,** 40–42.

Dienstag, J. L., Savarese, A. M., and Bhan, A. K. (1982). *Hepatology* **2,** 107S–115S.

Dudley, F. J., Fox, R. A., and Sherlock, S. (1972a). *Lancet 1,* 723–726.

Dudley, F. J., Giustino, V., and Sherlock, S. (1972b). *Br. Med. J.* **2,** 754–756.

Duscheiko, G. M., Hoofnagle, J. H., Cooksley, W. G., James, S. P., and Jones, E. A. (1983). *J. Clin. Invest.* **71,** 1104–1113.

Eddleston, A. L. W. F., and Williams, R. (1974). *Lancet 2,* 1543–1545.

Eddleston, A. L. W. F., Mondelli, M., Nieli-Vergani, G., and Williams, R. (1982). *Hepatology* **2,** 122S–127S.

Edgington, T. S., and Chisari, F. V. (1975). *Am. J. Med. Sci.* **270,** 213–227.

El Sheikh, N., Osman, C. G., Cullens, H., Eddleston, A. L. W. F., and Williams, R. (1978). *Clin. Exp. Immunol.* **31,** 158–165.

Galbraith, R. M., Eddleston, A. L. W. F., Williams, R., Zuckerman, A. J., and Bagshawe, K. D. (1975). *Lancet 2,* 528–530.

Gerber, M. A., Sarno, E., and Vernace, S. J. (1976). *N. Engl. J. Med.* **294,** 922–925.

Geubel, A. P., Keller, R. H., Summerskill, W. H. J., Dickson, E. R., Tomasi, T. B., and Shorter, R. G. (1976). *Gastroenterology* **71,** 450–456.

Gudat, F., and Bianchi, L. (1977). *Gastroenterology* **73,** 1194–1197.

Hodgson, H. J. F., Wands, J. R., and Isselbacher, K. J. (1978). *Proc. Natl. Acad. Sci. U.S.A.* **75,** 1549–1553.

Hopf, U., Meyer zum Buschenfelde, K. H., and Freudenberg, J. (1974). *Clin. Exp. Immunol.* **16,** 117–123.

Hopf, U., Arnold, W., Meyer zum Buschenfelde, K. H., Forster, E., and Bolte, J. P. (1975). *Clin. Exp. Immunol.* **22,** 1–8.

Hopf, U., Meyer zum Buschenfelde, K. H., and Arnold, W. (1976a). *N. Engl. J. Med.* **294,** 578–582.

Hopf, U., Meyer zum Buschenfelde, K. H., and Dierich, M. P. (1976b). *J. Immunol.* **117,** 639–645.

Hopf, U., Schaefer, E., Hess, G., and Meyer zum Buschenfelde, K. J. (1981). *Gastroenterology* **80,** 250–259.

Howlett, S. A., and McGuigan, J. E. (1975). *Gastroenterology* **69,** 960–964.

Husby, G., Strickland, R. G., Caldwell, J. L., and Williams, R. C. (1975). *J. Clin. Invest.* **56,** 1198–1209.

Hutteroth, T. H., and Meyer zum Buschenfelde, K. H. (1978). *Acta Hepato-Gastroenterol.* **25,** 243–247.

Ito, K., Nagawa, J., Okimoto, Y., and Nakano, H. (1972). *N. Engl. J. Med.* **286,** 1005.

Jensen, D. M., McFarlane, I. G., Portmann, B. S., Eddleston, A. L. W. F., and Williams, R. (1978). *N. Engl. J. Med.* **299,** 1–7.

Kakumu, S., Hara, T., Goji, H., and Sakamoto, N. (1978a). *Clin. Exp. Immunol.* **33,** 71–78.

Kakumu, S., Tateki, H., Goji, H., and Sakamoto, N. (1978b). *Cell. Immunol.* **36,** 46–53.

Kakumu, S., Arakawa, Y., Goji, H., Kashio, T., and Yata, K. (1979). *Gastroenterology* **76,** 665–672.

Kakumu, S., Yata, K., and Kashio, T. (1980). *Gastroenterology* **79,** 613–619.

Kawanishi, H., and MacDermott, R. P. (1979). *Gastroenterology* **76,** 151–158.

Kawanishi, H., Carter, W. N., Sheagren, J. N., Greenwood, J. M., MacDermott, R. P., and Ibrahim, M. (1978). *Gastroenterology* **78**, 1192 (abstr.).

Kawanishi, H., Greenwood, J. H., and Blackwell, W. H. (1980). *Gastroenterology* **78**, 1309 (abstr.).

Kawanishi, H., Tavassolie, H., MacDermott, R. P., and Sheagren, J. N. (1981). *Gastroenterology* **80**, 510–517.

Klingenstein, R. J., Savarese, A. M., Dienstag, J. L., Rubin, R. H., and Bhan, A. K. (1981). *Hepatology* **1**, 523 (abstr.).

Kohler, P. F., Trembath, J., Merrill, D. A., Singleton, J. W., and Dubois, R. S. (1974). *Clin. Immunol. Immunopathol.* **2**, 465–471.

Lavappa, K. S., Macy, M. L., and Shannon, J. E. (1976). *Nature (London)* **259**, 211–213.

Lee, W. M., Reed, E. D., Mitchell, C. G., Galbraith, R. M., Eddleston, A. L. W. F., Zuckerman, A. J., and Williams, R. (1975). *Br. Med. J.* **1**, 705–708.

McFarlane, I. G., Wojcicka, B. M., Zucker, G. M., and Eddleston, A. L. W. F. (1977). *Clin. Exp. Immunol.* **27**, 381–390.

McIntosh, R. M., Koss, M. M., and Gocke, D. J. (1976). *Q. J. Med.* **45**, 23–38.

Macnab, G. M., Alexander, J. J., and Lecatsas, G. (1976). *Br. J. Cancer* **34**, 509–515.

Meliconi, R., Miglio, F., Stancari, M. L., Baraldini, M., Stefanini, G. F., and Gasbarrini, G. (1983). *Hepatology* **3**, 155–161.

Meyer zum Buschenfelde, K. H. (1968). *Arch. Klin, Med.* **215**, 107–111.

Meyer zum Buschenfelde, K. H., and Hopf, U. (1974). *Br. J. Exp. Pathol.* **55**, 198–508.

Meyer zum Buschenfelde, K. H., and Miescher, P. A. (1972). *Clin. Exp. Immunol.* **10**, 89–102.

Meyer zum Buschenfelde, K. J., Kossling, F. K., and Miescher, P. A. (1972). *Clin. Exp. Immunol.* **10**, 99–108.

Meyer zum Buschenfelde, K. J., Manns, M., Hutteroth, T. H., Hopf, U., and Arnold, W. (1979). *Clin. Exp. Immunol.* **37**, 205–212.

Mieli-Vergani, G., Vergani, D., Portmann, B., White, Y., Murray-Lyon, I., Marigold, J. H., Woolf, I., Eddleston, A. L. W. F., and Williams, R. (1982). *Gut* **23**, 1029–1036.

Miller, D. J., Dwyer, J. M., and Klatskin, G. (1977). *Gastroenterology* **72**, 1199–1203.

Miller, D. J., Dwyer, J. M., and Klatskin, G. (1978). *Clin. Res.* **26**, 323A.

Miller, J., Smith, M. G. M., Mitchell, C. G., Reed, W. D., Eddleston, A. L. W. F., and Williams, R. (1972). *Lancet 2*, 296–297.

Mondelli, M., Mieli-Vergani, G., Alberti, A., Vergani, D., Portmann, B., Eddleston, A. L. W. F., and Williams, R. (1982). *J. Immunol.* **129**, 2773–2778.

Montano, L., Aranguibel, F., Boffill, M., Goodall, A. H., Janossy, G., and Thomas, H. C. (1983). *Hepatology* **3**, 292–296.

Mutchnik, M. G., Kawanishi, H., and Hopf, U. (1978). *Clin. Immunol. Immunopathol.* **10**, 398–402.

Naumov, N. V., Mondelli, M., Alexander, G. J. M., Tedder, R. S., Eddleston, A. L. W. F., and Williams, R. (1984). *Hepatology* **4**, 63–68.

Nelson-Rees, W. A., and Flandermeyer, R. R. (1976). *Science* **191**, 96–98.

Nowoslawski, A., Kraczynski, K., Nazarewicz, T., and Slusarczynk, J. (1975). *Am. J. Med. Sci.* **270**, 229–239.

Ortona, L., Laghi, V., Cauda, R., and Nervo, P. (1979). *Clin. Exp. Immunol.* **38**, 231–234.

Pape, G. R., Rieber, E. P., Eisenburg, J., Hoffman, R., Balch, C. M., Paumgartner, G., and Reithmuller, G. (1983). *Gastroenterology* **85**, 657–662.

Parillo, J. E., and Fauci, A. S. (1978). *Clin. Exp. Immunol.* **31**, 116–125.

Paronetto, F., and Vernace, S. (1975). *Clin. Exp. Immunol.* **19**, 99–104.

Paronetto, F., Gerber, M., and Vernace, S. J. (1973). *Proc. Soc. Exp. Biol. Med.* **143,** 756–760.

Potter, B. J., Elias, E., Thomas, H. C., and Sherlock, S. (1980). *Gastroenterology* **78,** 1034–1040.

Prince, A. M., and Trepo, C. (1971). *Lancet 1,* 1309–1312.

Ray, M. B., Desmet, V. J., Bradburne, A. F., Desmyter, J., Fevery, J., and De Groote, J. (1976). *Gastroenterology* **71,** 462–467.

Realdi, G., Alberti, A., and Trevisan, A. (1979). *Gastroenterology* **77,** 605–606.

Reed, W. D., Eddleston, A. L. W. F., Cullens, H., Williams, R., Zuckerman, A. J., Peters, D. K., Gwyn-Williams, D. G., and Maycock, W. d'A. (1973). *Lancet 2,* 1347–1351.

Rubin, R. H., Carney, W. P., Schooley, R. T., Colvin, R. B., Burton, R. C., Hoffman, R. A., Hansen, W. P., Cosimi, A. B., Russell, P. S., and Hirsch, M. S. (1981). *Int. J. Immunopharmacol.* **3,** 307–312.

Sabesin, S. M. (1963). *Am. J. Pathol.* **42,** 743–757.

Schumacher, K., Maerker-Alzer, G., and Wehmer, U. (1974). *Nature (London)* **251,** 655–656.

Smith, C. I., Cooksley, W. G. E., and Powell, L. W. (1980a). *Clin. Exp. Immunol.* **39,** 607–617.

Smith, C. I., Cooksley, W. G. E., and Powell, L. W. (1980b). *Clin. Exp. Immunol.* **39,** 618–625.

Smith, M. G. M., Golding, P. L., Eddleston, A. L. W. F., Mitchell, C. G., Kemp, A., and Williams, R. (1972). *Br. Med. J.* **1,** 527–530.

Solley, G. O., Dickson, E. R., Gleich, G. J., and Stobo, J. D. (1979). *Mayo Clin. Proc.* **54,** 127–130.

Tage-Jensen, U., Arnold, W., Dietrichson, O., Hardt, F., Hopf, U., Meyer zum Buschenfelde, K. H., and Nielsen, J. O. (1977). *Br. Med. J.* **1,** 206–208.

Tavassolie, H., and Kawanishi, H. (1978). *Gastroenterology* **75,** 990 (abstr.).

Thomas, H. C., Chadwick, R. H., Jain, S., and Sherlock, S. (1977). *Gastroenterolgoy* **73,** A52.

Thomas, H. C., DeVilliers, D., Potter, B., Hodgson, H., Jain, S., Jewell, D. P., and Sherlock, S. (1978). *Clin. Exp. Immunol.* **31,** 150–157.

Thomas, H. C., Potter, B. J., Elias, E., and Sherlock, S. (1979). *Gastroenterology* **76,** 673–679.

Thomas, H. C., Brown, D., Routhier, G., Janossy, G., Kung, P. C., Goldstein, G., and Sherlock, S. (1982). *Hepatology* **2,** 202–204.

Thomson, A. D., Cochrane, M. A. G., McFarlane, I. G., Eddleston, A. L. W. F., and Williams, R. (1974). *Nature (London)* **252,** 721–722.

Tong, M. J., Wallace, A. M., Peters, R. L., and Reynolds, T. B. (1975). *N. Engl. J. Med.* **293,** 318–322.

Tong, M. J., Nies, K. M., and Redeker, A. G. (1977) *Gastroenterology* **73,** 1418–1421.

Tremolada, F., Fattovich, G., Panelbianco, G., Ongaro, G., and Realdi, G. (1980). *Clin Exp. Immunol.* **40,** 89–95.

Trevisan, A., Realdi, G., Alberti, A., and Noventa, F. (1979). *Gastroenterology* **77,** 209–214.

Trevisan, A., Realdi, G., Alberti, A., Ongaro, G., Pornaro, E., and Miliconi, R. (1982). *Gastroenterology* **82,** 218–222.

Vierling, J. M., Nelson, D. L., Strober, W., Bundy, B. M., and Jones, E. A. (1977). *J. Clin. Invest.* **60,** 1116–1128.

Vogten, A. J. M., Hadzic, N., Shorter, R. G., Summerskill, W. H. J., Taylor, W. F., and Nelson, D. L. (1978). *Gastroenterology* **74,** 883–889.

Waele, M., Thielemans, C., and Van Camp, B. K. G. (1981). *N. Engl. J. Med.* **304,** 460–462.

Wands, J. R., and Isselbacher, K. J. (1975). *Proc. Natl. Acad. Sci. U.S.A.* **72,** 1301–1303.

Wands, J. R., Alpert, E., and Isselbacher, K. J. (1975a). *Gastroenterology* **69,** 1286–1291.

Wands, J. R., Perrotto, J. L., Alpert, E., and Isselbacher, K. J. (1975b). *J. Clin. Invest.* **55,** 921–929.

Warnatz, H., Rosch, W., Gerlich, W., and Gutmann, W. (1979). *Clin. Exp. Immunol.* **35,** 133–140.

Webb, L. J., Ross, M., Markham, R. L., Webster, A. D. W., Thomas, H. C., and Sherlock, S. (1980). *Gastroenterology* **79,** 99–103.

Yeung-Laiwah, A. A. C., Chandhuri, A. K. R., and Anderson, J. R. (1973). *Clin. Exp. Immunol.* **15,** 27–34.

Zinkernagel, R. M., and Doherty, P. C. (1979). *Adv. Immunol.* **27,** 52–177.

Hepatitis B Virus
and Primary Hepatocellular Carcinoma

EDWARD TABOR
Division of Anti-Infective Drug Products
Office of Biologics Research and Review
Food and Drug Administration
Rockville, Maryland

I. Introduction and Clinical Aspects

The hepatitis B virus (HBV) is one of the first human viruses for which
an etiological association with a human cancer has been partially established. This association was first suggested by careful observation of
tissue specimens from patients with primary hepatocellular carcinoma
(PHC) years before the development of sensitive serologic tests to detect
HBV. The development of the radioimmunoassay (RIA), the adaptation
of that sensitive assay method to the study of the hepatitis viruses, and
the careful collection of serum samples from patients and matched controls for RIA testing led to the recognition of the close association between HBV and PHC. Further confirmation of this association has been
possible using techniques from molecular biology to show that the DNA
of HBV is integrated into the DNA of the hepatocytes and the PHC
tumor cells in patients with PHC. The development and use of a safe
and effective HBV vaccine may provide a definitive means to test
whether the association between HBV and PHC is causal. When tech-

247

Copyright © 1985 by Academic Press, Inc.
All rights of reproduction in any form reserved.
ISBN 0-12-280672-7

nological advances lead to the production of an inexpensive version of this vaccine so that it can be made available extensively in underdeveloped countries where both HBV and PHC are prevalent, its use may have a significant impact on the patterns of cancer mortality in those regions.

PHC is a common form of cancer in many parts of the world; in some areas, it is the most common cause of cancer in young adult men, although it may appear at any adult age. The male/female ratio among patients with this disease is ~7:1 in some areas. In underdeveloped countries, the course of the disease from diagnosis to death is rapid, usually 3–6 months; in contrast, the course of PHC may extend for a year or more in some cases in more developed countries. This probably reflects the delay in diagnosis in underdeveloped countries, since >20% of PHC patients in Zambia were found to have had symptoms for >6 months before coming to medical attention (Bayley, 1978).

Symptoms of PHC at the time of presentation often include weight loss and abdominal pain. The abdominal pain appears with gradually increasing severity, may be in the right upper quadrant of the abdomen or diffuse, and increases with food intake. Amenorrhea, abdominal fullness after eating, or a mass in the abdomen may be noted. Abdominal pain after alcohol ingestion has also been noted in 57% of PHC patients who drink alcoholic beverages (Bayley, 1978). Signs associated with PHC include hepatomegaly, right upper quadrant mass, right upper quadrant tenderness, severe muscle wasting, ascites (especially bloody ascites), and icterus.

PHC has been documented rarely in children and occasionally in adolescents in endemic areas (Bowry and Cameron, 1976; Kew *et al.*, 1982) as well as in nonendemic areas such as the United States (Fraumeni *et al.*, 1968). The presence of active HBV infection in six of six pediatric PHC cases has been reported in one of these studies (Kew *et al.*, 1982). Among hepatic carcinomas of children, hepatoblastoma occurs more frequently than PHC.

Many cases of PHC can be diagnosed early in the course or prior to the examination of a liver biopsy by testing the patient's serum for α-fetoprotein (AFP). AFP is a serum α-1-globulin that is synthesized by fetal organs; it is present at low levels in normal adults. Elevated levels (>18 IU/ml by RIA) may be found in 30–95% of patients with PHC (Alpert, 1976; Trichopoulos *et al.*, 1980a). Although elevated levels of AFP also occur in association with liver regeneration, for instance during recovery from hepatitis, the elevations do not reach the same high levels, which are often >1000 IU/ml in PHC patients (Trichopoulos *et al.*, 1980a; Chen and Sung, 1977). Significant elevations of AFP may occur as long as 2 years before the appearance of clinically recognized PHC (Heyward *et al.*, 1982).

In addition to an association between elevated levels of AFP and PHC, an association has been noted between elevated levels of AFP and the presence of hepatitis B surface antigen (HBsAg) in the serum of PHC patients by several groups of investigators (Prince *et al.*, 1975; Reed *et al.*, 1973; Vogel *et al.*, 1970; Trichopoulos *et al.*, 1980a), but not by others (Kew *et al.*, 1979a; Kubo *et al.*, 1977a). This association becomes apparent at moderate and high AFP elevations; its significance has never been established. It has been suggested that this is not due simply to hepatic regeneration, and may reflect the oncogenic potential of HBV (Alpert, 1976). The fact that elevation of AFP levels may precede the onset of PHC by as long as 2 years (Heyward *et al.*, 1982) suggests that its production is a characteristic of early carcinogenesis or of a particular course of HBV infection that later results in PHC.

II. Pathological Studies

Even before the discovery of serological markers for HBV, an association was recognized between what we now know as hepatitis B and PHC. Investigators noted a high incidence of PHC in sub-Saharan Africa and Southeast Asia, with rates in 25- to 34-year-old males in one area nearly 500 times that seen in the United States (Higginson, 1963). They noted that the type of cirrhosis found most frequently in livers of patients with PHC was characterized by findings similar to "post-hepatitic" or "post-necrotic" cirrhosis (Higginson, 1963), findings that were also noted following clinically or pathologically recognized viral hepatitis. An etiologic hypothesis was formulated in which damage to the liver in childhood by a virus (carcinogenic or noncarcinogenic) predisposed to carcinogenesis following a second hepatotoxic event later in life (Higginson, 1963). One theory suggested that the second event involved a carcinogen acting synergistically with a second noncarcinogenic infectious agent (Higginson, 1963).

One very interesting observation in 1961 presaged the discovery of PHC-inducing viruses related to HBV in nonprimate animals nearly two decades later, but was forgotten. This was the report of the development of PHC in ducks with autopsy evidence of long-standing viral hepatitis (Ratcliffe, 1961).

Cirrhosis is frequently observed in nontumorous liver tissue from patients with PHC, and its role in the etiology of PHC has remained a subject of scientific debate. Macronodular cirrhosis is one sequela of HBV infection; the association now known to exist between HBV and PHC makes it reasonable to find macronodular cirrhosis in association with PHC. In fact, macronodular cirrhosis is the type found in >80% of PHC patients who have cirrhosis (Akagi *et al.*, 1982). In a prospective study, HBV infection with cirrhosis was found to be associated with later development of PHC more often than HBV infection without cirrhosis, although the number of patients with cirrhosis in this study was not large (Obata *et al.*, 1980). The association between HBV serological markers and PHC is greater among patients with accompanying cirrhosis than among those without cirrhosis (Chainuvati *et al.*, 1975; Okuda *et al.*, 1982); in those with PHC and alcoholic cirrhosis, no association with HBV serological markers is found when compared to controls (Omata *et al.*, 1979). However, other investigators have found only a small (but statistically not significant) increased prevalence of HBsAg in PHC patients with cirrhosis compared to those with PHC and no cirrhosis (Akagi *et al.*, 1982). The percentage of PHC cases with cirrhosis varies, but may be as high as 85% (Akagi *et al.*, 1982); this variable percentage and the variable relationship between cirrhosis and HBsAg may reflect the cumulative effect of all hepatotoxic influences in different geographic areas.

It has been suggested that the pathogenesis of HBsAg-positive PHC with cirrhosis may differ from that of PHC without cirrhosis (Okuda *et al.*, 1982). The average age at diagnosis of PHC is significantly higher in patients with extensive cirrhosis compared to those with moderate or no cirrhosis, suggesting a longer preclinical phase (Okuda *et al.*, 1982).

The orcein staining method (Shikata *et al.*, 1974), in which HBsAg becomes detectable by light microscopy in paraffin-embedded tissues by a reaction involving a disulfide component of HBsAg, as well as an aldehyde fuchsin staining method have been used to evaluate the role of HBV in PHC. In a study of 19 cases of PHC, HBsAg was detected in 8 (42%) in nonneoplastic hepatocytes; HBsAg was not detected in any of the PHC cells (Shikata *et al.*, 1977). In another study, 8 of 24 (33%) patients with PHC and cirrhosis had HBsAg detected in nonneoplastic tissue by the aldehyde fuchsin stain, compared to 0 of 16 patients with PHC in the absence of cirrhosis (Swenson *et al.*, 1980). Seven of the 8 positive samples were confirmed by immunoperoxidase staining.

Immunoperoxidase staining of liver tissue from PHC patients using antibodies to the hepatitis B core and surface antigens (anti-HBc, anti-HBs) conjugated with horseradish peroxidase has been used to show the presence of HBsAg and/or the hepatitis B core antigen (HBcAg) in non-neoplastic hepatocytes in liver biopsies from patients with PHC. In one study, 65% (13 of 20) of PHC patients with macronodular cirrhosis had either HBsAg in the cytoplasm (11 patients, 55%) or HBcAg in the nuclei (10 patients, 50%; in one additional case, along cytoplasmic membranes and in the cytoplasm) of hepatocytes (Omata *et al.*, 1979). Two additional patients in the study had HBsAg in their serum, although HBsAg was not detected by immunoperoxidase staining in their liver tissue.

Direct immunofluorescence using fluorescent-labeled anti-HBs revealed HBsAg in the cytoplasm of hepatocytes in cirrhotic nodules of 4 of 12 (33%) patients with PHC (Nazarewicz *et al.*, 1977). HBcAg was not detected in any of 12 liver tissue samples in the same study using similarly labeled anti-HBc. The detection of HBsAg in the cytoplasm of neoplastic cells from 1 of these patients was also reported. Six of the 12 patients (50%) had serologic evidence of active HBV infection.

Several groups of investigators have reported the detection of HBsAg (and in some cases HBcAg) in PHC tissue as well as in the surrounding nonneoplastic tissue. Using direct and indirect immunofluorescence techniques, Trevisan *et al.* (1978) detected HBsAg in nonneoplastic tissue from 16 of 107 PHC patients (15%) and in the cytoplasm of the tumor cells as well in 8 (7%). HBcAg was found in the nuclei of nonneoplastic cells of 8 of the 16 with HBsAg in nonneoplastic cells; HBcAg was also detected in the nuclei of cancer cells in 8 of the sixteen, 2 of whom did not have HBcAg detectable in nonneoplastic cells. Serum samples from most of these patients were not tested. HBV markers were detected by these investigators mainly in the livers of patients with well-differentiated tumors, although they did not report histological findings in detail. Using a combination of immunofluorescence, immunoperoxidase, and orcein techniques in the study of paraffin-embedded liver tissue from 44 PHC patients, Kew *et al.* (1980) detected HBsAg in nontumor cells alone in 22% of patients, tumor cells alone in 12%, and in both types of cells in 10%. HBsAg was detected more frequently in tumor cells when the cells were moderately differentiated than when they were poorly differentiated. No difference in sensitivity was found between immunofluorescence and immunoperoxidase staining; however, the orcein stain was not capable of detecting HBsAg in any of the tumor cells. In 4 of the patients in their study (10%), HBsAg was present in liver tissue (3 in nontumor cells, one in tumor cells), but not in serum. Nayak *et al.* (1979) detected HBsAg in tumor tissue from 5 of 18 (28%) PHC patients and in nontumor tissue from all 18, using indirect immunofluorescence and indirect immunoperoxidase methods applied to paraffin-embedded tissues. HBcAg was not detected in any of the tumor cells using similar methods, but was detected in nontumor cells in an unspecified number of livers. Bréchot *et al.* (1981) detected HBsAg by direct immunofluorescence in tumor tissue from 4 of 10 PHC patients with integrated HBV DNA (see Section VI) in their PHC tissue, and HBcAg in none. Both HBsAg and HBcAg were detected by immunofluorescence in adjacent nontumor tissue from all 3 patients from whom nontumor tissue was available. In most of these studies, if HBsAg was detected in tumor cells, fewer cells were positive than if HBsAg was detected in nontumor cells; the positive tumor cells were often separated from each other, but were found in clusters separated by vast areas of negative cells (Doury *et al.*, 1978; Nayak *et al.*, 1979; Kew *et al.*, 1980; Trevisan *et al.*, 1978).

Although a few electron microscopic studies of PHC tissue have been published, only one has reported the presence of HBsAg particles (Campion *et al.*, 1972). Presumably, HBsAg particles and HBcAg particles would often be seen in thin sections in those tissues in which the antigens have been detected using immunohistochemical methods, although extensive efforts might be necessary to detect HBsAg particles in the sparsely HBsAg-positive tumor cells. Electron microscopy using ferritin- or radiolabeled antibodies to HBsAg or HBcAg has not been reported for examination of PHC tissues. However, electron microscopy using an indirect immunoperoxidase technique has been used to demonstrate the presence of HBsAg in a hepatoma cell line (PLC/PRF/5) along the nuclear envelope, on the rough endoplasmic reticulum surface, and in the cisternae of the rough endoplasmic reticulum (Aoki *et al.*, 1982).

III. Geographical Distribution

The geographical association between PHC and chronic hepatitis has been recognized for several decades. Higginson noted in 1963 that there was a high prevalence of PHC, cirrhosis, viral hepatitis, and malnutrition in Africa and Asia, including tribal areas of South Africa, compared to low prevalences of all of these factors in the United States, England, Guatemala, and urban portions of South Africa. This geographical association was confirmed and shown to be specific for hepatitis B when serologic tests for HBsAg became available. In northern Europe and the United States, low prevalence areas for HBV, PHC was found at autopsy in 0.2–1.6% of deaths of all causes compared to 2.4–6.8% in Africa and Asia, high prevalence areas for HBV (Szmuness, 1978). The indigenous populations in high prevalence areas have a high risk for both PHC and HBV; Europeans living there are not subject to a significantly increased risk. PHC patients in high PHC prevalence areas tend to be younger than those from low prevalence areas, suggesting either earlier exposure to the etiological agent(s) or a shorter latency period (Szmuness, 1978). The two regions of the world with HBsAg carrier rates of ~10%, sub-Saharan Africa, and Southeast Asia, are also the areas with the highest prevalences of PHC (Fig. 1).

Three studies have compared the incidence or prevalence of PHC and HBV in different geographical regions within one country. Tabor *et al.* (1985) examined serial serum specimens obtained from residents of five villages in rural Zambia for HBV markers. New HBV infections during the 5-year study were less frequent in one of two villages in which no new cases of PHC had been detected during the preceding 11 years, compared to three villages in each of which two new cases of PHC had been diagnosed during the same period. Trichopoulos *et al.* (1976) examined the prevalence of PHC and HBsAg in nine regions of Greece; in most of the nine regions there was a strong association between a high

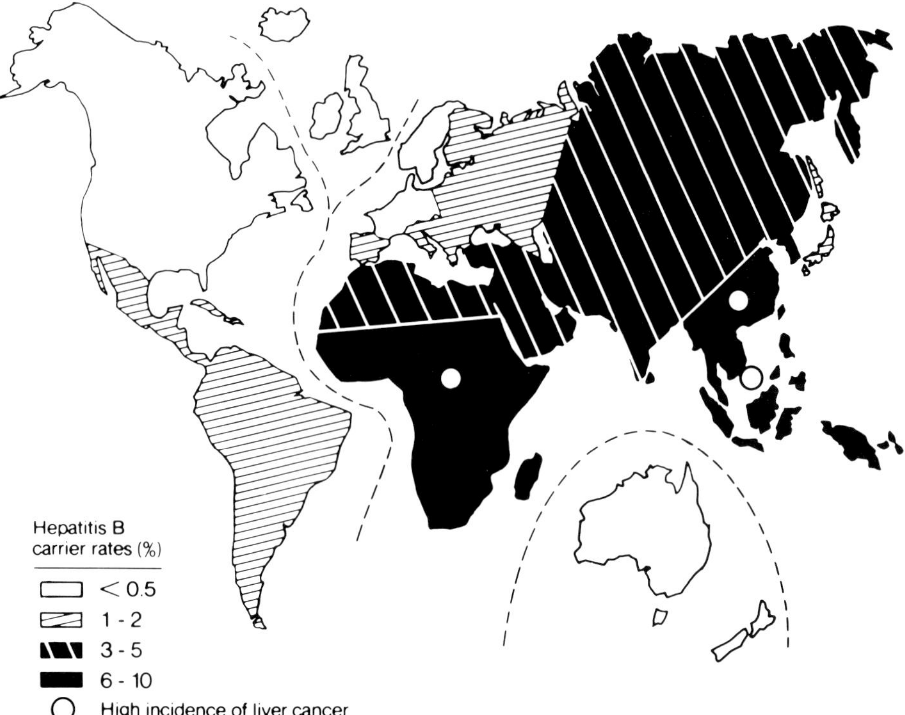

Figure 1. Geographic distribution of hepatitis B surface antigen (HBsAg) and primary hepatocellular carcinoma (PHC). [Reprinted from Szmuness (1978), with permission.]

prevalence of PHC and a high prevalence of HBsAg. Bagshawe *et al.* (1975) did not find any differences in HBsAg prevalence in a small number of patients (26) from two regions of Kenya with different prevalences of PHC.

IV. Serological Data

The association between HBsAg and PHC was first described by Sherlock *et al.* in 1970. During the early 1970s, numerous other investigators reported HBsAg in the serum of up to 50% of PHC patients from many geographical areas, using the relatively insensitive methods of agar gel diffusion and counterelectrophoresis. Higher prevalences of HBV markers were reported beginning in 1977, when the availability of RIAs for HBsAg and anti-HBs and various test methods for the detection of anti-HBc made it possible to detect HBV markers in up to 100% of PHC patients. Results using these tests also led to the realization that the association of HBV markers with PHC was limited to the markers of active HBV infection (HBsAg; in some studies, also anti-HBc in the absence of HBsAg or anti-HBs).

Tabor *et al.* (1977) documented the high prevalence of HBV markers that could be detected in PHC patients using the more sensitive assays, that this association could be demonstrated in white PHC patients from the United States as well as in black PHC patients from Africa, and that this association was limited to serological markers of active HBV infection. Sera from 93 patients with biopsy-proven PHC from Uganda, Zambia, and the United States were tested. Active HBV infection was present overall in 62% of PHC patients (58 of 93), compared to 10% of African controls (9 of 90) and <1% of U.S. controls. Active HBV infections were detected in 34 of 47 PHC patients from Uganda (72%, compared to 4 of 50 controls or 8%, $p < .0001$), 13 of 19 PHC patients from Zambia (68%, compared to 5 of 40 controls or 12%, $p < .0001$), and 11 of 27 U.S. patients (41%, compared to <1% of controls, $p < .0001$) (see Fig. 2).

Similar results were obtained in a study of white PHC patients and carefully matched controls from Greece (Trichopoulos *et al.*, 1978). The prevalence of serological markers of active or past HBV infection was determined in 80 Greek patients with PHC, in 160 age- and sex-matched controls, and in 40 patients with other tumors metastatic to the liver (MLC). Active infection with HBV indicated by HBsAg or anti-HBc (without anti-HBs) was more common in patients with PHC than in

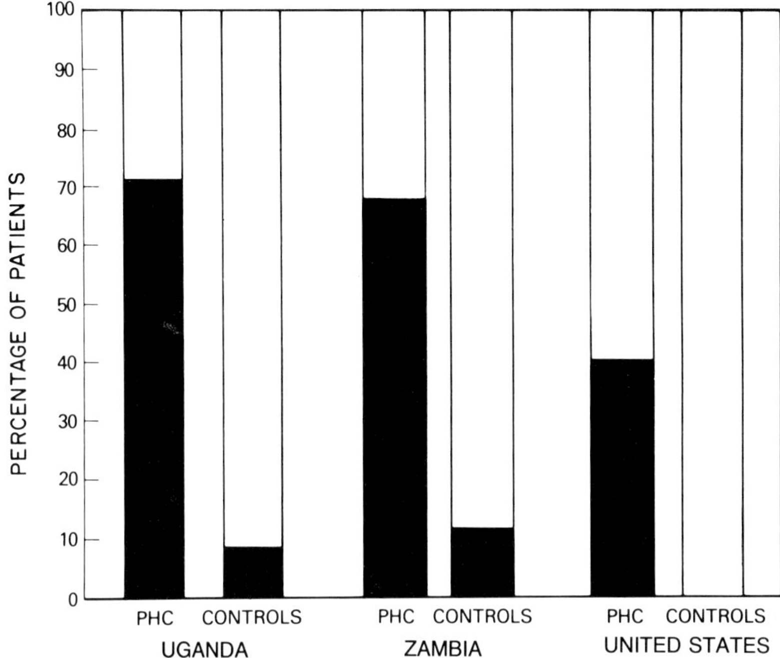

Figure 2. Serological evidence of active hepatitis B virus (HBV) infection in patients with primary hepatocellular carcinoma (PHC) and controls from Uganda, Zambia, and the United States. Active infection, indicated by the dark bar, is defined as the presence of hepatitis B surface antigen (HBsAg, with or without antibody to HBsAg, anti-HBs) or anti-HBc (without anti-HBs). [Reprinted from Tabor et al. (1977).]

controls or patients with MLC ($p < .001$); there was no significant difference between patients with MLC and controls (Table I). Patients with serological evidence of active HBV infection had a relative risk of PHC 10.4-fold greater than the risk in subjects without evidence of active infection. Patients who had recovered from prior HBV infection as indicated by anti-HBs had no greater risk for PHC than those lacking all three markers (estimated relative risk, 0.8). HBV serological markers were detected in 30 of 45 PHC patients with cirrhosis (67%), compared to 9 of 35 patients without cirrhosis (26%, $p < .001$). This study confirmed that the association between HBV and PHC seen in African and Asian populations could also be found in a white European population with different racial, environmental, and dietary circumstances.

The finding of an association between PHC and serological markers of active HBV infection was confirmed in studies by other investigators. These studies included findings of 70% of PHC patients with HBsAg compared to 10% of controls in the Philippines (Lingao et al., 1981); 67%

TABLE I
Hepatitis B Virus Markers in the Serum of Greek Patients and Controls[a]

HBsAg[b]	Anti-HBc	Anti-HBs	PHC	MLC	Controls
+	+	+	7	3	0
+	+	−	32	0	7
+	−	+	0	0	1
+	−	−	0	0	4
−	+	+	17	18	40
−	+	−	0	0	4
−	−	+	8	11	38
−	−	−	16	8	66
			80	40	160

[a]Reprinted from Trichopoulos et al. (1978) with permission.

[b]Abbreviations: HBsAg, hepatitis B surface antigen; anti-HBc, antibody to the hepatitis B core antigen; anti-HBs, antibody to HBsAg; PHC, primary hepatocellular carcinoma; MLC, other tumors metastatic to the liver.

with HBsAg or anti-HBs among PHC patients compared to 21% of controls in Japan (Kubo et al., 1977a); 79% of PHC patients with HBsAg compared to 11% of controls in Senegal (Larouzé et al., 1977); and 91% of PHC patients with HBsAg or anti-HBc alone compared to 39% of controls among blacks from several countries in southern Africa (Kew et al., 1979a).

The close association demonstrated between HBV and PHC is supported by the lack of an association between the serological markers of HBV and other cancers that have metastasized to the liver (Trichopoulos et al., 1978) and the lack of an association between serological evidence of prior hepatitis A virus (HAV) infection and PHC (Tabor et al., 1980). HAV is not related to the development of PHC, in marked contrast to the strong association between PHC and HBV, despite the fact that many regions with a high prevalence of PHC also have a high prevalence of HAV.

The hepatitis B e antigen (HBeAg) is uncommon among PHC patients. When tested by agar gel diffusion, HBeAg is detected in 0 to 5% of PHC patients; antibody to HBeAg (anti-HBe) is detected in 0 to 73% (Lingao et al., 1981; Kew et al., 1979a; Furuta et al., 1977; Trichopoulos et al., 1978; Tabor et al., 1977; Sankale et al., 1977; Coursaget et al., 1978). In two studies using the much more sensitive RIA, HBeAg was found in 12% and anti-HBe in 88% of small groups of HBsAg-positive patients with PHC (Viola et al., 1981; Heyward et al., 1982). Using RIA, HBeAg was detected in 38% and anti-HBe in 45% of a moderately large group of HBsAg-positive PHC patients from Korea (Chung et al., 1983). In studies in which all PHC patients were tested, including those negative for all other HBV markers, testing for HBeAg and anti-HBe did not permit the diagnosis of additional HBV infections in PHC patients (Coursaget *et al.*, 1978; Trichopoulos *et al.*, 1978; Tabor *et al.*, 1977). It has been suggested that the lower prevalence of HBeAg in PHC reflects the fact that active replication of HBV has become defective during the malignant process, or that active HBV replication has diminished in conjunction with the integration of the HBV genome into the hepatocyte DNA. This is consistent with the observation that seroconversion in an HBsAg carrier from HBeAg to anti-HBe can precede the clinical onset of PHC by 1 to 3 years (Heyward *et al.*, 1982).

The association between serological markers of HBV and PHC is supported by numerous reports of the development of PHC in prospectively followed HBsAg-positive patients. Dudley *et al.* (1972) reported the development of PHC in two HBsAg-positive patients whose earlier liver biopsies had shown only cirrhosis, although the precise intervals between the initial and the diagnostic biopsies were not reported. De Groote *et al.* (1978) reported three HBsAg-positive patients with biopsy evidence of chronic hepatitis who had received therapy with prednisone and azathioprine for a period of years and subsequently developed biopsy-proven PHC; the precise interval between the biopsies was not reported, but was stated to be >2 years. Kubo *et al.* (1978) reported 10 HBsAg-positive patients followed between 12 and 79 months for biopsy-proven cirrhosis or chronic hepatitis who subsequently developed PHC. They also reported the development of PHC in nine patients with biopsy-proven cirrhosis or chronic hepatitis who had anti-HBc or anti-HBs and in four patients who had no HBV serological markers following intervals of 24 to 168 months after their initial biopsies. Viola *et al.* (1981) reported an HBsAg-positive patient with cirrhosis in a liver biopsy who developed PHC an unspecified number of years later. In a prospective longitudinal study of 22,707 Chinese men in Taiwan, Beasley *et al.* (1981) observed the development of PHC in HBsAg carriers with an incidence of 1,158 per 100,000 population, compared to an incidence of 5 per 100,000 among noncarriers. The relative risk for the development of PHC among HBsAg carriers was 223 during an average follow-up period of 3.3 years per subject. A retrospective study of stored sera from men of Japanese ancestry in Hawaii found HBsAg in the serum of 10 of 16 (62%) PHC patients from 5 months to 3 years prior to the diagnosis of PHC (Nomura *et al.*, 1982). A retrospective study of stored serial sera from Alaskan Eskimos found HBsAg first appeared 9 and 12 years prior to the diagnosis of two cases of PHC (Heyward *et al.*, 1982).

Not all PHC patients have detectable HBV infections. PHC cases without detectable HBV serological markers have been evaluated (Bréchot *et al.*, 1981, 1982; Kiyosawa *et al.*, 1982). The possible role of integrated HBV DNA, toxins, and non-A, non-B hepatitis agents in some cases are discussed below (Sections VI, VIII, and IX).

Superinfection with the delta (δ) agent during HBV infection has been shown, in some cases of hepatitis B, to be associated with increased severity of liver damage; however, δ agent has rarely been found in association with PHC. In a series of 22 PHC patients with HBV infections in California, δ infection was found in one patient (4%), compared to 10 of 40 patients (25%) with chronic hepatitis without PHC from the same city (Govindarajan *et al.*, 1982). In studies in our laboratory conducted in collaboration with Drs. M. Rizzetto, J. Gerin, and D. Trichopoulos, no evidence of δ infection was found in 100 PHC patients from Greece; antibody to δ antigen was detected in 2 of 100 age- and sex-matched controls (E. Tabor, unpublished observations). Antibody to δ antigen also was not detected in 25 PHC patients from Uganda (E. Tabor, unpublished observations).

V. HBV and PHC in Families

Cases of PHC in patients with HBV serological markers occasionally occur in members of the same family. (The possible role of noninfectious environmental carcinogens to which families may also be exposed are discussed in Section VIII.) Tepfer (1972) and Denison *et al.* (1971) reported a family of three brothers who died from PHC with an interval of 4 years between the first two deaths and an interval of 4 months between the second and third deaths; two had been documented as HBsAg positive and one was not tested. The father of these brothers had died from PHC 23 years earlier, prior to the availability of tests for HBsAg. Johnson *et al.* (1976) reported another group of three brothers who were HBsAg carriers, two of whom had PHC. Ohbayashi *et al.* (1972) reported a mother, her two brothers, and a son who died from PHC; although these patients were not tested for HBV serological markers, most of their family were subsequently found to be either positive for HBsAg or anti-HBs. Sung and Chen (1978) reported two HBsAg-positive brothers whose PHC became clinically apparent simultaneously. Gilmore *et al.* (1981) reported three brothers with PHC (two HBsAg-positive, one not tested), two diagnosed ~7 years apart, and the third identified by subsequent screening. These findings appear unrelated to histocompatibility (HLA) antigens that might be shared by family members; HLA antigens do not differ between PHC patients and controls, or between PHC patients with and without HBsAg (Kew *et al.*, 1979b).

PHC patients often have family members with HBV markers; the high prevalence of HBsAg among mothers of PHC patients has been cited as evidence that the patients may have acquired their HBV infections from their mothers during the perinatal period. Larouzé *et al.* (1976) first reported this observation in 28 PHC patients in Senegal. They found that 71% of the mothers of PHC patients were HBsAg positive (an additional 10% had anti-HBs) compared to 14% of mothers of age- and sex-matched controls (an additional 53% had anti-HBs). None of the fathers of PHC patients had anti-HBs (18% had HBsAg); 48% of fathers of controls had anti-HBs (18% had HBsAg). Larouzé *et al.* suggested that the PHC patients were infected by their carrier mothers, and that the fathers had an inadequate or atypical rate of serological response to HBV despite apparently similar opportunities for exposure. Similar findings have been reported in parents of a group of 11 PHC patients in Taiwan, although no controls were reported (Sung and Chen, 1980). Fewer HBsAg-positive mothers were identified in families of 5 Eskimo patients with PHC, who differed from other series in the very young age range, 9–23 years (Boss *et al.*, 1981); cultural factors affecting transmission of HBV may be a possible explanation for the differences seen between these data and data from other studies.

Blumberg *et al.* (1975) suggested that the presence of HBsAg in either parent results in a greater male:female ratio in the offspring. If these male:female ratios are in fact a direct result of HBV, these circumstances may in part contribute to the greater prevalence of males among chronic carriers of HBsAg and among those PHC patients whose cancers are associated with HBV infections.

VI. Molecular Basis

The identification of HBV DNA integrated into the DNA of PHC tumor cells supports the possible etiological role of HBV and provides a possible mechanism by which its oncogenic potential could be expressed. HBV DNA has been identified by hybridization techniques to be integrated into the PHC tumor DNA in all (Bréchot *et al.*, 1981; Summers *et al.*, 1978b; Shafritz *et al.*, 1981) or most (Koshy *et al.*, 1981) PHC patients with HBsAg in their serum, as well as some patients with anti-HBc or anti-HBs in their serum (Shafritz *et al.*, 1981; Bréchot *et al.*, 1981, 1982), and occasional PHC patients with no HBV serum markers

(Bréchot *et al.*, 1981, 1982). Often it appears that several complete HBV DNA sequences are integrated in tandem with head-to-tail orientation (Bréchot *et al.*, 1981) or possibly in different locations within a given PHC cell population (Koshy *et al.*, 1981). The DNA in the tumors is usually integrated, but in occasional patients low molecular weight "extrachromosomal" DNA is also present (Shafritz *et al.*, 1981). In PHC cases, HBV DNA is often also detected in adjacent nontumorous liver tissue, with either the same or a different hybridization pattern from that of the tumor cells (Shafritz *et al.*, 1981; Bréchot *et al.*, 1981), and may be integrated and/or extrachromosomal (Shafritz *et al.*, 1981). However, it is always possible that detection of "extrachromosomal" DNA represents free intact HBV in blood in the hepatic sinusoids of the specimen in some cases (Shafritz *et al.*, 1981). Two well-studied PHC cell lines (PLC/PRF/5 and Hep 3B) producing HBsAg have been shown to have integrated HBV DNA sequences. Four cell lines not producing HBsAg did not have detectable HBV DNA sequences (Koshy *et al.*, 1981). It has been suggested, based on hybridization results on liver tissue from a small number of patients with acute hepatitis, that integration of HBV DNA occurs early in infection when it does occur (Bréchot *et al.*, 1981).

VII. Other Hepadna Viruses and PHC

Several viruses that resemble HBV but which infect nonprimate animals have been identified; one of these is closely associated with PHC in its host species. These viruses include the woodchuck hepatitis virus (WHV), which infects the woodchuck *Marmota monax* (Summers *et al.*, 1978a), the duck hepatitis virus, which infects the Pekin duck *Anas domesticus* (Mason *et al.*, 1980), and the ground squirrel hepatitis virus, which infects the Beechey ground squirrel *Spermophilus beecheyi* (Marion *et al.*, 1980). These viruses have been tentatively classified with HBV in a new category of viruses, the "hepadna viruses." These are double-stranded DNA viruses that are morphologically similar to HBV and whose antigens in some cases partially cross-react with those of HBV when detected in blood or liver tissue. WHV has been associated with a high death rate from PHC in woodchucks with integrated WHV DNA in tumor cells. Studies of these viruses, particularly WHV, and PHC may clarify the relationship between HBV and PHC in humans. The average age of captive woodchucks dying of PHC is 52 months, making this a useful model for the study of a tumor which may take decades to develop in humans.

VIII. Other Possible Etiologies

Several carcinogens have been suggested as causes of PHC in humans, either acting alone or with HBV. The most likely of these carcinogens is aflatoxin, a product of the mold *Aspergillus flavus* and of a few other saprophytic fungi. Aflatoxin is present in high concentration in the food in many areas where there is a high prevalence of PHC (Vogel and Linsell, 1972; Alpert *et al.*, 1968), and has been shown to be carcinogenic to the livers of experimental animals (Sun *et al.*, 1971; Kalengayi and Desmet, 1975a,b), including the rhesus monkey (Adamson *et al.*, 1973) and a species of marmoset (*Saguinus oedipomidas*) (Lin *et al.*, 1974). Other carcinogens suggested as possibly associated with the development of PHC include diethyl nitrosamine (DENA) (Kelly *et al.*, 1966), cycasin (Laqueur *et al.*, 1963), the mold *Penicillium islandicum* (Oettlé, 1964), and several alkaloids found in medicinal plants used in East Africa (Schoental, 1959; Tsega *et al.*, 1976). Only aflatoxin and DENA have been actively discussed as possible etiological factors in PHC in the years since the recognition of the association between HBV and PHC.

Other etiologies have also been discussed. One study suggested an association between tobacco smoking and PHC (Trichopoulos *et al.*, 1980b). Although exposure to certain steroidal hormones, such as those in birth control pills (Goodman and Ishak, 1982), and exposure to vinyl chloride (Makk *et al.*, 1976) have been associated with certain tumors of the liver, they have not been associated with PHC. Several reports have described PHC developing in persons with preexisting hepatitis unrelated to HBV (Ayoola *et al.*, 1982; Jenkins *et al.*, 1981). It is not clear whether these represent cases of non-A, non-B hepatitis of the type that is transmitted by blood transfusions. An attempt to transmit non-A, non-B hepatitis to a susceptible chimpanzee by inoculation of 1 ml serum from one such patient did not succeed; no non-A, non-B hepatitis occurred, and the chimpanzee remained susceptible to challenge with a known non-A, non-B hepatitis agent (E. Tabor, R. H. Resnick, and R. J. Gerety, unpublished data). The possibility that there is more than one agent responsible for cases of non-A, non-B hepatitis, the lack of sensitive universally accepted serological assays to identify cases caused by a single agent, and the possibility that integration of HBV may have occurred in these patients without HBV serological markers being detectable (perhaps in the presence of superinfection with non-A, non-B hepatitis) makes it impossible to determine whether the reported association between some cases of PHC and hepatitis unrelated to HBV is valid.

Type C RNA virus has also been suggested as a possible etiological agent in PHC, based on the isolation of this genus of virus from transformed mouse PHC cells (Rhim *et al.*, 1974). This finding remains to be confirmed; similar findings have not been reported in humans.

IX. A Unified Theory of the Etiology of PHC

Several versions of a unified theory of the etiology of PHC have been proposed, based on the strong association between HBV and PHC. A person with active HBV infection over a period of years has a markedly greater risk for developing PHC than someone who has never been or is no longer infected with this virus. It appears that someone never infected by HBV or who has recovered from HBV infection is unlikely to develop PHC. It is also probable that a person with chronic HBV infection would not develop PHC unless also affected by a second oncogenic event.

Alteration of the immune response permitting the HBsAg chronic carrier state to develop may interfere with the recognition and destruction of transformed liver cells. To explain the phenomenon of noninfectious PHC cells (PHC cell line PLC/PRF/5) that produce HBsAg (Tabor *et al.*, 1981) in the context of the known association between HBV and PHC, London and Blumberg (1982) proposed that the liver contains two populations of cells, those resistant to active infection ("R cells"), which are relatively immature and constitute a small proportion of adult hepatocytes, and those susceptible to active HBV infection ("S cells"), which are mature cells that predominate in the adult liver. Infection of S cells results in their destruction and the proliferation of R cells. Integration of HBV DNA may occur in either R or S cells, but integration in the already proliferating R cells, particularly at a propitious site in the gene, results in expansion of the R cell clone with neoplastic transformation. Stimulation of the R cell clone would require continued infection of S cells, presumably due to a failure of the host's immune system to eliminate the infection, until a point is reached when the R cell clone becomes autonomous. Independent growth of foci within the same liver having different integration patterns may explain the apparent multifocal origin of PHC in some patients (Shafritz, 1982) and the differing hybridization patterns in PHC cells compared to liver cells from the same patient.

It has been suggested that a second oncogenic agent may alter the immune response to transformed cells. Aflatoxin may interfere with lymphocyte morphology and lymphocyte transformation with consequent failure of the host to distinguish the transformed cells as foreign (Coady, 1977; Lutwick, 1979). A direct effect of aflatoxin on the virus itself has also been suggested as an alternative mechanism (Coady, 1977). It is also conceivable that chronic HBV infection may interfere with the immune response to aflatoxin-induced PHC, although no experimental evidence is available to support this.

It has been suggested that HBV may be carcinogenic via mechanisms similar to those of retroviruses, which have been shown to cause cancers in some animals (Summers and Mason, 1982). Although this similarity is only theoretical for HBV, reverse transcription has been demonstrated during replication of the duck hepatitis virus that resembles HBV. Confirmation and elaboration of those findings are eagerly awaited.

The precise relationship between HBV infection, integration of HBV DNA, and oncogenesis has not been demonstrated. Most theoretical models of the nature of this relationship have been based on animal models and tissue cultures infected with other tumor viruses. A few investigators have urged caution in drawing the conclusion that HBV is actually carcinogenic (Delong, 1982; Kew, 1978; Sabin, 1982). Criteria that should be met before concluding that HBV has an explicit oncogenic role have been outlined (Kew, 1978) (Table II). Clearly, even if HBV is oncogenic, it is probably not the etiology of all cases of PHC.

X. Future Prospects

It appears likely that advanced techniques of molecular biology will continue to provide additional evidence concerning the role of HBV in

TABLE II
Criteria Necessary to Prove the Oncogenic Role of HBV

Criterion	Proved	Not yet proved
HBV infection precedes tumor	+	
HBV antigens in tumor cells	+	
HBV integration in tumor cells	+	
Transformation of hepatocytes *in vitro* by HBV		+
Induction of PHC by HBV in experimental animals		+
Eradication of PHC by eradication of HBV		+

association with PHC. Whether this is a primary or secondary oncogenic role should become apparent with time. An explanation for those PHC cases without detectable HBV serological markers may be found at the same time, perhaps in terms of multiple etiologies, differing co-carcinogens with a single primary oncogenic event, or differing integration patterns of a single oncogenic virus.

Prevention of hepatitis B may lead to a reduction in the incidence of PHC. The availability of hepatitis B vaccines and the prospect of inexpensive mass-produced HBV vaccines made by recombinant DNA and synthetic techniques may provide future prophylaxis against HBV in many underdeveloped areas of the world where both HBV and PHC are prevalent. Intervention with hepatitis B vaccine may reduce the prevalence of PHC by preventing hepatitis B. However, the apparently long incubation period of PHC, from 9 years in some cases (Heyward *et al.*, 1982) to perhaps as long as 20–30 years after acquisition of chronic HBV infection, suggests that proof of this effect may take time.

The refinement of methods for laboratory study of PHC cell lines with integrated HBV DNA that produce HBsAg may provide systems in which to study treatments for PHC. A glimpse of such a system has been reported by Shouval *et al.* (1982), who studied the ability of monoclonal IgM anti-HBs to prevent and suppress the growth of the PHC cell line PLC/PRF/5 when transplanted into BALB/c nude mice. Confirmation of these findings will be eagerly awaited.

Because of the association between PHC and HBV, the rapid advances in HBV research have enabled investigators to obtain a better understanding of PHC. Future advances in HBV research will continue to provide preventive measures and model systems in which to develop treatments for PHC.

References

Adamson, R. H., Correa, P., and Dalgard, D. W. (1973). *J. Natl. Cancer Inst. (U.S.)* **50**, 549–553.

Akagi, G., Furuya, K., and Otsuka, H. (1982). *Cancer* **49**, 678–682.

Alpert, E. (1976). *In* "Hepatocellular Carcinoma" (K. Okuda and R. L. Peters, eds.), pp. 353–367. Wiley, New York.

Alpert, M. E., Wogan, G., and Davidson, C. S. (1968). *Gastroenterology* **54**, 149 (abstr.).

Aoki, N., Thung, S. N., and Gerber, M. A. (1982). *Lab. Invest.* **47**, 465–470.

Ayoola, E. A., Odelola, H. A., and Johnson, A. O. K. (1982). *Hepatology* **2**, 154 (abstr.).

Bagshawe, A. F., Gacengi, D. M., Cameron, C. H., Dorman, J., and Dane, D. S. (1975). *Br. J. Cancer* **31**, 581–584.

Bayley, A. C. (1978). *Proc. Assoc. Surg. E. Afr.* **1**, 33–37.

Beasley, R. P., Hwang, L. Y., Lin, C. C., and Chien, C. S. (1981). *Lancet 2*, 1129–1133.

Blumberg, B. S., Larouzé, B., London, W. T., Werner, B., Hesser, J. E., Millman, I., Saimot, G., and Payet, M. (1975). *Am. J. Pathol.* **81**, 669–682.

Boss, L. P., Bender, T. R., Schreeder, M. T., Lanier, A. P., Hardison, H. H., and Maynard, J. E. (1981). *Am. J. Epidemiol.* **114**, 95–101.

Bowry, T. S., and Cameron, H. M. (1976). *Trans. R. Soc. Trop. Med. Hyg.* **70**, 439–443.

Bréchot, C., Hadchouel, M., Scotto, J., Fonck, M., Potet, F., Vyas, G. N., and Tiollais, P. (1981). *Proc. Natl. Acad. Sci. U.S.A.* **78**, 3906–3910.

Bréchot, C., Nalpas, B., Couroucé, A., Duhamel, G., Callard, P., Carnot, F., Tiollais, P., and Berthelot, P. (1982). *N. Engl. J. Med.* **306**, 1384–1387.

Campion, E. C., Ludbrook, J., McLeod, G. M., Marshall, V. R., Mukherjee, T., and Wangel, A. G. (1972). *Br. Med. J.* **4**, 149–152.

Chainuvati, T., Viranuvatti, V., and Pongpipat, D. (1975). *Gastroenterology* **68**, 1261–1264.

Chen, D., and Sung, J. (1977). *Cancer* **40**, 779–783.

Chung, W. K., Sun, H. S., Park, D. H., Minuk, G. Y., and Hoofnagle, J. H. (1983). *J. Med. Virol.* **11**, 99–104.

Coady, A. (1977). *Trans. R. Soc. Trop. Med. Hyg.* **71**, 86–87 (lett.).

Coursaget, P., Maupas, P., Goudeau, A., and Drucker, J. (1978). *J. Clin. Microbiol.* **7**, 394–395.

De Groote, J., Fevery, J., and Lepoutre, L. (1978). *Gut* **19**, 510–513.

Delong, S. (1982). *In* "Viral Hepatitis" (W. Szmuness, H. J. Alter, and J. E. Maynard, eds.), pp. 253–259. Franklin Inst. Press, Philadelphia, Pennsylvania.

Denison, E. K., Peters, R. L., and Reynolds, T. B. (1971). *Ann. Intern. Med.* **74**, 391–394.

Doury, J. C., Roche, J. C., and Brisou, B. (1978). *Rev. Epidem. Santé Publ.* **26**, 161–170.

Dudley, F. J., Scheuer, P. J., and Sherlock, S. (1972). *Lancet 2*, 1388–1393.

Fraumeni, J. F., Miller, R. W., and Hill, J. A. (1968). *J. Natl. Cancer Inst. (U.S.)* **40**, 1087–1099.

Furuta, S., Kiyosawa, K., Nagata, A., Koike, Y., Sahara, T., Furukawa, K., Iijima, Y., Yamamura, S., Komatsu, H., Kawahara, K., Miura, M., Gibo, Y., Sodeyama, K., Oda, M., Tsuda, F., Akahane, Y., and Mayumi, M. (1977). *Gastroenterol. Jpn.* **12**, 460–465.

Gilmore, I. T., Harrison, J. M., and Parkins, R. A. (1981). *J. R. Soc. Med.* **74**, 843–845.

Goodman, Z. D., and Ishak, K. G. (1982). *Hepatology* **2**, 440–444.

Govindarajan, S., Ashcavai, M., and Peters, R. L. (1982). *Hepatology* **2**, 714 (abstr.).

Heyward, W. L., Bender, T. R., Lanier, A. P., Francis, D. P., McMahon, B. J., and Maynard, J. E. (1982). *Lancet 2*, 889–891.

Higginson, J. (1963). *Cancer Res.* **23**, 1624–1633.

Jenkins, P. J., Melia, W. M., Portmann, B., Longworth-Krafft, J. M., and Williams, R. (1981). *Gut* **22**, 332–335.

Johnson, P., Wansbrough-Jones, M., Eddleston, A. L. W. F., Williams, R., Calne, R. Y., and Maycock, W. d'A. (1976). *Digestion* **14**, 524 (abstr.).

Kalengayi, M. M., and Desmet, V. J. (1975a). *Cancer Res.* **35**, 2836–2844.

Kalengayi, M. M., and Desmet, V. J. (1975b). *Cancer Res.* **35**, 2845–2852.

Kelly, M. G., O'Gara, R. W., Adamson, R. H., Gadekar, K., Botkin, C. C., Reese, W. H., and Kerber, W. T. (1966). *J. Natl. Cancer Inst. (U.S.)* **36**, 323–351.

Kew, M. C. (1978). *In* "Viral Hepatitis" (G. N. Vyas, S. N. Cohen, and R. Schmid, eds.), pp. 439–454. Franklin Inst. Press, Philadelphia, Pennsylvania.

Kew, M. C., Desmyter, J., Bradburne, A. F., and MacNab, G. M. (1979a). *J. Natl. Cancer Inst. (U.S.)* **62**, 517–520.

Kew, M. C., Gear, A. J., Baumgarten, I., Dusheiko, G. M., and Maier, G. (1979b). *Gastroenterology* **77**, 537–539.
Kew, M. C., Ray, M. B., Desmet, V. J., and Desmyter, J. (1980). *Br. J. Cancer* **41**, 399–406.
Kew, M. C., Hodkinson, J., Paterson, A. C., and Song, E. (1982). *J. Med. Virol.* **9**, 201–207.
Kiyosawa, K., Akahane, Y., Nagata, A., Koike, Y., and Furuta, S. (1982). *Vox Sang.* **43**, 45–52.
Koshy, R., Maupas, P., Müller, R., and Hofschneider, P. H. (1981). *J. Gen. Virol.* **57**, 95–102.
Kubo, Y., Okuda, K., Shimokawa, Y., Arishima, T., Nagata, E., Hashimoto, M., Jinnouchi, S., Sawa, Y., Obata, H., and Hayashi, N. (1977a). *Gastroenterology* **72**, 1213–1216.
Kubo, Y., Okuda, K., Hashimoto, M., Nagasaki, Y., Ebata, H., Nakajima, Y., Musha, H., Sakuma, K., and Ohtake, H. (1977b). *Gastroenterology* **72**, 1217–1220.
Kubo, Y., Okuda, K., Musha, H., and Nakashima, T. (1978). *Gastroenterology* **74**, 578–582.
Laqueur, G. L., Mickelsen, O., Whiting, M. G., and Kurland, L. T. (1963). *J. Natl. Cancer Inst. (U.S.)* **31**, 919–951.
Larouzé, B., London, W. T., Saimot, G., Werner, B. G., Lustbader, E. D., Payet, M., and Blumberg, B. S. (1976). *Lancet* 2, 534–538.
Larouzé, B., Blumberg, B. S., London, W. T., Lustbader, E. D., Sankalé, M., and Payet, M. (1977). *J. Natl. Cancer Inst. (U.S.)* **58**, 1557–1561.
Lin, J. J., Liu, C., and Svoboda, D. J. (1974). *Lab. Invest.* **30**, 267–278.
Lingao, A. L., Domingo, E. O., and Nishioka, K. (1981). *Cancer* **48**, 1590–1595.
London, W. T., and Blumberg, B. S. (1982). *Hepatology* **2**, Suppl., 10s–14s.
Lutwick, L. I. (1979). *Lancet* 1, 755–757.
Makk, L., Delmore, F., Creech, J. L., Ogden, L. L., Fadell, E. H., Songster, C. L., Clanton, J., Johnson, M. N., and Christopherson, W. M. (1976). *Cancer* **37**, 149–163.
Marion, P. L., Oshiro, L. S., Regnery, D. C., Scullard, G. H., and Robinson, W. S. (1980). *Proc. Natl. Acad. Sci. U.S.A.* **77**, 2941–2945.
Mason, W. S., Seal, G., and Summers, J. (1980). *J. Virol.* **36**, 829–836.
Nayak, N. C., Sachdeva, R., Dhar, A., and Seth, H. N. (1979). *Indian J. Med. Res.* **69**, 161–167.
Nazarewicz, T., Krawczynski, K., Slusarczyk, J., and Nowoslawski, A. (1977). *J. Infect. Dis.* **135**, 298–302.
Nomura, A., Stemmerman, G. N., and Wasnich, R. D. (1982). *JAMA, J. Am. Med. Assoc.* **247**, 2247–2249.
Obata, H., Hayashi, N., Motoike, Y., Hisamitsu, T., Okuda, H., Kobayashi, S., and Nishioka, K. (1980). *Int. J. Cancer* **25**, 741–747.
Oettlé, A. G. (1964). *J. Natl. Cancer Inst. (U.S.)* **33**, 383–436.
Ohbayashi, A., Okochi, K., and Mayumi, M. (1972). *Gastroenterology* **62**, 618–625.
Okuda, K., Nakashima, T., Sakamoto, K., Ikari, T., Hidaka, H., Kubo, Y. Sakuma, K., Motoike, Y., Okuda, H., and Obata, H. (1982). *Cancer* **49**, 450–455.
Omata, M., Ashcavai, M., Liew, C., and Peters, R. L. (1979). *Gastroenterology* **76**, 279–287.
Prince, A. M., Szmuness, W., Michon, J., Demaille, J., Diebolt, G., Linhard, J., Quenum, C., and Sankalé, M. (1975). *Int. J. Cancer* **16**, 376–383.
Ratcliffe, H. L. (1961). *Cancer Res.* **21**, 26–30.
Reed, W. D., Eddleston, A. L. W. F., Stern, R. B., Williams, R., Zuckerman, A. J., Bowes, A., and Earl, P. M. (1973). *Lancet* 2, 690–694.
Rhim, J. S., Wuu, K. D., Vernon, M. L., Chen, H. W., Meier, H., Waymouth, C., and Huebner, R. J. (1974). *Cancer Res.* **34**, 484–490.

Sabin, A. (1982). *In* "Viral Hepatitis" (W. Szmuness, H. J. Alter, and J. E. Maynard, eds.), pp. 678–679. Franklin Inst. Press, Philadelphia, Pennsylvania.

Sankalé, M., Sow, A. M., and Thermos, M. (1977). *Afr. J. Med. Med. Sci.* **6,** 157–158.

Schoental, R. (1959). *J. Pathol. Bacteriol.* **77,** 485–580.

Shafritz, D. A. (1982). *Hepatology* **2,** Suppl., 35s–41s.

Shafritz, D. A., Shouval, D., Sherman, H. I., Hadziyannis, S. J., and Kew, M. C. (1981). *N. Engl. J. Med.* **305,** 1067–1073.

Sherlock, S., Fox, R. A., Niazi, S. P., and Scheuer, P. J. (1970). *Lancet* 1, 1243–1247.

Shikata, T., Uzawa, T., Yoshiwara, N., Akatsuka, T., and Yamazaki, S. (1974). *Jpn. J. Exp. Med.* **44,** 25–36.

Shikata, T., Yamazaki, S., and Uzawa, T. (1977). *Acta Pathol. Jpn.* **27,** 297–304.

Shouval, D., Wands, J. R., Zurawski, V. R., Isselbacher, K. J., and Shafritz, D. A. (1982). *Hepatology* **2,** Suppl., 128s–133s.

Summers, J., and Mason, W. S. (1982). *Cell* **29,** 403–415.

Summers, J., Smolec, J. M., and Snyder, R. (1978a). *Proc. Natl. Acad. Sci. U.S.A.* **75,** 4533–4537.

Summers, J., O'Connell, A., Maupas, P., Goudeau, A., Coursaget, P., and Drucker, J. (1978b). *J. Med. Virol.* **2,** 207–214.

Sun, S., Wei, R., and Schaeffer, B. T. (1971). *Lab. Invest.* **24,** 368–372.

Sung, J., and Chen, D. (1978). *Am. J. Gastroenterol.* **69,** 559–564.

Sung, J., and Chen, D. (1980). *Scand. J. Gastroenterol.* **15,** 321–324.

Swenson, P. D., Escobar, M. R., and Silverman, J. F. (1980). *Acta Biol. Acad. Sci. Hung.* **31,** 321–328.

Szmuness, W. (1978). *Prog. Med. Virol.* **24,** 40–69.

Tabor, E., Gerety, R. J., Vogel, C. L., Bayley, A. C., Anthony, P. P., Chan, C. H., and Barker, L. F. (1977). *J. Natl. Cancer Inst. (U.S.)* **58,** 1197–1200.

Tabor, E., Trichopoulos, D., Manousos, O., Zavitsanos, X., Drucker, J. A., and Gerety, R. J. (1980). *Int. J. Epidemiol.* **9,** 221–223.

Tabor, E., Copeland, J. A., Mann, G. F., Howard, C. R., Skelly, J., Snoy, P., Zuckerman, A. J., and Gerety, R. J. (1981). *Intervirology* **15,** 82–86.

Tabor, E., Bayley, A. C., Cairns, J., Pelleu, L., and Gerety, R. J. (1985). *J. Med. Virol.* **15** 113–120.

Tepfer, B. D. (1972). *Ann. Intern. Med.* **76,** 145–146 (lett.).

Trevisan, A., Realdi, G., Losi, C., Ninfo, V., Rugge, M., and Rampinelli, L. (1978). *J. Clin. Pathol.* **31,** 1133–1139.

Trichopoulos, D., Papaevangelou, G., Violaki, M., Vissoulis, C., Sparros, L., and Manousos, O. N. (1976). *Br. J. Cancer* **34,** 83–87.

Trichopoulos, D., Tabor, E., Gerety, R. J., Xirouchaki, E., Sparros, L., Munoz, N., and Linsell, C. A. (1978). *Lancet* 2, 1217–1219.

Trichopoulos, D., Sizaret, P., Tabor, E., Gerety, R. J., Martel, N., Munoz, N., and Theodoropoulos, G. (1980a). *Cancer* **46,** 736–740.

Trichopoulos, D., MacMahon, B., Sparros, L., and Merikas, G. (1980b). *J. Natl. Cancer Inst. (U.S.)* **65,** 111–114.

Tsega, E., Gold, P., Shuster, J., Whittemore, B., and Lester, F. T. (1976). *J. Trop. Med. Hyg.* **79,** 230–234.

Viola, L. A., Barrison, I. G., Coleman, J. C., Paradinas, F. J., and Murray-Lyon, I. M. (1981). *J. Med. Virol.* **8,** 169–175.

Vogel, C. L., and Linsell, C. A. (1972). *J. Natl. Cancer Inst. (U.S.)* **48,** 567–571.

Vogel, C. L., Anthony, P. P., Mody, N., and Barker, L. F. (1970). *Lancet* 2, 621–624.

Chapter 12

Histopathological Studies of Hepatitis B

LEONARDO BIANCHI AND HANS-PETER SPICHTIN
Department of Pathology
University of Basel
Basel, Switzerland

I. Introduction

In the last few years, a number of review papers on histopathology of acute and chronic hepatitis have appeared (Bianchi *et al.*, 1977; Mac-Sween, 1980; Peters, 1975; Phillips and Poucell, 1981; Popper, 1975). As a consequence of the exact serological definition of hepatitis B infection, progress has been made in the assessment of histopathological changes of hepatitis B. In addition to conventional histopathological features, tissue expression of viral antigens has been recognized as a useful additional tool in characterizing the type of hepatitis B infection. This chapter centers on histopathology associated with hepatitis B in humans, but

269

Copyright © 1985 by Academic Press, Inc.
All rights of reproduction in any form reserved.
ISBN 0-12-280672-7

reference will be made to morphological findings in the chimpanzee model of hepatitis B infection where relevant.

II. Tissue Expression of Hepatitis B Antigens

A. Introduction

It is generally accepted that both complete and incomplete synthesis of viral particles are not lethal for the liver cell in the absence of host-immune responsiveness. This classification of hepatitis B virus as a non-cytotoxic virus is compatible with its ability to produce persistent infections.

The assumption that liver cell damage in hepatitis B virus infections is mediated by host immunological reactions is substantiated by the following observations (for review, see Bianchi and Gudat, 1979; Levy and Chisari, 1981; also see Chapter 11 in this volume):

1. Hepatitis B virus carriers tolerate large numbers of virus-producing cells without substantial histological or biochemical cell damage
2. There is mild or even no inflammation despite the presence of generalized liver cell infection in immunologically compromised patients such as patients on hemodialysis, on cytotoxic treatment, or with malignant lymphoma
3. A carrier state can be induced by immunosuppression
4. There are no cytopathic effects seen in HBsAg-producing hepatocellular carcinoma cell lines
5. Many reports on nonspecific and virus-specific immunity indicate that there is an immune deficiency associated with spontaneously occurring chronic hepatitis B.

Based on this premise, we have suggested that the extent of viral antigen expression arbitrarily reflects the grade of "elimination insufficiency" of host defense mechanisms (Gudat *et al.*, 1975). An extensive review of hepatitis B virus antigen localization in liver tissue appears in Gerber and Thung (1979) and in Yamada *et al.* (1978).

B. Expression of HBcAg in Liver Tissue

The most instructive example for a fully tolerated hepatitis B virus replication is seen in kidney transplant recipients, who are immunosuppressed to the extent that they cannot reject the transplant. In this instance, HBcAg is found in almost every liver cell nucleus (Fig. 1A). This generalized HBcAg expression is usually associated with a nonaggressive type of inflammation (see Table I). Rarely and in extreme cases this accumulation of HBcAg particles may become visible in the light microscope as an eosinophilic, finely granular staining of single nuclei ("sanded nuclei;" Bianchi and Gudat, 1976) (Fig. 1B). In addition, HBcAg may be seen extruded from the nucleus; in occasional biopsies it has also been observed as a purely cytoplasmic fluorescence (Fig. 1C) with accumulation beneath the cell membrane suggesting a flow of particles from the nucleus toward the cell membrane (Gudat and Bianchi, 1977a).

Electron microscopy (Gudat *et al.*, 1975; Huang and Groh, 1973; Kamimura *et al.*, 1981), including immune ferritin or peroxidase methods (Gerber *et al.*, 1972; Huang *et al.*, 1972), has confirmed this distribution by the demonstration of 20- to 25-nm naked core particles in nuclei and the extracisternal space of the cytoplasm (Fig. 1D).

More recent immune electron microscopic studies (Yamada and Nakane, 1977) have revealed, in addition, nonparticulate HBcAg in nuclear and cytoplasmic ground substance, on free and membrane-bound ribosomes, and on cores associated with HBsAg filaments within the cisternae of the rough endoplasmic reticulum. Accordingly, Yamada *et al.* (1978) suggested the following steps for the formation of Dane particles: synthesis of nonparticulate HBcAg on ribosomes; transport through nuclear pores into the nucleus; assembly in core particles in the nucleus;

TABLE I

Histopathology of Hepatitis B: Histological Spectrum

Acute Hepatitis B
  Acute spotty necrotic hepatitis
  Acute hepatitis with piecemeal necrosis
  Acute hepatitis with bridging (confluent) necrosis
  Acute hepatitis with massive necrosis

Chronic Hepatitis B
  True HBV carrier
  Chronic nonaggressive hepatitis (chronic
    persistent hepatitis)
  Chronic aggressive (active) hepatitis
    With minimal activity [activity (a)]
    With moderate activity [activity (a)]
    With severe activity [activity (b)]

HBsAg-Positive Cirrhosis

HBsAg-Positive Hepatocellular Carcinoma

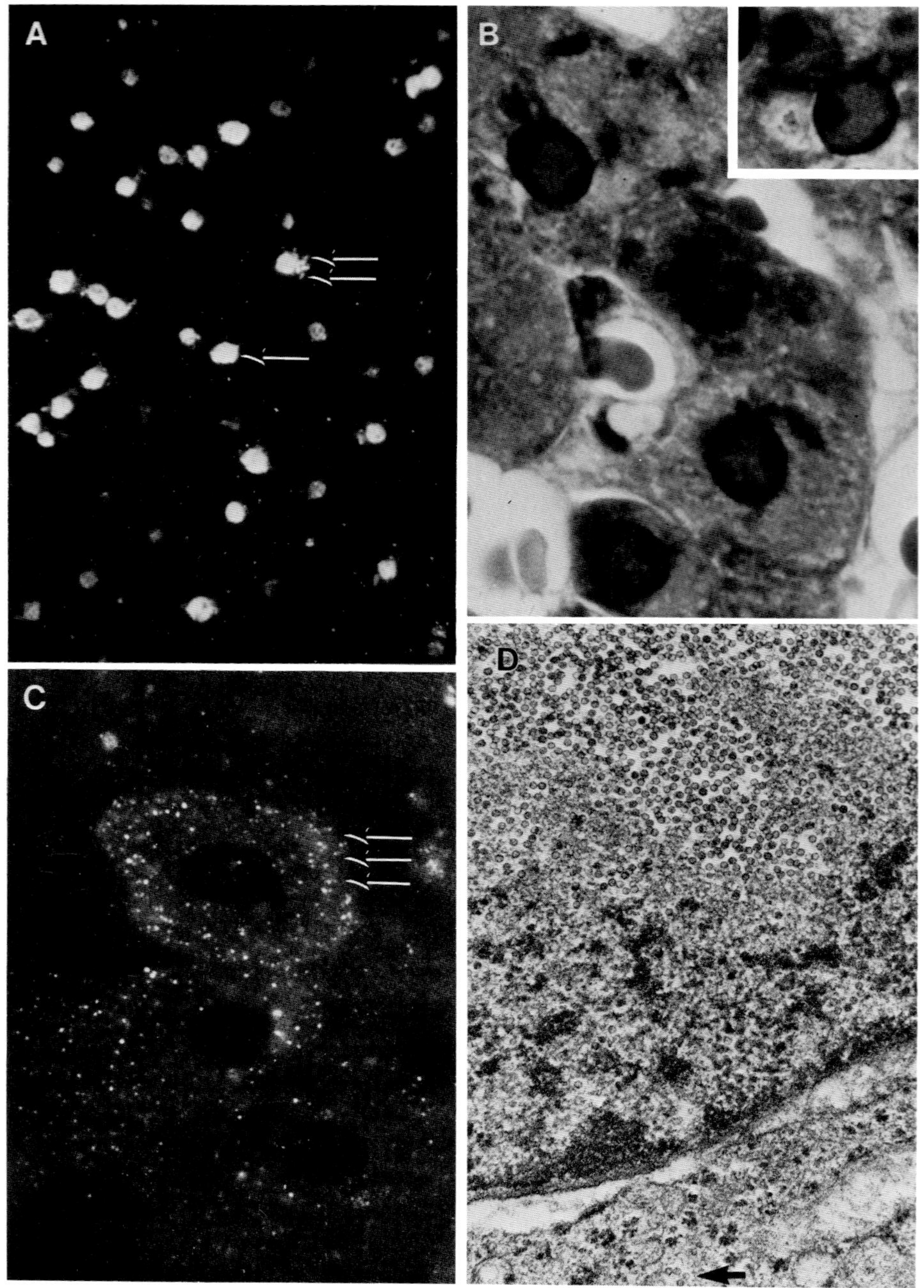

release of core particles into the extracisternal space; entry into the cister-nae of the rough endoplasmic reticulum; envelopment within the endo-plasmic reticulum to complete Dane particles; and release into extra-cellular space together with other excess HBsAg particles.

Our own observations suggest the extent of HBcAg expression ar-bitrarily reflects the degree of immune "elimination insufficiency." Three basic patterns are recognized in chronic hepatitis B (Gudat *et al.*, 1975; Bianchi and Gudat, 1979; Fig. 2). Besides the *generalized HBcAg type* exemplified by the kidney transplant recipient, there may be a focal nuclear positivity for HBcAg *(focal HBcAg type)*. This is most often associ-ated with chronic aggressive hepatitis or cases bordering on chronic persistent hepatitis (see Section III,B, and Table V). At the other end of the spectrum, HBcAg expression may be below immunohistological de-tection (sampling error), and recognizable only by the additional im-mune electron microscopic demonstration of Dane particles in blood. We now consider the presence of Dane particles in serum as a sign of active core replication, and thus such cases are considered to represent a focal HBcAg expression even in the absence of immunohistological find-ings. This may settle some discrepancies in the literature concerning the diagnostic significance of such patterns (Gerber and Thung, 1979). A true *HBcAg-free type*, expressing HBsAg only, is found in HBsAg carriers that circulate neither Dane particles nor HBeAg but antibodies specifical-ly directed against Dane particles (anti–Dane particle antibodies) and anti-HBe (see Section III,A, and Table V).

Finally, the effective elimination of virus-infected cells as seen in acute limited hepatitis B *(elimination type)* manifests itself by a lack of demon-strable viral antigens. Usually, this point is already reached at the height of acute hepatitis B (see Section II,A) and viral antigens are detectable in tissue only in the very early phase of hepatitis B (Arnold *et al.*, 1975).

It is our experience that fluctuations between neighbored expression patterns (e.g., between focal and generalized HBcAg type) may occur in chronic hepatitis B either spontaneously or following initiation or reduc-tion of immunosuppressive therapy.

In Fig. 2, a tentative scheme is shown in which it is assumed that an immune elimination insufficiency forms the basis of chronic hepatitis,

---

Figure 1. Demonstration of HBcAg in liver tissue. (A) Purely intranuclear HBcAg (arrow), demonstrated by immunofluorescence. Note outflow of HBcAg into cytoplasm in one place (two arrows). (B) Light microscopy of excess nuclear HBcAg ("sanded nuclei") in an immu-nosuppressed kidney transplant recipient. (C) Diffuse cytoplasmic pattern of HBcAg (three arrows). Nuclei emptied. (D) Electron microscopy of intranuclear naked HBcAg particles (24–27 nm) and some HBcAg particles in the cytosol (arrow).

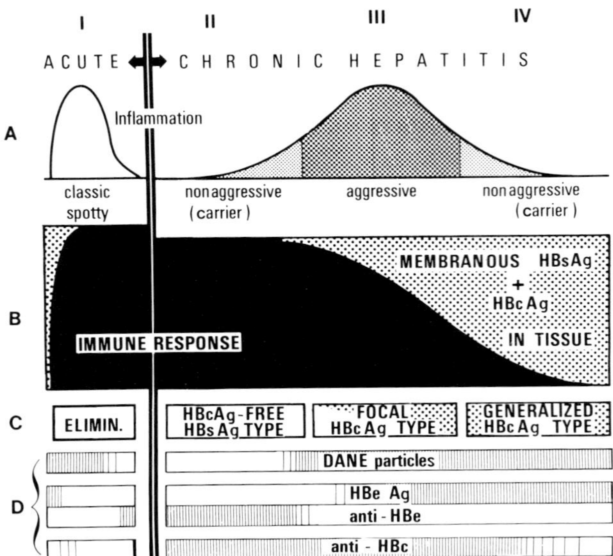

Figure 2. Hypothetical scheme of the four basic reaction types in a dynamic model of HB. (A) Type and severity of inflammatory reaction. (B) Extent of nuclear HBcAg and membrane-associated HBsAg in relation to efficiency of the immune response. (C) Integration of the four basic viral expression types (D) HB-associated antigens and antibodies in blood. Type-associated findings are read top to bottom: (I) classic acute hepatitis in the presence of a highly efficient immune response; (II) chronic persistent (nonaggressive) hepatitis, associated with HBcAg–free HBsAg type, lack of HBeAg, and presence of anti-HBe in serum; (III) chronic aggressive hepatitis, associated with a variable degree of HBcAg expression in accordance with the degree of histologic activity of the process; and (IV) chronic persistent (nonaggressive) hepatitis, associated with generalized HBcAg type, and exemplified by efficiently immunosuppressed patients (e.g., kidney transplant recipients). [From Bianchi *et al.* (1979), with permission of Churchill-Livingstone, Edinburgh.]

and that the gradual decrease of the elimination efficiency is inversely correlated to the extent of HBcAg expression in tissue. The prevailing inflammatory reaction and the virus-specific serology is correlated here with the HBcAg expression pattern.

C. Expression of HBsAg in Liver Tissue

By immunohistology and special stains (orcein, aldehyde thionine, and Victoria blue), HBsAg becomes visible in the cytoplasm of liver cells. All stages may be seen, from a faint localized perinuclear appearance to broad cytoplasmic involvement (Fig. 3A) with a margination along the cell membrane. The immunohistological incubation often reveals, in addition to these cytoplasmic patterns, a liver cell membrane-associated honeycomb pattern (Fig. 3B). The exact relation of the antigen to the liver cell membrane is not clear, but it may be related to HBsAg demonstrated on the surface of isolated liver cells incubated in suspension. In our material, a focal or generalized appearance of this membrane-associated fluorescence was closely related to active HBcAg formation in the same biopsy (Bianchi and Gudat, 1979).

The diffuse cytoplasmic excess deposition of HBsAg is visible by conventional light microscopy as a homogeneous ground-glass material in the cytoplasm of affected liver cells (Hadziyannis *et al.*, 1973), and it stains intensely brown with orcein (Fig. 3C). By electron microscope, ground-glass cells exhibit a marked proliferation of the smooth endoplasmic reticulum, with a dislocation of the cytoplasmic organelles toward the periphery of the cell. Within the cisternae of the endoplasmic reticulum, there are typical filaments (Fig. 3D) giving a positive reaction for HBsAg in immune electron microscopy (Gerber *et al.*, 1972; Yamada and Nakane, 1977).

D. Other HBV Markers in Liver Tissue

1. HBeAg. HBeAg, primarily detected as a nonparticulate HB-associated antigen in serum (Magnius and Espmark, 1972), has been identified as a HB core-associated antigen by Miyakawa and Mayumi (1982). In keeping with this, Arnold *et al.* (1977) could demonstrate HBeAg in liver cell nuclei, mostly co-occurring with HBcAg, but not in the cytoplasm as claimed by others (Trepo *et al.*, 1976).

2. Delta Antigen (δ). δ (Rizzetto *et al.*, 1977) is believed to represent a marker for a defective RNA virus coexisting with and depending on a replicating HBV infection. By immunofluorescence, δ is found mainly but not exclusively in liver cell nuclei (Fig. 4). Similar to HBcAg (Gudat and Bianchi, 1977a), a sequential nuclear–cytoplasmic flow of δ antigen has been observed (Stöcklin *et al.*, 1981).

It is suspected that δ infection may modulate the natural history as well as the histology of chronic HBV infections in chimpanzees and humans (Bonino *et al.*, 1981; Rizzetto *et al.*, 1977; Canese *et al.*, 1979). Superinfection of HBsAg carrier chimpanzees with the δ agent (Rizzetto *et al.*, 1980) results in the appearance of δ antigen in liver tissue, an acute hepatitis with histologic features of superimposed acute lobular changes including neutrophils (H. Popper, personal communication), which is paralleled by a reduction or disappearance of HB virus expression in liver tissue and blood (Rizzetto *et al.*, 1980). It is noteworthy, however, that intravenous drug abusers may be expressing both δ and circulating

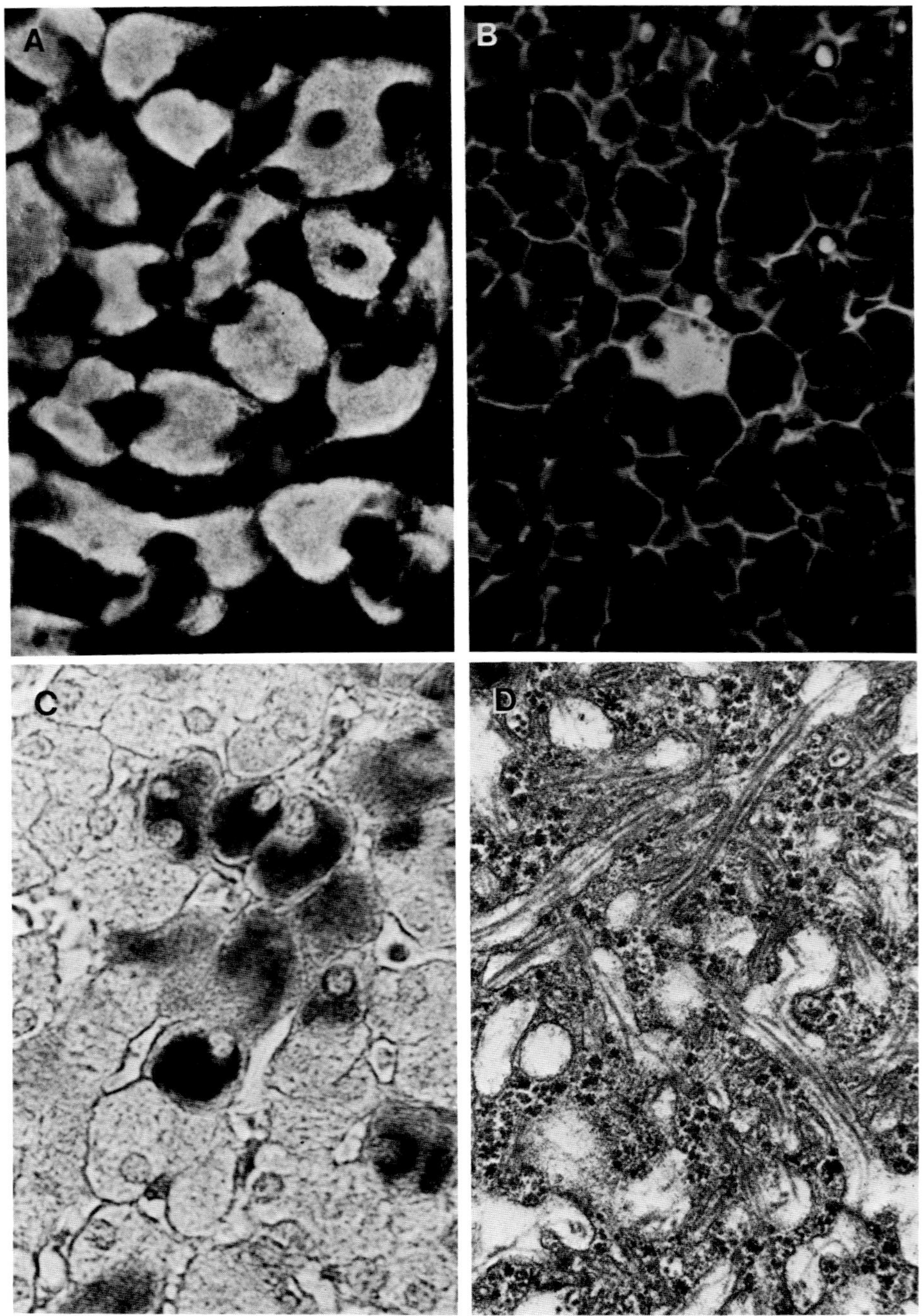

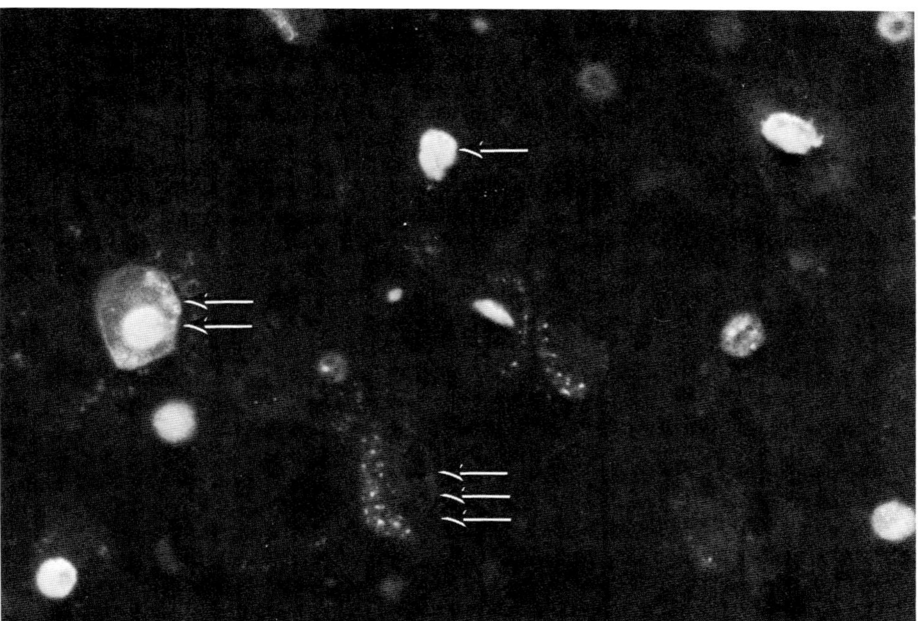

Figure 4. Differential distribution of δ antigen in liver cells: purely intranuclear fluorescence (arrow); as a second step, intranuclear and cytoplasmic localization (two arrows); and as a third step, purely cytoplasmic (mainly submembraneous) accumulation of δ antigen (three arrows), analogous to nuclear/cytoplasmic flow of HBcAg (compare with Fig. 1).

Dane particles in easily detectable numbers over long periods of time (Stöcklin *et al.*, 1981): Persistence of δ antigen over a period of 6 years could be demonstrated retrospectively on paraffin sections.

E. Hepatitis B Antigens on Liver Cell Surfaces

Essential for immunological killing of virus-infected cells is the expression of viral antigens on the liver cell surface. The most compelling evidence for such a target antigen on infected cells has been shown for HBsAg in tissue sections from patients with acute or chronic HBV infection (Gudat and Bianchi, 1977b; Ray *et al.*, 1976) and on isolated liver cells

---

Figure 3. Demonstration of HBsAg in liver tissue. (A) Specific immunofluorescence of purely intracytoplasmic HBsAg in an HBcAg–free HBsAg carrier. (B) Honeycomb-like membrane-associated pattern of HBsAg and focal intracytoplasmic HBsAg in a kidney transplant recipient. (C) HBsAg-positive liver cells in an orcein-stained paraffin section. (D) Electron microscopic demonstration of filamentous intracisternal HBsAg within a proliferated and distorted smooth endoplasmic reticulum.

(Alberti *et al.*, 1976; Realdi *et al.*, 1978), including immune electron microscopic demonstration (Yamada and Nakane, 1977). Realdi *et al.* (1978) reported that surface HBsAg could be capped by anti-HBs, suggesting an integration of the antigen into the plasma membrane.

Membrane-bound IgG can be demonstrated on isolated liver cells, mainly in chronic HBV infections with an inflammatory reaction, and less so in true chronic carriers. These IgG deposits are granular in contrast to the linear staining of liver cell surfaces in autoimmune type hepatitis (Hopf *et al.*, 1975). Elution studies (Trevisan *et al.*, 1982) with such cells revealed anti-HBc activity rather than anti-HBs. It cannot be excluded, however, that this represents antibody eluted from HBcAg-positive nuclei, which are known to harbor IgG, presumably anti-HBc (Arnold *et al.*, 1975; Gudat *et al.*, 1977).

By a double-marker technique, Trevisan *et al.* (1979) demonstrated a significant association between granular IgG on the cell surface and active nuclear HBcAg synthesis, but not with intracellular HBsAg. Further studies are needed to evaluate the immunopathological relevance of this humoral immune response, whether it has an effect on the inflammatory reaction (Hopf *et al.*, 1975) or whether it is a blocking effect for effective immune destruction causing persistence of actively replicating cells (Trevisan *et al.*, 1979).

Although there is circumstantial evidence for membrane-associated HBcAg (Gudat and Bianchi, 1977a; Ray *et al.*, 1976), its nature as target antigen has not been proven. Other antigen–antibody systems (Alberti *et al.*, 1978) are additional candidates for membrane-associated viral target antigens. Nothing is known about the occurrence of HBeAg at the level of the cell membrane.

F. Diagnostic Implications
of Immunohistological Findings

The demonstration of either HBsAg or HBcAg beyond the serum aminotransferase peak in acute infections is indicative of an elimination insufficiency, and a chronic course is most likely to occur, especially if viral antigens are present 3 months after onset of acute hepatitis B. The tissue localization of HBsAg is linked to circulating 20-nm spherical particles and tubular HBsAg, but not necessarily to circulating Dane particles. Even circulating HBsAg may be undetectable by radioimmunoassay, anti-HBc being the only detectable marker of infection (Omata *et al.*, 1978).

The demonstration of HBcAg is almost invariably correlated with circulating Dane particles, and thus may be taken as a marker for infectivity. The lack of demonstrable HBcAg, however, does not exclude the presence of circulating Dane particles, especially if HBeAg is positive in serum and/or if a rather effective active inflammation is present at the same time.

III. Histopathological Studies
of Acute Hepatitis B

Hepatitis B virus infection covers the entire clinical and histopathological spectrum of hepatitic liver disease, including different acute and chronic forms, cirrhosis, and hepatocellular carcinoma (Table I); the latter is discussed in Chapter 11.

Four types of acute hepatitis B with different biological behavior, diagnostic criteria, and prognostic implications are listed in Table I. All degrees of severity may be encountered.

A. Acute Classic Spotty Necrotic Hepatitis (Acute Lobular Hepatitis)

1. Histopathological Findings. In the chimpanzee, HBV infection results in acute hepatitis with diffuse lobular changes and tends to run a more prolonged course than hepatitis A infection (Popper *et al.*, 1980a,b). In humans, histology of acute HB is of the type generally described in text books (Bianchi *et al.*, 1971; Patrick and McGee, 1980; Scheuer, 1980).

In Table II, the main histological features of classic spotty necrotic hepatitis at the height of the disease are presented. A combination of and a balance between spotty liver cell necrosis, lymphohistiocytic intralobular reaction, and portal inflammation are the key features (Fig. 5). Degenerative and regenerative parenchymal changes coexist, giving rise to a typical variegated lobular picture. Two types of liver cell degeneration and necrosis, short-lived perivenular lytic necrosis and a long-lived randomly distributed eosinophilic type of necrosis, are always present. Intralobular and portal inflammation consists of about equal numbers of lymphocytes and histiocytes. Slight spillover of inflammatory cells from portal tracts into the parenchyma is common, but frank piecemeal necrosis is absent. The reticulin framework remains intact (Bianchi *et al.*, 1971, 1979).

Inconstant findings include small perivenular nonbridging confluent necroses that have no prognostic implications. Canalicular cholestasis of a variable degree may be present. Pigments from lysed hepatocytes may

TABLE II
Key Features of Acute Spotty Necrotic Hepatitis (at Height of Disease)

Constant Findings
 Lymphohistiocytic portal inflammation
  (every portal tract affected)
 Diffuse and/or focal intralobular lymphohistiocytic
  infiltration with centrilobular predilection (every lobule affected)
 Lobular disarray
 Cellular and nuclear pleomorphism
 Mitoses and binucleated cells increased
 Acidophilic bodies, randomly distributed
 Ballooning and lytic necrosis with pericentral
  predilection
 Reticulin framework intact

Inconstant Findings
 Cholestasis of variable degree
 Lipofuscin-like pigments and/or iron within
  intralobular and portal macrophages
 Pericentral (nonbridging) confluent necrosis
 Inflammatory bile duct lesions
 Ductular proliferation
 Minor degrees of portal connective tissue formation

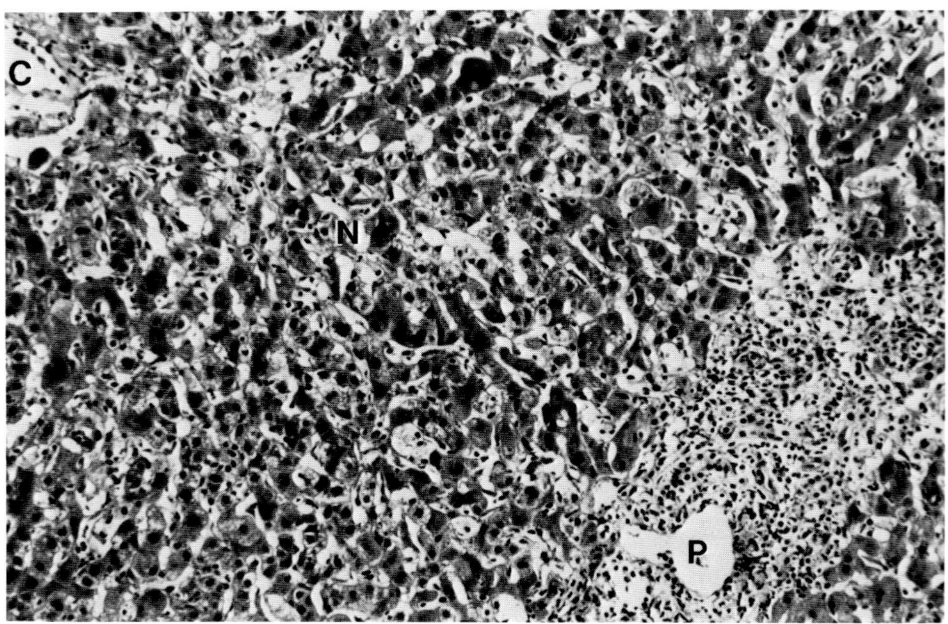

Figure 5. Fully developed acute spotty necrotic hepatitis. Portal tract infiltration (P), intra-lobular inflammatory changes, spotty necrosis (N), and lobular disarray; C, central vein.

be engulfed within swollen Kupffer cells and portal macrophages. Insignificant perivenular reticulin collapse and slight portal ductular proliferation may be found. Sometimes inflammatory bile duct lesions are present, which may predict a possible transition to chronicity (Christoffersen *et al.*, 1970).

2. Viral Antigens in Liver Tissue. At the height of acute spotty necrotic hepatitis, no viral antigens are detectable in liver tissue in most cases (elimination type). If viral expression is demonstrable at this stage, this may be taken as an indicator for impending chronicity.

3. Evolution of the Lesion. In accordance with immunological phenomena, a phasic evolution of histological changes is proposed (Bianchi, 1981). Based mainly on observations in experimental hepatitis B of chimpanzees, the following sequence of histological events may be designated: (1) viral infection, replication, and expression of viral and other proteins in liver cells, notably on the liver cell surface, without inflammation and necrosis; (2) sinusoidal and portal accumulation of lymphocytes followed by histiocytes, resulting in a lymphocyte predominance in early stages of disease (Fig. 6); and (3) further attraction of macrophages and appearance of spotty necrosis. Thus, a balanced lymphohistiocytic inflammation associated with spotty necrosis characterizes the *height of the disease.* It is not known whether virus-containing cells are eliminated by means of necrosis only. It is noteworthy, however, that at

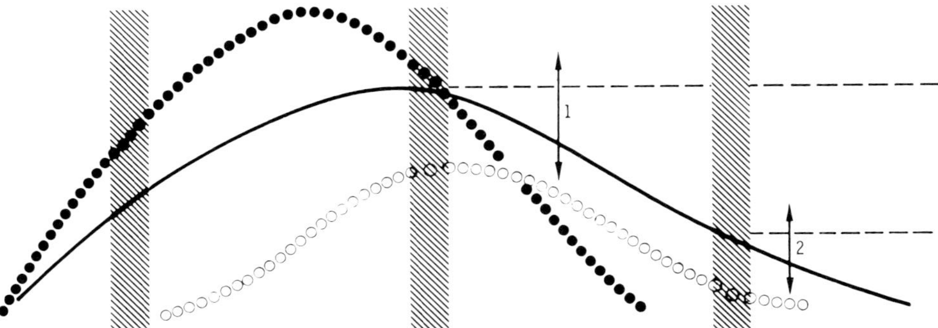

Figure 6. Diagrammatic representation of histological changes in the evolution of classic spotty necrotic hepatitis. Variation in the proportion of the morphological features allows differentiation of stages. Arrow 1: problem of differential diagnosis of later stages of acute hepatitis, acute hepatitis with possible transition to chronicity, and chronic aggressive hepatitis with acute exacerbation. Arrow 2: Problem of distinction between residual acute hepatitis, chronic persistent hepatitis, and nonspecific reactive hepatitis. Symbols: ●●●, parenchymal damage, necrosis; —, mesenchymal reaction; ○○○, pigmented macrophages. [From Bianchi *et al.* (1979) with permission, of Churchill-Livingstone, Edinburgh.]

the height of the disease viral antigens are no longer demonstrable in liver cells in the case of self-limited hepatitis B. Regeneration and restoration of the parenchyma is in concert with degeneration. (4) In *late and residual stages,* liver cell degeneration gradually subsides and lymphocytes disappear while macrophages persist. A net preponderance of mesenchymal over parenchymal alterations and a histiocytic predominance are characteristic features of these stages. (5) The net result of acute spotty necrotic hepatitis is complete virus elimination by means of necrosis and complete restoration of the parenchyma without sequelae.

B. Acute Hepatitis with Piecemeal Necrosis

1. Histopathological Findings. The main histological features are listed in Table III. Portal tracts are heavily widened by a disproportionately severe degree of portal and periportal inflammation. At the borders of portal tracts true piecemeal necrosis (Fig. 7) occurs, contrasting to mere spillover of inflammatory cells from portal tracts into the parenchyma (Bianchi *et al.,* 1977). The inflammatory infiltrate is composed predominantly of lymphocytes, often with conspicuous numbers of plasma cells (Dietrichson *et al.,* 1975). Spurs of newly formed connective tissue, rich in inflammatory cells (active septa), appear in periportal areas and may be rimmed by piecemeal necrosis (Desmet, 1973). Even portal–portal bridging by piecemeal necrosis ("sleeve necrosis") may be seen. As a rule, intralobular changes are less prominent.

This variant is most often seen in intravenous drug users, although it may occur spontaneously, particularly in the elderly (Bianchi *et al.,* 1979). In drug users, additional nonspecific granuloma formation and an abundance of eosinophilic leucocytes may be seen.

TABLE III
Key Features of Acute Hepatitis with Piecemeal Necrosis

In addition to features of spotty necrotic hepatitis
  Presence of variable degrees and extent of
    piecemeal necrosis
  Lymphocytic predominance over macrophages
    in portal tracts and parenchyma
  Portal lymph follicle formation
  Presence of plasma cells
  Granuloma formation in some cases
    (drug users)

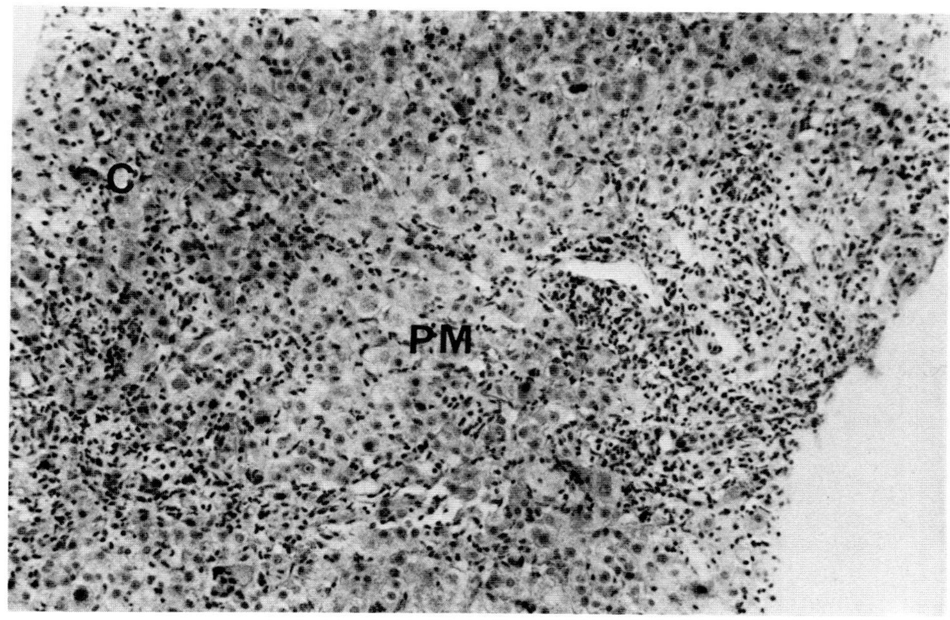

Figure 7. Acute hepatitis with piecemeal necrosis ("with possible transition to chronicity"). True piecemeal necrosis in a first acute hepatitic bout, together with features of acute spotty necrotic hepatitis in an intravenous drug user. Transition to chronic aggressive hepatitis documented after 3 years; to cirrhosis after 5 years. Abbreviations: PM, piecemeal necrosis; C, typical central hepatitis.

2. Viral Antigens in Liver Tissue. In many cases, a focal expression of HBcAg together with a variable degree of HBsAg expression (focal HBcAg type) as in chronic aggressive hepatitis is recognized. Persistence of this pattern has been documented in follow-up studies and transition into true chronic active or chronic persistent hepatitis has been verified in most patients (Aenishänslin *et al.*, 1975).

3. Evolution of the Lesion. The lesions thus combine features of the common type of spotty necrotic hepatitis with a periportal reaction typical of chronic active hepatitis. This has led to the term "acute hepatitis with possible transition to chronicity" (Bianchi *et al.*, 1971). In fact, piecemeal necrosis is regarded as the most predictive sign of impending chronic hepatitis (Bianchi *et al.*, 1977). Although the periportal lesion may regress spontaneously (Fauerholdt *et al.*, 1977), acute hepatitis with piecemeal necrosis more often evolves gradually into chronicity.

The interpretation of this variant of acute hepatitis and its pathogenesis is controversial. It has been suggested that the picture may result from a finely graded immune insufficiency in these patients (Gudat *et al.*, 1975).

C. Acute Hepatitis with Bridging (Confluent) Necrosis

1. Definitions. Necrosis affecting substantial groups of adjacent liver cells is referred to as confluent necrosis (Bianchi *et al.*, 1971). Bridging necrosis is a special form of confluent necrosis connecting different vascular structures in contrast to confluent necrosis limited to the perivenular (pericentral) region (Boyer and Klatskin, 1970). Bridging necrosis mainly occurs in three locations with respect to the liver acinus:

1. Central–central bridging, i.e., pericomplex acinar necrosis (Fig. 8)
2. Central–portal bridging, i.e., peri (simple) acinar necrosis (Fig. 8) (Bianchi *et al.*, 1979)
3. Portal–portal bridging is the result of piecemeal necrosis rather than of confluent necrosis and is seen in chronic aggressive hepatitis (Bianchi *et al.*, 1977).

2. Histopathological Findings. Main features of acute hepatitis with bridging confluent necrosis are summarized in Table IV. Bridging hepatic necrosis may vary in extent from lobule to lobule, and thus is often unevenly distributed. The alteration in the remaining parenchyma that is not affected by confluent necrosis may be extremely variable as well. Features of spotty necrotic hepatitis may be pronounced, focally accentuated, or may even be absent. The same is true for regenerative phenomena. Portal inflammation as a rule is mild. Cholestasis, if present, takes the form of ductular rather than canalicular bile deposition, and is accompanied by ductular proliferation and neutrophilic inflam-

---

TABLE IV
Key Features of Acute Hepatitis with Bridging (Confluent) Necrosis[a]

In addition to features of spotty necrotic hepatitis
   Confluent necrosis of varying degree and extent
     along acinar zone III (Rappaport)
       Central–central bridging (pericomplex acinar)
       Central–portal bridging (periacinar)
       Rarely, portal–portal bridging
   Ductular proliferation and cholestasis (very common)
   Variable degree of reticulin collapse, essentially
     reversible, except when associated with piecemeal
     necrosis and trapping of viable liver cells

---

[a]Features of acute hepatitis with bridging necrosis and piecemeal necrosis may occur simultaneously, superimposed on each other.

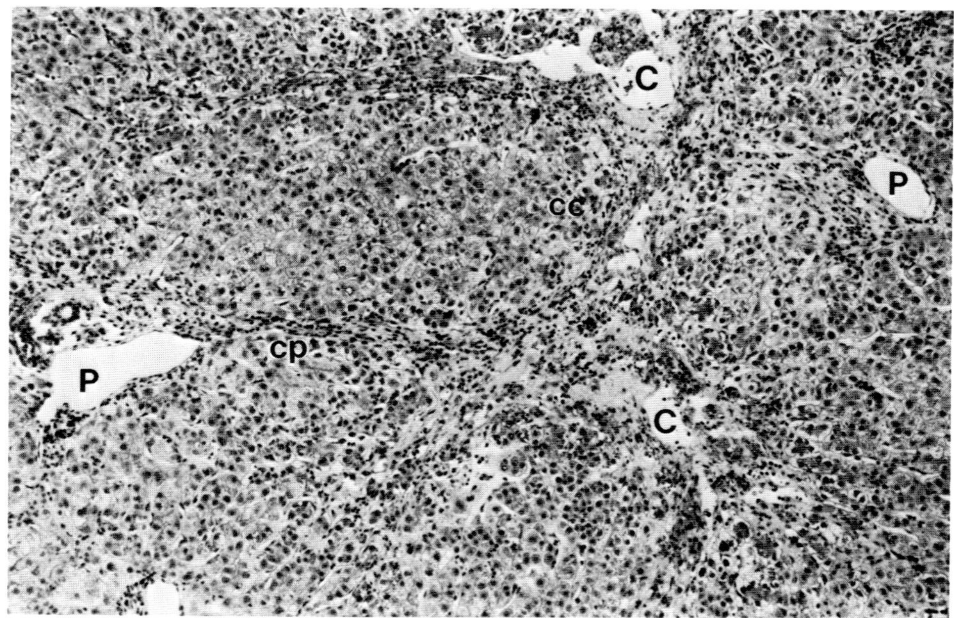

Figure 8. Acute hepatitis with bridging necrosis without piecemeal necrosis; C, central area; P, portal area; presence of both, central–central (cc) and central–portal (cp) bridging.

mation. The picture may thus simulate large bile duct obstruction (Schmid and Cueni, 1972), particularly later in the course when confluent necrosis has already been replaced by regeneration. Confluent necrosis may also be associated with piecemeal necrosis.

3. Viral Antigens in Liver Tissue. Bridging hepatic necrosis may or may not be accompanied by demonstrable viral antigens in liver tissue. There is preliminary evidence supporting the concept of virus elimination in cases not accompanied by piecemeal necrosis, while bridging necrosis associated with piecemeal necrosis tends to give the focal HBcAg pattern of viral expression. All these variable factors have bearing on the evolution of the lesion.

4. Evolution of the Lesion. Confluent necrosis results in a sudden dropout of extensive areas of liver cells, and thus contrasts sharply with spotty necrosis of acute hepatitis and piecemeal necrosis. Such a dropout of liver cells often is followed by collapse and condensation of the reticulin framework (passive septa). These septa contain few inflammatory cells, but portocaval shunts may form that compromise the hepatic microcirculation and promote the development of cirrhosis

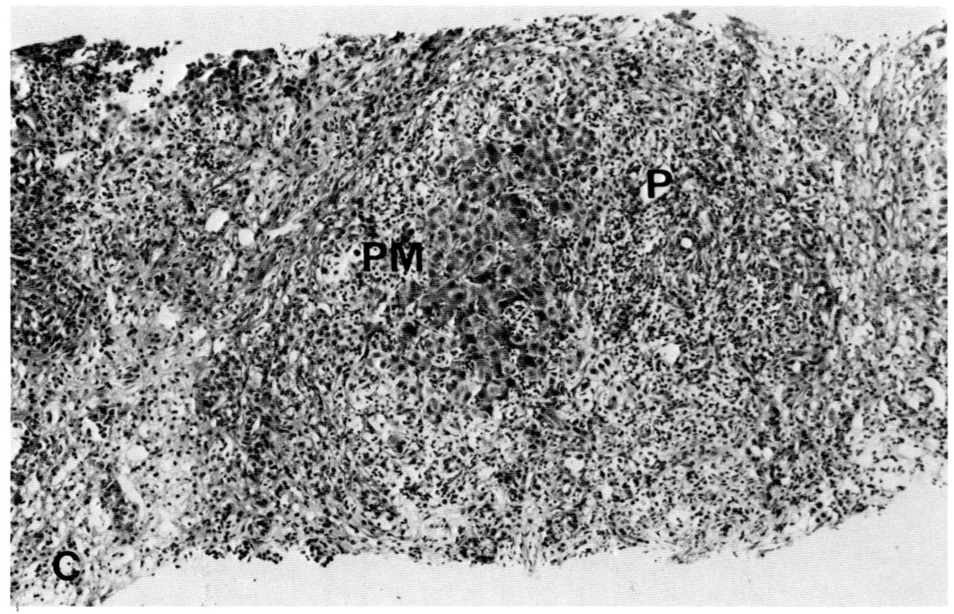

Figure 9. Acute hepatitis with bridging necrosis and piecemeal necrosis; P, portal tract; C, central area; PM, piecemeal necrosis at borders of necrotic bridges.

(Bianchi *et al.*, 1979). However, bridging confluent necrosis may as well be compensated by liver cell regeneration, leading to a substantially normal liver or to an insignificant scar (Desmet *et al.*, 1972).

Why some cases of hepatitis with bridging necrosis readily heal, while others lead to death in hepatic coma and others evolve to chronic aggressive hepatitis (Boyer and Klatskin, 1970), is still poorly understood and a matter of debate (Boyer, 1976; Conn, 1976: Scheuer, 1977).

In bridging necrosis, the state of parenchyma not affected by bridging is important in that severe spotty necrosis and/or severe cholestasis may lead to hepatic failure. The main factors responsible for progression to chronic aggressive hepatitis and cirrhosis are (1) presence of piecemeal necrosis (periportal, bordering confluent necrosis, or fibrous septa) (Fig. 9). For prognostic reasons it has been proposed to clearly differentiate cases of bridging hepatic necrosis without piecemeal necrosis from those with piecemeal necrosis (Bianchi *et al.*, 1977). The combination of bridging and piecemeal necrosis may also be the result of an acute bout of confluent necrosis superimposed on chronic aggressive hepatitis. (2) Presence of trapped liver cells; single or small islands of viable hepatocytes trapped within necrotic areas have been suspected to provide a continuing antigenic stimulus, perhaps in the form of neoantigens exposed on their cell membranes. Trapped liver cells as well as piecemeal necrosis might be regarded as the consequence of ineffective elimination of viral or cell membrane components and thus as the result of a disturbed immune response of the host. (3) Finally, the extent and topography of bridging necrosis are important in predicting cirrhosis. Central–portal bridging is a prerequisite for portocaval shunts that create the architectural scaffold for cirrhosis, particularly in the presence of piecemeal necrosis. Central–central bridging, however, does not affect hepatic microcirculation, and as a rule it is not accompanied by piecemeal necrosis and therefore readily heals.

D. Acute Hepatitis with Massive Necrosis

1. Histopathological Findings. Almost all liver cells in the lobule disappear, leaving only the reticulin framework. Sometimes a small periportal rim of surviving hepatocytes remains. According to the duration of the disease, periportal ductular proliferation may occur (Fig. 10). The degree

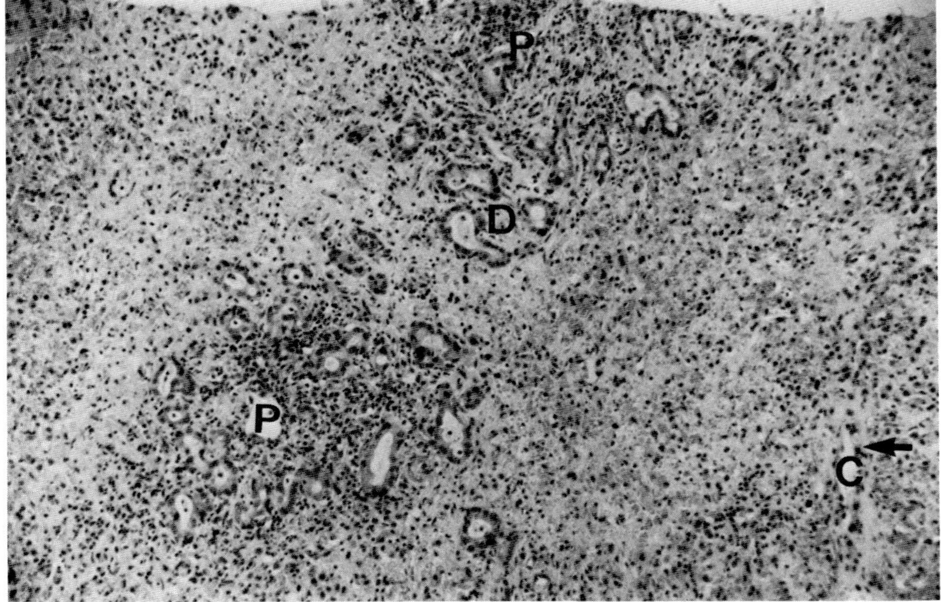

Figure 10. Acute hepatitis with massive necrosis. Note panlobular necrosis affecting two liver lobules. Ductular proliferation (D) and endophlebitis (arrow) are seen if survival is longer than 10 days. P, portal tracts; C, central vein.

of portal and intralobular infiltration is variable; little or no collapse is seen. Sinusoidal spaces often contain macrophages with or without engulfed pigments and cell debris. Endophlebitis may be observed, particularly in patients surviving longer than 10 days (Fig. 10; Ishak, 1973).

2. Viral Antigens in Liver Tissue. These could be searched for only in very few cases, so that no conclusive data are available.

3. Evolution of the Lesion. Mortality in acute hepatitis with massive necrosis (fulminant hepatitis) is >70%. Survival largely depends on the remaining intact liver mass capable of regeneration. It has been determined morphometrically that the mortality rate of massive necrosis is 100% if the total volume fraction of hepatocytes falls below 12% ($n = 85\%$) (Gazzard *et al.*, 1975). It is important to note that fulminant hepatitis, if survived, may heal without functional sequelae and without evolution to cirrhosis (Desmet *et al.*, 1972).

IV. Histopathological Studies of Chronic Hepatitis B

Definitions

An international group concerned with the definition and classification of liver disease (Fogarty International Center Criteria Committee, 1976) defined chronic hepatitis as "inflammation of the liver continuing without improvement for at least 6 months." This definition obviously is too broad, and merely describes a reaction pattern of the liver with a spectrum of clinical, biochemical, and histological features of inflammation due to a variety of causes. Moreover, it is a matter of debate whether cirrhosis is included or not. Another international group (De Groote *et al.*, 1968) proposed a subdivision of chronic hepatitis into chronic persistent hepatitis, with a generally good prognosis, and chronic aggressive (active) hepatitis, in which the outcome is doubtful. This classification is now widely accepted.

With respect to hepatitis B, a true HBV carrier state should be included. Thus, the classification depicted in Table V is proposed. Viral-induced chronic hepatitis results from persistence of antigens resistant to the attack of host defense systems. Chronicity has been observed in infection with the HBV as well as with agents of non-A, non-B hepatitis, but not with HAV. In chronic hepatitis B, the demonstration of viral antigens in liver tissue serves as a specific marker to characterize the type of chronic infection (see Section II).

TABLE V
Classification of Chronic Hepatitis B

	Infectivity
True HBV carrier	
Without HBcAg expression, HBcAg–free HBsAg type	Low
With generalized HBcAg, generalized HBcAg type	High
Chronic nonaggressive hepatitis (subtypes: chronic persistent hepatitis, chronic lobular hepatitis, chronic septal hepatitis)	
Without HBcAg expression, HBcAg–free HBsAg type	Low
With generalized HBcAg expression, generalized HBcAg type	High
With focal HBcAg expression, focal HBcAg type	High
Chronic aggressive (active) hepatitis (All with focal HBcAg expression) (= focal HBcAg type)	High
With minimal activity (a)	+++++[a]
With moderate activity (a)	+++
With severe activity (b)	+

[a]Number of pluses indicates degree of HBcAg expression.

A. True HBV Carrier

1. Definitions and Histopathological Findings. It should be noted that the term "HBV carrier," as used clinically, covers a variety of conditions associated with positivity for HBsAg in serum ranging from normal liver tissue to aggressive hepatitis and including even cirrhosis and hepatocellular carcinoma (Fig. 11). A true carrier state, however, is characterized by a combination of both; the lack of clinical symptoms, and histologically, the lack of inflammation or presence of a mild nonspecific reactive hepatitis only. The lobular architecture remains intact.

2. Viral Antigens in Liver Tissue. Two distinct types of HBV carriers are distinguished:

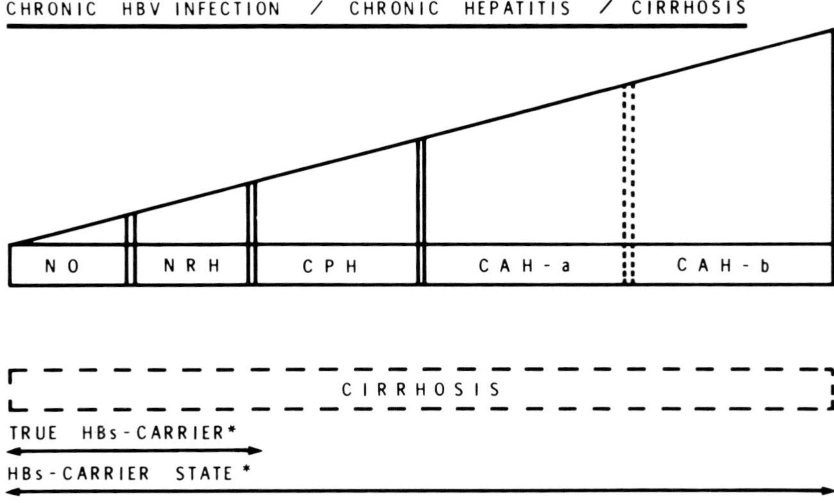

Figure 11. Diagrammatic presentation of the relation of the terms "chronic HBV infection," "chronic hepatitis," and "cirrhosis." The ascending line on the ordinate depicts the degree of inflammatory activity. In all types, HBV antigens are expressed in liver tissue with different patterns: NO, liver tissue without inflammation; NRH, nonspecific reactive hepatitis; CPH, chronic persistent hepatitis; CAH, chronic aggressive hepatitis. Note: (1) Cirrhosis may be associated with all patterns (NO, NRH, CPH, and CAH). (2) The true HBsAg carrier includes HBV expression in tissue without inflammation (NO) or with modest nonspecific inflammatory changes (NRH). (3) The clinically used term "HBs carrier state" is defined by absence of signs and symptoms of liver disease in the presence of seropositivity for HBsAg, and may include all patterns, even cirrhosis. The individual inflammatory patterns are not sharply delineated entities, but merge imperceptibly.

a. The *HBcAg–free HBsAg carrier* (Gudat *et al.*, 1975; Bianchi and Gudat, 1979) as a rule shows the highest numbers of hepatocytes expressing intracytoplasmic, but not membraneous, HBsAg in biopsies (Fig. 12); HBcAg expression is lacking or minimal. These patients are therefore considered low grade or not infective (see Table V). This type of carrier, common in the western world, seems to be stable for years. In the blood, are lacking and anti-e is positive.

b. The *generalized HBcAg carrier* represents the second type of true carrier with generalized HBcAg expression in tissue (Gudat *et al.*, 1975; Bianchi and Gudat, 1979) (Table V). This type is thus considered to be of high-grade infectivity. It preferentially occurs in immunosuppressed patients (e.g., kidney transplant recipients, and patients with malignant lymphoma) as well as in many cases in the Far East of HBV infection vertically transmitted from mother to child (Stevens *et al.*, 1975). This HBcAg carrier is less stable, and may become chronic persistent or even chronic active hepatitis.

The development of hepatocellular carcinoma is documented in carrier states, and may be explained by the incorporation of the HBV DNA into the human genome (Shafritz and Kew, 1981; see Chapter 11).

B. Chronic Persistent Hepatitis

1. Histopathological Findings. The main histological features are summarized in Table VI. The basic architecture is preserved. Portal tracts are expanded by a diffuse infiltrate that is predominantly lymphocytic with some plasma cells. Inflammation is confined to the portal tracts; the limiting plate remains intact (Fig. 13), and there is no necrosis of periportal hepatocytes (MacSween, 1980). There may be slight portal fibrosis

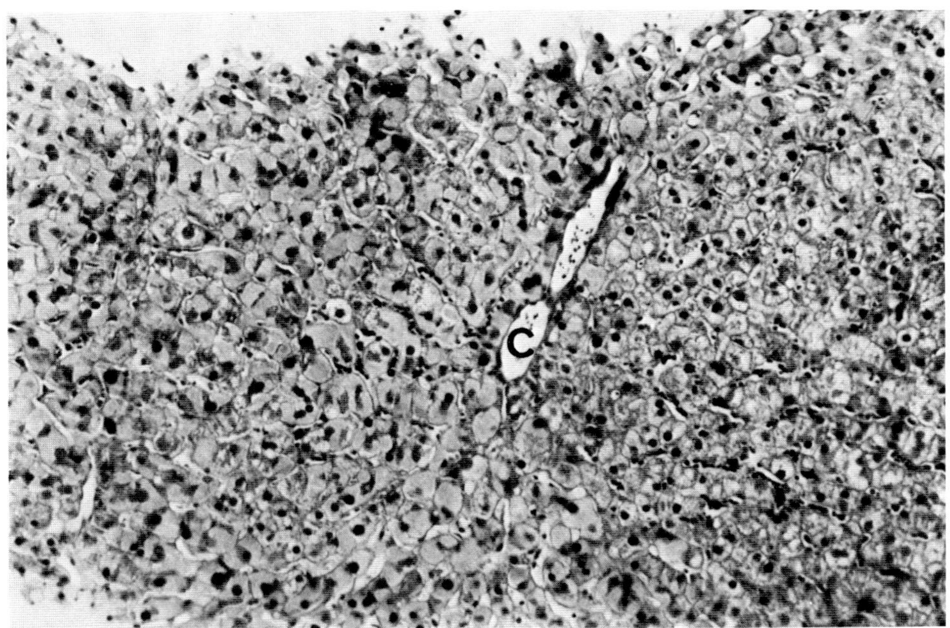

Figure 12. True HBcAg–free HBsAg carrier: (1) absence of inflammation and (2) presence of large numbers of HBsAg-containing ground-glass cells (left side) in an H + E-stained section. Right side, hepatocytes without HBsAg accumulation. C, central vein.

TABLE VI
Key Features of Chronic Persistent Hepatitis

Constant findings
    Lobular architecture preserved
    Chronic inflammation of portal tracts
    Portal fields sharply delineated
    Absence of piecemeal necrosis
    Slight focal intralobular inflammation

Inconstant findings
    Slight portal fibrosis
    Portal lymph follicles
    Bile duct lesions (rare in hepatitis B, but indicative of
        non-A, non-B hepatitis)
    HBsAg-containing ground-glass cells
    HBcAg-containing "sanded nuclei" (rare)
    Signs of superimposed acute hepatitis
    Cirrhosis

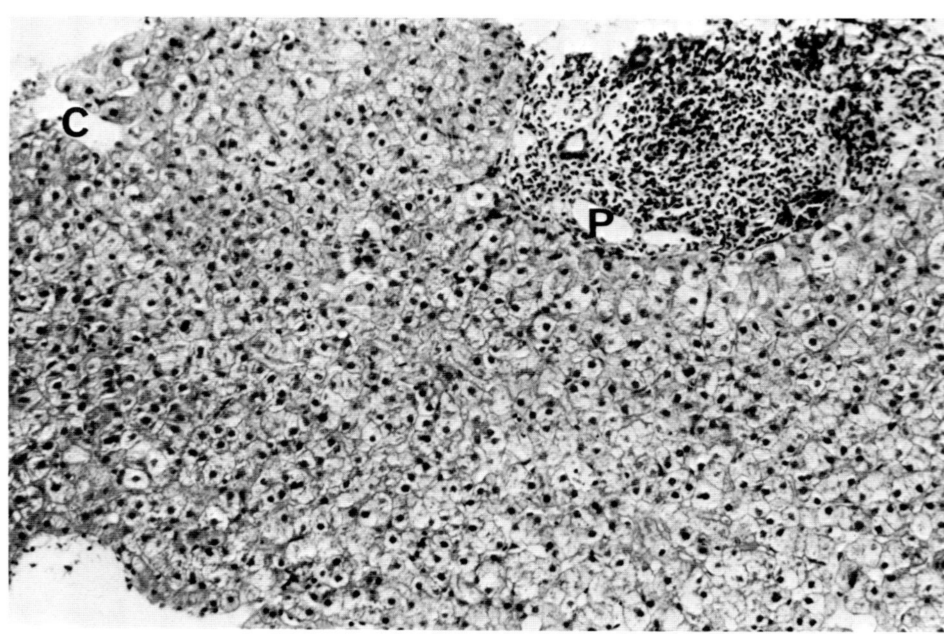

Figure 13. Chronic persistent hepatitis. Dense, predominantly lymphocytic portal inflammation without piecemeal necrosis. Slight parenchymal changes and slight focal intralobular inflammation. P, portal tract; C, central vein.

(De Groote *et al.*, 1968). Occasionally, lymph follicles with germinal centers may be recognized. Intralobular changes as a rule are minimal, and consist of small foci of liver cell necrosis with modest inflammatory reaction.

2. Viral Antigens in Liver Tissue. Chronic persistent hepatitis B may be associated with the generalized, the focal, or the HBcAg-free type of viral antigen expression (see Section II, and Figure 2). A shift from one type to another with concomitant change of the inflammatory activity occurs with considerable frequency.

3. Evolution of the Lesion. In general, chronic persistent hepatitis is considered to have a good prognosis. In many cases, the histological features persist for years without deterioration to a more aggressive form (De Groote *et al.*, 1968). It must be borne in mind, however, that chronic persistent hepatitis may be complicated by acute exacerbations, even with confluent necrosis, and in these cases progression to chronic active hepatitis may ensue. In some instances, features of the late and residual stage of acute spotty necrotic hepatitis may be seen in addition to the predominantly portal hepatitis typical of chronic persistent hepatitis ("unresolved hepatitis": Edmondson and Peters, 1971). In other cases, acute lobular alterations may be pronounced, with histological features seen at the height of the acute disease persisting for >6 months. For this, the term "chronic lobular hepatitis" seems appropriate (Popper and Schaffner, 1976). Another variant, said to have a much poorer prognosis, is "chronic septal hepatitis" (Gerber and Vernace, 1974), characterized by the formation of extensive portal–portal septa with conspicuous inflammatory activity. Chronic persistent hepatitis, particularly the "chronic septal" form, may also represent a regressive state of chronic active hepatitis after immunosuppressive therapy (Czaja *et al.*, 1981).

C. Chronic Aggressive (Active) Hepatitis

1. The Phenomenon of Piecemeal Necrosis. Piecemeal necrosis was originally described as an immunological type of necrosis by Popper *et al.* (1965). It represents chronic and gradual inflammatory destruction of small groups of liver cells at the mesenchymal–parenchymal interphase or a confluent necrosis associated with mononuclear inflammatory cells (Fig. 14). A close contact between lymphocytes/macrophages and hepatocytes (= peripolesis) is the hallmark of piecemeal necrosis. Liver cells in piecemeal necrosis show degenerative phenomena such as swelling, shrinkage, or gradual disintegration by sequential fragmentation of

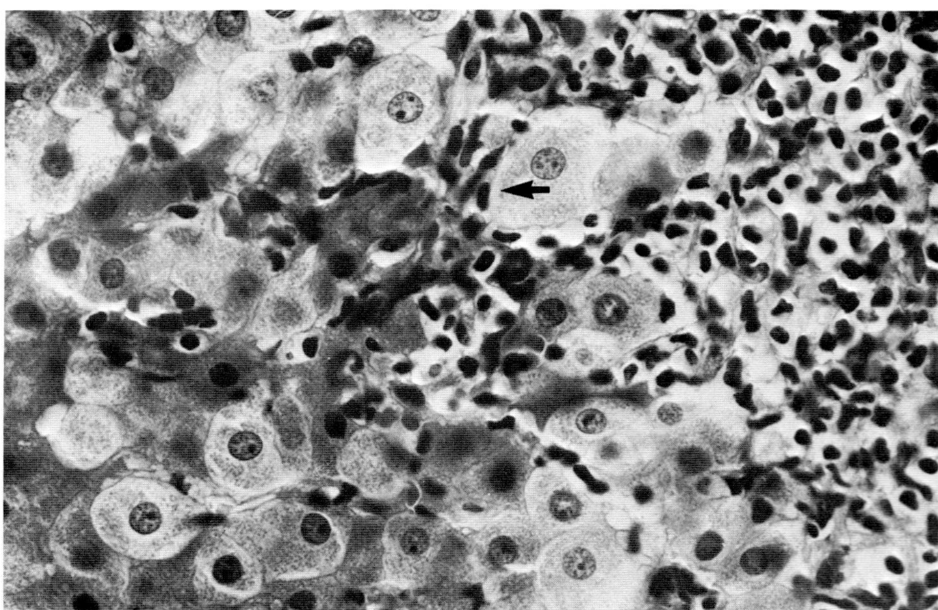

Figure 14. Piecemeal necrosis at border of portal tract including peripolesis (close contact between lymphocytes/histiocytes and membrane of hepatocyte) (arrow).

cytoplasm (apoptosis). Other liver cells in piecemeal necrosis may survive, become hyperplastic, and arrange in a tubular fashion (rosetting). As a result of piecemeal necrosis, the limiting plate may be broken; the peripherolobular parenchyma is progressively destroyed, and is replaced by newly formed connective tissue arranged in active fibrous septa (Bianchi *et al.*, 1977).

2. Histopathological Findings. The key histologic features of chronic aggressive hepatitis are summarized in Table VII. Portal tracts are markedly enlarged with a lymphohistiocytic infiltrate, intermixed with plasma cells in varying numbers. Limiting plates are eroded, with piecemeal necrosis of periportal hepatocytes accompanied by fibrous septum formation. For prognostic and therapeutic reasons, a gradation of activity of the inflammatory process has been proposed (Bianchi *et al.*, 1977; see also Tables V and VIII):

a. Activity (a) or moderate activity. This is characterized by dense inflammatory portal infiltration including piecemeal necrosis restricted to periportal areas, without significant intralobular septum formation (Fig. 15). It has proven useful to further subdivide "activity (a)" by defining cases of minimal activity (De Groote *et al.*, 1974). In these cases border-

TABLE VII
Key Features of Chronic Aggressive (Active)
Hepatitis

Constant Findings
    Chronic portal and periportal inflammation
    Periportal piecemeal necrosis
    Focal intralobular inflammation

Inconstant findings
    Lobular architecture disturbed
    Active and passive septa
    Signs of acute spotty necrotic hepatitis
    Bridging necrosis
    Liver cell rosetting at parenchymal/mesenchymal
      interphase
    Bile duct lesions (rare in hepatitis B)
    HBsAg-containing ground-glass cells
    HBcAg-containing "sanded nuclei" (rare)

---

ing on chronic persistent hepatitis, periportal piecemeal necrosis may not be present in all portal tracts or in a given portal tract and may be seen only in a segment of the perimeter of the portal area. These cases may often be mistaken for chronic persistent hepatitis; their unstable course with a high frequency of deterioration towards more aggressive forms justifies their classification into chronic active hepatitis (Czaja *et al.*, 1981). These cases may be recognized as such by their focal HBcAg expression in tissue (see below).

b. Activity (b) or severe activity. This includes cases with piecemeal necrosis in the periportal region and along fibrous septa (periseptal piecemeal necrosis; Fig. 16A) or cases that show bridging hepatic necrosis in addition to features of periportal or periseptal piecemeal necrosis (Fig. 16B). In contrast to the autoimmune type of chronic aggressive hepatitis, severe activity (b) is much less frequent in chronic hepatitis B. In chronic hepatitis B, inflammatory bile duct lesions may be present

TABLE VIII
Grading of Histological Activity in Chronic Aggressive Hepatitis

Activity (a) Minimal	Slight periportal piecemeal necrosis	
Moderate	Marked periportal piecemeal necrosis	
Activity (b) Severe	In addition to features of activity (a): periseptal piecemeal necrosis and/or bridging (confluent) necrosis with or without piecemeal necrosis at borders of necrotic bridges	

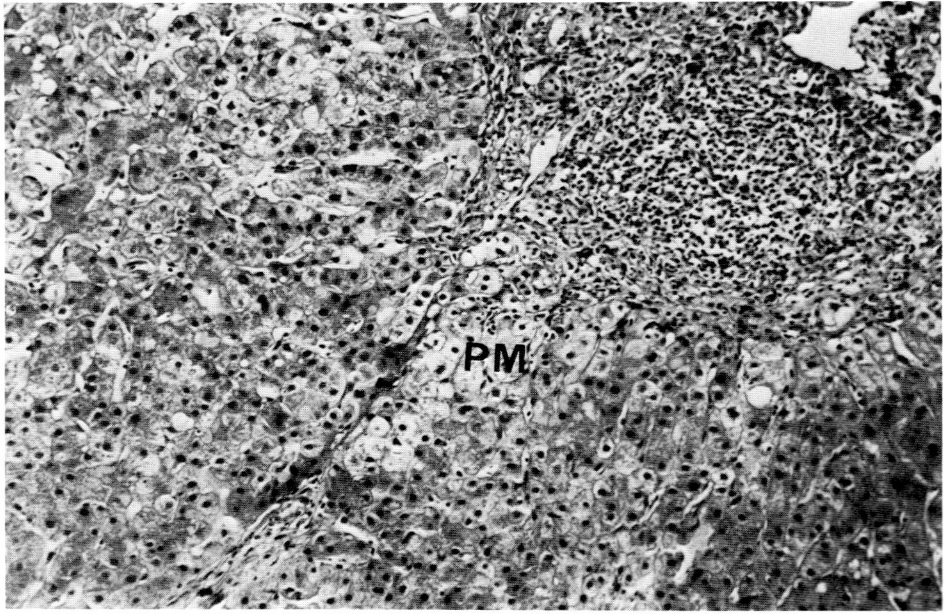

Figure 15. Chronic aggressive hepatitis, moderate activity (a). Piecemeal necrosis (PM) is restricted to periportal area.

(Christoffersen *et al.*, 1972), but they are far less common than in non-A, non-B hepatitis (see below).

3. Viral Antigens in Liver Tissue. Chronic aggressive hepatitis is usually accompanied by a focal expression of HBcAg (and HBsAg), often together with membraneous HBsAg expression (compare with Fig. 2). Interestingly, the same pattern is seen in acute hepatitis with piecemeal necrosis (see Section II,B), whereas the classical acute spotty necrotic hepatitis at the height of the disease exhibits no viral antigens. An inverse relationship between the amount of HBcAg expression in tissue and activity of the inflammatory process has been stressed (Bianchi *et al.*, 1979). In few cases of chronic aggressive hepatitis, particularly in intravenous drug users, δ antigen could be detected in liver cell nuclei (Stöcklin *et al.*, 1981).

Figure 16. Chronic aggressive hepatitis, severe activity (b). (A) Note periseptal piecemeal necrosis (PMs) in addition to periportal piecemeal necrosis (PMp). (B) Note piecemeal necrosis (PMc) at borders of bridging necrosis (BN), in addition to periportal piecemeal necrosis (PMp).

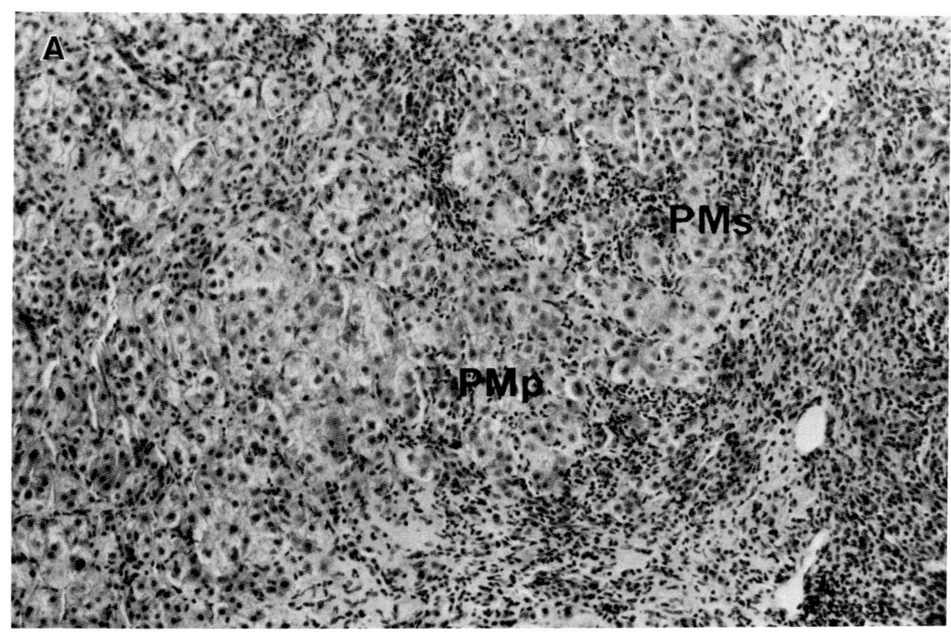
A
PMs
PMp

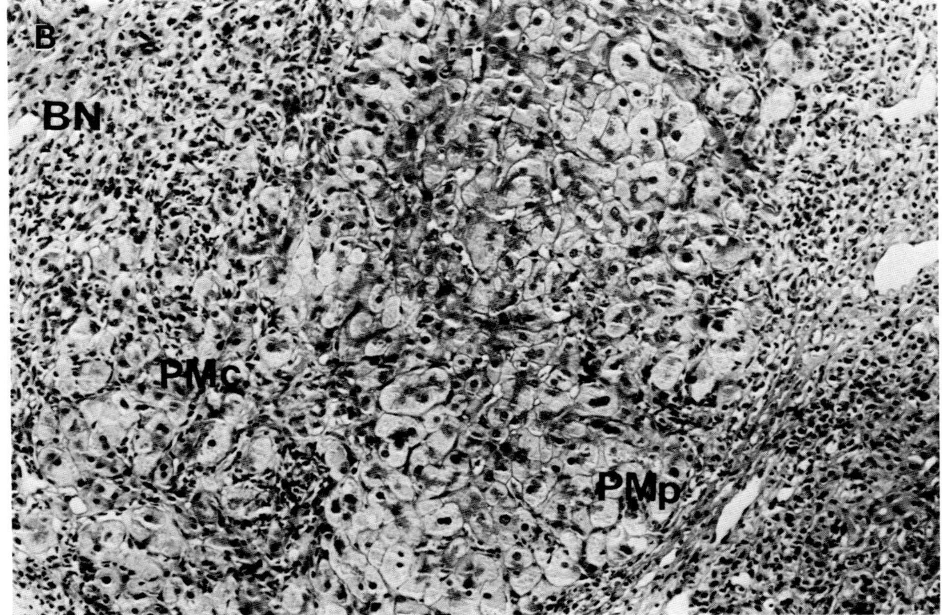
B
BN
PMc
PMp

4. Evolution of the Lesion. By definition, chronic aggressive hepatitis is mainly a progressive destructive inflammatory disease that ultimately ends in cirrhosis with high frequency. However, remissions, whether spontaneous or as an effect of therapy, may occur in some instances; the histological presentation is a regression to chronic persistent hepatitis (Czaja *et al.,* 1981). The speed of evolution is extremely variable. Several factors may be responsible for a poorer prognosis (MacSween, 1980): (1) superimposed acute bouts of spotty necrosis or even more of bridging confluent necrosis; (2) the presence of inflammatory bile duct lesions of the hepatitic type (Christoffersen *et al.,* 1972); or (3) the appearance of histological signs of cholestasis.

D. HBsAg-Positive Cirrhosis

Progression of chronic aggressive hepatitis to cirrhosis is gradual, resulting from continuing hepatocellular degeneration, architectural disturbances, fibrosis, and regenerative activity with nodule formation. But hepatic cirrhosis does not necessarily go through a phase recognizable as chronic aggressive hepatitis (MacSween, 1980). It should be appreciated that the term "cirrhosis" mainly refers to architectural disturbances, while the term "chronic aggressive hepatitis" is appropriate to characterize the inflammatory activity of the process. The terms may thus be used independently to characterize a given condition: "chronic aggressive hepatitis with cirrhosis" may describe a condition in which the activity of the disease dominates the clinical picture; "cirrhosis with features of chronic aggressive hepatitis" is the term characterizing a situation in which cirrhosis and its sequelae are the dominant clinical problem (Bianchi *et al.,* 1977). Furthermore, hepatitic cirrhosis that is mostly of the macronodular type may present with basically all types of inflammatory activity—no inflammation at all, minor nonspecific inflammatory changes, chronic persistent hepatitis, or chronic aggressive hepatitis (Fig. 11). Quite often in the evolution of cirrhosis, the inflammatory activity declines (note the shift to the left in Fig. 11).

Expression of viral antigens in cirrhosis is in keeping with the degree of inflammatory activity. All expression patterns may be found (see Fig. 2). When inflammatory activity declines in late stages of cirrhosis, the HBcAg–free HBsAg type of viral antigen expression may be found, with the loss of HBcAg in tissue, the disappearance of Dane particles from blood, and the appearance of anti-HBe. Intracytoplasmic HBsAg in tissue is then as a rule present in a very irregular distribution. Some cirrhotic nodules appear stuffed with HBsAg, while others are devoid of

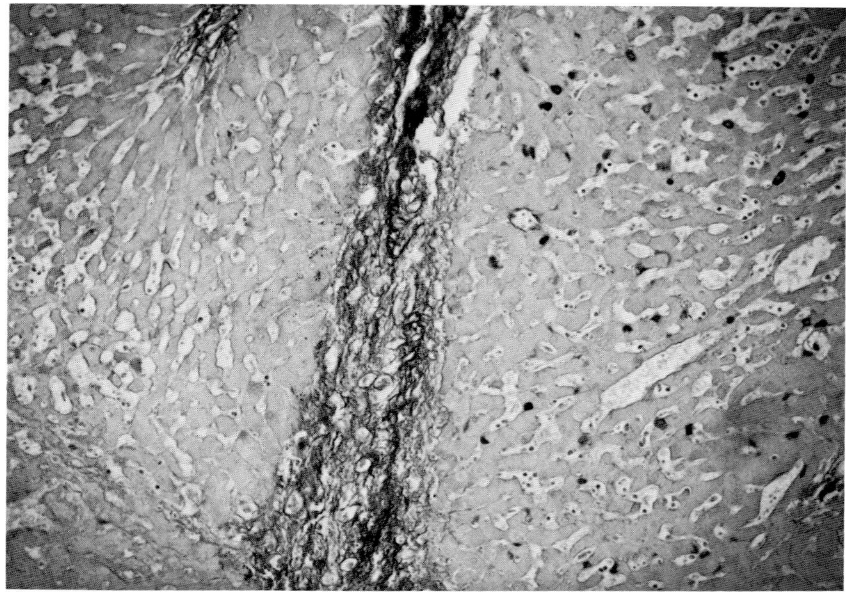

Figure 17. HBsAg-positive hepatitic cirrhosis. Note uneven distribution of HBsAg-containing cells, indicating autonomy of cirrhotic nodules. At right, note fairly extensive HBsAg expression; the nodule at the left is made up of hepatocytes devoid of HBsAg. Center, fibrous septum with collagen fibers and almost no inflammation. Orcein staining.

the antigen (Fig. 17). This stage of cirrhosis is regarded as at particularly high risk for developing hepatocellular carcinoma.

E. Hepatocellular Carcinoma

Hepatocellular carcinoma, as associated with HBV infection, is discussed in Chapter 11.

References

Aenishänslin, H. W., Stalder, G. A., Bianchi, L., Gudat, F., and Carmann, H. (1975). *Dtsch. Med. Wochenschr.* **100,** 857.

Alberti, A., Realdi, G., Tremolada, F., and Spina, G. P. (1976). *Clin. Exp. Immunol.* **25,** 396.

Alberti, A., Diana, S., Sculard, G. H., Eddleston, A. L. W. F., and Williams, R. (1978). *Br. Med. J.* **2,** 1056.

Arnold, W., Meyer zum Büschenfelde, K. H., Hess, G., and Knolle, J. (1975). *Klin. Wochenschr.* **53,** 1069.

Arnold, W., Nielsen, J. O., Hardt, F., and Meyer zum Büschenfelde, K. H. (1977). *Gut* **19,** 994.

Bianchi, L. (1981). *Springer Semin. Immunopathol.* **3,** 421.

Bianchi, L., and Gudat, F. (1976). *Lab. Invest.* **35,** 1

Bianchi, L., and Gudat, F. (1979). *Prog. Liver Dis.* **6,** 371.

Bianchi, L., De Groote, J., Desmet, V. J., Gedigk, P., Korb, G., Popper, H., Poulsen, H., Scheuer, P. J., Schmid, M., Thaler, H., and Wepler, W. (1971). *Lancet 1,* 333.

Bianchi, L., De Groote, J., Desmet, V. J., Gedigk, P., Korb, G., Popper, H., Poulsen, H., Scheuer, P. J., Schmid, M., Thaler, H., and Wepler, W. (1977). *Lancet 2,* 914.

Bianchi, L., Zimmerli-Ning, M., and Gudat, F. (1979). *In* "Pathology of the Liver" (R. N. M. MacSween, P. P. Anthony, and P. J. Scheuer, eds.), p. 164. Churchill-Livingstone, Edinburgh and London.

Bonino, F., Hoyer, B., Ford, E., Shih, J. W. K., Purcell, R. H., and Gerin, J. L. (1981). *Hepatology* **1,** 127.

Boyer. J. L. (1976). *Gastroenterology* **70,** 1161.

Boyer, J. L., and Klatskin, G. (1970). *N. Engl. J. Med.* **283,** 1063.

Canese, M. G., Rizzetto, M., Arico, S., Crivelli, O., Zanetti, H. R., Machiorlatti, E., Ponzetto, A., Leone, L., Mollo, F., and Verme, G. (1979). *J. Pathol.* **128,** 175.

Christoffersen, P., Poulsen, H., and Winkler, K. (1970). *Scand. J. Gastroenterol.* **5,** 117.

Christoffersen, P., Dietrichson, O., Faber, V. and Poulsen, H. (1972). *Acta Pathol. Microbiol. Scand., Sect. A* **80A,** 294.

Conn, H. O. (1976). *Gastroenterology* **70,** 1182.

Czaja, A. J., Ludwig, J., Baggenstoss, A. H., and Wolf, A. (1981). *N. Engl. J. Med.* **304,** 5.

De Groote, J., Desmet, V. J., Gedigk, P., Korb, G., Popper, H., Poulsen, H., Schmid, M., Uehlinger, E., and Wepler, W. (1968). *Lancet 2,* 626.

De Groote, J., Fevery, J., Verbrugghe, J., Desmet, V., and Vandenbroucke, J. (1974). Less active chronic hepatitis. A follow-up of 59 patients. *World Congr. Gastroenterol. 1974,* Abstract.

Desmet, V. J. (1973). *In* "The Liver" (E. A. Gall and F. K. Mostofi, eds.), IAP Monogr. No. 13, p. 286. Williams & Wilkins, Baltimore, Maryland.

Desmet, V. J., De Groote, J., and Van Damme, B. (1972). *Hum. Pathol.* **3,** 167.

Dietrichson, O., Juhl, E., Christoffersen, P., Elling, P., Faber, V., Iversen, K., Nielsen, J. O., Petersen, P., and Poulsen, H. (1975). *Acta Pathol. Microbiol. Scand., Sect. A* **83A,** 183.

Edmondson, H. A., and Peters, R. L. (1971). *In* "Liver" (W. A. D. Anderson, ed.), p. 1180. Mosby, St. Louis, Missouri.

Fauerholdt, L., Asnaes, S., Ranek, L., Schiodt, T., and Tygstrup, N. (1977). *Gastroenterology* **73,** 543.

Fogarty International Center Criteria Committee (1976). *In* (C. M. Leevy and N. Tygstrup, eds.), pp. 9–11. U.S. Govt. Printing Office, Washington, D.C.

Gazzard, B. G., Portmann, B., Murray-Lyon, I. M., and Williams, R. (1975). *Q. J. Med.* **44,** 615.

Gerber, M. A., and Thung, S. N. (1979). *Int. Rev. Exp. Pathol.* **20,** 49.

Gerber, M. A., and Vernace, S. (1974). *Virchows Arch. A. Pathol. Anat Histol.* **363,** 303.

Gerber, M. A., Schaffner, F., and Paronetto, F. (1972). *Proc. Soc. Exp. Biol. Med.* **140,** 1334.

Gudat, F., and Bianchi, L. (1977a). *Gastroenterology* **73,** 1194.

Gudat, F., and Bianchi, L. (1977b). *In* "Membrane Alterations as Basis of Liver Injury" (H.

Popper, L. Bianchi, and W. Reutter, eds.), p. 171. MTP Press, Ltd., Lancaster, England.

Gudat, F., Bianchi, L., Sonnabend, W., Thiel, G., Aenishänslin, W., and Stalder, G. A. (1975). *Lab. Invest.* **32**, 1.

Gudat, F., Bianchi, L., Finch. M., Krey, G., and Endo, Y. (1977). *Klin. Wochenschr.* **55**, 329.

Hadziyannis, S., Gerber, M. A., Vissoulis, C., and Popper, H. (1973). *Arch. Pathol.* **96**, 327.

Hopf, U., Arnold, W., Meyer zum Büschenfelde, K. H., Förster, E., and Bolte, J. P. (1975). *Clin. Exp. Immunol.* **22**, 1.

Huang, S. N., and Groh, V. (1973). *Lab. Invest.* **29**, 353.

Huang, S. N., Millman, I., O'Connell, A., Aronoff, A., Gault, H., and Blumberg, B. S. (1972). *Am. J. Pathol.* **67**, 453.

Ishak, K. G. (1973). *In* "The Liver" (E. A. Gall and F. K. Mostofi, eds.), IAP Monogr. No. 13, p. 218. Williams & Wilkins, Baltimore, Maryland.

Kamimura, T., Yoshikawa, A., Ichida, F., and Sasaki, H. (1981). *Hepatology* **1**, 392.

Levy, G. A., and Chisari, F. V. (1981). *Springer Semin. Immunopathol.* **3**, 439.

MacSween, R. N. M. (1980). *Clin. Gastroenterol.* **9**, 23.

Magnius, L. O., and Espmark, J. A. (1972). *J. Immunol.* **109**, 1017.

Miyakawa, Y., and Mayumi, M. (1982). *In* "Viral Hepatitis" (W. Szmuness, H. J. Alter, and J. E. Maynard, eds.), p. 183. Franklin Inst. Press, Philadelphia, Pennsylvania.

Omata, M., Afroudakis, A., Liew, C. T., Ashcavai, M., and Peters, R. L. (1978). *Gastroenterology* **75**, 1003.

Patrick, R. S., and McGee, J. O'D. (1980). "Biopsy Pathology of the Liver." Chapman & Hall, London

Peters, R. L. (1975). *Am. J. Med. Sci.* **270**, 17.

Phillips, M. J., and Poucell, S. (1981). *Hum. Pathol.* **12**, 1060.

Popper, H. (1975). *Am. J. Pathol.* **81**, 609.

Popper, H., and Schaffner, F. (1976). *Prog. Liver Dis.* **5**, 531.

Popper, H., Paronetto, F., and Schaffner, F. (1965). *Ann. N.Y. Acad. Sci.* **124**, 781.

Popper, H., Dienstag, J. L., Feinstone, S. M., Alter, H. J., and Purcell, R. L. (1980a). *In* "Virus and the Liver" (L. Bianchi, W. Gerok, K. Sickinger, and G. A. Stalder, eds.), p. 137. MTP Press, Ltd., Lancaster, England.

Popper, H., Dienstag, J. L., Feinstone, S. M., Alter, H. J., and Purcell, R. H. (1980b). *Virchows Arch. Pathol. Anat. Histol. A* **387**, 91.

Ray, M. B., Desmet, V. J., Bradburne, A. F., Desmyter, J., Fevery, J., and De Groote, J. (1976). *Gastroenterology* **71**, 462.

Realdi, G., Trevisan, A., Alberti, A., Losi, C., Rigoli, A. M., Rugge, M., and Pornaro, E. (1978). *J. Clin. Lab. Immunol.* **1**, 201.

Rizzetto, M., Canese, M. G., Arico, S., Crivelli, O., Trepo, C., Bonino, F., and Verme, G. (1977). *Gut* **18**, 997.

Rizzetto, M., Canese, M. G., Gerin, J. L., London, W. T., Sly, D. L., and Purcell, R. H. (1980). *J. Infect. Dis.* **141**, 590.

Scheuer, P. J. (1977). *Histopathology* **1**, 5.

Scheuer, P. J. (1980). "Liver Biopsy Interpretation." Baillière, London.

Schmid, M., and Cueni, B. (1972). *Hum. Pathol.* **3**, 209.

Shafritz, D. A., and Kew, M. C. (1981). *Hepatology* **1**, 1.

Stevens, C. E., Beasley, R. B., Tsui, J., and Lee, W. C. (1975). *N. Engl. J. Med.* **292**, 771.

Stöcklin, E., Gudat, F., Krey, G., Dürmüller, U., Gasser, M., Schmid, M., Stalder, G. A., and Bianchi, L. (1981). *Hepatology* **1**, 238.

Trepo, C., Vitvitski, L., Neurath, R., Hashimoto, N., Schaefer, R., Nemoz, G., and Prince, A. M. (1976). *Lancet 1*, 486.
Trevisan, A., Realdi, G., Alberti, A., and Noventa, F. (1979). *Gastroenterology* **77**, 209.
Trevisan, A., Realdi, G., Alberti, A., Ongaro, G., Pornaro, E., and Meliconi, R. (1982). *Gastroenterology* **82**, 218.
Yamada, G., and Nakane, P. K. (1977). *Lab. Invest.* **36**, 649.
Yamada, G., Feinberg, L. E., and Nakane, P. K. (1978). *Hum. Pathol.* **9**, 93.

Chapter 13

Chimpanzee Model for the Study of Hepatitis B

EDWARD TABOR
Division of Anti-Infective Drug Products
Office of Biologics Research and Review
Food and Drug Administration
Rockville,Maryland

I. Introduction

Development of a safe and effective hepatitis B vaccine, a specific immune globulin (hepatitis B immune globulin), and inactivation procedures to reduce the risk of transmission of hepatitis B by clotting factor concentrates were made possible by the use of the chimpanzee (*Pan troglodytes*) model for hepatitis B. Hepatitis B virus (HBV) has not yet been successfully cultivated in cell cultures or transmitted to nonprimate animals. Although gorillas (*Gorilla gorilla*), Celebes apes (*Cynopithecus niger*), and woolly monkeys (*Brachyteles arachnoides*) have been said to acquire HBV infections (Zuckerman *et al.*, 1978), and antibody to hepatitis B surface antigen (anti-HBs) has been detected in the serum of orangutans (*Pongo pygmaeus*), baboons (*Papio cynocephalus*), and squirrel

303   Copyright © 1985 by Academic Press, Inc.
All rights of reproduction in any form reserved.
ISBN 0-12-280672-7

monkeys (*Saimiri sciureus*) (Eichberg and Kalter, 1980; Shulman and Barker, 1969), successful experimental infection of these species by inoculation of HBV has not been reported. Experimental infection of gibbons (*Hylobates lar*) has been reported (Bancroft *et al.*, 1977); however, HBV may not be transmissible to 100% of gibbons (E. Tabor and R. J. Gerety; FDA; unpublished data) and the infectivity of inocula containing HBV has not been titered in gibbons (Tabor *et al.*, 1983c).

II. Characteristics of Suitable Chimpanzees

Of the two species of chimpanzees, *Pan troglodytes* and *P. paniscus*, only *P. troglodytes* has been reported to be susceptible to HBV infection. There are no published data concerning the relative susceptibility of the three subspecies of *P. troglodytes;* most studies have utilized the common or masked subspecies. Variant or strain differences among chimpanzees of the masked subspecies do not appear to affect susceptibility to HBV.

Equal susceptibility to HBV has been observed in male and female chimpanzees, and in chimpanzees of all ages, provided they have had no prior exposure to this virus. Infant chimpanzees, 18 months of age, and adult chimpanzees believed to be older than 25 years of age have been shown to be susceptible.

Infant chimpanzees born in captivity usually have anti-HBs in their serum that has been passively acquired from their immune mothers. Anti-HBs is common among adult chimpanzees in captivity. When passively transferred to an infant, these antibodies usually disappear between 6 and 12 months of age, although the pattern of disappearance has not been systematically studied. Rarely, an infant chimpanzee may have detectable maternal anti-HBs until 13 months of age.

Transmission of HBV from chronically infected chimpanzee mothers to their newborn infants would be expected since this type of transmission is common among humans. However, prospective observation of such transmission has not been reported, since chimpanzees that are chronically infected with HBV are not usually permitted to have close contact with other chimpanzees and are not included in organized breeding programs. Family groups of chimpanzees have been observed in which both adults and juvenile chimpanzees were chronically infected with HBV, although the source of the HBV infections was not determined (Zuckerman *et al.*, 1978).

Early attempts to transmit HBV to chimpanzees were conducted using chimpanzees that had been captured in their jungle habitat. The extent to which HBV is endemic among wild chimpanzees is not known (Deinhardt, 1976). However, patterns of commerce in captured chimpanzees have resulted in their close contact with humans residing in and near the jungle, among whom HBV is endemic. In some cases, pooled human serum was administered to chimpanzees in transit to "protect" them from a variety of human diseases, and this must certainly have resulted in inadvertent transmission of hepatitis B to many susceptible chimpanzees. Chimpanzees studied in captivity often were either no longer susceptible to HBV or were chronically infected and transmitted HBV to other chimpanzees housed with them. These factors delayed the recognition of the susceptibility of the chimpanzee to HBV, and made the provision of susceptible chimpanzees difficult after their susceptibility was recognized.

In the early 1970s, prohibition of the importation of chimpanzees into the United States for reasons of conservation of this endangered species led to the establishment of breeding colonies for chimpanzees there. The establishment of breeding colonies was also intended to provide a more reliable supply of seronegative chimpanzees than had been available from other sources. At the present time, all studies of HBV conducted in chimpanzees in the United States are done using chimpanzees that have been born and raised in breeding colonies, with the exception of some studies of antiviral compounds in chimpanzee chronic carriers that were imported from jungle areas in prior decades. The fact that chimpanzees have thrived in these colonies may one day lead to the anomalous situation of an extensive population of chimpanzees born in the United States, while the chimpanzee approaches extinction in Africa due to industrial and agricultural development of jungle lands. No difference has been found in the susceptibility to HBV between seronegative chimpanzees born in African jungles or in breeding colonies in the United States.

Chimpanzees used for the study of HBV infection must have no preexisting serological markers of HBV. They should not have been inoculated previously with any material containing HBV. Where possible, their prior close contact with humans and their prior inoculation with human blood, blood products, or plasma derivatives should have been minimal, in order to reduce the chance that a serologically undetectable HBV infection may have occurred or that prior inoculation of blood or its derivatives may have conferred immunity to HBV in the absence of detectable HBV antigens or antibodies. In this regard, colony-born chimpanzees provide the most reliable source for studies of HBV infection.

III. Procedures in Chimpanzees

Inoculating chimpanzees experimentally with hepatitis viruses, and obtaining serum and tissue specimens from them, must be done while the chimpanzees are anesthetized. The safety of the anesthesia is of primary importance because of the scarcity and value of the chimpanzees, and because the long incubation periods for human hepatitis necessitate repeated use of the anesthetic drug during the study. Cyclohexylamine (ketamine) is the most commonly used anesthetic drug for such studies; in some cases it is used in combination with xylazine. Neither of these is known to cause detectable hepatic toxicity or to interfere with liver metabolism (April *et al.*, 1982), and they have been shown to be safe when used weekly for periods up to 2 years (April *et al.*, 1982) or longer (E. Tabor, unpublished data).

Weekly blood samples of 25 ml can be obtained over periods up to 4 years in chimpanzees as young as 1 year of age with no reduction in hematocrit levels. Larger samples may be obtained weekly even from very young chimpanzees if the hematocrit is monitored. Samples can be obtained up to three times per week for periods of several months. Safe volumes may be estimated in proportion to the estimated total blood volume.

When antigens or antibodies suitable for reagent use are detected in a chimpanzee's serum, plasmapheresis may be performed. In adult chimpanzees, weekly or biweekly plasmapheresis over periods of many months can be safely performed. In young chimpanzees, plasmapheresis volumes must be reduced in proportion to the total blood volume of the chimpanzee. Pediatric blood bags should be used for chimpanzees <5 years of age. In chimpanzees under age 3 years, blood in volumes approaching that which would be safe for plasmapheresis (for instance, 50–60 ml from a 2-year-old chimpanzee weighing ~8 kg) may be withdrawn with simultaneous replacement in a second intravenous site using physiological saline with less stress for the chimpanzee and without exceeding the chimpanzee's ability to maintain its normal plasma volume.

It is essential to obtain liver tissue during studies of hepatitis B. For most studies of HBV in chimpanzees, monthly percutaneous liver biopsies are adequate. In some cases it is necessary to obtain more frequent samples, or larger samples for reagent use by means of laparotomy. Percutaneous liver biopsies can be obtained 1–2 times weekly for periods of 1 year or longer without harm to the chimpanzee. Biopsy by laparotomy is known to be safe when performed infrequently; the frequent use of this procedure has not been reported.

IV. Hepatitis B: A Comparison of Infections in Chimpanzees and Humans

Hepatitis B is characterized by identical serological events in humans and chimpanzees, although overall it is clinically and histologically a milder disease in chimpanzees. Following the inoculation of HBV using inocula of known infectivity, 100% of chimpanzees develop serological evidence of infection (Tabor *et al.*, 1983a). The end-point titers of infectivity of comparable but nonidentical infectious sera appear to be similar in humans (Barker and Murray, 1972) and chimpanzees (Tabor *et al.*, 1983a). The serological markers of HBV become detectable at comparable times and reach comparable titers in humans and chimpanzees.

Chimpanzees usually do not have clinically recognized signs and symptoms of hepatitis. A single case report of one chimpanzee with anorexia, lethargy, icterus, and right upper quadrant abdominal tenderness during HBV infection (Sly *et al.*, 1979) perhaps may have involved simultaneous infection with another virus as well, for instance an agent of non-A, non-B hepatitis. The only other published report of icterus in a chimpanzee (that was otherwise asymptomatic) with hepatitis B occurred during simultaneous acute hepatitis A and hepatitis B infections (Drucker *et al.*, 1978). In contrast, symptoms of hepatitis are noted in 20 (Aach *et al.*, 1978) to 45% (Hoofnagle *et al.*, 1978) of humans with hepatitis B, with 20 (Aach *et al.*, 1978) to 40% (Hoofnagle *et al.*, 1978) being icteric.

Aspartate and alanine aminotransferase (AST and ALT) serum levels in chimpanzees infected by HBV are usually elevated. From 70 to 100% of experimentally infected chimpanzees have some elevation of AST and ALT levels (Tabor *et al.*, 1983a); this is similar to the prevalence of AST and ALT elevations in humans with hepatitis B (Aach *et al.*, 1978). The mean peak level of AST and ALT in infected chimpanzees tends to be lower than the mean for infected humans, although peak levels as high as 500 IU/liter have been observed in some infected chimpanzees.

The frequency with which histological evidence of acute hepatitis is detected in liver biopsy specimens from chimpanzees with HBV infection has been well documented (Tabor *et al.*, 1983a). Similar prospective evaluation of the frequency of these findings has not been reported for humans, since liver biopsies are usually performed in humans with hepatitis B only when clinical indications of chronic hepatitis, cirrhosis, or hepatocellular carcinoma are present.

Histological evidence of acute hepatitis in serial liver biopsies from chimpanzees with serologically documented HBV infection may occur in as few as 33% of cases (Barker *et al.*, 1973; Tabor *et al.*, 1983a). Certain inocula may result in histological evidence of acute hepatitis in biopsies from 82% of chimpanzees with serologically documented hepatitis B infections (Tabor *et al.*, 1983a). These differences in severity were unrelated to the dilutions of the inocula (and hence the concentration of virus) with which the chimpanzees were infected, but were related to the particular inoculum administered. The δ agent, a defective virus that requires helper functions of HBV and may result in increased severity of HBV infections, did not play a role in the differences observed in these studies (Tabor *et al.*, 1983a). At the present time it is not possible to ascribe these "inoculum-associated" differences in severity to inherent differences among the subtypes of HBV. Nor does the presence or absence of histological abnormalities appear to be related to progression to chronicity, since histological abnormalities may be absent even in chronic carriers of HBV (Barker *et al.*, 1973).

When histological abnormalities in the liver are found in chimpanzees with acute hepatitis B, they include disorganization of the hepatic cords, hydropic changes, ballooning degeneration, eosinophilic changes, and a diffuse increase of lymphocytes scattered among the parenchymal cells. Periportal lymphocytic accumulation is usually present as well. Acidophilic bodies may be present, in some cases extruded into the sinusoids.

Fulminant hepatitis B has not been documented in chimpanzees. This phenomenon, characterized by massive hepatocyte destruction leading rapidly to coma and in many cases to death due to liver failure, occurs in ~0.5% of humans infected with HBV. The possibility that fulminant hepatitis, uncommon even among infected humans, might be observed if sufficient numbers of chimpanzees were inoculated with HBV cannot be ruled out. The hypothesis that co-infection by HBV plus other agents may contribute to the development of fulminant hepatitis B, if valid, may explain why fulminant hepatitis B does not occur in chimpanzees in the relatively controlled environment of the laboratory.

Chronic HBV infections result from ~4% of experimental infections in chimpanzees. Although chronicity is usually defined in humans by the persistence of HBsAg in serum for >6 months, persistence for >1 year has often been used as the definition of chronicity in chimpanzees, because clearance of infections between 6 and 12 months after the first appearance of HBsAg has been observed in approximately two-thirds of chimpanzees whose HBsAg is still detectable at 6 months (Tabor *et al.*, 1983a). Liver biopsies from chimpanzees with chronic HBV infection never have more severe alterations than those of mild chronic persistent hepatitis.

V. Inocula Containing the Hepatitis B Virus

A. Sources and End-Point Titers of Infectivity

Seven inocula containing the hepatitis B virus (HBV) and consisting of serum or plasma from chronically infected humans have been evaluated in chimpanzees (Table I). These inocula represent the four subtypes of HBsAg; the complete subtype profiles of two of the inocula have not been determined. The inocula designations and the laboratories that performed the infectivity studies are shown in Table I; they include inocula from the Center for Drugs and Biologics (CDB, formerly the BoB) and the National Institute of Allergy and Infectious Diseases (NIAID) (Tabor *et al.*, 1983a,c; Barker *et al.*, 1975), the Centers for Disease Control (Dr. D. Bradley, personal communication), the New York Blood Center

TABLE I

Titered Infectivity of Hepatitis B Virus Inocula in Chimpanzees

Laboratory	Designation (source)	HBsAg subtype	Chimpanzee infectious doses (CID) per ml
CDB(BoB)/NIAID[a,b]	CDB(BoB)/NIAID (human serum)	**adw**	$10^{7.0}$
		ayw	$10^{7.5}$
		adr	$10^{8.0}$
		ayr	$10^{0}(< 10^{4})$
CDC[a]	HLD (human plasma)	Unknown	$10^{8.0}$
NYBC[a]	NYBC challenge virus (human plasma)	**ad**	$\geq 10^{7.0}$
Nihon/Tokyo[a]	JHB 001 (human serum)	**adr**	$\geq 10^{8.0}$

[a]CDB(BoB), Center for Drugs and Biologics (previously called Bureau of Biologics); NIAID, National Institute for Allergy and Infectious Diseases; CDC, Centers for Disease Control; NYBC, New York Blood Center; Nihon/Tokyo, Nihon University and Tokyo Metropolitan Institute of Medical Science.

[b]These inocula were evaluated by CDB(BoB), NIAID, and CDC.

(Dr. A. Prince, personal communication), and Tokyo Metropolitan Hospital (Shikata *et al.*, 1977). In each of these inocula, the infectivity titer was between 10^7 and 10^8 CID_{50}/ml, except for the uncommon **ayr** inoculum, which had an end-point titer of infectivity of 10^0 ($<10^4$) CID_{50}/ml. End-point titers of infectivity are usually calculated using the Reed–Muench method because of the relatively small number of chimpanzees inoculated with each dilution of any inoculum (Hawkes, 1979). With all inocula reported, 100% of chimpanzees have been infected by every dilution except, with certain inocula, those dilutions near the end-point, which infected either one of two or two of three inoculated chimpanzees (Tabor *et al.*, 1983a). By defining 1 ml of the end-point dilution as containing 1 infectious unit or one chimpanzee infectious dose$_{50}$ (CID_{50}), the infectivity of the starting sera were calculated.

B. Relationship between End-Point Titers of Infectivity and Serological Markers of Hepatitis B

In detailed studies of three inocula containing HBV (Tabor *et al.*, 1983a), the end-point titers of infectivity exceeded the end-point titers of HBsAg as determined by radioimmunoassay (RIA). However, the difference between the end-point titer of infectivity and the end-point titer of HBsAg was different for each inoculum. The end-point titer of infectivity for the **adw** inoculum was 10^{-7}, while the end-point titer of HBsAg was 10^{-5} (a 100-fold difference); the end-point titer of infectivity for the **ayw** inoculum was $10^{-7.5}$, while that of HBsAg was 10^{-4} (a difference $>1,000$-fold); the end-point titer of infectivity for the **adr** inoculum was 10^{-8}, while that of HBsAg was 10^{-4} (a 10,000-fold difference).

No significant differences in the end-point titers of anti-HBc (10^{-3}, **adw**; 10^{-2}, **ayw** and **adr**) or HBeAg (10^{-3} for all three inocula) were detected by RIA. Neither anti-HBs nor anti-HBe was detected by RIA in any of the inocula. Forty-two-nm HBV were seen in all three inocula by electron microscopy. HBV DNA polymerase titers of 10^0 to 10^{-1} and HBV DNA titers of 10^{-2} to $10^{-2.5}$ are present in these three inocula (Berninger *et al.*, 1982).

C. Relationship between Incubation Period and End-Point Titers of Infectivity

With each of the three major inocula evaluated at CDB(BoB)/NIAID, an inverse relationship was observed between the amount of virus present in the dilution inoculated and the length of the incubation period (defined as the time from inoculation to the appearance of HBsAg) (Fig. 1) (Tabor *et al.*, 1983a; Barker *et al.*, 1975). However, this relationship is only approximate; incubation periods for infections caused by a given dilution vary, and substantial overlap in the range of incubation periods is observed between dilutions of inocula varying by a factor of 10 or 100. With the inocula containing HBsAg subtypes **ayw** and **adr,** fairly steep infectivity curves were observed (Fig. 1), with no incubation periods >15 weeks. With the inoculum containing subtype **adw,** however, the curve was steep only for dilutions between 10^0 and 10^{-3}; thereafter the incubation periods were longer and more variable, and the curve was less steep. However, the longest incubation period observed was 19 weeks. Although the reason for the difference between the **adw** infectivity curve and those of the **ayw** and **adr** inocula is not known, it has been shown that it is probably not due to instability of the **adw** inoculum during storage (Tabor *et al.*, 1983a). There are no data at the present time to suggest that inherent differences in infectivity patterns between HBV with different subtypes account for these observations; this possibility can only be ruled out by the titration of additional **adw** inocula.

D. Interpretation of Results

Caution should be used in applying the inverse relationship between the incubation period and the end-point titer of infectivity to the evaluation of the infectivity remaining after the application of procedures to inactivate HBV or to remove HBV from blood or plasma derivatives. Moderate changes in incubation period may not indicate a reduction in infectivity following such procedures, since the incubation period produced by a given dilution of an HBV-containing inoculum may vary to some extent independently of the effect of the treatment (Fig. 1). In addition, prolongation of the incubation period may not necessarily reflect a reduction in infectivity.

Extreme caution should be used in drawing conclusions about HBV infectivity on the basis of HBsAg titers after inactivation procedures. Attempts to remove or inactivate HBV may remove or alter the 22-nm HBsAg particles and leave residual infectious HBV. In addition, the relationship between the end-point titer of HBsAg and the end-point titer of infectivity varied among the inocula evaluated by CDB(BoB)/ NIAID and may be different from that found in other sera. Therefore, the inactivation of HBV by procedures applied to blood or plasma derivatives should not be extrapolated from the destruction of detectable HBsAg unless confirmed by the inoculation of susceptible chimpanzees.

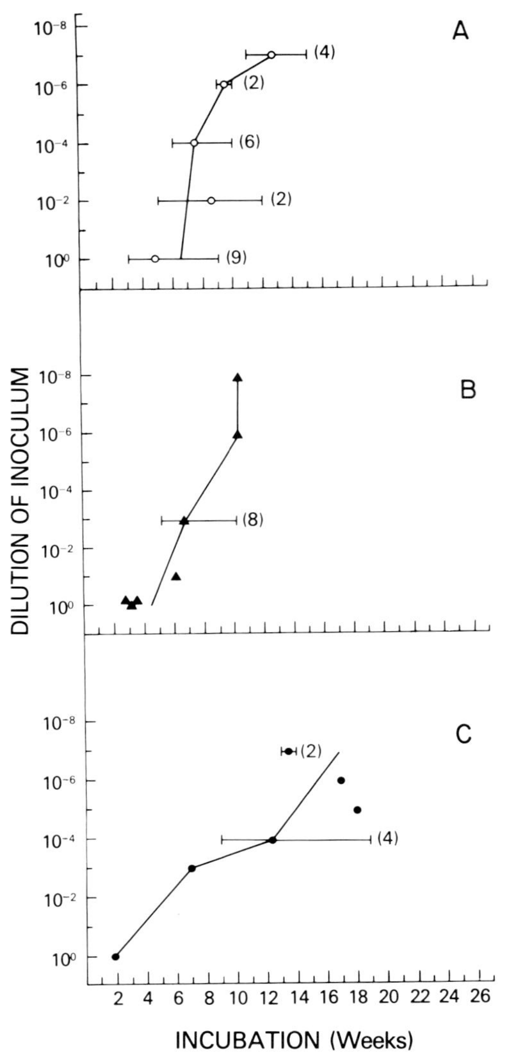

Figure 1. Relationship between dilution of three hepatitis B virus-containing inocula and incubation period in 47 chimpanzees. (A) **ayw;** (B) **adr;** (C) **adw.** Seven additional chimpanzees not infected following inoculation with dilutions of the inocula near or beyond the end points of infectivity are not shown. Incubation period shown in weeks. Points on bars indicate mean incubation period for the dilution; bars indicate the range of incubation periods for the dilution. Numbers adjacent to bars indicate the number of chimpanzees inoculated with that dilution; points without bars indicate that only 1 chimpanzee was inoculated with the dilution. Slope represents "best fit" slope for mean incubation periods for each dilution.

VI. Application of the Chimpanzee Model

A. Special Considerations

The longest incubation period observed in chimpanzees experimentally inoculated with titered inocula containing HBV is 19 weeks (Tabor *et al.*, 1983a). For this reason, as well as observations following transfusion or needle-stick transmission in humans, the chimpanzee safety test for the evaluation of hepatitis B vaccines has been set at 6 months, with weekly serological evaluation and monthly liver biopsy evaluation. While this is suitable for formalin-inactivated vaccines, a longer follow-up may be necessary for safety tests of other types of materials. Globulin preparations containing anti-HBs have been shown to prolong the incubation period of HBV in some situations, and studies evaluating such products in chimpanzees should include 12 months of follow-up. In one study, antihemophilic factor (AHF) containing experimentally added HBV, stabilized and heated at 60°C for 10 hr, resulted in a prolongation of the incubation period of HBV to 7–9 months in two chimpanzees, in a situation in which the infectivity was not completely eliminated. This did not occur in other situations in which different stabilizing procedures were used to permit heating AHF at 60°C for 10 hr. Nor has it occurred when albumin or plasma protein fraction are heated at 60°C for 10 hr, a procedure that has consistently inactivated HBV in these products. It appears that alteration of the virus by the heat may occur in a way that prolongs the process of virus attachment, entry, or replication. Thus, heat inactivation of HBV in any plasma derivative other than albumin or plasma protein fraction should be evaluated with a 12-month safety test in experimentally inoculated chimpanzees until more is known about the HBV-inactivation kinetics of this method.

Because the value and small numbers of chimpanzees make it necessary to use them sequentially for the study of more than one hepatitis agent, the possible interference by prior non-A, non-B hepatitis infection with subsequent HBV infections has been evaluated. Viral interference between non-A, non-B hepatitis and HBV has been shown in certain situations. Transmission of an agent of non-A, non-B hepatitis to chimpanzees with preexisting chronic HBV infections has been shown to result in reduction of the titer of HBsAg in serum and reduction of HBV DNA polymerase (Tsiquaye *et al.*, 1983; Bradley *et al.*, 1983), although actual clearance of chronic HBV infection has not been experimentally induced in this way. Clearly, most humans with chronic HBV infection do not clear HBV when they acquire non-A, non-B hepatitis, considering the high prevalence of co-existing HBV and non-A, non-B hepatitis infections and low incidence of clearance of chronic HBV infections. Although interference with transmission of HBV to chimpanzees has been claimed to occur in chimpanzees with prior acute or chronic non-A, non-B hepatitis, as evidenced by prolongation of HBV incubation periods (Brotman *et al.*, 1983), the validity of this observation is not clear.

Other investigators have reported, at international conferences, the interference of simultaneous acute non-A, non-B hepatitis with HBV infection in chimpanzees, but without full publication of the data. Some investigators, however, have observed the simultaneous transmission of hepatitis B and non-A, non-B hepatitis to a chimpanzee by a single inoculum containing both agents, with an interval of a few weeks between the infections and no apparent interference (Tabor, 1981). In studies conducted at CDB, no interference with HBV infections transmitted by carefully documented inocula occurred when chimpanzees were inoculated with HBV subsequent to apparent recovery from acute non-A, non-B hepatitis infections, or when those acute non-A, non-B hepatitis infections had progressed to apparent chronic non-A, non-B hepatitis infections. In fact, in every case the observed incubation period of HBV was less than or equal to the median incubation period of the HBV inoculum dilution used (Tabor *et al.*, 1983c).

The different findings reported with regard to viral interference between HBV and non-A, non-B hepatitis may reflect the existence of more than one non-A, non-B hepatitis agent, one that is capable of interfering and one that is not. Or they may reflect marked variations in the pathogenicity or expression of different non-A, non-B infections. When attempts are made to evaluate viral interference between two agents that require an *in vivo* system for transmission, one of which has no generally accepted serological markers and is likely to be caused by more than one agent, it is not surprising that the results are diverse.

When chimpanzees are selected for safety or efficacy tests, they must be fully susceptible to HBV. No HBV serological markers should be present in their serum, and where possible, chimpanzees should be used whose serology has been tested continuously from birth to the onset of the study. Chimpanzees born and raised in a breeding colony are better than those captured in the jungle, because of better observation and less chance for sporadic infection with HBV. Jungle-caught chimpanzees are acceptable if they are evaluated serologically for at least 6 months prior to the study. No chimpanzee that has ever been inoculated with material thought to contain HBV or HBsAg, even if no infection resulted, should be used for a hepatitis B safety or efficacy test. Even the use of such a chimpanzee as a positive control is inadvisable, except where a second positive control chimpanzee is available in the event the first proves not to be susceptible.

B. Evaluation of Hepatitis B Vaccines

The chimpanzee model for hepatitis B has made possible the development of vaccines to prevent this disease, despite the inability to propagate HBV *in vitro* (see Chapter 16). The safety, immunogenicity, and efficacy of these vaccines were first proved in chimpanzees (Purcell and Gerin, 1975, 1978; Hilleman *et al.*, 1975, 1978). The challenge inoculations of the vaccinated chimpanzees utilized some of the inocula with titered infectivity described above. The cross-protection afforded by antibodies induced by different HBsAg subtypes was first shown in chimpanzees (Gerety *et al.*, 1979; Maynard *et al.*, 1975; Purcell and Gerin, 1978). The possibility that hepatitis B vaccines might be useful for postexposure administration to prevent HBV infection was first suggested by chimpanzee studies (Purcell and Gerin, 1978). The successful inactivation of HBV for vaccine production was shown by inoculation of susceptible chimpanzees (see Section VI,C) and inoculation of chimpanzees continues to be required by most nations to evaluate the successful inactivation of HBV in the initial manufacture of vaccine and, in some, in each lot of hepatitis B vaccine.

As new forms of hepatitis B vaccines are developed, chimpanzees will probably be required for the initial evaluation of their safety, and perhaps also of their immunogenicity and efficacy, before they are used in humans. This may be true even for some vaccines produced by recombinant DNA techniques and those which result from the synthesis of HBV polypeptides. Whether individual lots of newer vaccines will have to be tested in chimpanzees prior to release will have to be decided individually for each form of vaccine, depending on its manufacturing procedure.

C. Evaluation of Procedures to Inactivate Hepatitis B Virus

Methods to inactivate the hepatitis B virus for vaccine production or for ensuring the safety of plasma derivatives have been proven effective by the inoculation of susceptible chimpanzees. Using titered inocula and susceptible chimpanzees, it has been shown that one can inactivate 10^5 CID_{50} of HBV/ml by means of 1:4000 formalin at 37°C for 72 hr (Tabor *et al.*, 1983b); 10^5 CID_{50}/ml by 1 μg/ml pepsin at pH 2.0 for 18 hr (Tabor *et al.*, 1983b); 10^5 CID_{50}/ml by 8 M urea for 4 hr (Tabor *et al.*, 1983b); $10^{3.5}$

CID$_{50}$/ml by heating at 60°C for 10 hr (Tabor *et al.*, 1981); 10^6 CID$_{50}$/ml by a process of three precipitation steps followed by heating at 60°C for 10 hr (Heimburger *et al.*, 1980, 1981); or 10^3 CID$_{50}$/ml by the addition of high-titer anti-HBs (Tabor *et al.*, 1980). These inactivation studies have resulted in a safe hepatitis B vaccine, and have contributed to the development of clotting factor concentrates with a reduced risk of transmitting hepatitis B.

References

Aach, R. D., Lander, J. J., Sherman, L. A., Miller, W. V., Kahn, R. A., Gitnick, G. L., Hollinger, F. B., Werch, J., Szmuness, W., Stevens, C. E., Kellner, A., Weiner, J. M., and Mosley, J. W. (1978). *In* "Viral Hepatitis" (G. N. Vyas, S. N. Cohen, and R. Schmid, eds.), pp. 383–396. Franklin Inst. Press, Philadelphia, Pennsylvania.

April, M., Tabor, E., and Gerety, R. J. (1982). *Lab. Anim.* **16,** 116–118.

Bancroft, W. H., Snitbhan, R., Scott, R. M., Tingpalapong, M., Watson, W. T., Tanticharoenyos, P., Karwacki, J. J., and Srimarut, S. (1977). *J. Infect. Dis.* **135,** 79–85.

Barker, L. F., and Murray, R. (1972). *Am. J. Med. Sci.* **263,** 27–33.

Barker, L. F., Chisari, F. V., McGrath, P. P., Dalgard, D. W., Kirschstein, R. L., Almeida, J. D., Edgington, T. S., Sharp, D. G., and Peterson, M. R. (1973). *J. Infect. Dis.* **127,** 648–662.

Barker, L. F., Maynard, J. E., Purcell, R. H., Hoofnagle, J. H., Berquist, K. R., London, W. T., Gerety, R. J., and Krushak, D. H. (1975). *J. Infect. Dis.* **132,** 451–458.

Berninger, M., Hammer, M., Hoyer, B., and Gerin, J. L. (1982). *J. Med. Virol.* **9,** 57–68.

Bradley, D. W., Maynard, J. E., McCaustland, K. A., Murphy, B. L., Cook, E. H., and Ebert, J. W. (1983). *J. Med. Virol.* **11,** 207–213.

Brotman, B., Prince, A. M., Huima, T., Richardson, L., van den Ende, M. C., and Pfeifer, U. (1983). *J. Med. Virol.* **11,** 191–205.

Deinhardt, F. (1976). *Adv. Virus Res.* **20,** 113–157.

Drucker, J., Tabor, E., Gerety, R. J., Jackson, D., and Barker, L. F. (1979). *J. Infect. Dis.* **139,** 338–342.

Eichberg, J. W., and Kalter, S. S. (1980). *Lab. Anim. Sci.* **30,** 541–543.

Gerety, R. J., Tabor, E., Purcell, R. H., and Tyeryar, F. (1979). *J. Infect. Dis.* **140,** 642–648.

Hawkes, R. A. (1979). *In* "Diagnostic Procedures for Viral, Rickettsial, and Chlamydial Infections" (E. H. Lennette and N. J. Schmidt, eds.), 5th ed., pp. 32–35. Am. Public Health Assoc., Washington, D. C.

Heimburger, N., Schwinn, H., and Mauler, R. (1980). *Gelben Hefte* **20,** 165–174.

Heimburger, N., Schwinn, H., Gratz, P., Luben, G., Kumpe, G., and Herchenhan, B. (1981). *Arzneim.-Forsch.* **31,** 619–622.

Hilleman, M. R., Buynak, E. B., Roehm, R. R., Tytell, A. A., Bertland, A. U., and Lampson, G. P. (1975). *Am. J. Med. Sci.* **270,** 401–404.

Hilleman, M. R., Bertland, A. U., Buynak, E. B., Lampson, G. P., McAleer, W. J., McLean, A. A., Roehm, R. R., and Tytell, A. A. (1978). *In* "Viral Hepatitis" (G. N. Vyas, S. N. Cohen, and R. Schmid, eds.), pp. 525–537. Franklin Inst. Press, Philadelphia, Pennsylvania.

Hoofnagle, J. H., Seeff, L. B., Bales, Z. B., Gerety, R. J., and Tabor, E. (1978). *In* "Viral

Hepatitis" (G. N. Vyas, S. N. Cohen, and R. Schmid, eds.), pp. 219–242. Franklin Inst. Press, Philadelphia, Pennsylvania.

Maynard, J. E., Krushak, D. H., Bradley, D. W., and Berquist, K. R. (1975). *Dev. Biol. Stand.* **30**, 229–235.

Purcell, R. H., and Gerin, J. L. (1975). *Am. J. Med. Sci.* **270**, 395–399.

Purcell, R. H., and Gerin, J. L. (1978). *In* "Viral Hepatitis" (G. N. Vyas, S. N. Cohen, and R. Schmid, eds.), pp. 491–505. Franklin Inst. Press, Philadelphia, Pennsylvania.

Shikata, T., Karasawa, T., Abe, K., Uzawa, T., Suzuki, H., Oda, T., Imai, M., Mayumi, M., and Moritsugu, Y. (1977). *J. Infect. Dis.* **136**, 571–576.

Shulman, N. R., and Barker, L. F. (1969). *Science* **165**, 304–306.

Sly, D. L., London, W. T., and Purcell, R. H. (1979). *J. Am. Vet. Med. Assoc.* **175**, 987–988.

Tabor, E. (1981). *In* "Non-A, Non-B Hepatitis" (R. J. Gerety, ed.), pp. 189–206. Academic Press, New York.

Tabor, E., Aronson, D. L., and Gerety, R. J. (1980). *Lancet* 2, 68–70.

Tabor, E., Murano, G., Snoy, P., and Gerety, R. J. (1981). *Thromb. Res.* **22**, 233–238.

Tabor, E., Purcell, R. H., London, W. T., and Gerety, R. J. (1983a). *J. Infect. Dis.* **147**, 531–534.

Tabor, E. Buynak, E., Smallwood, L. A., Snoy, P., Hilleman, M., and Gerety, R. J. (1983b). *J. Med. Virol.* **11**, 1–9.

Tabor, E. Purcell, R. H., and Gerety, R. J. (1983c). *J. Med. Primatol.* **12**, 305–318.

Tsiquaye, K. N., Portmann, B., Tovey, G., Kessler, H., Hu, S., Lu, X., Zuckerman, A. J., Craske, J., and Williams, R. (1983). *J. Med. Virol.* **11**, 179–189.

Zuckerman, A. J., Thornton, A., Howard, C. R., Tsiquaye, K. N., Jones, D. M., and Brambell, M. R. (1978). *Lancet* 2, 652–654.

Chapter 14

The Molecular Biology of Hepatitis B Virus and Related Viruses of Animals

WILLIAM S. ROBINSON
Department of Medicine
Stanford University School of Medicine
Stanford, California

I. Introduction

Hepatitis B virus (HBV) is found in human populations all over the world, and is of great medical importance because it is probably the most common cause of chronic liver disease (including hepatocellular carcinoma) in humans (Szmuness, 1978). This virus and three close relatives found in lower animal species [woodchucks (Summers *et al.*, 1978a), ground squirrels (Marion *et al.*, 1980), and Pekin ducks (Mason *et al.*, 1980)] have unusually interesting molecular and biological features that distinguish them from members of all of the previously recognized virus groups. These viruses represent a new virus group that has been called the hepadna virus group (Marion and Robinson, 1983; Robinson, 1980; Robinson *et al.*, 1982). Since these viruses have been identified relatively recently and have not yet been propogated in tissue culture, many details of their mechanism of replication are still not known. Several unique features of these viruses are apparent, however. One of the most notable features is the structure of their DNA. These viruses con-

319   Copyright © 1985 by Academic Press, Inc.
All rights of reproduction in any form reserved.
ISBN 0-12-280672-7

tain small circular DNA molecules (Robinson *et al.*, 1974) that are partly single stranded, and a DNA polymerase in the virion (Kaplan *et al.*, 1973; Robinson and Greenman, 1974) can repair the DNA to make it fully double stranded (Summers *et al.*, 1975; Landers *et al.*, 1977; Hruska *et al.*, 1977). Recent information also suggests that the mechanism of replication of the viral DNA may be unique and involve an RNA intermediate (Summers and Mason, 1982; Miller and Robinson, 1984a).

Important biological features include a striking tropism of the viruses for hepatocytes, very narrow host ranges, and the common occurrence of persistent infection with viral antigen and infectious virus in high concentrations in the blood and lower concentrations in certain other body fluids continuously for years. This pattern of infection accounts for the common transmission of HBV by percutaneous transfer of serum and serum-containing material, and when circulating immune complexes containing viral antigens are formed, immune complex disease sometimes results. In parts of the world where HBV infection rates are high, such as in eastern Asia, Oceania, and sub-Saharan Africa, the prevalence of persistent infection (HBsAg carriers) may exceed 10% in some populations (Szmuness, 1978). In the United States and northern Europe, the prevalence of persistent infection is closer to 0.1%. It has been estimated that there are >170 million HBsAg carriers in the world today (Szmuness, 1978). This large population of persistently infected individuals appears to be the main source or reservoir of virus for new human infections, since no important animal or environmental reservoir of HBV is known.

Acute hepatitis, often severe, was the first manifestation of primary HBV infection to be recognized. It is now clear that many primary infections are subclinical and not associated with significant liver disease. Persistent infection may be associated with a nearly normal liver or with chronic hepatitis. The latter may be severe and progressive, and may lead to cirrhosis and in some cases to hepatocellular carcinoma (Szmuness, 1978).

Current knowledge of the basic properties of hepatitis B and related viruses, their molecular structure and mechanism of replication, the state of virus in blood and in liver cells at different stages of infection, and the role of virus in liver disease are reviewed here.

II. Viral Forms in Serum

Hepatitis B viral forms in the blood of infected patients were identified and characterized after the discovery of the antigen on the surface of these particulate forms. Hepatitis B surface antigen (HBsAg) was discovered in 1965 by Blumberg, Alter, and Visnich (1965) while they were investigating human serum protein polymorphism. The antigen was first found in the serum of an Australian aborigine when a precipitin line formed in agar gel diffusion between that serum and the serum of a patient with hemophilia who had received multiple blood transfusions. Thus the antigen was first named Australia antigen (Alter and Blumberg, 1966). It was not immediately recognized to be a viral antigen. Several years of investigation led to its eventual association with acute hepatitis B (Blumberg *et al.*, 1967; Okochi and Murakami, 1968; Prince, 1968), and it was then named hepatitis-associated antigen (HAA), and later was given the current name, hepatitis B surface antigen. Hepatitis B surface antigen (HBsAg) in the blood remains the most useful marker of active HBV infection. It appears in the blood exclusively as a component of virions and incomplete particulate viral forms; no soluble or low molecular weight form has been detected (LeBouvier and McCollum, 1970; Bayer *et al.*, 1968). The serum of infected patients has been the principal source of viral material for physical characterization of HBV, since this virus has not been grown in cell culture systems.

Small spherical particles, heterogeneous in size and appearance (diameters approximately from 16 to 25 nm; they are called 22-nm particles), and filamentous or rod-shaped particles (~22 nm wide and up to several hundred nanometers in length) (Fig. 1) were the first HBsAg particulate forms observed in electron micrographs by Bayer *et al.* in 1968. These are the most numerous HBsAg-bearing particles in the serum of most HBV-infected patients, and they consist of protein, carbohydrate, and lipid. No nucleic acid has been found in them, and they are now considered to be incomplete viral coat particles. In 1970 a larger and more complex HBsAg-bearing particle was described by Dane *et al.* (1970). Strong evidence now indicates that this so-called Dane particle is the complete hepatitis B virion. The virion has a diameter of ~42 nm, with a lipid-containing outer layer or envelope ~7 nm in width and an electron-dense 28-nm diameter spherical internal core or nucleocapsid (Fig. 2, A) (Dane *et al.*, 1970). The surface of the virion shares antigenic determinants (HBsAg) with the incomplete viral forms (22-nm spherical and filamentous particles) (Dane *et al.*, 1970; Almeida *et al.*, 1971). The outer envelope of the virion with HBsAg can be removed by treatment with nonionic detergents such as Nonident P-40 (NP-40) leaving free core particles (Fig. 2B) containing the virus-specified hepatitis B core antigen (HBcAg), which is antigenically distinct from HBsAg (Almeida *et al.*, 1971). The viral core also contains the viral DNA (Robinson *et al.*, 1974) with a covalently attached polypeptide (Gerlich and Robinson, 1980), DNA polymerase activity (Kaplan *et al.*, 1973; Robinson and

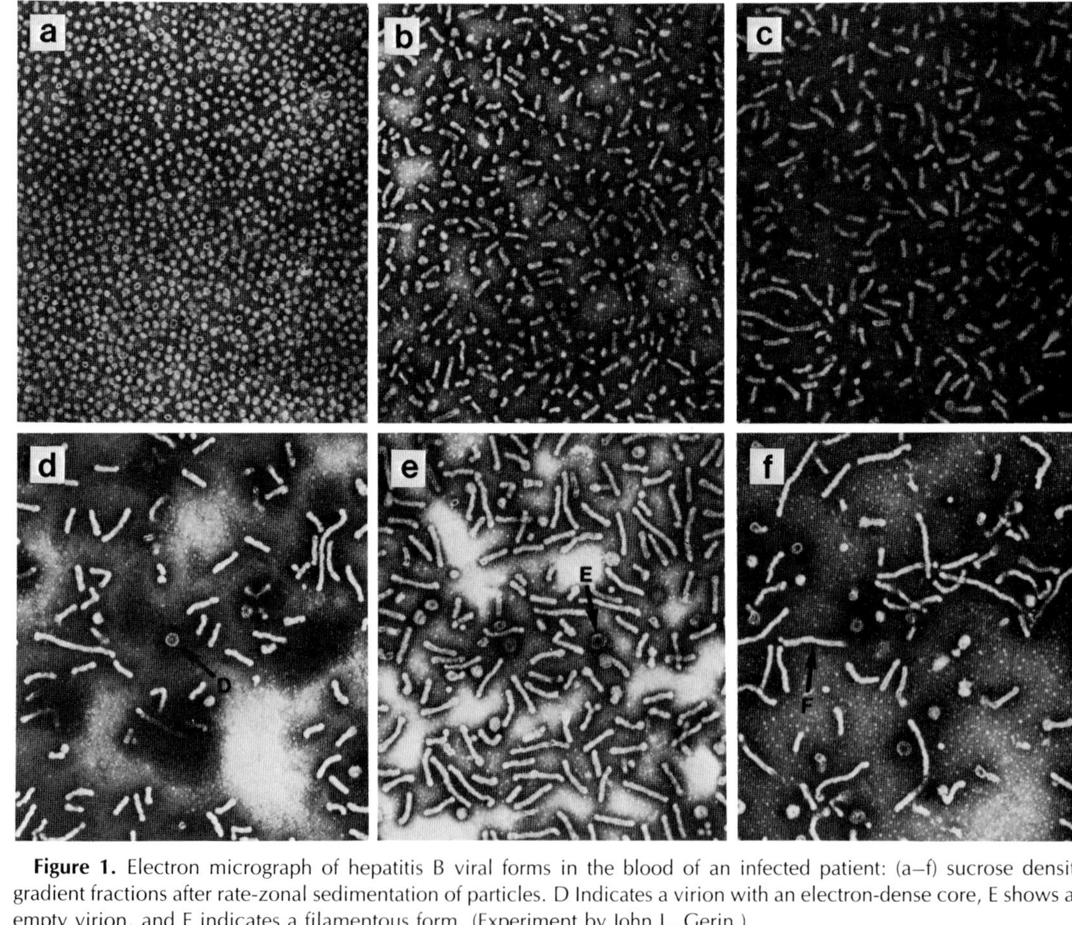

Figure 1. Electron micrograph of hepatitis B viral forms in the blood of an infected patient: (a–f) sucrose density gradient fractions after rate-zonal sedimentation of particles. D Indicates a virion with an electron-dense core, E shows an empty virion, and F indicates a filamentous form. (Experiment by John L. Gerin.)

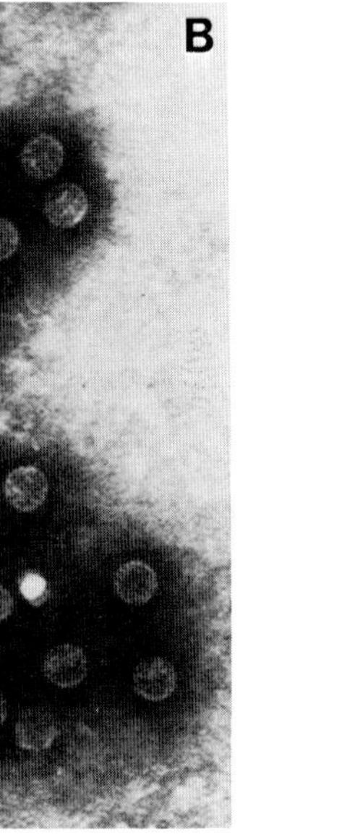
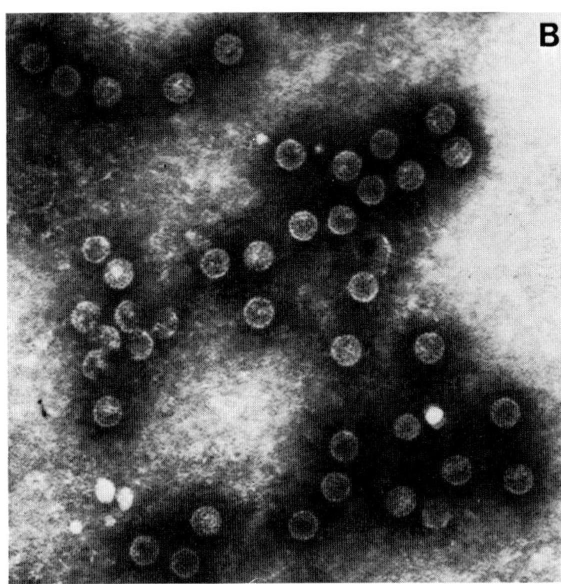
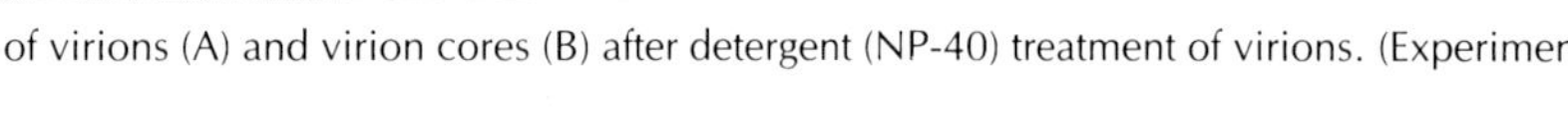
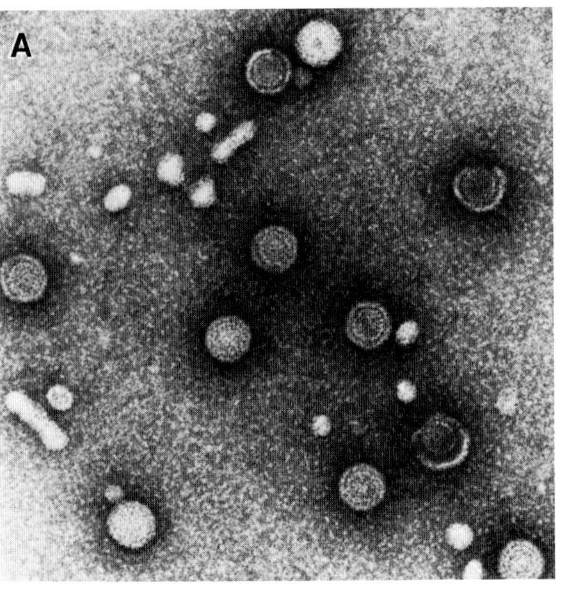

Figure 2. Electron micrograph of virions (A) and virion cores (B) after detergent (NP-40) treatment of virions. (Experiment by June Almedia.)

Greenman, 1974), protein kinase activity (Albin and Robinson, 1980), and apparently the third antigen associated with hepatitis B virus infection, hepatitis B e antigen (HBeAg), in a cryptic form (Takahashi *et al.*, 1979b); all are described in detail in this chapter. In addition to virions with electron-dense centers, virions with empty cores (Fig. 1) are found in all preparations. Figure 3 summarizes the viral forms found in the blood of HBV-infected patients.

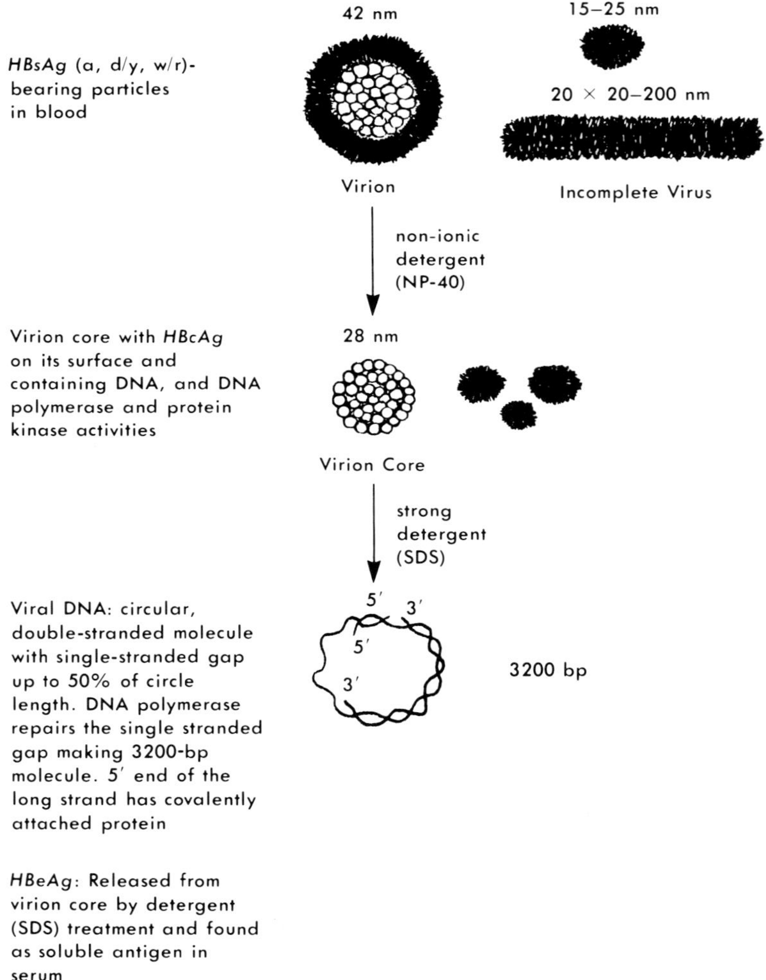

Figure 3. Schematic representation of hepatitis B viral forms found in the blood of infected patients.

The size of the hepatitis B virion estimated by electron microscopy (42 nm in diameter) is consistent with ultrafiltration studies showing that the infectious agent passes through Seitz filters with an average pore diameter of 52 nm (McCollum, 1952). The concentrations of physical virions in serum measured by electron microscopy (undetectable in some sera, up to 10^5–10^9 particles per milliliter in other sera, see Almeida, 1972) are consistent with directly measured concentrations of infectious HBV (Scullard *et al.*, 1982; Barker and Murray, 1972; Shikata *et al.*, 1977; Barker *et al.*, 1975; Hoofnagle, 1980). Inoculation of 1 ml of some undiluted HBsAg-reactive sera has failed to infect chimpanzees (Scullard *et al.*, 1982), suggesting that such patients circulate HBsAg only in the form of incomplete particles and not complete virions. Sera from other patients, on the other hand, have infected humans or chimpanzees in dilutions up to 10^{-7} (Barker and Murray, 1972) or 10^{-8} (Scullard *et al.*, 1982; Shikata *et al.*, 1977), indicating the presence of high concentrations of infectious virions. There have been few reported direct comparison of carefully measured physical virion particle concentrations with quantitative infectious HBV titers in the same sera (see Chapter 13). It has been shown that physical concentration and partial purification of virions result in preparations that are infectious at a higher dilution (10^{-10}) than has been reported for unconcentrated serum (Thomssen *et al.*, 1977).

The concentrations of incomplete viral forms in serum usually greatly exceed the concentrations of complete virions. Concentrations of 10^{13} 22-nm spherical particles/ml or higher have been found in some sera (Kim and Tilles, 1970), indicating that these particles outnumbered virions by 10^4-fold or more in most sera (see also Chapter 13).

Hepatitis B virus has been shown to retain infectivity for humans for 6 months when stored in serum at 30–32°C (Redeker *et al.*, 1968), and 15 years when frozen at −20°C. All infectivity for human volunteers is not lost at 60°C for up to 4 hr (Murray and Diefenbach, 1953), but it is lost at 60°C after 10 hr when in albumin (Gellis *et al.*, 1948), although not completely in whole serum (Soulier *et al.*, 1972; Shikata *et al.*, 1978). Infectivity in serum was destroyed at 90°C after 1 (Krugman *et al.*, 1970) or 20 min (Wewalka, 1953). Infectivity has also been destroyed by dry heat at 160°C after 1 hr (Salaman *et al.*, 1944).

Woodchuck hepatitis virus (WHV) was discovered by Summers, Smolec, and Snyder in 1978 (Summers *et al.*, 1978a) in a *Marmota monax* colony in the Philadelphia Zoo in the serum of animals commonly found to have hepatitis and hepatocellular carcinoma. Ground squirrel hepatitis virus (GSHV) was discovered by Marion *et al.* in 1980 in the serum of wild-caught *Spermophilus beecheyi* in northern California. The duck hepatitis B virus (DHBV) was discovered in 1981 by J. Summers, W. T. London, T. Sun, B. S. Blumberg (unpublished) in sera of domestic ducks from a geographical region of the Peoples Republic of China where hepatocellular carcinomas occurred commonly in these animals. The same spectrum of viral forms described above for HBV has been found in the blood of animals infected with WHV, GSHV, and DHBV. The complete virions of WHV (Summers *et al.*, 1978a) and GSHV (Marion *et al.*, 1980) appear, however, to be slightly larger (47 nm in diameter) than hepatitis B virions, and those of DHBV (Mason *et al.*, 1980) are more pleomorphic.

III. Viral Surface Antigen

Hepatitis B surface antigen (HBsAg) has at least five antigenic specificities. A group-specific determinant (**a**) is shared by all HBsAg preparations, and two pairs of subtype determinants (**d,y** and **w,r**) (the determinants of each pair are for the most part mutually exclusive and thus usually behave as alleles) have been demonstrated (LeBouvier, 1971; Bancroft *et al.*, 1972). Antigenic heterogeneity of the **w** determinants and additional determinants such as **q** and **x** or **g** have also been described (Couroucé-Pauty and Soulier, 1974; Couroucé *et al.*, 1976). The eight HBsAg subtypes **ayw$_1$, ayw$_2$, ayw$_3$, ayw$_4$, ayr, adw$_2$, adw$_4$,** and **adr** have been identified (Couroucé *et al.*, 1976). Isolated and usually single cases from the Far East with unusual combinations of HBsAg subtype determinants such as **awr, adwr, adyw, adyr,** and **adywr** have been reported (Mazzur *et al.*, 1974). The subtype determinants in these cases are found on the same particles, suggesting that phenotypic mixing or unusual genetic recombinants have formed during mixed infections. There is an uneven geographic distribution of HBsAg subtypes in infected populations (Mazzur *et al.*, 1974; Bancroft *et al.*, 1976). Subtypes **adw, ayw,** and **adr** are found in extensive geographical regions of the world. Subtype **ayr** occurs much less frequently in most of the world, but is commonly found in a few isolated populations in Oceania. The geographical distributions of subtypes probably reflect the locations of their origins and the migrations of infected human populations.

Immunization with highly purified HBsAg particles results in protection against HBV infection (Purcell and Gerin, 1975), as does administration of immune globulin preparations with a high titer of antibody against HBsAg (anti-HBs) (Seeff *et al.*, 1975; Redeker *et al.*, 1975), suggesting that it is the immune response to this antigen during infection that provides protection against reinfection (see Chapters 15 and 16). Strong evidence indicates that HBsAg is a virus-specified antigen. The first evidence suggesting this was the finding that the antigenic subtype found in secondary cases of hepatitis B virus infection is regularly the same as the subtype of the index case or the original source used in experimental infection (LeBouvier, 1972; Mosley *et al.*, 1972), indicating that the subtype determinants are specified by the viral genome and not by the host. In this way, HBsAg subtypes have provided very useful markers for epidemiological studies of the spread of virus in populations and in individual cases of transmission. More direct evidence that the viral genome codes for HBsAg comes from HBsAg polypeptide amino acid sequence and viral DNA base sequence studies (Peterson *et al.*, 1978; Charnay *et al.*, 1979), and studies of HBsAg expression in bacteria (Charnay *et al.*, 1980; Burrell *et al.*, 1979; Edman *et al.*, 1981b; Mackay *et al.*, 1981a) and yeast (Miyanohara *et al.*, 1983; Valenzuela *et al.*, 1982) transformed with recombinant plasmid vectors containing HBV DNA. HBsAg produced in bacterial and yeast cells may prove useful as a reagent for diagnostic testing and as antigen for an HBV vaccine, although the amount of this antigen produced by bacteria has generally been very small. Yields in yeast appear much greater than in bacteria; HBsAg expression probably results in toxicity to bacterial cells.

For chemical characterization of HBsAg, 22-nm spherical and filamentous particles can be purified by gel filtration, rate-zonal sedimentation, and equilibrium centrifugation in CsCl density gradients (e.g., see Gerin *et al.*, 1971). Centrifugation in CsCl density gradients separates these particles from virions because of a difference in buoyant density. The buoyant density of 22-nm spherical and filamentous particles in CsCl is ~1.18 g/ml (Kaplan *et al.*, 1976), reflecting a significant lipid content (~30% by weight). The higher buoyant density of virions [~1.28 g/ml for virions with DNA-containing nucleocapsids and 1.24 g/ml for those with empty cores (Hruska and Robinson, 1977)] reflects the contribution of their high buyoant density nucleocapsids. Lipid analysis of highly purified preparations of 22-nm HBsAg particles has revealed a mixture of lipids (Kim and Bissell, 1971; Steiner *et al.*, 1974) similar to that found in enveloped viruses and suggesting a host-cell origin for the lipid.

Seven or more polypeptides with apparent molecular weights between 25,000 and 100,000 have been isolated from purified preparations of 22-nm HBsAg particles of subtypes **adw, ayw,** and **adr** by sodium dodecylsulfate–polyacrylamide gel electrophoresis (SDS–PAGE) (Shih and Gerin, 1977a). A pair of the smallest polypeptides has been described as major components, and the larger polypeptides as minor components, by several investigators (reviewed in Robinson, 1977). Although estimates of the sizes of the major polypeptides have varied in different studies, 25,000 (P-25) and 29,000 daltons (P-29) are generally average apparent size estimates for the two polypeptides determined by SDS–PAGE. The major polypeptide with an apparently larger size (P-29) and one or two of the larger minor components appear to be glycopeptides, on the basis of periodic acid–Schiff staining (Chairez *et al.*, 1973; Shih and Gerin, 1977b) and radiolabeling with sugar (Marion *et al.*, 1979). P-25 and P-29 may consist of identical polypeptide chains, since they have identical amino acid compositions (Peterson *et al.*, 1978; Shih and Gerin, 1977a) and identical sequences for 19 amino acid residues at the amino terminus and the same sequence of three residues at the carboxy terminus (Charnay *et al.*, 1979). P-29 is glycosylated, and thus it is possible that the presence of carbohydrate in P-29 alone accounts for its apparent larger size. Recently the two polypeptides have been shown to have tryptic peptide maps that differ in only 1 of 27 spots (Gerlich *et al.*, 1980). This small difference could be due to glycosylation, some other posttranslational modification of one of the two polypeptides, or a difference in amino acid sequence, but clearly the two have very similar primary structures.

The isolated major polypeptides contain the group- and type-specific determinants of HBsAg (Gerin, 1974; Dreesman *et al.*, 1975) and induce anti-HBs when used to immunize animals (Gerin, 1974; Dreesman *et al.*, 1975; Shih and Gerin, 1975). Interestingly, several of the higher molecular weight minor polypeptides that have been isolated also appear to contain the same group- and type-specific HBsAg determinants (Dreesman *et al.*, 1975; Shih and Gerin, 1975, 1977a; Gold *et al.*, 1976), suggesting that the polypeptides are not unique but must share at least some amino acid sequences with the smaller major polypeptides. This is supported by recent tryptic peptide mapping, which has shown that the larger polypeptides contain tryptic peptides identical to most of those found in the smaller peptides (Feitelson *et al.*, 1981). Additional tryptic peptides indicate the presence of unique amino acid sequences in the larger polypeptides not present in the smaller ones. How the different polypeptides arise, and their exact amino acid sequence relationships, will require further studies including sequence analysis. The subtype determinants found in the polypeptides are the same as those present on the HBsAg particles for which they were isolated. Multiple polypeptides of different apparent size, all of which contain the same antigenic determinants, have not been described for other viruses.

Since polypeptides not containing carbohydrate induce anti-HBs, it is clear that the virus-specified antigenic determinants are contained in the polypeptide rather than in the carbohydrate of the glycoproteins. It is also clear that both group- and type-specific determinants reside on the same polypeptide. Thus, polypeptides of different HBsAg subtypes may contain a region of constant amino acid sequence specifying the group-specific determinant **a**, and a variable region specifying the type-specific determinants, for example, **d** or **y**. The exact structural basis of the subtype differences is not yet clear, however. The amino acid compositions of P-25 and P-29 from particles of HBsAg subtype **adw** and **ayw** are essentially indistinguishable (Peterson *et al.*, 1978). The amino-terminal sequence for nine residues and the single carboxy-terminal residue (isoleucine) for P-25 of HBsAg subtypes **ayw** and **adw** have been shown to be identical (Peterson *et al.*, 1977, 1978). Any sequence differences in the P-25 polypeptide of these subtypes must therefore exist in other regions of the polypeptides. Recently, tryptic peptide maps of the major non-glycosylated polypeptides (P-25) from HBsAg particles of different subtypes have been found to be substantially different (Feitelson *et al.*, 1981), as are the restriction endonuclease cleavage patterns of DNA from viruses of different HBsAg subtypes (Siddiqui *et al.*, 1979), suggesting significant differences in primary structure.

The recent molecular cloning of HBV DNA in bacterial cells and determination of the nucleotide sequences of the DNA of viruses of HBsAg subtype **ayw** (Charnay *et al.*, 1979) and **adw** (Valenzuela *et al.*, 1979) have led to the identification of the coding sequence for the major HBsAg-containing polypeptide (P-25). The ends of the conjectured DNA coding sequence would specify the known amino- and carboxy-terminal amino acid sequences of P-25. The included DNA base sequence would code for a polypeptide of 226 amino acids with a molecular weight of 25,422 (Charnay *et al.*, 1979), in close agreement with the apparent size of P-25 estimated by SDS–PAGE. The amino acid composition deduced from the nucleotide sequence of this gene is close to that reported for P-25 (Peterson *et al.*, 1978; Shih and Gerin, 1977a). The conjectured polypeptide has a high content of proline residues (10%) spread throughout the molecule, so that long alpha-helical regions would be prevented. Several hydrophobic regions are present. The polypeptide also has a high cysteine content (6%), and all of these residues occur in a central region of the polypeptide.

Since chemical reduction and alkylation have been shown to greatly reduce the HBsAg reactivity of HBsAg particles (Vyas *et al.*, 1972; Dreesman *et al.*, 1973), disulfide bonds in this region of the polypeptide would appear to be necessary for optimum HBsAg reactivity. When polypeptides are recovered after chemical reduction and SDS–PAGE, they must be reoxidized to obtain maximum HBsAg reactivity. High percentages of serine (10%) and threonine (8%), amino acids, to which sugar residues are commonly attached, are also present (Charnay *et al.*, 1979). Three of five asparagine residues are contained in Asn-X-serine (or threonine) tripeptides, found to be necessary for *N*-glycosidic bond formation (Struck *et al.*, 1978). The tryptophan (6%) and tryosine (3%) contents are consistent with the ultraviolet absorption spectrum of P-25 (Gerlich and Thomssen, 1975), which suggests a high trytophan/tryosine ratio.

Several regions of the major HBsAg polypeptide (P-25) made up of hydrophilic amino acids have been chemically synthesized and shown to induce antibodies in rabbits that immunoprecipitate the free HBsAg polypeptide and HBsAg particles from serum (Dreesman *et al.*, 1982; Vyas, 1981; Prince *et al.*, 1982). Synthetic peptides consisting of amino acid residues 2–16, 22–35, 48–81, and 95–109 (Lerner *et al.*, 1981), 117–137 and 122–137 cyclized through a disulfide bond (Dreesman *et al.*, 1982), 134–146 (Vyas, 1981), and 138–149 (Prince *et al.*, 1982), respectively (numbered from the amino terminus of the 226 amino acid P-25), have been shown to have this property. Nine synthetic peptides representing other regions of P-25 have failed to elicit reactive antibodies. These results suggest that the amino acid domains that elicited reactive antibodies are on the surface of HBsAg particles and carry HBsAg determinants. DNA base sequencing and construction of synthetic peptides on the basis of such base sequence data is an approach that may lead to a detailed understanding of the basis of HBsAg subtype differences, but for this the DNA of multiple viruses of different defined HBsAg subtypes will have to be cloned in bacterial cells and the HBsAg coding regions sequenced.

While HBsAg determinants clearly reside in polypeptide chains, the isolated polypeptides are significantly less reactive with anti-HBs and less immunogenic than intact HBsAg particles. Treatment of intact HBsAg particles with periodate or glycosidases and neuraminidase results in a significant loss of HBsAg reactivity (Burrell *et al.*, 1976), suggesting that in some way carbohydrate is necessary for full antigenicity of intact particles. The binding of HBsAg particles to lectins suggests that carbohydrate is on the particle surface and permits purification of the particles, for example, by affinity chromatography on concanavalin A columns (Neurath *et al.*, 1978a). The binding of HBsAg particles to a sialic acid-specific lectin and to a β-galactosidase-specific peanut lectin before and after neuraminidase digestion, respectively (Neurath *et al.*, 1975, 1978b), suggests that these two sugars may be the terminal and subterminal residues of the surface carbohydrate. Protease treatment does not destroy the HBsAg reactivity of intact HBsAg particles (Burrell *et al.*, 1976) as it does that of free polypeptides, suggesting that critical parts of the HBsAg-reactive polypeptides are unavailable to proteases in assembled particles.

Preparations of 22-nm particles consistently appear to contain small amounts of serum protein components (Millman *et al.*, 1971; Neurath *et al.*, 1974; Burrell, 1975) that have not been removed by extensive purification. Whether these are minor intrinsic constituents of the particles, or alternatively, only avidly bound to the particle surface, or just contaminating the preparation and co-purifying with HBsAg in some cases is not clear. The only serum component present in amounts large enough in purified HBsAg preparations to be detected by Coomassie Blue staining on SDS gels is apparently human serum albumin, which co-migrates as a separate polypeptide with one of the virus-specific polypeptides (Shih *et al.*, 1980). In this regard it is of interest that several laboratories have reported that HBsAg particles contain receptors for polymerized albumin (Hollinger and Dreesman, 1979; Imai *et al.*, 1979; Neurath and Strick, 1979a) and avid binding of serum albumin to such sites might account for the finding of significant amounts of this protein in purified HBsAg preparations.

Because the outer envelope of hepatitis B virions contains HBsAg and apparently lipid, it has been assumed that its chemical composition is similar to that just described for 22-nm HBsAg particles. However, there has been no direct chemical analysis of the virion envelope. It has been claimed that virions may have surface antigenic determinants (e.g., HBeAg) not present on the other particulate HBsAg forms (Neurath *et al.*, 1976), but others have failed to confirm this (Takahashi *et al.*, 1978a; Gerin *et al.*, 1978).

The surface antigens of WHV (Werner *et al.*, 1979) and GSHV (Marion *et al.*, 1980; Gerlich *et al.*, 1980) demonstrate significant although minimal specific cross-reaction with HBsAg. The two major polypeptides of the GSHV surface antigen are similar to, although distinctly smaller in size than, those of HBsAg, and only one-third of the tryptic peptides of the polypeptides of GSHV surface antigen and HBsAg are identical and two-thirds are distinct (Gerlich *et al.*, 1980). These results indicate that although WHV and GSHV are related to HBV, they are not the same virus, and the three probably diverged from a common ancestor in the distant past. The surface antigen of DHBV does not show serologic cross-reaction with those of any of the mammalian viruses (Mason *et al.*, 1980; Marion and Robinson, 1983). It contains a single major polypeptide of somewhat different apparent size (17,500 daltons) and much less homology, by tryptic peptide mapping (Marion *et al.*, 1984), indicating that DHBV is more distantly related to the mammalian viruses than the mammalian viruses are to each other. No subtype or other antigenic variation is known for the surface antigens of WHV, GSHV, or DHBV.

IV. Viral Nucleocapsid

The virion core or nucleocapsid bears the hepatitis B core antigen (HBcAg). HBcAg is found in the blood only as an internal component of virions and no free HBcAg has been detected in serum. The virion core is illustrated in Figs. 2B and 3. HBcAg-bearing particles with the electron microscopic appearance of virion cores have also been isolated from homogenates of HBV-infected liver (Hoofnagle *et al.*, 1973). A significant fraction of HBcAg particles isolated from virions (Hruska and Robinson, 1977) and a smaller fraction of these from infected liver (Robinson and Lutwick, 1976) have been shown to have a high buoyant density in CsCl (1.38 g/ml) and to contain DNA and DNA polymerase activity. However, most HBcAg particles from infected liver tissue (Hruska and Robinson, 1977; Robinson and Lutwick, 1976) and many from virions (Kaplan *et al.*, 1976; Hruska and Robinson, 1977) appear to have lower buoyant densities (1.33 g/ml) and to be empty particles with little or no DNA, and they manifest no DNA polymerase activity. The core particles of WHV and GSHV have similar ultrastructure to those of HBV, but DHBV cores differ in that spike-like structures protrude from the particle surface (Mason *et al.*, 1980).

Highly purified Dane particle cores and liver-derived HBcAg particles contain a single predominant polypeptide and an apparent weight of ~19,000 daltons (Hruska and Robinson, 1977; Budkowska *et al.*, 1977). Smaller amounts of higher molecular weight polypeptides have also been found. The antigenic specificity of these polypeptides is not well defined, although recent evidence suggests that the 19,000-dalton polypeptide may react with antibody to the hepatitis B e antigen (anti-HBe) (see Chapters 3 and 4). The free isolated polpeptide does not appear to react with anti-HBc (Hruska and Robinson, 1977).

Protein kinase activity has been found in virion cores and HBcAg particles from HBV-infected hepatic tissue (Albin and Robinson, 1980). The major 19,000-dalton polypeptide of core particles (and not other polypeptides) is heavily phosphorylated by this activity. This is similar to the protein kinase activities found in other enveloped viruses, which phosphorylate virion polypeptides closely associated with the viral nucleic acid. The role of this activity in virus infection and replication is not yet clear.

Although the antigenic specificity of HBcAg from different sources has not been carefully compared, no antigenic heterogeneity or variation has been described. Hepatitis B core antigen is considered to be a virus-specified antigen because it has been found only during hepatitis B virus infection, there is an early and brisk antibody response to HBcAg during infection (Krugman *et al.*, 1974), and it is an internal component of the virion (Almeida *et al.*, 1971). More direct evidence is the finding that bacterial cells transformed by a hybrid plasmid containing HBV DNA may express HBcAg (Burrell *et al.*, 1979; Edman *et al.*, 1981b; Valenzuela *et al.*, 1979; Pasek *et al.*, 1979; Hardy *et al.*, 1981; Mackay *et al.*, 1981b; Cohen and Richmond, 1982). HBcAg produced in this way has been used as a reagent for diagnostic serologic testing (Mackay *et al.*, 1981b).

The core antigens of WHV (Werner *et al.*, 1979) and GSHV (Feitelson *et al.*, 1982a) cross-react to a small extent with each other and with HBcAg, but not with antigens in DHBV. Like cores from HBV, GSHV cores contain protein kinase activity that phosphorylates the major core polypeptide (Feitelson *et al.*, 1982b).

V. e Antigen

Hepatitis B e antigen (HBeAg) was discovered in 1972 as a soluble antigen in serum that was physically and antigenically distinct from HBsAg and HBcAg (Magnius and Espmark, 1972). Its molecular weight was estimated to be 300,000 (Magnius, 1975). However, it proved difficult to purify and it is still not well characterized chemically. Recent evidence indicates that HBeAg is a complex of antigens, and up to three precipitin lines designated e_1, e_2, and e_3 may be detected by agar gel diffusion in sera from individual patients (Williams and LeBouvier, 1976; Tabor *et al.*, 1977; Miller *et al.*, 1978; Courucé-Pauty and Plancon, 1978). More recent evidence suggests that the original high molecular weight (300,000) form represents a complex of HBeAg with immunoglobulin IgG, and a separate 35,000-dalton component also present in serum is considered to be the free form of HBeAg (Takahashi *et al.*, 1978b,1979a). The 35,000-dalton form is said to be dissociable into 17,500-dalton polypeptides (Neurath *et al.*, 1978c). It is possible that e_1, e_2, and e_3 represent different complexes of HBeAg with or without immunoglobulin, but further investigation will be needed to determine the actual chemical and structural differences among them.

An intriguing feature of HBeAg is the high correlation of its occurrence in sera of HBV-infected patients with high concentrations of physical virions (Hindman *et al.*, 1976; Alter *et al.*, 1976; Takahashi *et al.*, 1976; Nordenfeldt and Andren-Sandberg, 1976) and infectious HBV (Scullard *et al.*, 1982; Shikata *et al.*, 1977), suggesting that HBeAg and virions are produced together during infection and raising the possibility of a direct physical relationship between the two. In this regard evidence is accumulating that HBeAg is a component of virion cores. Hepatitis B e antigen appears to be released when virion cores are disrupted with detergents (Takahashi *et al.*, 1979b; Neurath and Strick, 1979b; Budkowska *et al.*, 1979; Ohori *et al.*, 1979), and the isolated major polypeptide of core particles (19,000 daltons) appears to react with anti-HBe (Takahashi *et al.*, 1979b). Recently HBcAg produced in bacterial cells transformed with an HBV-plasmid vector DNA recombinant was converted to HBeAg by treatment with protease in the presence of detergent (Mackay *et al.*, 1981b). This suggests that the polypeptides of Dane particle cores manifest different antigenic specificities before (HBcAg) and after (HBeAg) detergent and/or protease treatment (see Chapter 3). Antigens cross-reacting with HBeAg have not been described for WHV, GSHV, or DHBV.

VI. Viral DNA

Hepatitis B virions contain small circular DNA molecules (Robinson *et al.*, 1974) that are partially double stranded (schematically illustrated in Fig. 4). The single-stranded portion varies in length from approximately 15 to 60% of the circle length in different molecules (Summers *et al.*, 1975; Landers *et al.*, 1977; Houska *et al.*, 1977). Thus the DNA consists of a long strand, *L*, of constant length (~ 3200 bases) in all molecules and a short strand, *S*, which varies in length between 1700 and 2800 bases (Landers *et al.*, 1977) in different molecules. The DNA polymerase activity in the virion repairs the single-stranded region in the viral DNA to make fully double-stranded molecules of ~3200 base pairs (bp). DNA synthesis is initiated for this reaction at the 3' end of the short strand, which occurs at different sites within a specific region (50%) of the DNA in different molecules. DNA synthesis is terminated when the uniquely located 5' end of the short strand is reached. The long strand is not a closed circle; a nick exists at a unique site ~300 bp from the 5' end of the short strand (Summers *et al.*, 1975; Sattler and Robinson 1979; Siddiqui *et al.*, 1979). The circular DNA can be converted to a linear form with single-stranded cohesive ends by selectively denaturing the 300-bp region between the 5' end of the short strand and the nick in the long

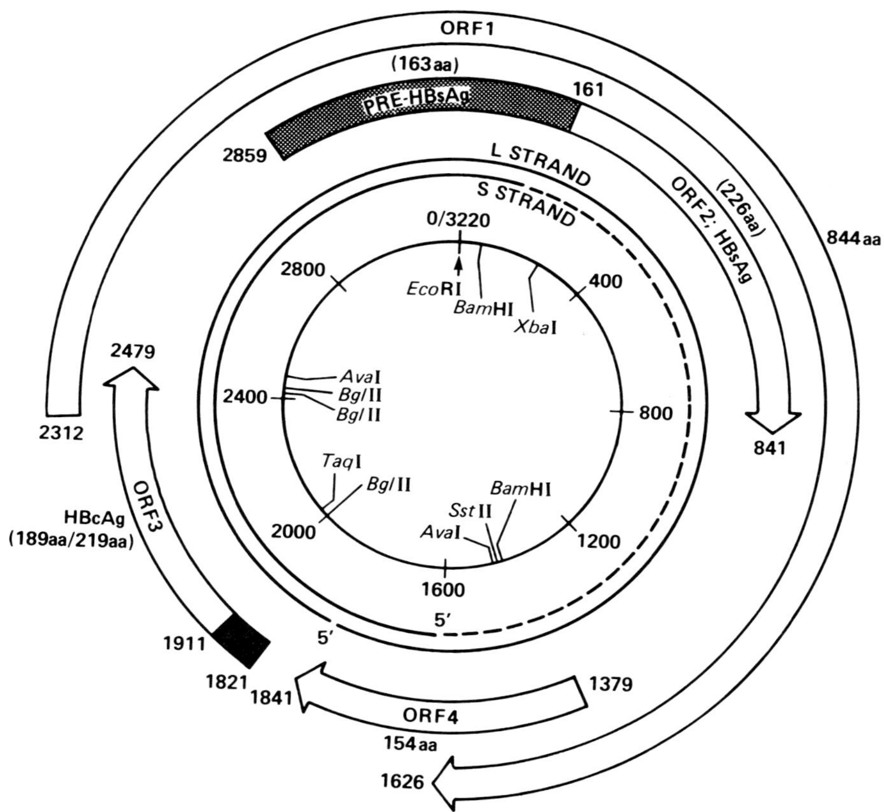

Figure 4. Physical and genetic map of HBV DNA (HBs Ag, **adw₂**). The broken line in the short (S) DNA strand represents the region within which the 3' end of the S strand may occur in different molecules, and the corresponding region of the long (L) strand is that which may be single stranded in different molecules. The restriction sites and locations of the nick in the L strand, the 5' end of the S strand, and the location of the single-stranded region are as reported by Siddiqui *et al.* (1979), and the open reading frames (large arrows) are those described by Galibert *et al.* (1979).

strand by heating under appropriate conditions (Sattler and Robinson, 1979). The linear form can be recircularized by reassociation of the complementary single-stranded ends. The 5' ends of both the long and short strands of HBV DNA appear to be blocked in a manner that prevents phosphorylation with polynucleotide kinase (Gerlich and Robinson, 1980). The chemical nature of the blocked 5' end of the short strand is unknown. A polypeptide is covalently atatched to the 5' end of the long strand of the DNA isolated from virions, and this undoubtedly prevents phosphorylation of this strand (Gerlich and Robinson, 1980).

HBV DNA has been cloned in bacterial cells and the complete nucleotide sequence determined (Galibert *et al.*, 1979; Valenzuela *et al.*, 1980). HBV DNA has four open reading frames in the complete or long DNA strand, which is therefore the minus strand (by convention, a viral DNA plus strand has the same nucleotide sequence as the viral messenger RNA, and the minus strand is complementary to messenger RNA). The coding sequences for the two major virion polypeptides have been identified. Open reading frame 2 (see ORF-2, Fig. 4) contains the nucleotide sequence specifying the major surface antigen reactive polypeptide. This coding sequence is 681 nucleotides long and specifies a polypeptide of 25,422 daltons. The sequence upstream from the initiation codon for this polypeptide in ORF-2 is called the pre-*S* region, and if translated *in vivo* could give rise to a large P-25 precursor with a C-terminal sequence identical to that of P25. Whether such a precursor is actually made *in vivo* or whether this pre-*S* region has some other function remains to be determined. ORF-3 (Fig. 4) contains the nucleotide sequence that specifies the major polypeptide of the virion core. This sequence codes for a polypeptide of 183 amino acids. Polypeptides coded by the two other open reading frames on the long DNA strand (ORF-1 and -4, Fig. 4) have yet to be identified. ORF-1 completely overlaps ORF-2 and could potentially code for a polypeptide of 95,000 daltons. ORF-4 is the smallest potential coding sequence in the long strand and could specify a polypeptide of ~16,000 daltons or 154 amino acids. HBV and WHV DNAs have a sequence within the smallest open reading frame on the long strand (ORF-4) and near the nick in that strand that can form a stable hairpin structure, and it has been speculated (Galibert *et al.*, 1982) that this sequence might function as the origin of replication.

VII. The State of Virus in Infected Cells, Expression of Viral Genes, and the Mechanism of Virus Replication

The earliest studies of HBV in infected hepatocytes revealed that HBcAg could be detected only in the nuclei of hepatocytes by immunofluorescent staining, and HBsAg in the cytoplasm and on cell surfaces (Barker *et al.*, 1973, Gudat *et al.*, 1975; Ray *et al.*, 1976). Consistent with this, electron microscopy demonstrated particles with the appearance of virion cores exclusively in hepatocyte nuclei (Almeida *et al.*, 1970; Huang, 1971; Camamia *et al.*, 1972). Particles resembling HBsAg forms have not been readily detected in cells, and the morphogenesis of these particles including complete virions is unclear. During persistent infection, a variable number of cells contain detectable viral antigens by immunofluorescent staining (from <1% to virtually all hepatocytes in different patients) (Barker *et al.*, 1973; Gudat *et al.*, 1975; Ray *et al.*, 1976). Interestingly, the pattern of viral antigen expression appears to be different in different cells of the same chronically infected liver. Commonly, most positive cells stain only for HBsAg; fewer have only detectable HBcAg, and even fewer cells contain both HBsAg and HBcAg. In the liver of some chronic carriers, HBsAg is the only detectable viral antigen. In all chronic carriers producing relatively high concentrations of viral DNA and DNA polymerase-containing virions, significant numbers of HBcAg positive cells can be found. The different patterns of viral antigen synthesis in individual cells of the same chronically infected liver indicate that individual viral genes are expressed differently in different cells (see also Chapter 12).

More recently, the forms of viral DNA and synthesis of viral DNA strands in DHBV-infected duck liver (Mason *et al.*, 1982; Summers and Mason, 1982) and HBV-infected human liver (Miller and Robinson, 1984a,b) have been studied. Results suggested that the DNAs of these viruses replicate in a unique and interesting way. HBV DNA is present in infected liver cells of HBsAg carriers in several distinct forms. The predominant form is the 3200-bp closed circular (form I) DNA, which is found exclusively in the cell nucleus (Miller and Robinson, 1984a). Several HBV DNA forms are present in liver cell cytoplasm, and these appear to be contained in particles with DNA polymerase activity (Miller and Robinson, 1984a,b). In DHBV-infected duck liver, similar particles have been shown to have properties of viral cores (Summers and Mason, 1982). The particles from HBV-infected human liver contain 3200-bp relaxed circular (form II) and linear (form III) viral DNA, 3200-nucleotide single viral DNA strands, and viral DNA–RNA hybrid molecules (Almeida *et al.*, 1970; Huang, 1971). In the DHBV system, the hybrid molecules appear to contain full length (3200-nucleotide) plus strands of viral RNA containing a polyA sequence (Summers and Mason, 1982). The endogenous DNA polymerase activity in the particles catalyzes the incorporation of nucleoside triphosphates into viral DNA, minus strands of the DNA–RNA hybrid molecules, in the presence or absence of actinomycin D, which inhibits DNA-dependent DNA synthesis. This suggested that the plus DNA strand is synthesized on an RNA template by a reverse transcriptase mechanism analogous to that known for retroviruses. In the DHBV system, the RNA strand of the DNA–RNA hybrid molecules appeared to be degraded as the DNA strand length increased, reminiscent of the RNase H activity of retro-viruses. Evidence in the DHBV system suggests that a protein serves as a primer for minus DNA strand synthesis, and growing minus DNA strands of the DNA–RNA hybrid are found to be covalently attached to the protein primer. Nucleoside triphosphates were also incorporated into the plus strand of the relaxed circular DNA molecules in a DNA-dependent DNA synthetic reaction in the liver particles.

These findings in HBV-infected human liver and DHBV-infected duck liver suggested the following working model for replication of viruses of this group. Following virus entry into liver cells, 3200-bp closed circular viral DNA is formed in the cell nucleus; this may function as a template for viral messenger RNA synthesis and synthesis of the 3200-nucleotide RNA plus strand, which will serve as a template for minus strand DNA synthesis. The full length plus RNA strand, newly synthesized viral DNA polymerase (reverse transcriptase), and the protein primer for minus DNA strand synthesis, are assembled with the major structural polypeptide of the viral core into core particles or viral nucleocapsids. Viral minus strand DNA is then synthesized within the core particles, utilizing the protein primer and the RNA template that is degraded by RNase H activity as DNA synthesis proceeds. The viral DNA plus strand is synthesized utilizing the minus strand DNA as template in a circular conformation. Core particles are then assembled into complete virions with HBsAg and cell membrane lipid-containing envelopes. In the case of HBV (Miller and Robinson, 1984a,b), virus formation and release from the cell can apparently take place at any step after assembly of the core particle, since virions (Dane particles) can be found in the blood that contain DNA–RNA hybrid molecules as well as partly single-stranded circular DNA molecules. Endogenous DNA polymerase activity in the virions catalyzes the incorporation of nucleotides into minus DNA strands of the former and plus DNA strands of the latter.

Results of restriction endonuclease digestion of DNA from HBV-infected liver and Southern blot analysis suggest that viral DNA sequences are also integrated in cellular DNA in at least many and possibly all HBV-infected livers. Evidence for this in some studies (Brechot *et al.*, 1981; Kam *et al.*, 1982b) was the finding of one or more DNA fragments containing viral DNA sequences that are larger than unit length viral DNA (3200 bp) after but not before digestion of cell DNA with a restriction enzyme (e.g., *Hind*III) for which no recognition sites exist in the viral DNA. The specific high molecular weight *Hind*III DNA fragments containing viral sequences have been found to be different in liver of different chronically infected patients. The ability to detect such DNA fragments by Southern blotting has been interpreted to mean that viral

DNA is integrated in the same site in many different cells of the liver of each chronically infected patient with this finding, but the site is different in different patients. Direct evidence proving this conclusion is not yet available. Other viruses such as retroviruses, which readily integrate in cellular DNA, appear to do so at many and possibly random sites in the cellular DNA; specific integration sites are not detected in tissue DNA by the experimental strategy just described for HBV unless the cells are of clonal origin (e.g., as are cells in most viral-induced tumors) (reviewed in Varmus and Swanstrom, 1982). Integration of viral DNA at specific sites (although apparently at different sites in different patients) in HBV-infected liver appears to be unprecedented.

Other studies (Miller and Robinson, 1984b; Koshy *et al.*, 1981) have obtained evidence for random integration by detecting subgenomic--sized DNA fragments with HBV DNA sequences after digestion of infected liver DNA with a restriction enzyme that cleaves HBV DNA at more than one site, and no fragments containing HBV DNA greater than genome length after *Hin*dIII digestion. No evidence of integrated HBV DNA has been found in other infected livers.

Although viral DNA thus appears to integrate in cellular DNA of some infected livers, the integrated sequences have not been characterized in detail. It is clear, however, that the integrated viral DNA is present in much smaller amounts (e.g., <1 copy per cell) than the free viral DNA forms (e.g., >500 copies per cell) in liver in which HBV is replicating (Miller and Robinson, 1984b; Kam *et al.*, 1982b). Although the role of integrated viral DNA in virus replication has not been established, HBsAg has been shown to be expressed in cells in which the only detectable viral DNA is apparently integrated in cellular DNA. Expression of no other viral gene in an integrated form has been observed. It is not known whether the entire viral genome or only part is integrated in such infected liver cells, whether the integrated sequences retain the order of viral sequences in virion DNA (except that the HBsAg gene must be intact when this gene is expressed as an integrated sequence), or whether integration occurs at unique sites in the viral DNA. Further investigation including cloning and sequencing of integrated viral DNA will be needed to provide more direct evidence for integration, and to answer the above questions about the state of integrated viral DNA and its role in the virus life cycle.

More detailed information is available concerning the state of integrated viral DNA in hepatocellular carcinomas (hepatomas) of man and woodchucks and in human hepatoma cell lines in tissue culture, many but not all of which appear to contain integrated viral DNA. Restriction endonuclease *Hin*dIII digestion of tumor DNA and Southern blot analysis (Southern, 1975) have revealed DNA fragments apparently containing viral DNA sequences that are larger than unit length (3200 bp) viral DNA, similar to those described above for nontumorous infected liver and suggesting integration of viral DNA at a few (usually 1–4) specific cellular DNA sites in such hepatocellular carcinoma tissue, but always at different sites in different tumors (Brechot *et al.*, 1981, 1982; Koshy *et al.*, 1981; Marion *et al.*, 1979b; Shafritz *et al.*, 1981; Shafritz, 1982; Chen *et al.*, 1982; Miller and Robinson, 1983; Chakraborty *et al.*, 1981; Edman *et al.*, 1981a; Twist *et al.*, 1981). Cloning and sequence analysis of integrated viral DNA with flanking cellular DNA sequences has proven that viral sequences are integrated in host DNA of hepatocellular carcinomas. In all cases of woodchuck (Ogston *et al.*, 1982) and human tumors and tumor cell lines studied to date, the viral DNA contains extensive deletions and rearrangements that are different for each integrated viral sequence, and the site in the viral DNA which joins cellular DNA is also different for each integrated viral sequence. At this time there is no demonstrated difference between the state of integrated viral DNA in hepatocellular carcinoma and infected nontumorous liver.

HBV DNA sequences appear to be integrated in at least eight specific cellular DNA sites in one hepatoma cell line, and these have been shown to be extensively methylated, unlike HBV DNA forms in virions and nontumorous liver in which there is no detectable methylation (Miller and Robinson, 1983). The more extensive methylation of the coding sequences for the core polypeptide than of sequences coding for the HBsAg polypeptide is correlated with the expression of HBsAg, but not of HBcAg or other viral gene products by this cell line. This finding raises the possibility that methylation of viral DNA may be involved in regulation of viral gene expression in hepatomas.

Although hepatitis B virus in serum has not been made to successfully infect cells in culture, the availability of large quantities of cloned viral DNA produced in bacterial cells transformed with HBV–plasmid vector DNA recombinants has permitted DNA transfection studies utilizing a variety of cultured mammalian cell types. Introduction of the entire viral genome (Hirschman *et al.*, 1980; Dubois *et al.*, 1980; Gough and Murray, 1982; Wang *et al.*, 1982; Pourcel *et al.*, 1982; Colbere-Garapin *et al.*, 1983) or subgenomic fragments containing coding sequences for the surface antigen polypeptide (Pourcel *et al.*, 1982; Colbere-Garapin *et al.*, 1983; Moriarty *et al.*, 1981; Stratowa *et al.*, 1982; Siddiqui, 1983; Crowley *et al.*, 1983; Stenlund *et al.*, 1983; Wang *et al.*, 1983; Laub *et al.*, 1983) or the major core polypeptide (Yoakum *et al.*, 1983) has resulted in expression of HBsAg (Hirschman *et al.*, 1980; Dubois *et al.*, 1980; Gough and Murray, 1982; Wang *et al.*, 1982,1983; Pourcel *et al.*, 1982; Colbere-Garapin *et al.*, 1983; Moriarty *et al.*, 1981; Stratowa *et al.*, 1982; Siddiqui, 1983; Crowley *et al.*, 1983; Stenlund *et al.*, 1983; Laub *et al.*, 1983), HBcAg (Gough and Murray, 1982) or HBeAg (Gough and Murray, 1982; Colbere-Garapin *et al.*, 1983). HBV DNA either without (Hirschman *et al.*, 1980; Dubois *et al.*, 1980; Gough and Murray, 1982; Wang *et al.*, 1982; Pourcel *et al.*, 1982; Colbere-Garapin *et al.*, 1983) or within (Moriarty *et al.*, 1981; Stratowa *et al.*, 1982; Siddiqui, 1983; Crowley *et al.*, 1983; Stenlund *et al.*, 1983; Wang *et al.*, 1983; Laub *et al.*, 1983; Yoakum *et al.*, 1983) specific eukaryotic expression vectors containing SV40 (Moriarty *et al.*, 1981; Siddiqui, 1983; Crowley *et al.*, 1983; Laub *et al.*, 1983; Yoakum *et al.*, 1983) papilloma virus (Stenlund *et al.*, 1983; Wang *et al.*, 1983), or Moloney sarcoma virus (Stratowa *et al.*, 1982) regulatory elements has been successfully used. HBV gene expression has been demonstrated in mouse (Dubois *et al.*, 1980; Gough and Murray, 1982; Wang *et al.*, 1982,1983; Pourcel *et al.*, 1982; Colbere-Garapin *et al.*, 1983; Stratowa *et al.*, 1982; Stenlund *et al.*, 1983; Hirschman and Garfinkel, 1982), rat (Gough and Murray, 1982), monkey (Moriarty *et al.*, 1981; Siddiqui, 1983; Crowley *et al.*, 1983; Laub *et al.*, 1983), and human (Hirschman *et al.*, 1980; Yoakum *et al.*, 1983) cells. HBsAg appears to be released from these cells in the form of particles similar to those found in serum of HBV-infected patients. Such experiments offer approaches for investigating HBV gene expression and its regulation, and for the production of HBV gene products for diagnostic or therapeutic uses.

Perhaps the most interesting experiments achieving expression of HBsAg in a foreign host were those by Smith *et al.* (1983) in which vaccinia virus–HBV recombinants were isolated after transfection of vaccinia virus infected CV-1 cells with a plasmid vector containing a 1.35-kb HBV DNA fragment that included the HBsAg polypeptide coding sequence. Subsequent infection of CV-1 cells with the vaccina virus–HBV recombinants led to HBsAg production, and HBsAg particles purified from the culture medium contained characteristic HBsAg polypeptides. When rabbits were vaccinated intracutaneously with recombinant virus, an anti-HBs response indicated that HBsAg was expressed in the infected animals. This interesting result provides an important approach with potential for developing a "live" vaccine for HBV.

Transcription of HBV genes in several cell lines containing all or part of the HBV genome integrated in cellular DNA, and 2.0- to 2.5-kb mRNAs containing the HBsAg polypeptide coding sequence have been described (Pourcel *et al.*, 1981; Gough, 1983; Edmond *et al.*, 1980; Chakraborty *et al.*, 1980). Transcription of the *S* gene was found to be initiated at more than one site in COS cells transfected with HBV DNA contained in an SV40 vector (Laub *et al.*, 1983). A study of viral specific

RNA in infected chimpanzee liver, perhaps a more natural system than the above cell culture systems, revealed a major *S* gene transcript that had been initated near the start codon of the *S* gene and within the pre-*S* region, and it was polyadenylated at a site within the core polypeptide gene (Cattaneo *et al.*, 1983). Much more work will be required to better understand transcription of all HBV genes and its regulation during natural infections.

VIII. The State of HBV Replication at Different Stages of Infection, and the Mechanism of Associated Liver Disease

Almost all patients with primary HBV infection and clinically apparent acute hepatitis B have been shown to have detectable HBsAg (Hoofnagle *et al.*, 1978), HBeAg (Fields *et al.*, 1978; Murphy *et al.*, 1975; Ling *et al.*, 1979; Aldershvile *et al.*, 1980), and DNA and DNA polymerase containing (complete) virions (Kaplan *et al.*, 1974; Krugman *et al.*, 1974) in the blood, at least transiently. During the late incubation period and early during the acute disease, almost all hepatocytes have been reported to be positive by immunofluorescent staining for HBsAg and HBcAg (Barker *et al.*, 1973; Gudat *et al.*, 1975; Ray *et al.*, 1976). The state of viral DNA in liver during acute hepatitis B has not been adequately studied, although evidence for integrated viral DNA has been reported for two patients (Brechot *et al.*, 1981). However, the forms of virus in blood and antigen expression in liver suggest that almost all hepatocytes are replicating virus during early stages of primary infection.

No studies have been done on virus replication in liver of those patients with primary HBV infections detected only by anti-HBs and anti-HBc seroconversion and who have subclinical hepatitis without detectable HBsAg in the blood (Hoofnagle *et al.*, 1978). Of the patients who fail to terminate acute HBV infections and who become chronic HBsAg carriers (serum HBsAg-positive for 6 months or more), a fraction continue to have HBeAg and DNA and DNA polymerase containing virions in their blood for prolonged periods. Such patients have high concentrations of infectious virus in their blood (Scullard *et al.*, 1982; Shikata *et al.*, 1977; Thomssen *et al.*, 1977) and are highly contagious for contacts (Okada *et al.*, 1976; Tong *et al.*, 1981; Stevens *et al.*, 1975; Alter *et al.*, 1976; Grady *et al.*, 1976; Perrillo *et al.*, 1979). A variable number of liver cells contain HBsAg and/or HBcAg detected by immunofluorescent staining (Barker *et al.*, 1973; Gudat *et al.*, 1975; Ray *et al.*, 1976), and free replicating forms of viral DNA (closed and relaxed circular, and linear double-stranded, single-stranded and DNA–RNA hybrids) and possibly integrated viral DNA are present (Miller and Robinson, 1984b; Brechot *et al.*, 1981; Kam *et al.*, 1982b; Koshy *et al.*, 1981) indicating complete virus replication is proceeding in at least some cells. Such patients frequently but not always have chronic persistent or chronic active hepatitis (Gudat *et al.*, 1975; Hess *et al.*, 1977; Norkrans *et al.*, 1980).

Other carriers appear to have HBsAg and often anti-HBe but no detectable DNA and DNA polymerase-containing virions or HBeAg in the blood, and have HBsAg and integrated viral DNA sequences but no detectable free viral DNA forms or HBcAg in the liver cells (Miller and Robinson, 1984b; Brechot *et al.*, 1981; Kam *et al.*, 1982b; Koshy *et al.*, 1981). As described above, not all cells (and frequently only a small fraction of cells) are HBsAg positive by immunofluorescent staining. Such patients have been shown to be much less contagious than carriers with HBeAg and DNA polymerase-containing virions in serum (Okada *et al.*, 1976; Tong *et al.*, 1981; Stevens *et al.*, 1975; Alter *et al.*, 1976; Grady *et al.*, 1976; Perrillo *et al.*, 1979), and at least some appear to have no detectable infectious virus in the blood (Scullard *et al.*, 1982). These patients must be replicating complete virus at a very low level or not at all, and the only viral gene expressed appears to be the HBsAg gene in an integrated state. Many but not all of these patients appear to have little or no liver disease (Gudat *et al.*, 1975; Hess *et al.*, 1977; Norkrans *et al.*, 1980), and are considered to be "healthy carriers" (see also Chapter 12).

Although the natural history of persistent HBV infection has not been completely defined, titers of HBsAg, HBeAg, and complete virions have been shown to fall with time in many chronic carriers with these markers in the blood, and in 10–20% of such patients per year HBeAg and complete virions become undetectable (Scullard *et al.*, 1981; Realdi *et al.*, 1980), although most such patients remain HBsAg positive for many months or years. In 1–2% of HBsAg carriers per year, HBsAg in serum becomes undetectable (Scullard *et al.*, 1981; Szmuness *et al.*, 1973; Helske, 1974; Sampliner *et al.*, 1979) so that no serological markers of active infection remain. Thus many persistent infections appear to wind down with time as complete virus replication and associated contagiousness wane even though HBsAg production continues. In some patients HBsAg expression eventually ceases.

The mechanism of liver cell injury in acute and chronic hepatitis B has not been established, but there has been much conjecture about the role of the cellular immune response. Much of the evidence for this has been reviewed (Edgington and Chisari, 1975; Drenstag *et al.*, 1982) (Chapter 10). The failure to date to clearly demonstrate, in patients with hepatitis

B, the presence of cells that are cytotoxic for target cells bearing HBsAg suggests that this antigen is not one to which a cytotoxic response is directed. Because (as reviewed above) complete virus replication appears to proceed more often in patients with active hepatitis B than in healthy carriers who appear more often to express only HBsAg, it is possible that a cellular immune response directed at HBcAg or HBeAg (or some as yet undescribed viral antigen) rather than at HBsAg is responsible for hepatic injury during HBV infection. In this regard a recent study has provided evidence for cytotoxicity of peripheral blood cells for autologous hepatocytes in chronic hepatitis B that is blocked by anti-HBc, suggesting that HBcAg may be the target antigen for the cytotoxic cell (Eddleston *et al.*, 1982).

A prominent reason often given to support the hypothesis that liver cell injury in hepatitis B is caused by immune attack is the belief that HBV is not a cytopathic virus. Evidence given for this is the observation that hepatoma cell lines in culture that contain the entire HBV genome in an integrated state and express HBsAg, but are not replicating complete virus (i.e., contain no detectable HBcAg, replicating viral DNA or infectious virus), have no apparent impairment in growth or function (Macnab *et al.*, 1976; Marion *et al.*, 1979a). Also, healthy carriers producing only HBsAg may have little or no liver injury (Hess *et al.*, 1977). These observations do not exclude the possibility, however, that when HBV-infected cells express HBcAg, HBeAg, and other viral gene products in addition to HBsAg and are replicating viral DNA, the infection is cytopathic. Again, the association of HBeAg in serum and HBcAg in liver with active hepatitis as described above is consistent with such a mechanism. Additional evidence supporting this possibility is the recent finding that introduction of a viral DNA fragment containing the HBcAg polypeptide coding sequence into a human hepatoma cell line already producing HBsAg without impairment of cell growth or function resulted in a significant cytopathic effect when HBcAg was expressed (Stenlund *et al.*, 1983). Thus a direct cytopathic effect by replicating virus must still be considered a possible mechanism for hepatic injury by HBV.

A second form of liver disease associated with hepadna virus infection is hepatocellular carcinoma (PHC). There is a strong association between long-standing hepadna virus infection and PHC formation in humans (Szmuness, 1978; Beasley *et al.*, 1981; Obata *et al.*, 1980) and woodchucks (Summers *et al.*, 1978a; Marion and Robinson, 1983; Popper *et al.*, 1981), and viral DNA is found integrated in the cellular DNA of many tumors as described above. Exactly how these viruses are involved in PHC formation, however, is not clear. Any role of the virus must be consistent with the observations that integrated viral DNA can apparently not be detected in some tumors in man (Lutwick and Robinson, 1977; Summers *et al.*, 1978b; Kam *et al.*, 1982a; R. H. Miller, S.-C. Lee, and W. S. Robinson, unpublished results) and woodchucks (Mitamura *et al.*, 1982), and as described above, integration sites appear to be different in every tumor containing viral DNA, and the integrated viral DNA is differently rearranged at different integration sites (see Chapter 11).

Concerning the role of virus in PHC formation, it is of interest that at least superficially these viruses appear to share some features with RNA tumor viruses or retroviruses, although as described above many features of HBV and the related viruses are unique and define this virus group. Among the common features are similarities in genome structure, although the nucleic acid type in virions is different for the two virus groups, that is, DNA in the case of hepadna viruses and RNA in retroviruses. Separation and repair of the cohesive ends of hepadna virus DNAs results in linear molecules with direct, repeat terminal sequences of ~300 bp (Sattler and Robinson, 1979), as described above, and similar to those of retroviruses (reviewed in Varmus and Swanström, 1982). All of the viral messenger RNAs appear to be transcribed from the same DNA strand and thus in the same direction for viruses of both groups. In addition, the hepadna viral DNA appears to replicate through an RNA intermediate utilizing a reverse transcriptase (Summers and Mason, 1982; Miller and Robinson, 1984a) as described above, a mechanism with some analogy to retrovirus replication (reviewed in Varmus and Swanström, 1982). Viruses of both groups cause persistent infection with virus and viral antigen in the blood for periods as long as many years. A fourth similarity is that viruses of both groups appear to integrate readily in cellular DNA. However, it has yet to be shown that hepadna virus DNA integration is a regular and integral event in virus replication, that the viral genome in the integrated state retains its organization, that integration occurs at a specific site in the viral DNA, or that integration is essential to the mechanism of cell transformation, all of which appear to be features of retroviruses (reviewed in Varmus and Swanström, 1982).

A fifth similarity is that when exclusively integrated in the DNA of infected cells, both hepadna viruses (Marion *et al.*, 1979a) and retroviruses (Robinson *et al.*, 1981) may express only the gene for their envelope protein. A sixth similarity is tumor formation during infection by at least some members of each group. The clear association between HBV and WHV infections and hepatocellular carcinomas is among the more intriguing features of these viruses, and it will be of great interest to investigate in more detail their role in formation of these tumors. It will be important to determine whether they may integrate in sites adjacent to oncogenes and function as some retroviruses are thought to function in cell transformation and tumor induction (Hayward *et al.*, 1981), cause tumors by a "hit and run" mechanism (Galloway and McDougall, 1983), or relate to PHC formation in some other way. Although it has been speculated that some environmental factor such as a chemical carcinogen in addition to virus may be necessary for PHC formation (Popper, 1978) there is no evidence for such a mechanism at this time (see Chapter 11).

References

Albin, C., and Robinson, W. S. (1980). *J. Virol.* **34**, 297–302.
Aldershvile, G. G., Frösner, J., Nielsen, O., Hardt, E., Deinhardt, F., and Skinhoj, P. (1980). *J. Infect. Dis.* **141**, 293.
Almeida, J. D. (1972). *Am. J. Dis. Child.* **123**, 303.
Almeida, J. D., Waterson, A. P., Trowel, J. M., and Neale, G. (1970) *Microbios* **2**, 145–153.
Almeida, J. D., Rubenstein, D., and Stott, E. J., (1971). *Lancet* 2, 1225–1227.
Alter, H. J., and Blumberg, B. S. (1966). *Blood* **27**, 297.
Alter, H. J., Seeff, L. B., Kaplan, P. M., McAuliffe, V. J., Wright, E. C., Gerin, J. L., Purcell, R. H. Holland, P. V., and Zimmerman, H. J. (1976). *N. Engl. J. Med.* **295**, 909–913.
Bancroft, W. H., Mundo, F. K., and Russel, P. K. (1972). *J. Immunol.* **109**, 842–848.
Bancroft, W. H., Holland, P. B., Mazzur, S., Couroucé, A. M., and Madalinski, K. (1976). *Bibl. Haematol. (Basel)* **42**, 42.
Barker, L. F., and Murray, R. (1972). *Am. J. Med. Sci.* **263**, 27.
Barker, L. F., Chisari, F., McGrath, P. P., Dalgard, D. W., Kirschstein, R. L., Almeida, J. D., Edgington, T. S., Sharp, D. C., and Peterson, W. R. (1973). *J. Infect. Dis.* **127**, 648–662.
Barker, L. F.; Maynard, J. E., and Purcell, R. H. (1975). *J. Infect. Dis.* **134**, 451.
Bayer, M. E., Blumberg, B. S., and Werner, B. (1968). *Nature (London)* **218**, 1057–1059.
Beasley, R. P., Lin, C. C., Hwang, L. Y., and Chien, C. S. (1981). *Lancet* 2, 1129–1133.
Blumberg, B. S., Alter, H. J., and Visnich, S. (1965). *JAMA, J. Am. Med. Assoc.* **191**, 541.
Blumberg, B. S., Gerstley, B. J. S., Hungerford, D. A., London, W. T., and Sutnick, A. I. (1967). *Ann. Intern. Med.* **66**, 924.
Brechot, C., Hadchouel, M., Scotto, J., Fonck, M., Potet, F., Vyas, G. N., and Piollais, P. (1981). *Proc. Natl. Acad. Sci. U.S.A.* **78**, 3906–3910.
Brechot, C., Pourcel, C., Hadchouel, M., Dejean, A., Louise, A., Scotto, J., and Tiollais, P. (1982). *Hepatology* **2**, 275–345.
Budkowska, A., Shih, J. W.-K., and Gerin, J. L. (1977). *J. Immunol.* **118**, 1300–1350.
Budkowska, A., Kalinowska, B., and Nowoslowski, A. (1979). *J. Immunol.* **123**, 1415–1416.
Burrell, C. J. (1975). *J. Gen. Virol* **27**, 117–126.
Burrell, C. J., Leadbetter, G., Mackay, P., and Marmion, B. P. (1976). *J. Gen. Virol.* **33**, 41–50.
Burrell, C. J., Mackay, P., Greenway, P. J., Hofschneider, P. H., and Murray, K. (1979). *Nature (London)* **279**, 43–47.
Camamia, F., DeBac, C., and Ricci, G. (1972). *Am. J. Dis. Child.* **123**, 309.

Cattaneo, R., Will, H., Hernandez, N., and Schaller, H. (1983). *Nature (London)* **305**, 336–338.

Chairez, R., Steiner, S., Melnick, J. L., and Dreesman, G. R. (1973). *Intervirology* **1**, 224–228.

Chakraborty, P. R., Ruiz-Opazo, N., Shouval, D., and Shafritz, D. A. (1980). *Nature (London)* **286**, 531–533.

Chakraborty, P. R., Ruiz-Opazo, N., Shouval, D., and Shafritz, D. A. (1981). *Nature (London)* **286**, 531–533.

Charnay, P., Mandart, E., Hampe, A., Fitoussi, F., Tiollais, P., and Galibert, F. (1979). *Nucleic Acids Res.* **7**, 335–345.

Charnay, P., Gervais, M., Louise, A., Galibert, F., and Tiollais, P. (1980). *Nature (London)* **286**, 893.

Chen, D. S., Hoyer, B. H., Nelson, J., Purcell, R. H., and Gerin, J. L. (1982). *Hepatology* **2**, 425–465.

Cohen, B. J., and Richmond, J. E. (1982). *Nature (London)* **296**, 677–678.

Colbere-Garapin, F., Horodniceanu, F., Kourilsky, P., and Garapin, A. C. (1983). *EMBO J.* **2**, 21–25.

Couroucé, A. M., Holland, P. V., Muller, J. Y., and Soulier, J. P. (1976). *Bibl. Haematol. (Basel)* **42**, 1–158.

Couroucé-Pauty, A. M., and Plancon, A. (1978). *Vox Sang.* **34**, 231–238.

Couroucé-Pauty, A. M., and Soulier, J. P. (1974). *Vox Sang.* **27**, 533–549.

Crowley, C. W., Liu, C.-C., and Levinson, A. D. (1983). *Mol. Cell. Biol.* **3**, 44–55.

Dane, D. S., Cameron, C. H., and Biggs, M. (1970). *Lancet* 2, 695–698.

Dienstag, J. L., Khan, A. K., Klingenstein, R. J., and Savarese, A. M. (1982). *In* "Viral Hepatitis (W. Szmuness, H. J. Alter, and J. E. Maynards, eds.), pp. 221–236. Franklin Inst. Press, Philadelphia, Pennsylvania.

Dreesman, G. R., Hollinger, F. B., McCombs, R. M., and Melnick, J. L. (1973). *J. Gen. Virol.* **19**, 129–134.

Dreesman, G. R., Chairez, R., Suarez, M., Hollinger, F. B., Courtney, R. J., and Melnick, J. L. (1975). *J. Virol.* **16**, 508–515.

Dreesman, G. R., Sanchez, Y., Ionescu-Matiu, I., Sparrow, J. T., Six, H. R., Peterson, D. L., Hollinger, F. B., and Melnick, J. L. (1982). *Nature (London)* **295**, 158–160.

Dubois, M.-F., Pourcel, C., Rousset, S., Chany, C., and Tiollais, P. (1980). *Proc. Natl. Acad. Sci. U.S.A.* **77**, 45–49.

Eddleston, A. L. W. F., Mondelle, M., Mieli-Vergani, G., and Williams, R. (1982). *Hepatology* **2**, 122s.

Edgington, T. S., and Chisari, F. V. (1975). *Am. J. Med. Sci.* **270**, 213–227.

Edman, J. C., Gray, P., Valenzuela, P., Rall, L. B., and Rutter, W. J. (1981a). *J. Virol.* **37**, 238–243.

Edman, J. C., Hallewell, R. A., Valenzuela, P., Goodman, H. M., and Rutter, W. J. (1981b). *Nature (London)* **291**, 503.

Edmond, J. C., Gray, P., Valenzuela, P., Rall, L. B., and Rutter, W. J. (1980). *Nature (London)* **286**, 535–538.

Feitelson, M. A., Marion, P. L., and Robinson, W. S. (1981). *J. Virol.* **39**, 447–454.

Feitelson, M. A., Marion, P. L., and Robinson, W. S. (1982a). *J. Virol.* **43**, 687–696.

Feitelson, M. A., Marion, P. L., and Robinson, W. S. (1982b). *J. Virol.* **43**, 741–748.

Fields, H. A., Bradley, D. W., Davis, C. L., Murphy, B. L., Schable, C. A., and Maynard, J. E. (1978). *J. Immunol.* **121**, 930–935.

Galibert, F., Mandart, E., Fitoussi, F., Tiollais, P., Charnay, P. (1979). *Nature (London)* **281**, 646–650.

Galibert, F., Chen, T. N., and Mandart, E. (1982). *J. Virol.* **41**, 51–65.

Galloway, D. A., and McDougall, J. K. (1983). *Nature (London)* **302,** 21–24.

Gellis, S. S., Neefe, J. R., Stokes, J., Jr., Strong, L. E., Janeway, C. A., and Scatchard, G. (1948). *J. Clin. Invest.* **27,** 239.

Gerin, J. L. (1974). *In* "Mechanisms of Virus" (W. S. Robinson, and C. F. Fox, eds.), pp. 215–224. Benjamin, Menlo Park, California.

Gerin, J. L., Holland, P. V., and Purcell, R. H. (1971). *J. Virol.* **7,** 569–576.

Gerin, J. L., Shih, J. W.-K., McAuliffe, V. J., and Purcell, R. H. (1978). *J. Gen. Virol.* **38,** 561–566.

Gerlich, W., and Robinson, W. S. (1980). *Cell* **21,** 801.

Gerlich, W., and Thomssen, R. (1975). *Dev. Biol. Stand.* **30,** 78–87.

Gerlich, W. H., Feitelson, M. A., Marion, P. L., and Robinson, W. S. (1980). *J. Virol.* **36,** 787–795.

Gold, J. W. M., Shih, J. W.-K., Purcell, R. H., and Gerin, J. L. (1976). *J. Immunol.* **117,** 1404–1406.

Gough, N. M. (1983). *J. Mol. Biol.* **165,** 683–699.

Gough, N. M., and Murray, K. (1982). *J. Mol. Biol.* **162,** 43–67.

Grady, G. F., Gitnick, G. L., and Prince, A. M. (1976) *Lancet 2,* 492.

Gudat, F., Bianchi, O., and Sonnabend, W. (1975). *Lab. Invest.* **32,** 1.

Hardy, K., Stahl, S., and Kupper, H. (1981). *Nature (London)* **293,** 481–483.

Hayward, W., Neel, B. G., and Astrin, S. M. (1981). *Nature (London)* **290,** 475–480.

Helske, T. (1974). *Scand. J. Haematol., Suppl.* **22,** 1.

Hess, G., Arnold, W., Shih, J. W., Kaplan, P., Purcell, R., Gerin, J., and Buschenfelde, M.-Z. (1977). *Infect. Immun.* **17,** 550–554.

Hindman, S. H., Gravelle, C. R., Murphy, B. L., Bradley, D. W., Budge, W. R., and Maynard, J. E. (1976). *Ann. Intern. Med.* **85,** 458–460.

Hirschman, S. Z., and Garfinkel, E. (1982). *Hepatology* **2,** 79s–84s.

Hirschman, S. Z., Price, P., Garfinkel, E., Christman, J., and Acs, G. (1980). *Proc. Natl. Acad. Sci. U.S.A.* **77,** 5507–5511.

Hollinger, F. B., and Dreesman, G. R. (1979). *Gastroenterology* **76,** 641–643.

Hoofnagle, J. H. (1980). *In* "Virus and the Liver" L. Bianchi, W. Gerok, K. Sickinger, and G. A. Stalder, eds.), p. 27. MTP Press, Ltd., Lancaster, England.

Hoofnagle, J. H., Gerety, R. J., and Barker, L. F. (1973). *Lancet 2,* 869–873.

Hoofnagle, J. H., Seeff, L. B., Bales, Z. B., Gerety, R. J., and Tabor, E. (1978). *In* "Viral Hepatitis" (G. N. Vyas, S. N. Cohen, and R. Schmid, eds.), pp. 219–242. Franklin Inst. Press, Philadelphia, Pennsylvania.

Hruska, J. F., and Robinson, W. S. (1977). *J. Med. Virol.* **1,** 119–131.

Hruska, J. F., Clayton, D. A., Rubenstein, J. L. R., and Robinson, W. S. (1977). *J. Virol.* **21,** 666–672.

Huang, S. a. (1971). *Am. J. Pathol.* **64,** 783.

Imai, M., Yanase, Y., Nojiri, T., Miyakawa, Y., and Mayumi, M. (1979). *Gastroenterology* **76,** 242–247.

Kam, W., Rall, L., Schmid, T., and Rutter, W. J. (1982a). *In* "Viral Hepatitis" (W. Szmuness, H. J. Alter, and J. E. Maynard, eds.), p. 809. Franklin Inst. Press, Philadelphia, Pennsylvania.

Kam, W., Rall, L., Smuckler, E., Schmid, R., and Rutter, W. (1982b). *Proc. Natl. Acad. Sci. U.S.A.* **79,** 7522–7526.

Kaplan, P. M., Greenman, R. L., Gerin, J. L., Purcell, R. H., and Robinson, W. S. (1973). *J. Virol.* **12,** 995–1005.

Kaplan, P. M., Gerin, J. L., and Alter, H. J. (1974). *Nature (London)* **249,** 762.

Kaplan, P. M., Ford, E. C., Purcell, R. H., and Gerin, J. L. (1976). *J. Virol.* **17,** 885–893.

Kim, C. Y., and Bissell, D. M. (1971). *J. Infect. Dis.* **123,** 470–476.

Kim, C. Y., and Tilles, J. G. (1970). *J. Clin. Invest.* **52,** 1176.

Koshy, R., Maupas, P., Muller, R., and Hofschneider, P. H. (1981). *J. Gen. Virol.* **57,** 95–102.

Krugman, S., Giles, J. P., and Hammond, J. (1970). *J. Infect. Dis.* **122,** 432–436.

Krugman, S., Hoofnagle, J. H., Gerety, R. J., Kaplan, P. M., and Gerin, J. L. (1974). *N. Engl. J. Med.* **290,** 1331–1335.

Landers, T. A., Greenberg, H. B., and Robinson, W. S. (1977). *J. Virol.* **23,** 368–376.

Laub, O., Rall, L. B., Truett, M., Shaul, Y., Standring, D. N., Valenzuela, P., and Rutter, W. J. (1983). *J. Virol.* **48,** 271–280.

LeBouvier, G. L. (1971). *J. Infect. Dis.* **123,** 671–675.

LeBouvier, G. L. (1972). *In* "Hepatitis and Blood Transfusion" (G. N. Vyas, A. Perkins, and R. Schmid, eds.), p. 97. Grune & Stratton, New York.

LeBouvier, G. L., and McCollum, R. W. (1970). *Adv. Virus Res.* **16,** 357.

Lerner, R. A., Green, N., Alexander, H., Liu, F. T., Sutcliffe, J. G., and Shinnick, T. M. (1981). *Proc. Natl. Acad. Sci. U.S.A.* **78,** 3403.

Ling, C., Mushahwar, I. K., Overby, L. R., Berquist, K. R., and Maynard, J. E. (1979). *Infect. Immun.* **24,** 352–356.

Lutwick, L. I., and Robinson, W. S. (1977). *J. Virol.* **21,** 96.

Mackay, P., Pasek, M., and Magazin, M. (1981a). *Proc. Natl. Acad. Sci. U.S.A.* **78,** 4510–4514.

Mackay, P., Lees, J., and Murray, K. (1981b). *J. Med. Virol.* **8,** 237–243.

Macnab, G. M., Alexander, J. J., Lecatsas, G., Bey, E. M., and Urbanowicz, J. M. (1976). *Br. J. Cancer* **34,** 509.

Magnius, L. O. (1975). *Clin. Exp. Immunol.* **20,** 209–216.

Magnius, L. O., and Espmark, J. A. (1972). *J. Immunol.* **109,** 1017–1021.

Marion, P. L., and Robinson, W. S. (1983). *Curr. Top. Microbiol. Immunol.* **105,** 99–121.

Marion, P. L., Salazar, F. H., Alexander, J. J., and Robinson, W. S. (1979a). *J. Virol.* **32,** 796–802.

Marion, P. L., Salazar, F. H., Alexander, J. J., and Robinson, W. S., (1979b), *J. Virol.* **33,** 795–806.

Marion, P. L., Oshiro, L., Regnery, D. C., Scullard, G. H., and Robinson, W. S. (1980). *Proc. Natl. Acad. Sci. U.S.A.* **77,** 2941–2945.

Marion, P. L., Knight, S. S., Feitelson, M. A., Oshiro, L. S., and Robinson, W. S. (1984). *J. Virol.* **48,** 534–541.

Mason, W. S., Seal, G., and Summers, J. (1980). *J. Virol.* **36,** 829–836.

Mason, W. S., Aldrich, C., Summers, J., and Taylor, J. M. (1982). *Proc. Natl. Acad. Sci. U.S.A.* **79,** 3997–4001.

Mazzur, S., Burget, S., and Blumberg, B. S. (1974). *Nature (London)* **247,** 38.

McCollum, R. W. (1952). *Proc. Soc. Exp. Biol. Med.* **81,** 157.

Miller, D. J., Williams, A. E., LeBouvier, G. L., Dwyer, J. M., Grant, J., and Klaskin, G. (1978). *Gastroenterology* **74,** 1208–1213.

Miller, R. H., and Robinson, W. S. (1983). *Proc. Natl. Acad. Sci. U.S.A.* **80,** 2534–2538.

Miller, R. H., Tran, C. T. and Robinson, W. S. (1984a). *Virology* **139,** 53–63.

Miller, R. H., and Robinson, W. S. (1984b). *Virology* **137,** 390–399.

Millman, I., Hutanen, H., Merino, F., Bayer, M. E., and Blumberg, B. S. (1971). *Res. Commun. Chem. Pathol. Pharmacol.* **2,** 667–686.

Mitamura, K., Hoyer, B., Ponzetto, A., Nelson, J., Purcell, R. H., and Gerin, J. L. (1982). *Hepatology* **2,** 47S–50S.

Miyanohara, A., Toh-E, A., Nozaki, C., Hamada, F., Ohtomo, N., and Matsubara, K. (1983). *Proc. Natl. Acad. Sci. U.S.A.* **80**, 1–5.

Moriarty, A. M., Boyer, B. H., Shih, J. W.-K., Gerin, J. L., and Hamer, D. H. (1981). *Proc. Natl. Acad. Sci. U.S.A.* **78**, 2606.

Mosley, J. W., Edwards, V. M., Meihaus, J. E., and Redeker, A. G. (1972). *Am. J. Epidemiol.* **95**, 529–535.

Murphy, B. L., Peterson, J. M., and Ebert, J. W. (1975). *Intervirology* **6**, 207–211.

Murray, R., and Diefenbach, W. C. (1953). *Proc. Soc. Exp. Biol. Med.* **84**, 230.

Neurath, A. R., and Strick, N. (1979a). *Interviriology* **11**, 128.

Neurath, A. R., and Strick, N. (1979b). *J. Gen. Virol.* **42**, 645–649.

Neurath, A. R., Prince, A. M., and Lippin, A. (1974). *Proc. Natl. Acad. Sci. U.S.A.* **71**, 2663.

Neurath, A. R., Hashimoto, N., and Prince, A. M. (1975). *J. Gen. Virol.* **27**, 81–91.

Neurath, A. R., Trepo, C., Chen, M., and Prince, A. M. (1976). *J. Gen. Virol.* **30**, 277–285.

Neurath, A. R., Prince, A. M., and Giacalove, V. (1978a). *Experientia* **34**, 414–415.

Neurath, A. R., Strick, N., and Huang, C. Y. (1978b). *Intervirology* **10**, 265–275.

Neurath, A. R., Szmuness, W., Stevens, C. E., Strick, N., and Harley, J. E. (1978c). *J. Gen. Virol.* **38**, 549.

Nordenfeldt, E., and Andren-Sandberg, M. (1976). *J. Infect. Dis.* **134**, 85–89.

Norkrans, G., Nordenfeldt, E., Hermondsson, S., and Iwarson, S. (1980). *Scand. J. Infect. Dis.* **12**, 159.

Obata, H., Hayashi, N., and Motoike, Y. (1980). *Int. J. Cancer* **25**, 741.

Ogston, C. W., Jonak, G. J., Rogler, C. E., Astrin, S. M., and Summers, J. (1982). *Cell* **29**, 385–394.

Ohori, H., Onodera, S., and Ishida, N. (1979). *J. Gen. Virol.* **43**, 423–427.

Okada, K., Kamiyama, I., Inomata, M., Imai, M., Miyakawa, Y., and Mayumi, M. (1976). *N. Engl. J. Med.* **294**, 746–749.

Okochi, K., and Murakami, S. (1968). *Vox Sang.* **15**, 374.

Pasek, M., Goto, T., Gilbert, W., Ziuk, B., Schaller, H., MacKay, P., Leadbetter, G., and Murray, K. (1979). *Nature (London)* **282**, 575–579.

Perrillo, R. P., Gelb, L., Campbell, C., Wellinghoff, W., Ellis, F. R., Overby, L., and Aach, R. D. (1979). *Gastroenterology* **76**, 1319–1325.

Peterson, D. L., Roberts, I. M., and Vyas, G. N. (1977). *Proc. Natl. Acad. Sci. U.S.A.* **74**, 1530–1534.

Peterson, D. L., Chien, D. Y., Vyas, G. N., Nitecki, D., and Bond, H. E. (1978). *In* "Viral Hepatitis" (G. N. Vyas, S. N. Cohen, and R. Schmid, eds.), pp. 569–573. Franklin Inst. Press, Philadelphia, Pennsylvania.

Popper, H. *In* "Viral Hepatitis (G. N. Vyas, S. N. Cohen, and R. Schmid, eds.), pp. 451–454. Franklin Inst. Press, Philadelphia, Pennsylvania.

Popper, H., Shih, J. W.-K., Gerin, J. L., Wong, D. C., Hoyer, B. H., London, W. T., Sly, D. L., and Purcell, R. H. (1981). *Hepatology* **1**, 91.

Pourcel, C., Louise, A., Gervais, M., Chenciner, N., Dubois, M.-F., and Tiollais, P. (1981). *J. Virol.* **42**, 100–105.

Pourcel, C., Sobzack, E., Dubolis, M.-F., Gervais, M., Drouet, J., and Tiollais, P. (1982). *Virology* **121**, 175–183.

Prince, A. M. (1968). *Proc. Natl. Acad. Sci. U.S.A.* **60**, 814.

Prince, A. M., Ikram, H., and Hopp, T. P. (1982). *Proc. Natl. Acad. Sci. U.S.A.* **79**, 579–582.

Purcell, R. H., and Gerin, J. L. (1975). *Am. J. Med. Sci.* **270**, 395–399.

Ray, M. B., Desmet, V. I., and Bradburne, A. F. (1976). *Gastroenterology* **71**, 462.

Realdi, G., Alberti, A., Rugge, M., Bortolotti, F., Rigoli, A. M., Tremolada, F., and Ruol, A. (1980). *Gastroenterology* **79**, 195–199.

Redeker, A. G., Hopkins, C. E., Jackson, B., and Peck, P. (1968). *Transfusion* **8**, 60.

Redeker, A. G., Mosley, J. W., Gocke, D. J., McKee, A. P., and Pollack, W. (1975). *N. Engl. J. Med.* **293**, 1055–1059.

Robinson, H. L., Astrin, S. M., Senior, A. M., and Salazar, F. H. (1981). *J. Virol.* **40**, 745–751.

Robinson, W. S. (1977). *Annu. Rev. Microbiol.* **31**, 357–377.

Robinson, W. S. (1980). *Ann. N.Y. Acad. Sci.* **354**, 371–378.

Robinson, W. S., and Greenman, R. L. (1974). *J. Virol.* **13**, 1231–1236.

Robinson, W. S., and Lutwick, L. I. (1976). *In* "Animal Virology" (D. Baltimore, A. Huang, and C. F. Fox, eds.), pp. 787–811. Academic Press, New York.

Robinson, W. S., Clayton, D. A., and Greenman, R. L. (1974). *J. Virol.* **14**, 384–391.

Robinson, W. S., Marion, P. L., Feitelson, M., and Siddiqui, A. *In* "Viral Hepatitis" (W. Szmuness, H. J. Alter, and J. E. Maynard, eds.), pp. 57–68. Franklin Inst. Press, Philadelphia, Pennsylvania.

Salaman, M. H., Williams, D. I., King, A. J., and Nico, C. S. (1944). *Lancet* 2, 7–8.

Sampliner, R. E., Hamilton, F. A., and Iseri, O. A. (1979). *Am. J. Med. Sci.* **277**, 17.

Sattler, F., and Robinson, W. S. (1979). *J. Virol.* **32**, 226–233.

Scullard, G. H., Pollard, R. B., Smith, J. L., Sacks, S. L., Gregory, P. B., Robinson, W. S., and Merigan, T. C. (1981). *J. Infect. Dis.* **143**, 772–783.

Scullard, G. H., Greenberg, H. B., Smith, J. L., Gregory, P. G., Merigan, T. C., and Robinson, W. S. (1982). *Hepatology* **2**, 39.

Seeff, L. B., Zimmerman, H. J., Wright, E. C., Finkelstein, J. D., Greenlee, H. B., Hamilton, J., Leevy, C. M., Tamburrow, C. H., Vlahcevic, Z., Zimmon, D. S., Felsher, B. F., Garcia-Pont, P., Dietz, A. A., Koff, R. S., Kierman, I., Schiff, E. R., Zemel, R., and Nath, N. (1975). *Lancet* 2, 939–941.

Shafritz, D. A. (1982). *Hepatology* **2**, 35S–41S.

Shafritz, D. A., Shouval, D., Sherman, H., Hadziyannis, S., and Kew, M. (1981). *N. Engl. J. Med.* **305**, 1067–1073.

Shih, J. W.-K., and Gerin, J. L. (1975). *J. Immunol.* **115**, 634–639.

Shih, J. W.-K., and Gerin, L. L. (1977a). *J. Virol.* **21**, 347–357.

Shih, J. W.-K., and Gerin, J. L. (1977b). *J. Virol.* **21**, 1219–1222.

Shih, J. W.-K., Tan, P. L., and Gerin, J. L. (1980). *Infect. Immun.* **28**, 459–463.

Shikata, T., Karasawa, T., Abe, K., Uzqwa, T., Suzuki, H., Oda, T., Imai, M., Mayumi, M., and Moritsugu, Y. (1977). *J. Infect. Dis.* **136**, 571.

Shikata, T., Karasawa, T., Abe, K., Takahashi, T., Mayumi, M., and Oda, T. (1978). *J. Infect. Dis.* **138**, 242–244.

Siddiqui, A. (1983). *Mol. Cell. Biol.* **3**, 143–146.

Siddiqui, A., Sattler, F. R., and Robinson, W. S. (1979). *Proc. Natl. Acad. Sci. U.S.A.* **76**, 4664–4668.

Smith, G. L., Mackett, M., and Moss, B. (1983). *Nature (London)* **302**, 490–495.

Soulier, J. P., Blatix, C., Couroucé, A. M., Benamou, D., Amouch, P., and Drouet, J. (1972). *Am. J. Dis. Child.* **123**, 429–433.

Southern, E. M. (1975). *J. Mol. Biol.* **98**, 503–517.

Steiner, S., Huebner, M. T., and Dreesman, G. R. (1974). *J. Virol.* **14**, 572–577.

Stenlund, A., Lamy, D., Moreno-Lopez, J., Ahola, H., Pettersson, U., and Tiollais, P. (1983). *EMBO J.* **2**, 669–673.

Stevens, C. E., Beasley, R. P., and Tsui, J. (1975). *N. Engl. J. Med.* **232**, 1231.

Stratowa, C., Doehmer, J., Wang, Y., and Hofschneider, P. H. (1982). *EMBO J.* **1**, 1573–1578.

Struck, D. K., Lennarz, W. J., and Brew, K. (1978). *J. Biol. Chem.* **253**, 5786–5794.

Summers, J. A., and Mason, W. S. (1982). *Cell* **29**, 403–415.

Summers, J. A., O'Connell, A., and Millman, I. (1975). *Proc. Natl. Acad. Sci. U.S.A.* **72,** 4597–4601.
Summers, J. A., Smolec, J. M., and Snyder, R. (1978a). *Proc. Natl. Acad. Sci. U.S.A.* **75,** 4533–4537.
Summers, J. A., O'Connell, A., Maupas, P., Goudeau, A., Coursaget, P., and Drucker, J. (1978b). *J. Med. Virol.* **2,** 207.
Szmuness, W. (1978). *Prog. Med. Virol.* **24,** 40–69.
Szmuness, W., Prince, A. M., and Brotman, B. (1973). *J. Infect. Dis.* **127,** 17.
Tabor, E., Gerety, R. J., and Barker, L. F. (1977). *J. Infect. Dis.* **136,** 541–547.
Takahashi, K., Imai, M., Tsuda, F., Takahashi, T., Miyakawa, Y., and Mayumi, M. (1976). *J. Immunol.* **117,** 102–105.
Takahashi, K., Yamashita, S., Imai, M., Miyakawa, Y., and Mayumi, M. (1978a). *J. Gen. Virol.* **38,** 431–436.
Takahashi, K., Imai, M., Miyakawa, Y., Iwakiri, S., and Mayumi, M. (1978b). *Proc. Natl. Acad. Sci. U.S.A.* **75,** 1952.
Takahashi, K., Miyakawa, Y., Gotanda, T., Mishiro, S., Imai, M., and Mayumi, M. (1979a). *Gastroenterology* **77,** 1193.
Takahashi, K., Akahane, Y., Gotanda, T., Mishiro, T., Imai, M., Miyakawa, Y., and Mayumi, M. (1979b). *J. Immunol.* **122,** 275–279.
Thomssen, R., Gerlich, W., Stamm, B., Bismas, R., Lorenz, P. R., Majer, M., Weinmann, E., Arnold, W., Hess, G., Wepler, W., and Linge, O. (1977). *N. Engl. J. Med.* **296,** 396.
Tong, M. J., Thursby, M., Rakela, J., McPeak, C., Edwards, V. M., and Mosley, J. W. (1981). *Gastroenterology* **80,** 999.
Twist, E. M., Clark, H. F., Aden, A. P., Knowles, B. B., and Plotkin, S. A. (1981). *J. Virol.* **37,** 239–243.
Valenzuela, P., Gray, P., Quiroga, M., Zaldivar, J., Goodman, H. M., and Rutter, W. J. (1979). *Nature (London)* **28,** 815–819.
Valenzuela, P., Quiroga, M., Zaldivar, J., Gray, P., and Rutter, W. J. (1980). *In* "Animal Virus Genetics" (B. Fields, R. Jaenisch, and C. F. Fox, eds.), pp. 57–70. Academic Press, New York.
Valenzuela, P., Medina, A., Rutter, W. J., Ammerer, G., and Hall, D. B. (1982). *Nature (London)* **298,** 347–350.
Varmus, H., and Swanström, R. (1982). *In* "RNA Tumor Viruses" (R, Weiss, N. Teich, H. Varmus, and J. Coffin, eds.), pp. 369–512. Cold Spring Harbor Press, Cold Spring Harbor, New York.
Vyas, G. N. (1981). *In* "Hepatitis B Vaccine" (P. Maupas and P. Guesry, eds.), pp. 227–237. Elsevier/North-Holland Press, Amsterdam.
Vyas, G. N., Rao, K. R., and Ibrahim, A. B. (1972). *Science* **187,** 1300–1301.
Wang, Y., Schafer-Ridder, M., Stratowa, C., Wong, T.-K., and Hofschneider, P. H. (1982). *EMBO J.* **1,** 1213–1216.
Wang, Y., Stratowa, C., Schaefer-Differ, M., Doehmer, J., and Hofschneider, P. H. (1983). *Mol. Cell. Biol.* **3,** 1032–1039.
Werner, B. G., Smolec, J. M., Snyder, R., and Summers, J. (1979). *J. Virol.* **32,** 314–322.
Wewalka, F. (1953). *Schweiz. Z. Allg. Pathol.* **16,** 307–312.
Williams, A., and LeBouvier, G. (1976). *Bibl. Haematol. (Basel)* **42,** 71–75.
Yoakum, G. H., Korba, B. E., Lechne, J. F., Tokiwa, T., Gazdar, A. F., Seeley, T., Siegel, M., Leeman, L., Autrup, H., and Harris, C. C. (1983). *Science* **222,** 385–389.

Chapter 15

Passive Immunoprophylaxis

LEONARD B. SEEFF
Gastroenterology/Hepatology Section
Veterans Administration Medical Center
and Georgetown University Medical Center
Washington, D.C.

I. Historical Perspectives

Effective prophylaxis of viral disease using immune globulin (gamma globulin, IG, formerly called ISG) first became a reality in the mid-1940s. This followed a report from Enders (1944) indicating that the γ-globulin fraction of human plasma contained antibodies directed against some viruses, and the development by Cohn and associates (1944) of a safe and effective means of mass producing this plasma product. By that time, a great deal of information had already been gathered regarding the etiology and epidemiology of viral hepatitis, but it was not yet possi-

353

Copyright © 1985 by Academic Press, Inc.
All rights of reproduction in any form reserved.
ISBN 0-12-280672-7

ble to identify the specific viral agents responsible for the disease. Indeed, the diagnosis of viral hepatitis had to depend on the occurrence of relatively nonspecific symptoms such as anorexia, nausea, loss of taste for cigarettes, and right upper quadrant pain, generally accompanied by overt icterus and by the development of nonspecific biochemical test abnormalities.

Thus, at the time that IG first became available, investigators faced the following dilemmas: (1) the precise distinction between the different viral agents could not be established; (2) the epidemiological assumptions used to separate the then-known forms of viral hepatitis were often in error (Bryan and Gregg, 1975); (3) the existence of a virus or viruses not associated with hepatitis A or B (i.e., non-A, non-B) had not been recognized; (4) asymptomatic disease identifiable only by the development of increased concentrations of serum enzymes (i.e., aminotransferases) could not be detected, since these enzymes had not yet been identified; (5) viral infection, defined as the occurrence of serological markers of hepatitis in the absence of biochemical evidence of disease could not be recognized; and (6) most important from the viewpoint of immunoprophylaxis, specific hepatitis antibodies could not be measured in IG.

Despite these handicaps, several studies were initiated in 1945, each involving the administration of IG for what almost certainly were outbreaks of hepatitis A (Gellis *et al.*, 1945; Havens and Paul, 1945; Stokes and Neefe, 1945). That they proved successful can be accounted for by the fact that hepatitis A was a common disease, and hence antibody (anti-HAV) would be expected to be present in high frequency in the general population and consequently in the donors who contributed the plasma from which the IG batches were prepared. In contrast, hepatitis B has always been less prevalent in the United States than hepatitis A, and conceivably was even less so in 1944, since the circumstances that are now known to enhance its spread (e.g., illicit parenteral drug abuse, widespread and promiscuous male homosexuality) presumably did not flourish to the same extent at that time as they do at present. Accordingly, it can be assumed that immune globulin produced in 1944 must have contained little or no antibody against hepatitis B (anti-HBs).

With the discovery in recent years of the specific viruses responsible for hepatitis A (Feinstone *et al.*, 1973) and hepatitis B (Blumberg *et al.*, 1965), and the development of highly sensitive tests that permit measurement of specific, protective antibodies, it has been possible to confirm some of these assumptions. Early studies of commercial immune globulin batches using these techniques demonstrated that all lots contained anti-HAV, albeit in widely varying titers, ranging from 1:220 to

1:16,000 (Froesner *et al.*, 1977a; Miller *et al.*, 1975). Similar results were noted in later studies conducted at the Bureau of Biologics (currently Office of Biologics Research and Review). Thus, Hoofnagle and Waggoner (1980), who examined 62 lots of IG that had been submitted to this agency in the years 1962 through 1977, found that they all contained anti-HAV with a reasonably consistent titer of ~1:1,000, regardless of the year of manufacture. Smallwood and co-workers (1980), on the other hand, in an evaluation of 201 lots received from six different manufacturers between 1967 and 1977, found that half the lots manufactured in 1967, 69% of lots manufactured in 1972, and 100% of those manufactured in 1977 contained anti-HAV in titers of 1:1,000. They speculated that the increase both in the mean titer of anti-HAV and in the percentage of lots found to contain these high titers was the result of the greater reliance that had developed over the years on paid plasmapheresis donors. It should be noted that even at the present time the minimum anti-HAV titer necessary to prevent hepatitis A has not been established.

Somewhat different results have emerged with regard to the anti-HBs content of IG preparations. In two separate reports published in 1975, one from the Bureau of Biologics and the other from the Massachusetts Department of Public Health, it was noted that the prevalence and titers of anti-HBs in preparations submitted to the Bureau of Biologics prior to 1972 were low, whereas lots manufactured subsequently showed marked increases both in prevalence and titer of anti-HBs (Grady *et al.*, 1975; Hoofnagle *et al.*, 1975). Because this change appeared to coincide with the introduction of mandatory screening, by highly sensitive assays, of all blood donors for HBsAg, both groups of investigators surmised that the prohibition of HBsAg-positive donors had permitted identification of anti-HBs that previously had been bound in complex to HBsAg. Later studies from the Bureau of Biologics indicated that the titer of anti-HBs in standard IG had continued to increase. Thus, Hoofnagle and Waggoner (1980) found that the mean titer of anti-HBs in 45 lots of IG manufactured between 1967 and 1971 was <1:10, whereas it was 1:500 in 12 lots manufactured between 1973 and 1977. Gerety *et al.* (1980) found that among 76 lots submitted to the Bureau of Biologics in 1979, all had anti-HBs present; 92% had titers of 1:100, although only 8% had titers exceeding 1:1,000. This information has an important bearing on the use of this product for the prevention of hepatitis B, as will be discussed.

The data pertaining to the presence of HBsAg in IG are also of importance in regard to its mode of action in the prevention of hepatitis B. Studies of early lots of IG preparations, namely those produced prior to 1965, demonstrated HBsAg in low titer only in occasional lots (Hoofnagle *et al.*, 1975). With the use of more sophisticated techniques, it was later shown that the majority of these earlier lots contained HBsAg, but that the presence of the antigen had been masked by having formed an immune complex with anti-HBs. Thus, 78% of the 45 lots manufactured between 1962 and 1971, all of them HBsAg negative as determined by conventional radioimmunoassay (RIA) or passive hemagglutination (PHA) tests, were in fact positive for HBsAg when the test was performed after ultracentrifugation of the IG through an acid–sucrose medium; the acid condition caused dissociation of the HBsAg–anti-HBs complexes (Hoofnagle and Waggoner, 1980). In contrast, none of 12 lots manufactured after 1973 had detectable HBsAg, regardless of the manner in which the test was performed. The implications of these findings will also be discussed.

II. Early Studies of Immunoprophylaxis against Hepatitis B

The first study directed specifically at evaluating the efficacy of IG for the prevention of presumed hepatitis B was undertaken in 1945 (Grossman *et al.*, 1945). In view of the vast amounts of plasma used during World War II, it had become apparent that blood transfusions often preceeded the development of viral hepatitis; the disease was presumed to be "serum" or hepatitis B. In this first study, alternate hospitalized battle casualties who had been transfused with either whole blood or plasma were given two injections of 10 ml of IG at a 1-month interval, and they and an untreated control group were followed for the development of jaundice. "Hepatitis" developed in 11.5% of the 384 untreated patients but in only 2.9% of the 384 patients who were immunized with IG, leading to the conclusion that IG had had a beneficial effect.

This "positive" study was, however, followed by three others that reached quite opposite conclusions. Duncan and co-workers, in 1947, conducted a study similar to that by Grossman involving transfused battle casualties, and found an incidence of posttransfusion hepatitis of 1.2% in treated patients and 0.9% in an untreated control group. They did note that there was a prolongation of the incubation period of hepatitis in the treated patients. In 1948, Stokes reported results from a series of studies among human volunteers (Stokes *et al.*, 1948). These involved the administration of varying doses of IG in differing schedules to volunteers who had first been inoculated parenterally with different strains of infectious serum; in one of the studies, prophylaxis was attempted with convalescent plasma. None of these series of studies showed IG to be protective, nor was there any evidence of prolongation of the incubation period in those receiving IG.

In 1953, Drake *et al.* performed yet another volunteer inoculation study using "convalescent" γ globulin. Twenty-eight healthy volunteers received an inoculum of the Fort Bragg strain of homologous serum hepatitis, and some were also given IG either intramuscularly or mixed with the infectious serum in the hope of neutralizing the infectious agent. Fifty percent of these individuals developed jaundice, and an additional 18%, anicteric hepatitis. Among the reasons offered for the failure of efficacy of the IG was the probablility that it had contained little or no specific antibodies, either because of poor immunogenicity of HBV or because the antibody had become tissue fixed or destroyed in the course of IG manufacture. Other explanations that might now be considered are (1) some of the donors might have been HBsAg positive, which could have resulted in HBsAg–anti-HBs complexes in the final plasma pool, or (2) the disease under study might not have been hepatitis B.

These latter considerations derive support from data from a study conducted more recently by Kuhns *et al.* (1976). In this study, patients undergoing cardiovascular surgery (having received an average of 18 units of blood each) were randomized to receive two 10-ml injections of IG, the first given within 7 days of transfusion and the second on the thirtieth day. The plasma used for preparation of the globulin had come from patients with a past history of anicteric hepatitis, presumed to be hepatitis B. Nevertheless, when tested by sensitive assay the IG revealed a very low titer of anti-HBs (1:4). Not surprisingly, the incidence of hepatitis B in this study was found to be the same in the IG and placebo recipients. What was surprising at that time, however, is that more than two-thirds of the cases of posttransfusion hepatitis could not be defined as hepatitis B. Thus, because of this series of negative results, until as recently as 1972 the Advisory Committee on Immunization Practices (1968) stated that IG should not be administered as a routine measure to individuals exposed to hepatitis B.

III. Early Studies using IG with Measurable Hepatitis B Antibodies (Anti-HBs)

The first study to suggest that IG containing moderate to high titers of hepatitis B antibody might be effective in the prevention of hepatitis B was one that involved U.S. servicemen stationed in Korea (Cooperative Study, 1971). In a trial conducted during a more than 2 year period from May 1967 to August 1969, 107,803 newly arrived soldiers received, by random selection, an intramuscular injection of either 2, 5, or 10 ml of IG, or a placebo. Sixty-five percent of them were given a second injection of the same material 5–7 months later. Compared with placebo recipients, the incidence of hepatitis was found to be significantly lower in those who received either 5 or 10 ml of IG, but not among those receiving the 2-ml dose. Of great interest is that protection against endemic hepatitis occurred regardless of whether the disease was HBsAg positive or HBsAg negative. Subsequent examination of the IG used in this study, which had been prepared from plasma of prison volunteers, demonstrated that it contained anti-HBs with a titer in excess of 1:1,280 (Ginsberg *et al.*, 1972). These results suggested that IG containing anti-HBs in only moderate titers appeared capable of preventing hepatitis B acquired via low-level exposure through the mechanism of passive immunoprophylaxis. A recent reanalysis of the IG used in the Korean trial has led to an alternative view regarding its mechanism of action (Lemon *et al.*, 1980). Lemon *et al.* examined two of the four original lots of IG, the placebo used in that trial, and two lots of contemporary IG, and found HBsAg in both of the two Korean IGs (identified in one by direct assay and in the other after centrifugation through a pH 2.5 sucrose gradient) as well as in one of the two albumin placebos, but not in the two contemporary IGs (both of which contained low-titer anti-HBs). These results suggested that the original IG had probably conferred immunity by active rather than passive immunization, thus simulating the effect of a vaccine.

Based on these data, and following the demonstration by Prince *et al.* (1971) that IG could be prepared to contain extremely high anti-HBs titers, a controlled study was undertaken by Krugman and colleagues (1971) to evaluate the efficacy of hyperimmune globulin against hepatitis B. This hepatitis B immune globulin (HBIG) had been prepared from a 5-liter plasma pool obtained from a single hemophiliac donor, and contained an anti-HBs titer of 1:260,000 as measured by PHA. A control globulin used in the study had an anti-HBs titer of 1:16. Ten children experimentally inoculated with MS-2 (HBsAg-positive) serum received the HBIG in a dose of 0.04 ml/kg 4 hr later. An additional 5 children exposed to MS-2 received the conventional IG 4 hr later, and a control group of 11 children were given the infectious serum alone. Six of the 10 children in the first group were completely protected, and an additional 1 developed attenuated disease (60–70% protection); 2 of 5 in the second group developed hepatitis B (40% protection). Also noted was a prolonged incubation period of hepatitis B in HBIG recipients as well as a reduced HBsAg carrier state (HBIG, 20%, versus controls, 45%). Because the passively administered anti-HBs disappeared within 14 to 94 days (mean, 42 days), the mechanism of action of HBIG was assumed to be that of passive–active immunization.

IV. Clinical Studies of the Efficacy of HBIG

Following the demonstration in an experimental setting of an apparent protective effect of HBIG against hepatitis B, a series of studies were undertaken to evaluate its efficacy in a variety of clinical situations. In summarizing these studies, it seems appropriate to consider them as those aimed at prevention prior to exposure (preexposure prophylaxis) and those evaluating administration following exposure (postexposure prophylaxis).

V. Preexposure Prophylaxis Studies

A. Endemic Hepatitis B

Only one additional study has been undertaken to evaluate the efficacy of HBIG in the prevention of endemically acquired hepatitis. Szmuness and colleagues (1974) initiated a trial in three separate institutions for the mentally retarded where it was known that naturally acquired hepatitis B was a common problem. Eighty-one newly admitted children under the age of 15 years were randomly assigned to receive HBIG (44 children) or standard IG (37 children). The HBIG contained an anti-HBs titer of 1:262,144 and the IG a titer of 1:16, both measured by PHA, and the doses used were 0.02 ml/kg given at 4-month intervals beginning 1–2 weeks after admission; the children received between three and six injections. They were then followed with montly serological and biochemical tests for an average of 20 to 21 months. Concurrently, 52 children at one of the institutions who did not enter the trial for one of several reasons were followed as a "control" group. This group was seen for an average of 25 months, with blood specimens obtained at 3- to 5-month intervals.

Evidence of hepatitis B infection (HBsAg or anti-HBs) occurred slightly less frequently in the HBIG recipients (32%) than in the other two groups (56 and 61%). However, the combined figures for the development of HBsAg and amminotransferase abnormalities accompanied by evidence of hepatitis B infection were 14% for the HBIG group, 8% for the IG group, and 25% for the "control" group. None of the globulin recipients became HBsAg carriers, but the carrier state did develop in one-half of the control patients; also, anti-HBs developed significantly more frequently in the IG than the HBIG group. The investigators interpreted these data as demonstrating an approximately equal efficacy of HBIG and IG in the prevention of hepatitis B. Furthermore, they suggested that HBIG had probably acted through passive immunization, while the IG had induced passive–active immunization. Unfortunately, the "control" group was not comparably selected and was not similarly followed, and hence the real benefit from either of the two globulins in this setting remain unclear. In addition, the authors agreed that the sample size was too small to reach a firm conclusion regarding the efficacy of HBIG in the prevention of hepatitis B.

B. Posttransfusion Hepatitis B

Numerous trials have been undertaken since 1945 to evaluate IG for the prevention of posttransfusion hepatitis (Creutzfeldt *et al.*, 1966; Csapo *et al.*, 1963; Duncan *et al.*, 1947; Grossman *et al.*, 1945; Holland *et al.*, 1966; Katz *et al.*, 1971; Knodell *et al.*, 1976; Kuhns *et al.*, 1976; Mirick *et al.*, 1965; Prospective Cooperative Study, 1972; Seeff *et al.*, 1977, 1978a; Soulier *et al.*, 1972; Spellberg and Berman, 1971). In retrospect, it is apparent that they were planned, designed, and conducted with varying degrees of skill and sophistication, depending in large measure on the period during which they were undertaken. Furthermore, the majority were initiated at a time when posttransfusion hepatitis was believed to be synonymous with hepatitis B. Prior to the discovery of HBsAg as an indicator of hepatitis B virus (HBV) infection, investigators had no means of distinguishing between hepatitis B and non-A, non-B hepatitis, an important handicap since the latter constituted as much as three-fourths of all cases of posttransfusion hepatitis even before HBsAg screening became available (Gocke *et al.*, 1970). Also, they could not define the HBV carrier or identify protective antibody in globulin products tested.

After the advent of HBsAg testing, one uncontrolled (Soulier *et al.*, 1972) and four controlled (Knodell *et al.*, 1976; Kuhns *et al.*, 1976; Seeff *et al.*, 1977, 1978a) trials were conducted that permitted evaluation of the efficacy of passive immunoprophylaxis against posttransfusion hepatitis B. In the single uncontrolled study, only high-titer IG was studied; in all of the four controlled trials, IG was tested, and in two of them, the efficacy of HBIG was evaluated also. The first of these studies, by Soulier *et al.*

(1972), involved the administration of γ globulin with an anti-HBs titer by PHA of 1:53,000 to 18 persons who had been transfused with HBsAg-positive blood. The doses received ranged from 0.06 to 0.2mg/kg. None of the recipients became HBsAg positive, and only two developed mild serum aminotransferase elevations. These tantalizing data were a stimulus for further study.

Kuhns *et al.* (1976) studied 195 patients undergoing cardiac surgery who had been transfused with an average of 18 units of blood each; testing of donor blood for HBsAg had been initiated at variable intervals during the study. The patients were randomized to receive either IG (derived from donors with a past history of icteric hepatitis, but which nevertheless had an anti-HBs titer of only 1:4), or an albumin placebo, in a dose of 20 ml [10 ml on the seventh (± 3) postoperative days and 10 ml on the thirtieth (± 5) days]. Patients were followed at regular intervals for 6 months with serological and biochemical tests. Hepatitis developed in 26% of placebo recipients and in 25% of IG recipients; the incidence of hepatitis B was almost identical in the two groups (7.8 versus 7.5%). Thus, this study showed no clear-cut effect of IG in preventing post-transfusion hepatitis B, but it did demonstrate that approximately two-thirds of cases of posttransfusion hepatitis were not HBV infections.

Knodell *et al.* (1976) also approached this problem through the study of cardiac surgery patients. A total of 279 patients was selected randomly to receive 10 ml of HBIG (anti-HBs titer, 1×10^6), IG (anti-HBs titer, 1×10^2) or a placebo (2.5% albumin) just before surgery. The blood that was used in surgery had been obtained from volunteer army donors. Patients were followed by blood specimen testing at weekly intervals while in the hospital, and then at 3, 6, and 9 months postoperatively. The total number of cases of hepatitis that developed was identical in the HBIG and IG recipients, and in both, hepatitis occurred significantly less frequently than it did among the placebo recipients. However, the numbers of cases that could be defined as hepatitis B were too few to permit any firm conclusions to be drawn (placebo, 1.1%; IG, 1.1%; HBIG, 0%).

The remaining two trials were both conducted as Veterans Administration Cooperative Studies (Seeff *et al.*, 1977, 1978a). The first involved 2204 patients who were transfused with an average of 3.3 units of blood, obtained from both volunteer and commercial donors (Seeff *et al.*, 1977). The patients were selected randomly to receive two 10-ml injections of either IG, devoid of anti-HBs, or an albumin placebo, the first injection given within 96 hr of transfusion and the second 28 $\pm$ 3 days later. Follow-up consisted of biochemical and serological analyses at 2-week intervals for a minimum of 22 weeks. The results suggested that the IG had reduced the incidence of icteric non-A, non-B posttransfusion hepatitis. However, no effect could be established with regard to the incidence of posttransfusion hepatitis B (placebo, 2.6%; IG, 2.1%).

Because the IG did not contain anti-HBs, a second Veterans Administration Cooperative Study was undertaken to evaluate the efficacy of HBIG (Seeff *et al.*, 1978a). This trial did not include a placebo group, in view of the fact that the first study had demonstrated apparent benefit from IG in reducing non-A, non-B posttransfusion hepatitis. Accordingly, HBIG (anti-HBs titer, 1:100,000 by PHA) was compared to the IG of the first trial (devoid of anti-HBs) in 969 transfused individuals who had received a mean of 3.7 units of blood from both volunteer and commercial donors. The dose schedule used for the globulins was the same as that of the original study. At the end of the trial, only 4 of the 123 patients who developed hepatitis could be defined as having HBV-related disease, and they occurred with equal frequency in the two globulin treatment groups. However, HBV infection (HBsAg alone or the late development of anti-HBs) did occur significantly more frequently in the IG than the HBIG recipients. The majority of those who developed antibody following IG administration had anti-HBs but not anti-HBc, the serological response known to follow vaccination (Purcell and Gerin, 1975). Thus, it was inferred that the IG, prepared in 1944, might have contained small amounts of HBsAg, which could have conferred vaccine-like properties. However, HBsAg could not be detected in the IG (perhaps because of complexing with anti-HBs), although anti-HBc was found.

In summary, these data have led to the conclusion that immunoprophylaxis for posttransfusion hepatitis B is unnecessary, because screening of blood donors for HBsAg, with interdiction of those found to be positive, has in itself virtually eliminated the disease in this setting. Nevertheless, occasional errors are committed in which donor blood, mistakenly reported to be HBsAg negative, is administered. In these instances, it seems prudent to administer HBIG (Telischi *et al.*, 1980), even though absolute proof of efficacy is still lacking.

C. Hemodialysis-Associated Hepatitis B

At least five separate groups have evaluated the efficacy of HBIG for the prevention of hemodialysis-acquired hepatitis B. Desmyter *et al.* (1975) randomly selected 29 hemodialysis patients to receive either HBIG (anti-HBs titer 1:25,000 by PHA), or IG (without detectable anti-HBs). The patients were given two 5-ml injections at a 6-month interval, and were followed for a 16-month period with biochemical and serological testing. HBsAg developed in 13.3% of HBIG and in 71.4% of IG recipients, accompanied by evidence of hepatitis in all the HBIG and in a little more than one-half the IG recipients. The protection rate in the study was calculated to be 80%. Because HBIG recipients developed anti-HBs or anti-HBc alone, it was suggested that the effect of HBIG was to induce passive–active immunization.

An uncontrolled study was reported in the same year by Courouce-Pauty *et al.* (1975) from France. They used a globulin with an anti-HBs titer of 1:64,000, and administered it in a single dose to patients exposed either through HBsAg-positive transfusions, to accidentally exposed medical personnel, or to hemodialysis staff. A single injection was used in the first two studies and repeated injections in the latter one. None of 90 hemodialysis staff given the repeated injections developed HBsAg or hepatitis, whereas the disease occurred in 37% of 8 persons who refused, or who were not given, the globulin. Clearly, the real meaning of these provocative results were clouded by the far-from-ideal study design.

Another study from the French group, on this occasion a controlled one, was reported by Kleinknecht *et al.* (1977). The investigators reasoned that consistently high levels of anti-HBs were needed in order to prevent hepatitis B. They thus arranged for hemodialysis patients, randomly selected, to receive HBIG (with an anti-HBs by PHA of 1:54,000) in a dose of 0.08 ml/kg every 5 weeks during a 6-month period and every 2 months thereafter until the study conclusion ~30 months later. Those not receiving HBIG received no other globulin material, but were followed in much the same fashion as the HBIG-treated group. Among the untreated "control" patients, 92% showed evidence of hepatitis B, and 77% developed clinical hepatitis. None of the treated patients developed clinical hepatitis, although 13% showed evidence of recent exposure to HBV. The evidence of minimal exposure to hepatitis B suggested that the HBIG had impaired passive–active immunization. Thus, multiple injections of HBIG appeared to afford complete protection, but at the expense of long-term immunity.

In 1977, Iwarson *et al.* reported results of a randomized, double-blind trial of globulins in Danish hemodialysis and laboratory staff members. They administered either HBIG (anti-HBs titer, 1:355,000 by PHA) or IG (anti-HBs titer, 1:100) on two occasions separated by 3 months, and followed the 110 recipients for a total of 28 months. They also evaluated a "control" group of 125 individuals from the same location who were unwilling to participate in the trial. Clinical hepatitis developed in 1.7% of the HBIG recipients, in 3.8% of IG recipients (no statistically significant difference between these two), and in 10.4% of the untreated group. Thus, both HBIG and IG appeared to afford protection, although, as pointed out by the authors, the control group was not a randomly selected one, a fact that might have adversely weighted the results.

The most ambitious and best-designed of the randomized, controlled trials was reported by Prince *et al.* (1978) from the United States. The study was designed to evaluate efficacy in both hemodialysis patients (284 patients) and staff members (280 staff). These individuals received 3 ml of either HBIG (anti-HBs titer, 1:500,000 by PHA), moderate-titer IG (anti-HBs titer, 1:5,000), or low-titer IG (anti-HBs titer, 1:50) on two occasions at 4-month intervals. The outcome differed somewhat between the patients and staff. The early results among the patients suggested that HBIG was highly effective; at 8 months, hepatitis B or HBsAg alone was detected in 5.5% of high-titer, 16.9% of intermediate-titer, and 18.5% of the low-titer globulin recipients. By the twelfth month, however, the frequencies had changed to the nonsignificant differences of 18.7, 20.8, and 21.7%, respectively. A similar trend was noted among the staff members, although a definite difference still existed at 12 months (HBIG, 12.5%, versus low-titer IG, 10.3%).

It thus appeared that the HBIG had either prolonged the incubation period or that reexposure to HBV had been responsible for futher cases. The investigators surmised that if the latter explanation was the correct one, then the use of more frequent injections might have proven effective. However, as they pointed out, this approach is prohibitively expensive, protentially dangerous, and probably unnecessary if careful surveillance and routine preventive measures are maintained, as has been shown in British hemodialysis units (Public Health Laboratory Service Report, 1974). The mechanism of action of HBIG in this study appeared to be that of passive–active immunization, since the incidence of hepatitis B and HBV infection combined was significantly lower in the HBIG than in the low-titer IG recipients. However, the similar effects of HBIG and of IG among patients in this study might have represented either equal benefit or equal lack of effect, an outcome that could not be established because of the absence of an appropriate control group.

D. Clotting Factor Concentrate-Related Hepatitis B

Clotting factor concentrates, such as factor VIII (antihemophilic factor, AHF) and Factor IX complex are made from the pooled plasma of a thousand or more donors. These labile factors, unless stabilized, cannot withstand the heating step applied to other plasma derivatives to inactivate HBV. Thus, although they may be HBsAg negative, it is probable that some of the preparations contain subdetectable levels of HBsAg, in view of the high frequency of HBV serological markers found in recipients. Accordingly, Tabor *et al.* (1980) undertook an experimental study aimed at removing HBV infectivity from these concentrates. Commercial factor IX complex was reconstituted, and to each of three samples $10^{3.5}$ chimpanzee infectious doses of HBV were added and the combination incubated for 1 hr. HBIG was then added to the two infected factor IX concentrates, and these were incubated for an additional 1 hr. The three samples (two infected, one uninfected) were then innoculated intravenously into three chimpanzees, who were followed for 52 weeks by weekly serological testing. Only the chimpanzee that received the infected inoculum without HBIG developed HBV infection, suggesting that products that may be infected with HBV, but cannot be heat treated because they contain labile factors, can possibly be "immune inactivated." It is noteworthy that the intravenous route of administration did not cause harm to the chimpanzees. Other investigators have suggested that this approach is neither feasible nor desirable because of potential side effects to the intravenous administration of IgG antibodies, the production of immune complexes, and the high cost (Sibinga *et al.*, 1980). In actuality, IgG antibodies are present in currently administered AHF and factor IX complex, and the amount of anti-HBs needed to "neutralize" HBV is small and relatively inexpensive.

VI. Postexposure Prophylaxis Studies

A. Transmission by Sexual Contact

In 1975, Redeker *et al.* reported results of a study that had been designed to evaluate the efficacy of HBIG for the prevention of secondary cases of hepatitis B in sexual contacts of persons with acute hepatitis B. Susceptible persons who had had regular sexual contact within 2 to 4 weeks of onset of acute disease in the index case were selected randomly to receive a single 5-ml injection of either HBIG (anti-HBs titer, 1:200,000 against **adw,** 1:500,000 against **ayw** subtypes of HBsAg), or a placebo globulin (prepared from plasma units without detectable anti-HBs) no later than 30 days after onset of the disease in the partner. The study participants were followed by both telephone questionnaire and spaced serological testing for a period of 40 weeks after the injection. The IG group received their injections between 7 days prior to 30 days following onset of jaundice in the contact (mean, 9.8 days), and the HBIG group, from 6 days before to 21 days after (mean, 10 days). Nine of 33 (27%)

control globulin-treated contacts followed for at least 150 days developed hepatitis B (6 icteric, 3 anicteric) as compared to 1 anicteric case among 25 (4%) HBIG recipients ($p = .02$). The HBIG recipients also showed a lower frequency of subclinical infection (i.e., anti-HBs development) than did the IG group (22% versus 5%), although this difference was not statistically significant ($p = .14$). Thus, these data suggested that HBIG was highly effective in preventing sexually transmitted hepatitis B, a well-documented means of spread of the disease (Judson, 1981). However, because in previous studies it had appeared that HBIG simply prolonged the incubation period of hepatitis B, and because the patients in this study had been followed for a period of only 5 months, the conclusions of this study were received with some scepticism. This concern was somewhat allayed by a later report from Mosley (1978) indicating that continued evaluation of the study participants for 7 to 12 months after injection had failed to reveal additional cases of hepatitis B.

A different conclusion has been reached in another randomized but not double-blinded trial that involved the participation of 60 subjects (Perrillo *et al.*, 1984). In this study, susceptible sexual partners of persons who had developed acute hepatitis B in the preceeding 6 weeks were given a single intramuscular injection either of HBIG or IG (anti-HBs titer, 1:32). The dose during the first year was 0.06 ml/kg body weight for both preparations, and follow-up was maintained for 1 year. During the second year, the dose of IG was increased approximately twofold, and the subjects were followed for 6 months. HBV events developed in 4 of 21 (19%) recipients of the low-dose IG; 2 of the 4 manifested as clinical hepatitis. Among the 19 HBIG recipients, 2 (11%) developed serological evidence of HBV infection, 1 of whom developed only anti-HBc 36 weeks after the injection, while in the 20 high-dose IG recipients, 3 (15%) developed an HBV event (HBsAg or anti-HBc only). In all instances, HBsAg disappeared rapidly. Thus, the HBV attack rates were not significantly different from one another, but they did differ significantly ($p < .002$) from the expected HBV infection rate that follows sexual contact of 33%, a figure derived by the authors from three previous studies. Although the number of individuals in the study was small, the data did show also that clinical illness in these globulin recipients occurred less frequently than would have been anticipated. The authors thus concluded that both conventional IG and HBIG appeared to provide passive–active immunization for sexual contacts of individuals with acute hepatitis B, and stated their view that IG in a dose of 0.12 ml/kg body weight is the preferred product for passive prophylaxis in this setting. It must be noted, however, that these conclusions are based on small numbers, that a concurrent placebo group was not studied (for ethical reasons, as stated), and that clinical hepatitis did occur even though only in the low-dose IG group.

B. Needle-Stick Studies

Several studies have been conducted to evaluate HBIG for the prevention of hepatitis B transmitted through accidental needle-stick exposure (British Medical Research Council/Public Health Laboratory Service Report, 1980; Grady *et al.*, 1978; Ichida *et al.*, 1980; Seeff *et al.*, 1978b); two were designed as double-blind, controlled trials (Grady *et al.*, 1978; Seeff *et al.*, 1978b).

One of these, a Veterans Administration Cooperative Study conducted between 1972 and 1975, included the participation of 11 hospitals (Seeff *et al.*, 1978b). A total of 419 susceptible persons exposed by accidental needle-stick to HBsAg-positive blood were selected randomly to receive two 5-ml injections of either HBIG (anti-HBs titer, 1:100,000 by PHA) or IG (anti-HBs titer, <1:8). The first injection was administered within 7 days of the accidental exposure, and the second ~28 days later. The study participants were followed thereafter at regular intervals for a total of 12 months. At the end of this period, hepatitis B had developed in 3 of 216 (1.4%) HBIG and in 12 of 203 (5.9%) IG recipients, a difference that was significant ($p = .016$). Two of the three cases in the HBIG group developed their disease beyond 22 weeks, while all 12 in the IG group were clustered between 9 and 14 weeks of exposure. The disease was icteric (i.e., serum bilirubin >2.4 mg%) in 14 of 15 cases. In contrast to the overt disease, the development of subclinical infection (i.e., anti-HBs without serum aminotransferase abnormalities) occurred significantly more frequently in the IG than the HBIG recipients.

In a later evaluation, it was determined that hepatitis had developed almost exclusively in individuals who had been exposed to HBsAg-positive material that was also positive for HBeAg (Alter *et al.*, 1976). Analysis of the effect of immunoprophylaxis in this group (i.e., those exposed to HBsAg-positive, HBeAg-positive blood) demonstrated a difference between HBIG and IG that was even more significant ($p < .001$). Of note is that among the IG recipients exposed to HBeAg-positive material (as identified by immunodiffusion), only 22% developed overt disease, while an additional 15.7% developed anti-HBs alone; this indicated that despite the positive history, not all of these individuals had suffered exposure to infectious material. These data suggested that HBIG was superior to a placebo-IG for the prevention of hepatitis B following small-volume percutaneous exposure, but the efficacy of currently available IG could not be ascertained from this study. The mechanism of action of the globulins in this study, as originally advanced (Seeff *et al.*, 1975), was that HBIG had prevented the disease by passive immunization while IG had induced passive–active immunity. However, a different interpretation emerged after stored sera from the study were restudied using more sensitive serological tests (Hoofnagle *et al.*, 1979). Among 296 individuals whose sera were available for reanalysis, hepatitis B occurred in 2% of those who had received HBIG and in 8% of those receiving IG, while subclinical HBV infection occurred in 10 and 4%, respectively, of these two groups. Thus, the total frequency of infection was equal in both groups. However, in light of the predominantly subclinical disease in the HBIG recipients, it appeared that HBIG had in fact permitted the occurrence of passive–active immunity.

An added finding was that anti-HBs without overt hepatic disease or other HBV serological markers had developed in 53 IG but in only 1 HBIG recipient. Because this is the serological pattern that follows active immunization (i.e., vaccination), the IG (manufactured in 1944 and thus predating HBsAg testing of plasma donors) was examined for the presence of HBsAg. No HBsAg could be detected, however, until the IG was ultracentrifuged through 30% acid–sucrose; HBsAg was then found in the supernatant. In contrast, no HBsAg was present in HBIG. Thus, it could be inferred that the IG had contained HBsAg–anti-HBs complexes, accounting for the lack of detectable HBsAg until the complexes were separated by the acid conditions, and that the released HBsAg was then presumably capable of inducing a vaccine-like response.

Support for this interpretation subsequently came from the reanalysis of two other postexposure prophylaxis studies in which IG of pre-1972 vintage had been evaluated. In the study by Szmuness *et al.* (1974) involving institutionalized mentally compromised individuals, 48% of the recipients of IG had developed anti-HBs without HBsAg or hepatitis B, which was attributed originally to passive–active immunity; however, this response can also be accounted for by active immunization. More direct evidence for this explanation was derived through the reexamination of the IG used in the study conducted earlier in Korea (Cooperative Study, 1971). Although originally reported to contain anti-HBs with a titer in excess of 1:1,280, repeat evaluation failed to identify anti-HBs, but occult HBsAg was found following acid–sucrose centrifugation (Lemon *et al.*, 1980). Thus, this globulin, like the one used in the VA study, appeared to behave as a moderately effective "vaccine," leading the investigators to conclude that this study should no longer be considered an example of one demonstrating efficacy of IG containing low-titer anti-HBs (i.e., equivalent to contemporary IG).

The second double-blind, controlled trial of immunoprophylaxis following accidental exposure, also a multicenter study, examined the relative efficacies of three globulins, one of high titer (anti-HBs, 1:500,000), one with an intermediate titer (1:5,000), and one with a titer equivalent to that of "normal-titer" globulin (1:50) (Grady *et al.*, 1978). A total of 435 susceptible medical personnel entered the trial. By the end of 4 months, no cases of hepatitis had occurred among the high-titer recipients, but almost 7% of intermediate- and low-titer globulin recipients had developed the disease. However, this significant difference disappeared by the end of the study when the incidence was noted to be 9.8, 10.2, and 12.3%, respectively. The late cases found in the high-titer group were attributed to reinfection in 20% of instances, and in the remainder, to prolongation of the incubation period induced by the HBIG. An extended incubation period had been noted also in the VA study as well as elsewhere (Froesner *et al.*, 1977b; Wauters and Leski, 1976). Another similarity to the VA study was that individuals with preexisting anti-HBs appeared to be completely protected, and that the presence of HBeAg defined particularly infectious HBsAg-positive inocula (U.S. National Heart and Lung Institute Collaborative Study Group, 1976). Indeed, they subsequently confirmed that this test discriminated adequately between infectious and noninfectious HBsAg-positive persons, since approximately one-fifth of persons exposed to HBeAg-positive sera developed hepatitis, whereas clinical hepatitis developed in only 2.5% of those exposed to anti-HBe positive sera and in none of those exposed to sera negative for both HBeAg and anti-HBe (Werner and Grady, 1982).

Thus, the results of these two studies differed. The precise reason is unclear, although one explanation offered is the possibility that the HBIG used in the latter study might have had compromised neutralizing ability in view of the discovery of fragmented anti-HBs (Grady *et al.*, 1982). In another effort to define a reason for the difference, retesting of the stored sera for anti-HBc was undertaken (similar to that performed in the VA study), but this only served to confirm and not explain the difference (Grady *et al.*, 1982). Of note is that the IG used in the National Cooperative Study also contained acid-dissociable HBsAg–anti-HBs complexes.

In other uncontrolled "needle-stick" studies, the conclusions reached were that HBIG was indeed protective. One of them, reported by the British Medical Research Council and Public Health Laboratory Service (1980), involved 322 persons who had been exposed to HBsAg-positive blood and had received a single 500-mg injection of high-titer globulin within 14 days of the accident. Three percent developed overt hepatitis

B, and an additional 2% seroconverted to anti-HBs without clinical illness. Because these figures resembled those of the VA study, the Working Party concluded that the globulin had been protective. Similar results were achieved in the other study, conducted in Japan (Ichida *et al.*, 1980).

C. Studies of Perinatally Transmitted (Maternal–Fetal; Vertical) Hepatitis B

Transmission of hepatitis B to infants from mothers who have acute hepatitis B in the third trimester (Schweitzer *et al.*, 1973) or who are HBsAg carriers (Beasley and Stevens, 1978) is well documented, and correlates strongly with the presence of HBeAg in the blood of the mother (Okuda *et al.*, 1976). Because these infants almost invariably become HBsAg carriers who are at great risk of developing hepatocellular carcinoma (Szmuness, 1978), interruption of HBV transmission at the time of birth is of extreme importance.

Kohler *et al.* (1974a) were the first investigators to attempt the prevention of perinatal transmission of hepatitis B with HBIG. They reported an uncontrolled study in which four neonates born to HBsAg-positive mothers were given HBIG within 1 to 6 days of delivery. All four remained HBsAg negative for 5 to 14 months, whereas six of seven untreated neonates born under the same circumstances became HBsAg carriers. Additional reports of uncontrolled studies followed involving the evaluation of both HBIG and IG. Dosik and Jhaveri (1978; Jhaveri *et al.*, 1980) found that HBIG administered on the day of birth and then at 5-week intervals for a period of 6 months prevented hepatitis B in an infant born to an HBsAg-positive mother; a sibling born a year earlier to the same mother had died at 2 months of age with fulminant hepatitis B.

In four subsequent studies, success was reported following the use of repetitive doses of HBIG. Reesink *et al.* (1979), in Holland, treated 21 children born to HBsAg carrier mothers (some also HBeAg positive) with HBIG in a dose of 0.05 ml/kg within 48 hr of birth, followed by 0.16 ml/kg at monthly intervals for 6 months. None of these infants developed HBsAg, whereas 5 of 20 children who were not treated, and 2 of 3 whose HBIG was not administered until the fourth or fifth day, became positive. A single case, reported from Sweden by Iwarson *et al.* (1979), involved an infant born to a drug addict mother positive for both HBsAg and HBeAg. The infant received the first HBIG injection on the day of birth, the second, 1 month later, and the third, 4 months after birth. The child remained HBsAg negative, but developed subclinical infection as indicated by the presence of anti-HBc and anti-HBs more than a year after the last injection, suggesting that passive–active immunization had been produced. The results of a study from the United States involving 13 infants born to HBsAg-positive mothers and treated "successfully" with five or six doses of HBIG presumably has limited meaning since all 13 mothers were HBeAg negative (Jhaveri *et al.*, 1980). However, encouraging results came from a study in Japan in which 44 neonates whose mothers were both HBsAg- and HBeAg-positive received repeated doses of HBIG (0.17 ml/kg), the first within 24-hr of birth and the others at 15-week intervals for an average of 3.7 doses (Yano *et al.*, 1980). One of these 44 infants (who had received only a single injection) became a carrier, while all of a group of untreated infants became carriers. The evidence suggesting that there is only limited value from a single injection of HBIG was confirmed in subsequent uncontrolled (Boxall *et al.*, 1980; Matsumoto *et al.*, 1979) and controlled (Beasley and Stevens, 1978) studies.

There have been two studies to evaluate conventional IG for the prevention of maternal–fetal transmission of hepatitis B, with conflicting results. Varma (1976) treated seven newborns of mothers with acute hepatitis in the third trimester (HBeAg status not reported) with 2 ml IG (equivalent to 0.06 ml/kg), the injection being administered within 1 week of delivery. None of the babies became carriers. A similar study was performed later by Tong *et al.*, (1979). These investigators studied infants born to carrier mothers (most of them positive also for HBeAg and/or DNA polymerase), as well as to mothers with acute hepatitis B. The infants received the same dose as that used by Varma, as a single injection within 7 days of birth (if the mother had had acute hepatitis), or two injections separated by 4 months (if the mother was a carrier and the infant did not develop HBV markers in the interim). Two-thirds of the infants in each category became HBsAg carriers.

The variability of these results underscored the need for a controlled trial. Thus far, two have been performed. The first of these, reported by Beasley and Stevens (1978), involved babies born to HBsAg carrier mothers in Taiwan. The babies were selected randomly to receive HBIG (with a titer of 1:200,000), IG, or an albumin placebo in a dose of 0.6 ml/kg. Although the intention was to treat the neonates as soon as possible after birth, the final data revealed that their mean age at the time of injection was 46 hr. The important findings of the study included the following: (a) at the end of a year, the overall frequency of HBsAg was slightly, although not significantly, lower in the HBIG than in the placebo group (60 versus ±70%); conversely, anti-HBs developed more frequently in the HBIG group (18 versus 3%), so that the overall frequency of HBV markers did not differ between the two groups; (b) among the placebo group who developed HBsAg, 90% did so within 5 months, as compared to 45% of the HBIG group (i.e, the development of HBsAg was delayed by HBIG); (c) antigenemia remained persistent a little less frequently in the HBIG (63%) than the placebo (83%) group, and conversely, was transient more frequently (38 versus 17%); and (d) the timing of HBIG administration played a critical role in the outcome, since 47% of the babies treated prior to 48 hr developed persistent antigenemia whereas *all* of those treated at 48 hr or later became persistently positive ($p = .03$). This suggested that future trials would require very early administration of HBIG.

Accordingly, the same investigators mounted a second double-blind, controlled trial in Taiwan that required that immunoprophylaxis be achieved immediately after birth (Beasley *et al.*, 1981). They also examined the effect of higher and of multiple doses. The study involved 117 infants who were born to HBsAg-, HBeAg-positive mothers, and who received one of three treatment regimens: (a) 1.0 ml saline at birth and again at 3 and 6 months; (b) 1.0 ml HBIG at birth, and saline at 3 and 6 months; and (c) 0.5 ml HBIG diluted in 0.5 ml IG at birth, 3, and 6 months. Evaluation of the infants continued for at least 15 months. The mean administration time was 36 min after birth, and 95% of the infants received their injection within 1 hr. HBsAg developed in 94, 79, and 75% of the three groups respectively, and remained persistently positive in 91, 30, and 23% of them. The efficacy rate for a *single* HBIG injection in reducing the carrier state was thus calculated to be 45%, and for the multiple injections schedule, 75%. Noteworthy is the fact that the majority of HBIG recipients developed active anti-HBs, an outcome that suggested the effect of passive–active immunization. Thus, this study demonstrated that early and repetitive injections of HBIG had a statistically highly significant effect in reducing HBsAg persistence, although this procedure did not prevent HBV infection.

The most recent study aimed at evaluating immunoprophylaxis for the interruption of perinatal transmission of hepatitis B was reported from California by Nair *et al.* (1984). To one group of 10 infants whose HBsAg-positive carrier mothers were also HBeAg positive, they administered, within 24 hr of birth, HBIG only in a dose of 0.15 ml/kg body weight. A second group of 20 neonates whose carrier mothers were anti-HBe positive received, by random selection, either HBIG or IG in the same dose. Both of these groups were given the same form and dose of immune globulin at 5-week intervals for a total of six injections. A third group, consisting of 4 newborns whose mothers had had acute hepatitis B during the third trimester, received only 2 doses of HBIG separated by

1 month. All three groups were followed for a period of 18 months for evidence of HBV infection. Three of the 10 infants in the first group developed HBsAg (at 10, 12, and 18 months of age), as did 1 of the 20 infants in the second group (an HBIG recipient, at 18 months) and 1 of the 4 in the third group (at 10 months). This outcome was interpreted to represent postnatal rather than perinatal (within 6 months of birth) infection, presumably a result of continued contact with their chronically infected mothers or siblings. The HBIG appeared to have conferred perinatal protection, but since most of the HBIG recipients retained anti-HBs only for the duration of the HBIG injections, they once again became susceptible to infection. The investigators thus concluded that both passive (with HBIG) and active (with vaccine) prophylaxis was needed in order to ensure prolonged protection, a topic that will be addressed subsequently.

VII. The Use of Globulin for the Treatment of Viral Hepatitis

Several groups of investigators have examined globulin products for their therapeutic value in patients with established viral hepatitis, but the results have been disappointing. Thus, in early studies, no benefit was found from the use of conventional IG in the treatment of either acute (Evans *et al.*, 1955) or chronic (Volwiler and Dealey, 1949) hepatitis. More recent studies have involved the evaluation of high-titer anti-HBs, administered as globulin or plasma, to patients with HBsAg-positive chronic hepatitis (Geffroy *et al.*, 1970; Kohler *et al.*, 1974b; Reed *et al.*, 1973) and fulminant hepatitis B (Acute Hepatic Failure Study Group, 1977; Gateau *et al.*, 1976), but these results, too have been negative, despite the initial encouraging reports regarding fulminant hepatitis (Cohen and Litt, 1972; Dupuy *et al.*, 1975; Gitnick *et al.*, 1974; Gocke, 1971). An important example is a national study conducted in the United States, in which a total of 63 patients with acute hepatitis B complicated by hepatic encephalopathy (Stages II–IV) were given an intravenous infusion of HBIG or an albumin placebo (Acute Hepatic Failure Study Group, 1977). The initial dose selected contained 1.32 g of immunoglobulin G protein in the belief that this was adequate to abolish viremia. However, the HBsAg level was not altered by this dose or by a later increase of the dose to 5.28g. Moreover, there was no significant difference noted in mortality between either of the two dosage groups or between them and the placebo recipients. Thus, current knowledge provides no support for the use of globulin products in the treatment of either acute or chronic hepatitis.

VIII. Combined Passive–Active Immunization

The data presented thus far suggest that passively administered anti-HBs is capable of preventing hepatitis B, albeit not completely; as defined in the postexposure studies involving a single exposure episode, the maximum protection rate has ranged between 75 and 78%. However, because administered anti-HBs has a relatively short half-life, passive immunoprophylaxis has only limited value in situations requiring preexposure prophylaxis, especially where contact with HBsAg persists. In these circumstances, the degree of protection appears to be enhanced by repeated injections of HBIG, but clearly this approach is inconvenient and time consuming, expensive, and potentially dangerous.

The advent of the hepatitis B vaccine appears to have provided a potential solution to this problem (Hilleman *et al.*, 1975; Redeker *et al.*, 1975). Early trials conducted among homosexual men chronically exposed to the hepatitis B virus had determined the vaccine to be highly immunogenic and protective (Francis *et al.*, 1982; Szmuness *et al.*, 1980). Furthermore, these studies suggested that the vaccine has a beneficial effect even among persons who have already been exposed to hepatitis B, a conclusion derived from the modified response noted in vaccinees during the early postinjection period; although the frequency of hepatitis B virus events was similar in the placebo and vaccine groups, the placebo recipients were more likely to have overt hepatitis B, and the vaccine recipients to have inapparent hepatitis or only an HBV-related serological response. Thus, the hepatitis B vaccine (like the rabies vaccine) appears to afford some degree of protection even when used after an exposure has already occurred.

To circumvent the problem of delayed immune response, Szmuness and co-workers (1981) undertook a study to evaluate the effect of combined passive–active immunization, using both HBIG and vaccine. Concerned that passive antibody from HBIG might interfere with or inhibit the development of vaccine-induced antibody, they studied three groups of age- and sex-matched medical personnel, each receiving a different treatment regimen. One group was administered an initial 3-ml injection of HBIG followed by the vaccine (20-μg dose) at 1 and 6 months, another was given both HBIG and vaccine at entry and then the vaccine alone at months 1 and 6, and the third received the vaccine only according to conventional protocol (0, 1, and 6 months). All persons of the first two groups were found to have detectable anti-HBs at the end of the first month, but anti-HBs was detected in only 52% of the third (vaccine alone) group at the comparable time. By the third month, the anti-HBs prevalence was still significantly higher in the first two groups as compared to the third, although the difference disappeared after the 6-month booster dose. Also of note is that the anti-HBs titer in the combined treatment groups exceeded that of the vaccine treatment group until after the 6-month injection, when the difference became nonsignificant. The study thus demonstrated the feasibility of immediate protection (passive–active immunity) from the simultaneous administration of HBIG and vaccine. Later, this group of investigators showed that the same effect could be achieved by the simultaneous administration of 20 μg of vaccine together with only 1.0 ml of HBIG (C. E. Stevens and W. Szmuness, personal communication).

Other investigators have also demonstrated a highly beneficial effect from passive–active immunization. Zachoval *et al.* (1982) found that anti-HBs could be identified within 2 hr in medical personnel who received combined HBIG and vaccine, with peak levels developing 2 to 4 days later. Goudeau *et al.* in France showed similar results in studies carried out in patients and staff in a hemodialysis unit (Goudeau *et al.*, 1982b), as well as among hospital staff members exposed accidently through a needle-stick injury to HBsAg-positive blood (Goudeau *et al.*, 1982a).

The most compelling of the passive–active immunization studies, however, is one conducted in Taiwan by Beasley *et al.* (1983) involving neonates born to mothers positive for both HBsAg and HBeAg. In this randomized, controlled trial, one group of 51 neonates received HBIG (0.5 ml) immediately after birth and again at 3 months of age, at which time they were also given hepatitis B vaccine (20 μg), followed by the same vaccine dose 1 and 6 months later. A second group of 50 neonates received a single injection of HBIG at birth and then began the same three-dose vaccine program starting at days 4 through 7. In a third group of 50 neonates, the HBIG was given immediately after birth and the vaccine program was initiated at 1 month of age. For all three groups, the mean time of administration of HBIG was 2.1 ± 4.8 hours. Among the total of 159 infants treated according to these various schedules, only 9 (5.7%) became chronic carriers, there being no significant differences between the three treatment groups. The remaining 150 neonates all developed anti-HBs, some in very high titer. These figures contrast with data acquired by these investigators from an earlier group of *untreated* infants, born to carrier mothers, in which it was found that 95.2% of them had developed evidence of HBV infection by 3 months of age, 92.5% of whom became HBsAg carriers. Thus, the protective efficacy of this combined prophylaxis program was 93.6%; this same group has found that the protective efficacy for HBIG alone is 72%, and for vaccine alone, 75%.

It is conceivable that future vaccines may be sufficiently immunogenic on their own to provide protection equal to that afforded by the combined passive–active immunization schedule using the current products. In the meantime, the combination of HBIG and hepatitis B vaccine represents an important and highly effective addition to the armamenterium available at present for postexposure prophylaxis.

IX. Current Recommendations for Prophylaxis of Hepatitis B

Official guidelines regarding the use of immune globulin for the prevention of hepatitis B have varied with the state of available knowledge at the time of their issuance. As recently as 1972, the view expressed by the Public Health Service Advisory Committee on Immunization Practices was that immune globulins were ineffective for this purpose and therefore could not be recommended. In 1977, the same committee, having by this time knowledge of hepatitis B virus serology, the availability of HBIG, and the benefit of numerous trials on which to base new conclusions, recommended that HBIG should be used following accidental needle-stick exposure to HBsAg-positive blood or secretions, as well as for infants born to mothers with acute HBsAg-positive hepatitis in the third trimester. They indicated also that since post-1972 IG contains detectable anti-HBs (albeit of low and variable titer), this product could be used, if HBIG were not available, for postexposure prophylaxis as outlined above, or for preexposure prophylaxis (if deemed advisable) of staff and patients in hemodialysis units and custodial institutions for the mentally retarded.

The most recent set of guidelines was issued by the Centers for Disease Control in 1981 (Public Health Service Advisory Committee on Immunization Practices, 1981). The basis for this new pronouncement appeared to be the continued uncertainty regarding the true benefit and place for the use of HBIG, the evidence that its efficacy is likely to be highest if used as soon as possible after exposure, the concerns about its high cost, the belief that conventional IG (containing low anti-HBs titers) has some protective value, and the logistical problems that surround the extended period needed to obtain the results of serological testing. Taking these items into account, and based on the evidence that exposure to blood *known* to contain HBsAg leads to clinical hepatitis B in ~1 in 20 instances, while exposure to blood of *unknown* HBsAg status is associated with a risk of ~1 in 2000, they constructed the following responses for nonimmune (anti-HBs-negative) exposed persons.

A. Postexposure Prophylaxis

1. Percutaneous (Needle-Stick) Exposure
   a. Known HBsAg-Positive Source. Immediate (within 24 hr) administration of HBIG (0.06 ml/kg) or of IG (only if HBIG is unavailable), followed by a second identical dose 1 month later.
   b. Known Source, Unknown HBsAg Status.
      i. High-risk source (e.g., acute unidentified viral hepatitis, persons with Downs' Syndrome, hemodialysis patients, persons from Asia, homosexual men and parenteral drug abusers): Immediate (within 24 hr) administration of IG (0.06 ml/kg), followed as soon as possible (but no later than 7 days) by HBIG (if blood tests demonstrate HBsAg), with a repeat dose 1 month later
      ii. Low-risk source (average hospital patient): HBsAg testing not recommended and prophylaxis optional; a single dose of IG, 0.06 ml/kg (within 24 hr) is suggested if prophylaxis is undertaken
   c. Both Source and HBsAg Status Unknown. Same approach as that described above for low-risk source
2. Perinatal Exposure
   Administer HBIG (total dose of 0.5 ml, given intramuscularly) as soon as possible after birth (no later than 24 hr), with the same dose repeated at 3 and 6 months of age.
3. Sexual Exposure to Persons with Acute Hepatitis B
   No specific recommendation, although HBIG is not precluded if prophylaxis is considered to be desirable.

B. Preexposure Prophylaxis

1. Hemodialysis Staff and Patients
   Routine prophylaxis is not recommended. However, if surveillance measures and general barrier precautions fail, IG (0.05–0.07 ml/kg) every 4 months can be considered.

2. Staff and Patients in Institutions for the Mentally Disabled
   The same approach is suggested as that advised for hemodialysis units. Finally, it must be emphasized that preexisting anti-HBs, representing evidence of past exposure, is protective, and hence precludes the need for immunoprophylaxis.

X. Additional Considerations Regarding Immunoprophylaxis

In the opinion of the present author, other approaches might be considered for some aspects of these guidelines. For example, it seems inappropriate to depend for protection entirely on IG for the person exposed to an apparent low-risk source if that source is HBsAg positive. An alternative strategy, therefore, is either to proceed with the steps taken following a high-risk exposure, as outlined above, or to select the appropriate immune globulin only after studying, at the earliest possible time, the serological status of the contaminating source and the exposed person. Obviously, if neither the source nor the HBsAg status is available, the use of IG alone does seem a rational approach.

With regard to the exciting data of the passive–active immunization studies, it is apparent that the combination of HBIG and vaccination provides the greatest likelihood for success for prophylaxis applied postexposure. At the time of this writing, no official recommendation has been forthcoming regarding the use of combined prophylaxis. This regime should receive official sanction, and, indeed, it is now being applied routinely for situations currently regarded as appropriate for postexposure prophylaxis, especially where the potential for continued exposure exists. Thus, a combination of HBIG (0.6 ml/kg) and hepatitis B vaccine (20 μg), followed by a second and third injection of the vaccine alone 1 and 6 months later, should be administered to nonimmune medical personnel who sustain a needle-stick exposure to HBsAg-positive blood, for neonates born to a mother who is positive for HBsAg at the time of delivery (particularly if she is also HBeAg-positive and is known to be a carrier), and for the sexual partner of a person who is an HBsAg-positive carrier.

The degree of benefit that can be expected for sexual contacts of an individual with *acute* hepatitis B is uncertain. There are three alternative approaches that may be considered in this situation: (a) to administer no treatment at all in view of the controversy regarding the benefits of immunoprophylaxis for sexual exposure; (b) to administer a single dose of HBIG; or (c) to employ combined prophylaxis on the basis that the emergence of a carrier state in a person with acute hepatitis B cannot be accurately predicted at the outset of the illness; the receipt of the remaining two doses of vaccine would then be predicated on the outcome of the acute disease in the index case.

Implicit in the currently available data documenting the remarkable immunogenicity and efficacy of the hepatitis B vaccine is that passive prophylaxis with HBIG for preexposure circumstances need no longer be an issue of debate. There is now little doubt that all nonimmune persons who work or reside in situations of high risk should receive the vaccine either before or as early as possible after entering this environment. Provided a successful active immune response results (i.e., anti-HBs develops), full protection against future exposure, at least for a period of ~5 years, can be anticipated; there is currently conjecture that an additional booster dose will be needed 5 years after the initial injection. It must be recalled, however, that 5–15% of vaccinees fail to develop anti-HBs. Accordingly, should a hepatitis B-positive needle-stick exposure occur subsequently, it is prudent to examine any such individual for anti-HBs so as to permit repeat immunization if it is not found.

It is evident that during the past decade, the ability to prevent hepatitis B has been remarkably facilited by the rapidly advancing knowledge regarding its epidemiology, the development of increasingly sensitive serological tests for markers of HBV, and the advent of HBIG and hepatitis B vaccine. There is now the exciting possibility that hepatitis B can, in the foreseeable future, be eliminated as a major public health problem in the United States.

References

Acute Hepatic Failure Study Group (1977). *Ann. Intern. Med.* **86,** 272.
Advisory Committee on Immunization Practices (1968). *Ann. Intern. Med.* **69,** 1009.
Alter, H. J., Seeff, L. B., Kaplan, P. M., McAuliffe, V. J., Wright, E. C., Gerin, J. L., Purcell, R. H., Holland, P. V., and Zimmerman, H. J. (1976). *N. Engl. J. Med.* **295,** 909.
Beasley, R. P., and Stevens, C. E. (1978). *In* "Viral Hepatitis" (G. N. Vyas, S. W. Cohen, and R. Schmid, eds.), pp. 333–345. Franklin Inst. Press, Philadelphia, Pennsylvania.
Beasley, R. P., Hwang, L.-Y., Lin, C.-C., Stevens, C. E., Wang, K.-Y., Sun, T.-S., Hsieh, F.-S., and Szmuness, W. (1981). *Lancet 2,* 388.
Beasley, R. P., Hwang, L.-Y., Lee, G. C.-Y., Lan, C.-C., Roan, C.-H., Huang, F.-Y., and Chen, C.-L. C. (1983). *Lancet 2,* 1099.
Blumberg, B. S., Alter, H. J., and Visnich, S. (1965). *JAMA, J. Am. Med. Assoc.* **191,** 541.

Boxall, E. H., Flewett, T. H., Derso, A., and Tarlow, M. J. (1980). *Lancet 1*, 419.

British Medical Research Council/Public Health Laboratory Service Report (1980). *Lancet 1*, 6.

Bryan, J. A., and Gregg, M. B. (1975). *Am. J. Med. Sci.* **270**, 271.

Cohen, M. I., and Litt, I. F. (1972). *J. Pediatr.* **80**, 851.

Cohn, E. J., Oncley, J. L., Strong, L. E., Hughes, W. L., Jr., and Armstrong, S. H., Jr. (1944). *J. Clin. Invest.* **23**, 417.

Cooperative Study. *Arch. Intern. Med.* **128**, 723.

Couroucé-Pauty, A.-M., Delons, S., and Soulier, J.-P. (1975). *Am. J. Med. Sci.* **270**, 375.

Creutzfeldt, W., Severidt, H.-J., Brachmann, H., Schmidt, G., and Tschaepe, V. (1966). *Dtsch. Med. Wochenschr.* **91**, 1905.

Csapo, J., Budai, J., Bartos, A., and Nyerges, G. (1963). *Acta Paediatr. Acad. Sci. Hung.* **4**, 195.

Desmyter, J., Bradburne, A. F., Vermylen, C., Daneels, R., and Boelaert, J. (1975). *Lancet 2*, 377.

Dosik, H., and Jhaveri, R. (1978). *N. Engl. J. Med.* **298**, 602.

Drake, M. E., Barondess, J. A., Bashe, W. S., Jr., Henle, G., Stokes, J. Jr., and Pennell, R. B. (1953). *JAMA, J. Am. Med. Assoc.* **152**, 690.

Duncan, G. G., Christian, H. A., Stokes, J. Jr., Rexer, W. F., Nicholson, J. T., and Edgar, A. (1947). *Am. J. Med. Sci.* **213**, 53.

Dupuy, J. M., Frommel, D., and Alagille, D. (1975). *Lancet 1*, 191.

Enders, J. R. (1944). *J. Clin. Invest.* **23**, 510.

Evans, A. S., Nelson, R. S., Sprinz, H., and Cantrell, F. P. (1955). *Am. J. Med.* **19**, 783.

Feinstone, S. M., Kapikian, A. Z., and Purcell, R. H. (1973). *Science* **182**, 1026.

Francis, D. P., Handler, S. C., Thompson, S. E., Maynard, J. E., Ostrow, D. G., Altman, N., Braff, E. H., O'Malley, P., Hawkins, D., Judson, F. N., Penley, K., Nylund, T., Christie, Q., Meyers, F., Moore, J. N., Gardner, A., Doto, I. L., Miller, J. H., Reynolds, G. H., Murphy, B. L., Schable, C. A., Clark, B. T., Curran, J. W., and Redeker, A. L. (1982). *Ann. Intern. Med.* **97**, 362.

Froesner, G. G., Haas, H., and Hotz, G. (1977a). *Lancet 1*, 432.

Froesner, G. G., Froesner, H.-R., Deinhardt, F., Haussman, W., and Knabf, U. H. (1977b). *Lancet 2*, 1023.

Gateau, P. H., Opolon, P., Nusinovici, V., Ropars, C., and Caroli, J. (1976). *Digestion* **14**, 304.

Geffroy, Y., Colin, R., Paillot, B., Heicketsweiler, P., Ropartz, C., Rivat, L., Laumonier, R., and Fordimare, A. (1970). *Presse Med.* **78**, 1578.

Gellis, S. S., Stokes, J. Jr., Brother, G. M., Hall, W. M., Gilmore, H. R., Beyer, E., and Morrissey, R. A. (1945). *JAMA, J. Am. Med. Assoc.* **128**, 1062.

Gerety, R. J., Smallwood, L. A., and Tabor, E. (1980). *N. Engl. J. Med.* **303**, 529.

Ginsberg, A. L., Conrad, M. E., Bancroft, W. H., Ling, C. M., and Overby, L. R. (1972). *N. Engl. J. Med.* **286**, 562.

Gitnick, G., Hartman, D. I., and Madden, S. C. (1974). *West. J. Med.* **120**, 241.

Gocke, D. J. (1971). *N. Engl. J. Med.* **284**, 919.

Gocke, D. J., Greenberg, H. B. V., and Kavey, N. B. (1970). *JAMA, J. Am. Med. Assoc.* **212**, 877.

Goudeau, A., Maupas, P., Dubois, F., and Coursaget, P. (1982a). *In* "Viral Hepatitis" (W. Szmuness, H. J. Alter, and J. E. Maynard, eds.), p. 579. Franklin Inst. Press, Philadelphia, Pennsylvania.

Goudeau, A., Geslin, N., Dubois, F., Pierre, D., Lesage, G., Yvonnet, B., Coursaget, P., and Maupas, P. (1982b). *In* "Viral Hepatitis" (W. Szmuness, H. J. Alter, and J. E. Maynard, eds.), pp. 758–759. Franklin Inst. Press, Philadelphia, Pennsylvania.

Grady, G. F., Rodman, M., and Larsen, L. H. (1975). *J. Infect. Dis.* **132**, 474.

Grady, G. F., Lee, V. A., Prince, A. M., Gitnick, G. L., Fawaz, K. A., Vyas, G. N., Levitt, K. P., Senior, J. D., Galambos, J. T., Bynum, T. E., Singleton, J. W., Clowdus, B. F., Akeemar, K., Aach, R. D., Winkelman, E. I., Schiff, G. M., and Hersh, T. (1978). *J. Infect. Dis.* **138**, 625.

Grady, G. F., Cyr, K. M., and Werner, B. G. (1982). *In* "Viral Hepatitis" (W. Szmuness, H. J. Alter, and J. E. Maynard, eds.), p. 753. Franklin Inst. Press, Philadelphia, Pennsylvania.

Grossman, E. B., Stewart, S. G., and Stokes, J. Jr. (1945). *JAMA, J. Am. Med. Assoc.* **129**, 991.

Havens, W. P., Jr., and Paul, J. R. (1945). *JAMA, J. Am. Med. Assoc.* **129**, 270.

Hilleman, M. R., Buynak, E. B., Roehm, R. R., Tytell, A. A., Bertland, A. U., and Lampsom, G. D. (1975). *Am. J. Med. Sci.* **270**, 401.

Holland, P. V., Rubinson, R. M., Morrow, A. G., and Schmidt, P. J. (1966). *JAMA, J. Am. Med. Assoc.* **196**, 471.

Hoofnagle, J. H., and Waggoner, J. G. (1980). *Gastroenterology* **78**, 259.

Hoofnagle, J. H., Gerety, R. J., and Barker, L. F. (1975). *Transfusion* **15**, 408.

Hoofnagle, J. H., Seeff, L. B., Bales, Z. B., Wright, E. C., and Zimmerman, H. J. (1979). *Ann. Intern. Med.* **91**, 813.

Ichida, F., Yoshikawa, A., Komina, K., Hirasawa, Y., Kanoh, H., Yano, M., and Kikuchi, K. (1980). *Gastroenterol. Jpn.* **15**, 407.

Iwarson, S., Ahlmen, J., Eriksson, E., Hermodsson, S., Kjellman, H., Ljunggren, C., and Selender, D. (1977). *J. Infect. Dis.* **135**, 473.

Iwarson, S., Norkrans, G., Hermodsson, S., and Nordenfelt, E. (1979).*Scand. J. Infect. Dis.* **11**, 167.

Jhaveri, R., Rosenfeld, W., Salazar, J. D., Dosik, H., Chang, C.-C., and Evans, H. E. (1980). *J. Pediatr.* **97**, 305.

Judson, F. N. (1981). *Sex. Transm. Dis.* **8**, Suppl., 336.

Katz, R., Rodriquez, R., and Ward, R. (1971). *N. Engl. J. Med.* **285**, 925.

Kleinknecht, D., Courouce, A. M., Delons, S., Naret, C., Adhemar, J. P., Ciancioni, C., and Fermaman, J. (1977). *Clin. Nephrol.* **8**, 373.

Knodell, R. G., Contrad, M. E., Ginsberg, A. L., and Bell, C. J. (1976). *Lancet, 1,* 557.

Kohler, P. F., Dubois, R. S., Merrill, D. A., and Bowes, W. A. (1974a). *N. Engl. J. Med.* **291**, 1378.

Kohler, P. F., Trembath, J., Merrill, D. A., Singleton, J. W., and Dubois, R. S. (1974b). *Clin. Immunol. Immunopathol.* **2**, 465.

Krugman, S., Giles, J. P., and Hammond, J. (1971). *JAMA, J. Am. Med. Assoc.* **218**, 1665.

Kuhns, W. J., Prince, A. M., Brotman, B., Hazzi, C., and Grady, G. F. (1976). *Am. J. Med. Sci.* **272**, 251.

Lemon, S. M., Gates, N., and Bancroft, W. H. (1980). *Ann. Intern. Med.* **92**, 869.

Matsumoto, S., Tomigashi, T., and Fujmoto, S. (1979). *Perinatology* **9**, 615.

Miller, W. J., Provost, P. J., McAleer, W. J., Ihensohn, O. L., Villarejos, V. M., and Hilleman, M. R. (1975). *Proc. Soc. Exp. Biol. Med.* **149**, 254.

Mirick, G. S., Ward, R., and McCollum, R. W. (1965). *N. Engl. J. Med.* **273**, 59.

Mosley, J. W. (1978). *In* "Viral Hepatitis" (G. N. Vyas, S. N. Cohen, and R. Schmid, eds.), p. 603. Franklin Inst. Press, Philadelphia, Pennsylvania.

Nain, P. V., Weissman, J. Y., Tong, M. J., Thursby, M. W., Paul, R. H., and Henneman, C. E. (1984). *Gastroenterology* **87,** 293.

Okuda, K., Kamijama, I., Inomata, M., Imai, M., Miyakawa, Y., and Mayumi, M. (1976). *N. Engl. J. Med.* **294,** 746.

Perrillo, R., Campbell, C., and Castigan, D. (1978). *Hepatology* **1,** 536.

Perrillo, R. P., Campbell, C. R., Strang, S., Bodicky, C. J., and Costigan, D. J. (1984). *Arch. Intern. Med.* **144,** 81.

Prince, A. M., Szmuness, W., Woods, K. P., and Grady, G. F. (1971). *N. Engl. J. Med.* **285,** 933.

Prince, A. M., Szmuness, W., Mann, M. K., Vyas, G. N., Grady, G. F., Shapiro, F. L., Suki, W. N., Freidman, E. A., Avram, M. M., and Stenzel, K. H. (1978). *J. Infect. Dis.* **137,** 131.

Prospective Cooperative Study (1972). *JAMA, J. Am. Med. Assoc.* **220,** 692.

Public Health Laboratory Service Report (1974). *Br. Med. J.* **4,** 751.

Public Health Service Advisory Committee on Immunization Practices (1972). *Ann. Intern. Med.* **77,** 427.

Public Health Service Advisory Committee on Immunization Practices (1977). *Mortal. Morbid. Week. Rep.* **26,** 425–442.

Public Health Service Advisory Committee on Immunization Practices (1981). *Mortal. Morbid. Week. Rep.* **30,** 423–435.

Purcell, R. H., and Gerin, J. L. (1975). *Am. J. Med. Sci.* **270,** 395.

Redeker, A. G., Mosley, J. W., Gocke, D. J., McKee, A. P., and Pollack, W. (1975). *N. Engl. J. Med.* **293,** 1055.

Reed, W. D., Eddleston, A. L. W. F., Cullens, H., Williams, R., Zuckerman, A. J., Peters, D. K., Williams, D. G., and Maycock, W. D. A. (1973). *Lancet* **2,** 1347.

Reesink, H. W., Reerink-Brongers, E. E., Lafeber-Schut, B. J. T., Kalshoven-Benschop, J., and Brummehuis, H. G. J. (1979). *Lancet* **2,** 436.

Schweitzer, I. L., Dunn, A. E. G., Peters, R. L., and Spears, R. L. (1973). *Am. J. Med.* **55,** 762.

Seeff, L. B., Zimmerman, H. J., Wright, E. C., Felsher, B. F., Finkelstein, J. D., Garcia-Pont, P., Greenlee, H. P., Dietz, A. A., Hamilton, J., Koff, R. S., Leevy, C. M., Kiernan, T., Tamburro, C. H., Schiff, E. R., Vlahcevic, Z., Zemel, R., Zimmon, D. S., and Nath, N., (1975). *Lancet* **2,** 939.

Seeff, L. B., Zimmerman, H. J., Wright, E. C., Finkelstein, J. D., Garcia-Pont, P., Greenlee, H. B., Dietz, A. A., Leevy, C. M., Tamburro, C. H., Schiff, E. R., Schimmel, E. M., Zemel, R., Zimmon, D. S., and McCollum, R. W. (1977). *Gastroenterology* **72,** 111.

Seeff, L. B., Wright, E. C., Zimmerman, H. J., Hoofnagle, J. H., Dietz, A. A., Felsher, B. F., Garcia-Pont, P., Gerety, R. J., Greenlee, H. B., Kiernan, T., Leevy, C. M., Nath, N., Schiff, E. R., Schwartz, C., Tabor, E., Tamburro, C. H., Vlahcevic, Z., Zemel, R., and Zimmon, D. S. (1978a). *In* "Viral Hepatitis" (G. N. Vyas, S. N. Cohen, and R. Schmid, eds.), pp. 371–381. Franklin Inst. Press, Philadelphia, Pennsylvania.

Seeff, L. B., Wright, E. C., Zimmerman, H. J., Alter, H. J., Dietz, A. A., Felsher, B. F., Finkelstein, J. D., Garcia-Pont, P., Gerin, J. L., Greenlee, H. B., Hamilton, J., Holland, P. V., Kaplan, P. M., Kiernan, T., Koff, R. S., Leevy, C. M., McAuliffe, V. J., Nath, N., Purcell, R. H., Schiff, E. R., Schwartz, C. C., Tamburro, C. H., Vlahcevic, Z., Zemel, R., and Zimmon, D. S. (1978b). *Ann. Intern. Med.* **88,** 285.

Sibinga, C. T. S., Das, P. C., and Nieweg, H. O. (1980). *Lancet* **2,** 537.

Smallwood, L. A., Tabor, E., Finlayson, J. S., and Gerety, R. J. (1980). *Lancet* **2,** 482.

Soulier, J.-P., Blatix, C., Couroucé, A. M., Benamon, D., Amouch, P., and Drouet, J. (1972). *Am. J. Dis. Child.* **123,** 429.

Spellberg, M. A., and Berman, P. M. (1971). *Am. J. Gasteoenterol.* **55,** 564.

Stokes, J., Jr., and Neefe, J. R. (1945). *JAMA, J. Am. Med. Assoc.* **127,** 144.

Stokes, J., Jr., Blanchard, M., Neefe, J. R., Gellis, S. S., and Wade, C. R. (1948). *JAMA, J. Am. Med. Assoc.* **138,** 336.

Szmuness, W. (1978). *Prog. Med. Virol.* **24,** 40.

Szmuness, W., Prince, A. M., Goodman, M., Ehrich, C., Pick, R., and Ansari, M. (1974). *N. Engl. J. Med.* **290,** 701.

Szmuness, W., Stevens, C. E., Harley, E. J., Zang, E. A., Oleszko, W. R., Williams, D. C., Sodowsky, R., Morrison, J. M., and Kellner, A. (1980). *N. Engl. J. Med.* **303,** 833.

Szmuness, W., Stevens, C. E., Oleszko, W. R., and Goodman, A. (1981). *Lancet 1,* 575.

Tabor, E., Aronson, D. L., and Gerety, R. J. (1980). *Lancet 2,* 68.

Telischi, M., Ziyai, M., Steigmann, F., and Ling, C. M. (1980). *JAMA, J. Am. Med. Assoc.* **244,** 2312.

Tong, M. J., McPeak, C. M., Thursby, M. W., Schweitzer, I. L., Henneman, C. E., and Ledger, W. J. (1979). *Gastroenterology* **76,** 536.

U. S. National Heart and Lung Institute Collaborative Study Group (1976). *Lancet 2,* 492.

Varma, R. R. (1976). *JAMA, J. Am. Med. Assoc.* **236,** 2302.

Volwiler, W., and Dealey, J. P., Jr. (1949). *Gastroenterology* **12,** 87.

Wauters, J. P., and Leski, M. (1976). *Br. Med. J.* **2,** 19.

Werner, B. G., and Grady, G. F. (1982). *Ann. Intern. Med.* **97,** 367.

Yano, M., Koga, M., Sato, A., Masumoto, T., and Kubota, K. (1980). *Gastroenterology* **79,** 1131.

Zachoval, R., Deinhardt, F., Frösner, H., and Frösner, G. (1982). *In* "Viral Hepatitis" (W. Szmuness, H. J. Alter, and J. E. Maynard, eds.), pp. 757–758. Franklin Inst. Press, Philadelphia, Pennsylvania.

Chapter 16

Active Immunization/HBsAg Particle Vaccines

ROBERT J. GERETY
Center for Drugs and Biologics
Office of Biologics Research and Review
Food and Drug Administration
Bethesda, Maryland

I. Introduction

During acute and chronic hepatitis B infections, hepatitis B virus (HBV), in addition to excess, noninfectious hepatitis B surface antigen (HBsAg) particles, are released into the blood from infected liver cells. Routinely, noninfectious HBsAg particles including "tubules" 20–22 nm in cross-section that are variable in length and "spheres" 20–22 nm in diameter far outnumber infectious HBV in the blood. In plasma selected from certain asymptomatic HBsAg carriers, the ratio of noninfectious

385

Copyright © 1985 by Academic Press, Inc.
All rights of reproduction in any form reserved.
ISBN 0-12-280672-7

HBsAg particles to infectious HBV can be 10,000 to 1 (Tabor *et al.*, 1983a). The concentration of HBsAg in such plasma can reach 100–200 μg/ml of protein.

After the discovery of HBsAg in 1964 and the determination that it represented the outer coat (capsid) of HBV later in the 1960s, it became clear that noninfectious 20- to 22-nm spheres of HBsAg visible by electron microscopy could be effectively separated from among the larger, more dense HBV by ultracentrifugation (Bond and Hall, 1972). The ability to separate these noninfectious HBsAg spheres from HBV, the high concentrations of HBsAg in plasma, and the knowledge that HBV could be inactivated by heat and other methods permitted the development of plasma-derived HBsAg particle vaccines for the prevention of hepatitis B. Early studies of Krugman and co-workers (1970) had shown that serum containing HBV–HBsAg, when boiled and injected into humans prior to exposure to HBV, was immunogenic and provided protection against hepatitis B.

To produce plasma-derived HBsAg particle vaccines, the small, less dense HBsAg spheres in the plasma of asymptomatic carriers of HBsAg are separated by ultracentrifugation (and/or precipitation, chromatography, or solid-phase immunoadsorption) from among the larger, more dense HBV (Fig. 1). The spheres, once separated, are treated first for the purpose of purification and later to inactivate viruses (including HBV) that might be present in the starting plasma and co-purify with the HBsAg spheres. Data concerning the inactivation of viruses by steps in the manufacture of the United States-licensed hepatitis B vaccine, as well as a discussion of the general safety of this vaccine, appear in Gerety and Tabor (1982) and in Sections III,B, IV,A, and IV,C below. The plasma-derived HBsAg particle vaccine of Merck, Sharp & Dohme (MSD) was licensed in the United States after being tested in chimpanzees and humans. It has proved safe and effective at preventing hepatitis B, and has been recommended routinely for use in certain high-risk populations. To date, it has been given to hundreds of thousands of recipients.

HBsAg particles similar to the spheres observed in and purified from plasma are produced by a cell line derived from a human hepatocellular carcinoma (PLC/PRF 5) and by genetically engineered systems including yeast, mammalian cells, and vaccinia virus. In the case of the PLC/PRF 5 cells, the entire HBV genome was apparently inserted into the cellular DNA under conditions existing in the infected liver cells during HBV infection. In the case of the yeast and the mammalian cell lines, a piece of the HBV genome coding for HBsAg was intentionally inserted into the cellular DNA or via suitable vectors. In all but the vaccinia (here an HBV genome fragment is inserted into the virus), "spheres" of HBsAg

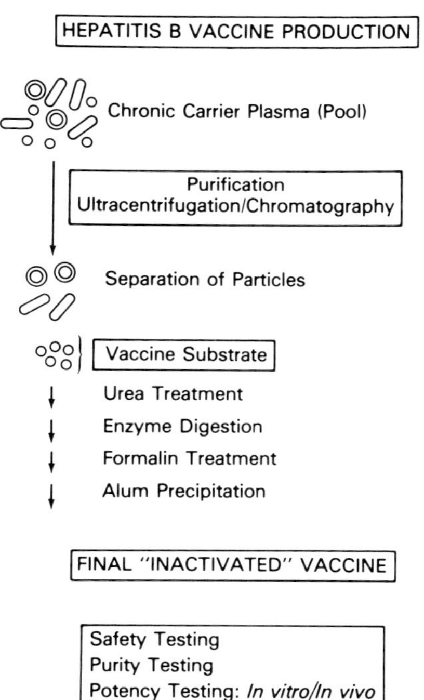

Figure 1. The manufacture of plasma-derived HBsAg particle vaccine (MSD). The "spheres" are separated from "tubules" and HBV by ultracentrifugation and subjected to procedures to accomplish purification and virus inactivation. The "spheres" are then adsorbed to alum to yield the final alum-adsorbed, inactivated, plasma-derived HBsAg particle vaccine.

are harvested and purified either from cell culture supernatants or after breakage of the cells to release the HBsAg. With the vaccinia, vaccinated recipients infected with virus recombinants produce HBsAg in their infected cells resulting in immunity to variola and also to HBV.

Unlike HBsAg purified from plasma, genetically derived HBsAg spheres should be free from infectious HBV, since only that portion of the HBV genome coding for HBsAg has been inserted. In the case of the PLC/PRF 5 cells, complete copies of the HBV genome have been "naturally" inserted during HBV infection, but no complete HBV appear to be produced by these cells (Tabor *et al.*, 1981).

Immunity against different HBsAg–HBV subtypes ("broad-spectrum HBV immunity") has been provided by immunization with plasma-derived HBsAg particle vaccines produced from large pools of human plasma from asymptomatic chronic carriers of HBsAg. Whether a "homogeneous" pool of HBsAg particles (as opposed to the "heterogeneous" HBsAg particles present in large pools of carrier plasma) can

also provide similar broad-spectrum immunity against diverse HBV subtypes has not yet been determined with certainty. Preliminary data suggest that genetically derived HBsAg particles can provide this type of
immunity, however.

II. Early Studies

A. HBsAg

The discovery of HBsAg (the first HBV-associated antigen to be recognized) and the determination that it was specifically associated with
hepatitis B (Blumberg *et al.*, 1965, 1967; Prince, 1968; Giles *et al.*, 1969;
Okochi and Murakami, 1968) permitted systematic studies to determine
its physical and chemical as well as antigenic makeup. Intense efforts in
a number of laboratories to characterize HBsAg employed purification
methods including isopycnic and rate-zonal ultracentrifugation, sometimes in combination with precipitation steps, gel filtration, and solid-
phase immunoadsorption. When either plasma or semipurified concentrated preparations of HBsAg was viewed by electronmicroscopy, three
morphologically distinct particles could be identified. These particles are
filaments (20–22 nm in width and variable in length), 20- to 22-nm
spheres, and a complex double-shelled particle 40–42 nm in diameter.
The former two particles clearly represented noninfectious HBV capsid
material, while the latter, first described by Dane *et al.* (1970) and often
referred to as "Dane" particles, are almost certainly HBV particles.

Studies of HBsAg purified from human plasma have provided a great
deal of information about the physical and chemical properties of this
lipoprotein antigen and its constituent polypeptides (see Chapters 2, 17,
and 18). The buoyant density of HBsAg "spheres" is ~1.21 g/cm^3. Amino acid analyses reveal a high proportion of acidic amino acids, accounting for the acidic isoelectric pH of HBsAg (Dreesman *et al.*, 1972). Compared to other viral coat proteins, HBsAg has higher concentrations of
cysteine (or cystine), proline, leucine, and phenylalanine, and lower
concentrations of lysine, arginine, aspartate, and glutamate. Although it
is predominantly protein, lipid, mostly in the form of phospholipids
(phosphatidylcholine and sphingomyelin) are a part of HBsAg (Alter
and Blumberg, 1966; Steiner *et al.*, 1974). Carbohydrate is also present as
glycoprotein and perhaps as glycolipid (Chairez *et al.*, 1973; Burrell *et al.*,
1973).

Early studies suggested that HBsAg is largely dependent on intact
disulfide bonds to retain its immunogenicity (Sukeno *et al.*, 1972; Vyas *et
al.*, 1972). Recent studies using either polypeptides derived from intact

HBsAg or chemically synthesized (see Chapter 18) indicate that the immunogenicity of HBsAg may be independent of both carbohydrate and lipid as well as somewhat independent of secondary structure.

As well as being morphologically heterogeneous, HBsAg is antigenically heterogeneous. It possesses a group determinant **a** (common to all HBsAg), and at least two pairs of allelic subgroup determinants designated **d/y** and **w/r** (LeBouvier and Williams, 1975). Immunity to all HBV is associated with actively acquired antibody (anti-HBs) directed against the a determinant of HBsAg. Anti-HBs, or other immune mediators directed to subgroup determinants, probably participate in immunity to HBV infection when the potentially infecting virus bears these determinants; anti-**a** antibodies alone, however, can provide immunity.

B. Studies in Laboratory Animals

Prior to the availability of specific serological tests capable of detecting HBsAg and anti-HBs, attempts to transmit hepatitis B to laboratory animals or nonhuman primates were unsuccessful. Using available serological tests, it was soon found that chimpanzees frequently had HBsAg or anti-HBs in their sera, as did gibbons and gorillas; laboratory animals were routinely devoid of HBsAg–anti-HBs. Occasionally, serological markers of hepatitis B have also been reported in woolly monkey and rhesus monkey sera. Serological evidence of natural infection with HBV in chimpanzees was soon followed by the demonstration that this species provided a highly sensitive animal model for experimental hepatitis B infection. Inoculation of serologically negative chimpanzees with materials containing infectious HBV routinely produces mild disease characterized by serological evidence of infection including the appearance of HBsAg, anti-HBc, mildly elevated serum aminotransferase activity, histological evidence of hepatitis in liver biopsies, and eventually anti-HBs upon recovery.

Serological identification of chronically infected chimpanzees was also accomplished. HBsAg obtained from such chimpanzee plasma and HBcAg obtain from chimpanzee liver specimens contributed greatly to the characterization of these two HBV-associated antigens. In addition, high-titer anti-HBs and anti-HBc obtained from infected or immunized chimpanzees provided reagents for *in vitro* serological tests for HBsAg–HBcAg and for reagents to subtype a variety of different HBsAg determinants. Chimpanzees are the animal of choice for studies of hepatitis B because of their availability, equivalent susceptibility to humans, and data accumulated using this species (Barker *et al.*, 1975; Tabor *et al.*, 1983a).

C. Studies in Humans

Early studies in humans set the stage not only for well-designed, purposeful use of chimpanzees and inocula with known HBV infectivity ("titered inocula"), but also for the production of vaccine from human plasma containing HBsAg. The transmission of hepatitis B to humans using infective human serum was proved before the discovery of HBsAg. In studies conducted in the 1950s, sera from asymptomatic blood donors thought previously to have transmitted hepatitis to recipients of their blood were documented to be infectious when inoculated into human volunteers (Neefe *et al.*, 1954; Murray *et al.*, 1954). Sera from these early studies, when reanalyzed in the 1970s, confirmed the transmission of hepatitis B (and also non-A, non-B hepatitis; see Hoofnagle *et al.*, 1977) to recipient volunteers in these studies. Reinoculation of the same infectious serum into recovered individuals failed to cause hepatitis B a second time, providing good evidence for acquired immunity to HBV infection. As the infectious sera used in these studies were obtained retrospectively from blood donors previously implicated in the transmission of hepatitis to recipients of their blood, long-term chronic infections with persistent HBV viremia appeared to occur with some frequency. Murray and his colleagues also demonstrated that HBV could be inactivated by heating at 60°C for 10 hr (and not by heating at 60°C for <10 hr). This procedure of heating at 60°C for 10 hr is still applied today to plasma derivatives including albumin that are able to withstand this treatment.

Studies conducted at the Willowbrook State School by Krugman and his colleagues in the 1950s and 1960s confirmed the transmissibility and identity of hepatitis B and HBV, and helped characterize the epidemiology of the virus and the disease (Krugman *et al.*, 1962, 1967). Krugman *et al.* also demonstrated that HBV can be inactivated by boiling in distilled water, and that injection of the inactivated virus followed by exposure to infectious HBV resulted in protection against infection (Krugman *et al.*, 1970, 1971). This observation proved the feasibilty of preparing an inactivated HBsAg vaccine from infectious human plasma.

III. Chimpanzee Studies

A. Pedigreed Infectious Inocula

Following the documentation of susceptibility of chimpanzees to HBV infection at a level of sensitivity equivalent to that of humans, HBV inocula were evaluated in this species to provide for the later evaluation of procedures to inactivate HBV and to produce vaccines to prevent hepatitis B. The Office of Biologics Research and Review (formerly Bureau of Biologics) and the National Institute of Allergy and Infectious Diseases of the National Institutes of Health prepared three HBV inocula with the most common subtypes of HBsAg: **adw, ayw,** and **adr** (Barker *et al.*, 1975; Tabor *et al.*, 1983a). The infectivity of these inocula was documented by the intravenous inoculation of 54 chimpanzees. End-point infectivity titers are $10^{-7.0}$ (**adw**), $10^{-7.5}$ (**ayw**), and $10^{-8.0}$ (**adr**). The mean incubation period for infections transmitted by each dilution of each of the inocula was inversely proportional to the amount of infectious virus in the dilution (Fig. 2). These inocula have been made available to investigators and manufacturers around the world to evaluate experimental methods for inactivating HBV in plasma derivatives manufactured from large pools of human plasma. They have also been used to evaluate passive and active immunization against HBV by challenging chimpanzees treated with hyperimmune globulin or vaccine.

B. Vaccine Safety Testing

Data accumulated from the inoculation of chimpanzees with HBV confirmed the sensitivity and reproducibility of this animal model for the study of hepatitis B (Tabor *et al.*, 1983a). Of 47 chimpanzees inoculated with "titered" HBV-containing sera, all acquired infections detectable by serological tests for HBV-associated antigens and antibodies; most could also be detected by elevated serum aminotransferase activity or histopathological changes of hepatitis in liver biopsy specimens (Table I). Observations of chimpanzees inoculated with these infectious sera provided background data for initial safety testing of inactivated

TABLE I

Hepatitis B Infections in Chimpanzees Inoculated with One of Three Human Sera (Inocula) Containing HBV[a]

HBV/HBsAg subtype	Number infected	Number with elevated serum aminotransferase activity[b]	Number biopsied	Number with acute hepatitis in liver biopsy specimen[b]
ayw	23	20 (87)	17	14 (82)
adr	14	14 (100)	12	4 (33)
adw	10	7 (70)	6	2 (33)

[a]All chimpanzees also developed serological evidence of HBV infection.
[b]Numbers in parentheses indicate percentages.

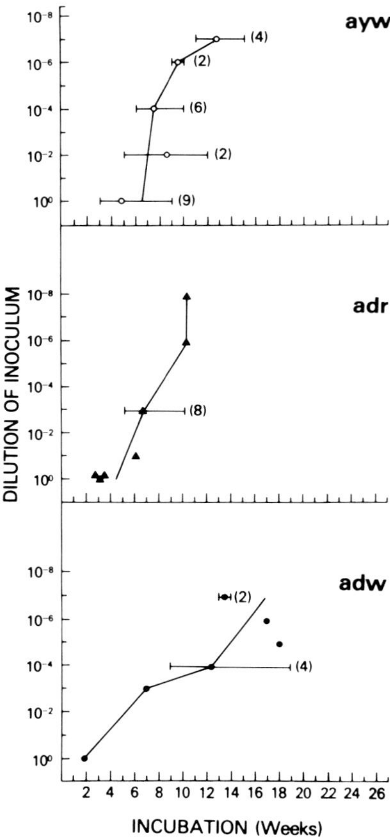

Figure 2. Relationship between the dilution of three HBV-containing inocula (**ayw, adr,** and **adw**) and the incubation period in 47 chimpanzees. The incubation period (in weeks) is the time from inoculation until the appearance of HBsAg. The bars and points on the bars indicate the range of and mean incubation period, respectively, for each dilution. The numbers in parentheses indicate the number of chimpanzees inoculated with that dilution. Individual points indicate 1 chimpanzee was inoculated with the dilution. Slopes represent the "best-fit" slopes for the mean incubation periods for each dilution.

hepatitis B vaccines in chimpanzees. The Office of Biologics Research and Review proposed requirements for inactivated hepatitis B vaccines require that initial lots of vaccine be safety tested by the intravenous inoculation of 1 dose of vaccine into each of 2 chimpanzees and 10 doses into 2 additional chimpanzees. All 4 chimpanzees are evaluated using sensitive serological and biochemical tests and liver biopsies for a period of 6 months (Gerety *et al.*, 1979). An identical safety test was later endorsed by the World Health Organization (WHO) (1980) to apply to all inactivated plasma-derived hepatitis B vaccines worldwide. The 6-month follow-up of inoculated chimpanzees during safety tests derives from data indicating that the incubation period of HBV infections is never longer than 6 months (Tabor *et al.*, 1983a).

During extensive studies of titered HBV inocula in chimpanzees, no infection appeared beyond 18 weeks, irrespective of how little infectious virus was contained in the inoculum. The choice of 1 and 10 doses of vaccine for chimpanzee safety tests is to maximize the volume of vaccine tested while limiting the amount of HBsAg, since too much could "immunize" the inoculated chimpanzees, leading to failure to detect small amounts of infectious HBV. Tabor *et al.* (1980) clearly demonstrated that large quantities of vaccine antigen when employed in a safety test can result in failure to detect small amounts of residual infectious HBV. In their study, 100 ml of vaccine antigen (HBsAg, 40 μg/ml) was injected intravenously, followed thereafter by a small amount of HBV at a second site. No evidence of hepatitis B virus infection was detected in chimpanzees inoculated in this manner, despite assurance that the HBV was infectious and that there was adequate follow-up for 6 months. To date, each lot of U.S.-licensed hepatitis B vaccine has been safety tested intravenously in four seronegative chimpanzees as described above; none have shown evidence of HBV infection.

C. Vaccine Immunogenicity

Once HBsAg was recognized, preparations purified from the plasma of chronic carriers of HBsAg were inoculated into a variety of laboratory animals and into nonhuman primates. Anti-HBs could be induced readily by injecting HBsAg into mice, guinea pigs, rabbits, sheep, goats, horses, and several species of monkeys, including rhesus monkeys. Early plasma-derived HBsAg particle vaccines were assessed for immunogenicity in a variety of laboratory animals prior to the acceptance of the currently employed mouse potency test (see Sections IV,B and VII). It was shown early on that 0.1–1.0 μg of HBsAg without adjuvant could induce anti-HBs response in 50% of random strains of guinea pigs (Gerety *et al.*, 1979).

Early studies of the immunogenicity of plasma-derived HBsAg particle vaccine (lot 559, Merck, Sharp, & Dohme) were reported by Hilleman *et al.* (1978). In one, six seronegative chimpanzees received three doses subcutaneously of 20 μg of unadjuvanted vaccine in 1-ml volumes administered at 1-month intervals. Four of the six made anti-HBs after a single dose of vaccine, and five of six after two doses. The sixth chimpanzee failed to make anti-HBs despite receiving three doses of vaccine.

Purcell and Gerin (1975) reported similar data in chimpanzees using two HBsAg particle vaccines produced at the National Institutes of Health. In their studies, one **ayw** and one **adw** plasma-derived HBsAg particle vaccine was administered to seronegative chimpanzees. Each animal received 20-µg doses of unadjuvanted vaccine subcutaneously on day 1 and again on day 30. Two chimpanzees that received the **ayw** vaccine and one that received the **adw** vaccine made anti-HBs; the latter was only detectable by a sensitive radioimmunoassay, however.

Both early studies of vaccine immunogenicity in chimpanzees indicated that HBsAg was far less immunogenic in chimpanzees than it had been in laboratory animals. These findings, when confirmed in early clinical studies in humans, resulted in a hepatitis B vaccine adjuvanted with alum being developed and eventually licensed.

D. Vaccine Efficacy

To determine whether vaccination with purified plasma-derived HBsAg particle vaccines protected against HBV infection, each of two groups inoculated both vaccinated and control chimpanzees with titered, pedigreed HBV-containing inocula. Purcell and Gerin (1975) inoculated three vaccinated and two unvaccinated control chimpanzees intravenously with $10^{3.5}$ chimpanzee infections doses of HBV (HBsAg subtype **ayw**). Both unvaccinated chimpanzees developed hepatitis B as evidenced by elevated serum aminotransferase activity, HBsAg, anti-HBc, and eventually anti-HBs. Two chimpanzees vaccinated with two 20-µg doses of **ayw** vaccine 1 month apart did not show any evidence of HBV infection. One chimpanzee that received two 20-µg doses of **adw** vaccine, while not developing hepatitis B, did show serological evidence of HBV infection in the form of an active anti-HBc response. The protection provided by these vaccines was not attributable to the "homologous" nature of the **ayw** vaccine (antigenically identical to the challenge inoculum) but to the better immune response to the **ayw** vaccine in these chimpanzees than to the **adw** vaccine. Data from clinical trials in man (detailed below) confirmed that "heterologous" HBsAg particle vaccines (antigenically dissimilar to the challenge HBV) are effective at preventing HBV infections on the basis of anti-HBs response to the **a** determinant common to all HBsAg–HBV.

A similar study of vaccine efficacy was carried out in chimpanzees and reported by Hilleman *et al.* (1978). Six chimpanzees vaccinated with three 20-μg doses of HBsAg particle vaccine (HBsAg **ayw** + **adw,** predominantly **adw**) and five unvaccinated chimpanzees were challenged intravenously with 1000 chimpanzee infectious doses of HBV. All five unvaccinated chimpanzees developed hepatitis B, as evidenced by elevated serum aminotransferase activity, HBsAg, anti-HBc, or anti-HBs. By contrast, none of six vaccinated chimpanzees showed elevations of serum aminotransferase activity, HBsAg, or anti-HBc. One chimpanzee, which failed to produce detectable anti-HBs following vaccination, was also protected against HBV infection following challenge with the infectious HBV. Studies of the ability of plasma-derived HBsAg particle vaccines to prevent HBV infection in chimpanzees provided the scientific basis for the initial clinical trials in human discussed in detail below.

Prior to the vaccine studies outlined above, data on "cross-protection" following recovery from experimental HBV infection (antigenically dissimilar HBV first inoculated during initial infection and later inoculated following recovery) and challenge were reported (Gerety *et al.*, 1979). In this study nine chimpanzees that had recovered from HBV infection acquired 6 to 88 weeks earlier were challenged with HBV-bearing HBsAg of a second subtype contained in inocula with known infectivity. Following a total of 12 challenges, no reinfections by HBV were detected using sensitive serological tests on samples collected for >12 months.

IV. Plasma-Derived HBsAg Particle Vaccines

A. Plasma Source

Plasma-derived HBsAg particle vaccines are unique among human vaccines, as they are manufactured solely from human plasma obtain by plasmapheresis from asymptomatic individuals with chronic hepatitis B. Plasma from donors selected for vaccine manufacture contains high concentrations of noninfectious HBsAg and lesser concentrations of infectious HBV. The ratio of HBsAg to HBV can be as great as 10,000:1 (Tabor *et al.*, 1983a).

Vaccine plasma donors are selected for their high titers of HBsAg. Of necessity, the majority of plasma donors are from among previously identified groups at high risk for acquiring hepatitis B. In the general population, there are <2 acceptable (high HBsAg titer) vaccine plasma donors among each 10,000 individuals. Among certain high-risk populations for hepatitis B (e.g., sexually active male homosexuals), there are ~80 acceptable plasma donors per 10,000 individuals (Gerety and Tabor,

1982). By U.S. federal regulation, all vaccine plasma donors must be asymptomatic and in apparent good health. They must meet all federal requirements for acceptable plasmapheresis donors, except that their serum aminotransferase activity may exceed the level permitted "normal" donors (but it must be stable). Each donor provides a complete history, receives a complete physical examination (repeated at least once each year), undergoes laboratory tests before his or her initial plasma donation, and must maintain normal levels of hemoglobin and serum protein and a normal hematocrit value throughout the course of plasma donations (Code of Federal Regulations, 1979; Office of Biologics Research and Review Guidelines, 1977).

Data confirm that circulating HBeAg in plasma correlates with higher plasma HBV levels when compared with plasma donors who either lack HBeAg or who have anti-HBe. Initially, it was felt that HBeAg-positive plasma should not be used to produce vaccine. As knowledge accumulated regarding the feasibility of vaccine manufacture from HBeAg-negative plasma and the inactivation of HBV, recommendations were modified to permit the use of HBeAg-positive plasma (Gerety *et al.*, 1979).

Although plasmapheresis is common in the United States as a method for obtaining plasma for the manufacture of plasma derivatives, this is not true throughout the world. Vaccine source material, however, can be obtained by whole blood donations as well. The source material for a variety of hepatitis B plasma-derived particle vaccines appears in Table

TABLE II
Source Material for Plasma-Derived HBsAg Particle Vaccines[a]

Investigator(s)	Source material	HBsAg titer (concentration)[b]	HBsAg subtype(s)	HBeAg	Anti-HBe
Gerin-Purcell					
(NIAID)	Plasma	≥ 1:50	adw	+	−
	Plasma	≥ 1:50	adw	+	−
Hilleman (MSD)	Plasma	≥ 1:128	adw + ayw	+	−
Cabasso	Plasma	1:1024	adw + ayw	+	−
Okochi	Blood	c	adr + adw	−	+
Thomssen	Plasma	8 μg/ml	adw + ayw	−	+
Maupas	Serum	≥ 1:4	ayw	−	+
Brummelhuis	Blood	2 μg/ml	adw	+	−
Takahashi	Plasma	c	adr	−	+

[a]Adapted from Gerety *et al.* (1979).

[b]Protein concentration (Lowrey or HBsAg reciprocal end-point titration by counterelectrophoresis).

[c]Unspecified.

II. Initially, a variety of HBsAg subtypes were included in these vaccines. Subsequent data proved the efficacy of a single subtype of HBsAg as vaccine against a variety of potentially infectious HBV. This resulted in vaccines with a single HBsAg subtype (usually **adw** due to its ready availability). As vaccines are manufactured and licensed in more restricted areas and smaller countries, the HBsAg subtype will most likely be that which is most readily available locally.

B. Production and Standardization of Vaccine

The source material for vaccine can differ, as shown in Table II. The philosophy of the production of plasma-derived HBsAg particle vaccine, as well as the methods, also differ. The U.S.-licensed vaccine of Merck, Sharpe, & Dohme (MSD) will be highlighted here. It should, however, be known that there are plasma-derived vaccines produced by Institut Pasteur in France, and others in Japan, England, Germany, and the Netherlands that may be licensed by the time this book is published.

The MSD vaccine is manufactured as shown in Fig. 1. To isolate the 20- to 22-nm HBsAg spheres, acceptable plasma pools are treated with ammonium sulfate (concentration step) followed by isopycnic ultracentrifugation in sodium bromide, and finally rate-zonal ultracentrifugation in sucrose. The purified spheres are then treated with pepsin (1 μg/ml, pH 2.0, at 37°C for 18 hr) to remove residual plasma proteins, with 8 M urea at 37°C for 4 hr followed by dialysis, and finally with 1:4000 formaldehyde solution at 37°C for 72 hr.

The various methods available and used for purification of HBsAg particles for vaccine include ultracentrifugation, chromatography, fractional precipitation such as with polyethylene glycol, enzyme digestions, and solid-phase immunoadsorption. The methods used for the purification of the source materials in Table II appear in Gerety *et al.* (1979). Some may have been modified or changed since these data were published.

Vaccine is standardized with regard to protein content, absence of extraneous materials (including blood group substances, immunoglobulins, and other plasma proteins), absence of adventitious agents, general safety, and absence of infectious HBV. In addition, the HBsAg content is compared to a reference vaccine both *in vitro* (radioimmunoassay) and *in vivo* (mouse potency assay) (see WHO, 1980, and below). There is currently a U.S. vaccine reference for the latter two assays; a great deal of study is underway to provide WHO reference materials for this purpose.

C. Vaccine Safety

Steps in the manufacture of plasma-derived HBsAg particle vaccines have been shown to remove or inactivate HBV and other infectious viruses. Ultracentrifugation procedures designed to isolate HBsAg spheres from among the larger, more dense HBV have been shown by chimpanzee inoculation studies to remove 10,000 infectious doses of HBV (Gerety *et al.*, 1979). In addition, each of three steps employed during vaccine manufacture by MSD (see Fig. 1) has been individually shown to inactivate 100,000 infectious doses of HBV per milliliter by chimpanzee inoculation (Tabor *et al.*, 1983b). Briefly, in this study between 10^3 and 10^5 chimpanzee infectious doses of HBV per milliliter, subtypes **adr** or **ayw,** were treated either with 1 μg/ml pepsin at pH 2.0 for 18 hr at 37°C, 8 M urea for 4 hr at 37°C, or 1:4000 formalin at 37°C for 72 hr. One milliliter of each HBV inoculum subjected individually to one of these procedures was inoculated intravenously into one or two susceptible chimpanzees (a total of eight chimpanzees). No evidence of HBV infection was detected in weekly serum samples from the chimpanzees during 6 months of observation, and liver biopsy specimens showed no evidence of hepatitis.

Procedures used in the manufacture of hepatitis B vaccine when applied individually to representatives of each virus group have also been shown to inactivate them. The pepsin treatment has been shown to inactivate rhabdoviruses represented by vesicular stomatitis virus, poxviruses represented by vaccinia, togaviruses represented by sindbis, herpes viruses represented by herpes simplex (type 1), coronaviruses represented by infectious bronchitis virus, and reovirus (Gerety and Tabor, 1982). The urea treatment, in addition to inactivating the previously mentioned viruses, also inactivates myxoviruses, represented by Newcastle disease virus, and picornaviruses, represented by mengovirus; lesser concentrations of urea when applied to less highly purified material than hepatitis B vaccine inactivates viruses in the slow virus category represented by the scrapie agent. Formalin inactivates a wide variety of viruses including parvoviruses, and has been shown in two studies to inactivate agents of human non-A, non-B hepatitis (Gerety and Tabor, 1982).

In 1979, Zuckerman voiced reasonable concerns regarding the safety of a vaccine for use in man and obtained from the plasma of infected persons. The entire scientific community including this author demanded extreme caution to ensure the freedom of this unique vaccine from all contaminating materials or agents. Concerns regarding viruses, their nucleic acids, oncogenic potential, and autoimmune consequences were looked for in early studies in recipient chimpanzees and humans; none were found then or now.

As outlined in detail in Section VII of this chapter, each lot of MSD vaccine released by the Office of Biologics Research and Review is tested for sterility, injected into suckling and adult mice, guinea pigs, the allantoic and yolk sac of embryonated eggs, and into animal (Vero cells) and human-derived cell lines (WI-38 cells) to confirm the absence of infectious viruses. In addition, 22 doses of vaccine are injected intravenously into chimpanzees, which are followed for 6 months as outlined above. To date, >25 lots of vaccine have been tested in this manner with no evidence of residual infectious agents.

During initial trials of the MSD hepatitis B vaccine, 19,000 vaccinees experienced only minor immediate adverse reactions, primarily soreness at the injection site (Szmuness *et al.*, 1981a; Francis *et al.*, 1982). At this time, >400,000 doses of vaccine have been distributed, and no serious adverse reactions in recipients have been proved to be vaccine related.

Beginning in 1978, a disease manifested by susceptibility to Kaposi's sarcoma and opportunistic infections was identified and associated with an acquired, specific defect in cell-mediated immunity. This disease has been termed *acquired immune deficiency syndrome* (AIDS). Because AIDS occurs among populations that are sources of HBsAg-positive plasma for vaccine manufacture, this syndrome had to be considered when discussing hepatitis B vaccine safety. For AIDS to be transmitted by the MSD hepatitis B vaccine, HTLV III (the likely causative agent) would need to chronically infect humans who would continue to circulate the agent while appearing healthy. In addition, HTLV III would have to have physical characteristics permitting it to copurify with HBsAg spheres and to resist inactivation by all three procedures (inactivating procedures) applied to the vaccine. This is not the case for HTLV III. This fact has been borne out by data resulting in reassurances concerning the vaccine from the scientific community (Centers for Disease Control, 1981a,b) and supported by data documenting inactivation of retroviruses, including HTLV III, by procedures routinely applied to MSD vaccine and described above.

D. Clinical Evaluation of Vaccine

Following the completion of many small clinical trials employing hepatitis B vaccine, which provided the necessary safety and immunogenicity data, several large, controlled, randomized, double-blind, and placebo-controlled clinical trials of vaccine efficacy were conduced in the United States using the MSD vaccine. Using 40-μg doses of an **adw** vaccine (lot 751) administered at 0, 1, and 6 months, Szmuness *et al.* (1981a) conducted a vaccine efficacy study among sexually active male homosexuals in New York City. This group was chosen for this study because of their high attack rate of hepatitis B. Participants were chosen from among 13,000 homosexual men, and matched to equalize exposures to HBV in a vaccinated and a control group. The vaccine proved to be safe, immunogenic, and effective (Szmuness *et al.*, 1981a). Over 95% of vaccinees developed anti-HBs, which persisted throughout the 2-year follow-up. The attack rate of HBV infection was 3.2% among vaccinees and 25.6% among recipients of the placebo material (vaccine diluent) ($p < .0001$). The majority of hepatitis B cases in vaccinees occurred either prior to completion of the vaccination regime or among those who did not make anti-HBs despite receiving three 40-μg doses of vaccine. This study, in addition to unequivocally documenting the efficacy of the MSD vaccine at preventing hepatitis B infections, also documented that vaccine immunogenicity equated with efficacy.

A similarly designed, randomized, double-blind, placebo-controlled vaccine trial of MSD vaccine was conducted by the Centers for Disease Control (Francis *et al.*, 1982). It was carried out in five U.S. cities among 1,402 homosexual males, using three 20-μg doses of vaccine administered at 0, 1, and 6 months. In this study, 85% of vaccinees made anti-HBs after three doses of vaccine. Hepatitis B infections were far less among vaccinees than among placebo recipients ($p = .0004$). Once again, 10 of 11 infections among vaccinees occurred either in nonresponders to vaccine or in those who made little anti-HBs after vaccination. Francis *et al.* (1982) concluded that three 20-μg doses of vaccine were safe, immunogenic, and efficacious in preventing HBV infections.

Additional studies reported by Krugman *et al.* (1981) and Szmuness *et al.* (1981b) in 202 and 336 vaccine recipients, respectively, showed the patterns of anti-HBs responses to 40-μg or 20-μg doses of MSD hepatitis B vaccine to be similar if not the same. It was on the basis of the four studies described here and a number of smaller, earlier studies that the 20-μg dose of MSD vaccine was licensed in November, 1981 by the Office of Biologics Research and Review.

Although I have concentrated on hepatitis B plasma-derived vaccine manufactured in the United States, it must be noted that other groups have been equally active in this area. They include those listed in Table II, the Institute Pasteur, and Zuckerman and co-workers (see Chapter 17).

Researchers at the Institute of Virology at Tours, France, and finally at the Institut Pasteur, Paris, France have been very active in this area (Barin *et al.*, 1978; Crosnier *et al.*, 1981; Maupas *et al.*, 1976). In randomized, placebo controlled trials of a plasma-derived HBsAg particle vaccine produced by the Institut Pasteur, this vaccine has been shown to be safe, immunogenic, and effective at preventing HBV infections (Crosnier *et al.*, 1981); it is licensed for use in France and no doubt will be available elsewhere when this volume is published.

E. Risk–Benefit Considerations, High-Risk Groups, and Vaccine Use Policy

As with any vaccine, considerations of the benefit(s) of vaccination compared to both real and potential risks associated with vaccination have to be considered. There is little doubt that the licensed U.S. plasma-derived HBsAg vaccine is highly effective in preventing hepatitis B (Szmuness *et al.*, 1981a; Francis *et al.*, 1982). There are ~200,000 new cases of hepatitis B reported each year in the United States; 10,000 of these cases require hospitalization, up to 1,000 die with fulminant hepatitis B, and 10,000–20,000 remain chronically infected and serve as a human reservoir for additional HBV transmission. It has been estimated that one-half of the reported cases of hepatitis B in the United States occur among those in designated high-risk groups. Therefore, one-half of all cases of hepatitis B could theoretically be prevented by vaccinating all persons at high risk of hepatitis B. An added benefit would be the prevention of 10,000 to 20,000 new chronic infections each year. Despite the fact that a very large body of data has not yet been accumulated from long-term follow-up of hepatitis B vaccine recipients (MSD vaccine, first licensed in November, 1981), it is clear that the risk of hepatitis B among persons in high-risk groups far exceeds the risk of vaccination with a highly purified, multiply inactivated viral antigen administered in 20-µg amounts intramuscularly. This opinion is shared by the Office of Biologics Research and Review, the National Institutes of Health, the American College of Physicians, and the Centers for Disease Control Advisory Committee on Immunization Practices (Centers for Disease Control, 1981a,b).

The estimated lifetime risk of acquiring an HBV infection is ~5% for the U.S. population, but approaches 100% for the highest risk groups. The expected prevalences of HBV infection, as defined by serological markers of active (HBsAg) or past HBV infection (anti-HBs/anti-HBc), appear in Table III. The high prevalence of HBV infections among dental and medical workers relate to the frequency with which they are exposed to blood and also to the population groups that they serve (Gerety, 1981). The Centers for Disease Control has compiled standardized prevalences of seropositivity, and has ranked occupational catego-

TABLE III
Risk of HBV Infection Evaluated by Risk Category and Prevalences of Serological Markers[a]

| | | Serological marker of HBV infection | |
Group studied	Risk category	HBsAg (%)	Serological markers (%)
Immigrants from endemic areas	High	13	70–85
Institutionalized mentally retarded		10–20	35–80
Intravenous drug users		7	60–80
Active homosexual males		6	35–80
Household contacts of carriers		3–6	30–60
Hemodialysis patients		3–10	
Prisoners	Intermediate	1–8	10–80
Staff in institutions for the mentally retarded		1	10–25
Health care workers with frequent exposure to blood		1–2	15–30
Health care workers with little or no contact with blood	Low	0.3	3–10
Healthy first-time volunteer blood donors		0.3	3–5

[a]Adapted from Centers for Disease Control, 1981a.

ries among health care workers, as shown in Table IV, with regard to relative risk. These data represent the best information that is available. Clearly, time in a particular subcategory or previous employment in another subcategory may have influenced this ranking, as did the socioeconomic status of persons in certain subcategories of employment.

The vaccine use policy in the United States dictates preexposure prophylaxis by vaccine for all individuals in the high-risk populations as defined above. The United States is clearly a country categorized as having a "low endemicity" of hepatitis B. In areas with "high endemicity," depending on vaccine availability and cost, hepatitis B vaccine might be used to vaccinate susceptibles in the younger age categories or to vaccinate all newborns. Clearly, hepatitis B vaccine use in the near future either alone or with hepatitis B immune globulin will also extend to postexposure situations including newborns delivered to infected mothers, sexual partners of HBsAg-positive individuals, and perhaps even to individuals suffering accidental percutaneous exposures to HBV-containing materials.

Prevaccination screening for serological markers of ongoing or past hepatitis B infections is not necessary (vaccine produces no adverse

TABLE IV

Risk of Hepatitis B in Health Care Personnel Ranked by Standardized
Prevalences of Serological Positivity[a]

Standardized prevalence	Occupational subcategory
27	Medical technologists
26	Blood bank and hemodialysis technicians
19	EKG and pulmonary technicians
18	Attending physicians
17	Dentists, nurses, anaesthetists, and surgical technicians
15	Aides and orderlies, administrative assistants, and those employed in the laundry, housekeeping, and supply departments
13	Lab assistants, inhalation therapists, and food service workers
12	Chemists, microbiologists, and radiation and nuclear medicine technicians
11	Nurses, cytology technicians, and those in building maintenance
10	Hygienists, social workers, dieticians, and clerical workers
9	Research technicians, dental hygienists, administrators, pharmacists, and their assistants

[a]Compared to control population where the prevalence was from 4 to 6%.
Information provided by the Centers for Disease Control.

effects if administered either to chronic carriers of HBsAg or to those
with actively acquired anti-HBs), but may be cost effective if the population subgroup to be vaccinated has a large proportion of immune individuals (see Centers for Disease Control, 1981a).

V. HBsAg Particle Vaccine from a Human Hepatocellular Carcinoma Cell Line

Although HBV–HBsAg has never been induced to replicate in cell
culture systems by inoculation with infectious HBV, a human hepatoma
cell line (PLC/PRF 5) isolated by Alexander *et al.* (1976) produces spherical HBsAg particles and releases them into the cell culture supernatant.
The PLC/PRF 5 cell line possesses multiple, apparently complete copies
of the HBV genome in each cell, but does not appear to produce infec-

tious HBV (Tabor *et al.*, 1981). The ability of these cells to synthesize HBsAg is apparently preserved as a stable phenotypic trait during their propagation in culture. These cells also produce α-anti-trypsin in a perinuclear distribution while neither HBcAg nor albumin have been detected (Gerber and Thung, 1981).

HBsAg particles have been purified from PLC/PRF 5 cell culture supernatants (Lu *et al.*, 1984). Quantitative recovery of HBsAg spheres was obtained from cell culture supernatants by concentration with a Pellicon Ultrafilter, followed by either isopycnic and rate-zonal ultracentrifugation or solid-phase immunoadsorption with mouse monoclonal anti-HBs coupled to Sepharose 2B. The purity of these HBsAg preparations was examined by polyacrylamide gels and by electron microscopy. In addition, the purity of the preparations was confirmed by the constant ratio of protein to antigenic activity relative to a serum-derived HBsAg standard.

The immunogenicity of these PLC/PRF 5-derived HBsAg particles when adsorbed to alum was compared in mice to that of a standard alum-adsorbed, serum-derived, ultracentrifugally purified HBsAg particle vaccine. The concentration of HBsAg resulting in the seroconversion to anti-HBs positive of 50% of groups of 15 mice (ED_{50}) was 0.91 and 0.88 μg for the PLC/PRF 5-derived HBsAg purified by centrifugation and by solid-phase immunoadsorption, respectively. The ED_{50} for the plasma-derived HBsAg vaccine standard was 0.93 μg. This study clearly indicates that HBsAg vaccine can be produced from PLC/PRF 5 cell supernatants. Concerns regarding the use of human cancer cells to produce vaccine, however, will most likely dictate that other alternative sources for HBsAg particle vaccines be evaluated first to find a replacement for human plasma-derived HBsAg vaccine.

VI. HBsAg Particle Vaccines from Genetically Engineered Systems

The manufacture of HBsAg particle vaccines from human plasma is restricted somewhat by the availability of high-titer HBsAg-containing plasma and greatly by the cost of both purification and inactivation procedures necessary to assure the absence of adventitious agents that might be present in the starting plasma. Alternatively, genetically engineered HBsAg particle-producing systems have been described, including SV-40-infected monkey kidney cells, mouse L cells, bacteria, yeast, Chinese hamster ovary cells, and vaccinia virus (Moriarty *et al.*,

1981; Burrell *et al.*, 1979; Hitzeman *et al.*, 1983; McAleer *et al.*, 1984; Smith *et al.*, 1983). SV-40-infected monkey kidney cells and mouse L cells as producers of HBsAg particles have not been pursued for a variety of reasons, and expression of HBsAg by bacteria with HBV genome inserts have yielded unsatisfactory expression of HBsAg particles.

Valenzuela *et al.* (1982) first showed that a portion of the HBV genome, when inserted into the yeast *Saccharomyces cerevisiae*, could result in the production of HBsAg "spheres" similar to those isolated and purified from human plasma (see also Hitzeman *et al.*, 1983). Yeast-produced HBsAg spheres are not released into the yeast culture medium, and therefore must be released from the yeast cells by homogenization,

TABLE V

Steps in the Manufacture of Plasma-Derived HBsAg Particle Vaccines and Applicable Federal Regulations

Step	Applicable federal regulations
I. Plasmapheresis of HBsAg-positive individuals	a. 21 CFR,640,subpart G b. 21 CFR,606, Good Manufacturing Practices c. Office of Biologics Guidelines for the Plasmapheresis of HBsAg-Reactive Donors (5/23/77) d. 21 CFR,610.40 e. 21 CFR,610.41
II. Shipment of HBsAg-reactive plasma	a. 49 CFR,173.387 b. 42 CFR,72.25 c. NIH Guide, Volume 4, No. 1, 2/10/75
III. Sterility and inocuity testing, and testing for adventitious agents applied to plasma pool	a. 21 CFR,640,74 b. 21 CFR,630,35a(1),(2),(3),(4),(5)
IV. Testing for extraneous substances	a. 21 CFR,610.11
V. Release testing of vaccine lots	a. All applicable requirements in III and IV b. Potency testing [Parallel-line assay (RIA) and Mouse Potency Assay compared with vaccine reference standard as defined by Office of Biologics Research and Review]

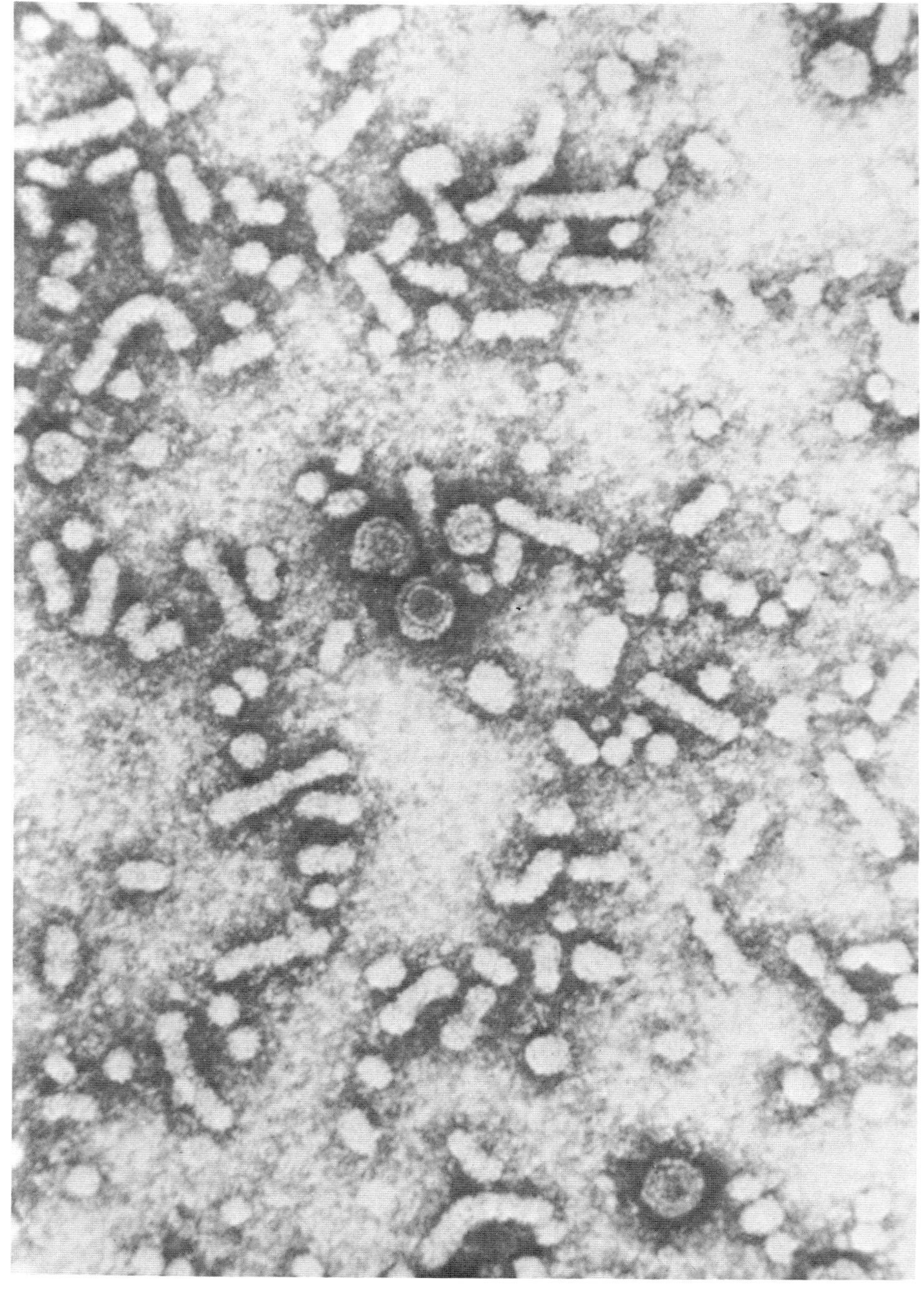

sonication, or fracture by glass beads. When isolated, the nonglycosylated HBsAg spheres (unlike plasma-derived HBsAg which is glycosylated) have been shown to be immunogenic in mice (McAleer *et al.*, 1984), and in rabbits and guinea pigs (Hitzeman *et al.*, 1983). McAleer *et al.* (1984) expanded their studies of yeast-derived HBsAg by documenting the immunogenicity of purified yeast-derived HBsAg in Grivet monkeys and in chimpanzees. In addition, four chimpanzees were vaccinated with three 40-μg doses of alum-adjuvanted yeast-derived HBsAg in 1-ml volumes at 1-month intervals; all developed anti-HBs (reciprocal end-point titers between 1:540 and 1:18,300). When challenged with 1000 chimpanzee infectious doses of HBV (either **adr** or **ayw** subtype) intravenously, four unvaccinated control chimpanzees developed HBV infections while none of the "vaccinated" chimpanzees showed any evidence of HBV infection. It is thus clear that anti-HBs responses induced to this yeast-derived HBsAg can protect against virus challenge by "heterologous" HBsAg-bearing virus. Yeast-derived HBsAg particle vaccine would appear at this time to represent a good candidate to replace plasma-derived HBsAg particle vaccines.

Recently, that portion of the HBV genome coding for HBsAg has been inserted into the vaccinia virus genome, resulting in a potential live virus vaccine against hepatitis B (Smith *et al.*, 1983). The HBsAg particles produced by vaccinia recombinant virus-infected CV-1 cell monolayers exhibited physical, chemical, and electron microscopic characteristics identical with those of plasma-derived HBsAg spheres. They induced anti-HBs when injected into rabbits (10^8 PFU of "recombinant" vaccinia virus at either one or four intradermal sites) (Smith *et al.*, 1983). Studies to evaluate the safety and efficacy of this vaccine in chimpanzees have been initiated.

VII. U.S. Regulation of Vaccine

The federal regulation of plasma-derived HBsAg particle vaccine begins with the control of facilities in which HBsAg-containing plasma is obtained by plasmapheresis, and ends with a variety of tests required to be accomplished on each lot of vaccine prior to its release for sale. Many of the requirements for this vaccine also apply to and are required for release of other vaccines; some are applicable to and have been developed specifically for this vaccine.

Figure 3. Electron photomicrograph of plasma from HBsAg carrier. Note the 20- to 22-nm "spheres" among the tubular HBsAg and the intact, double-shelled HBV (×200,000).

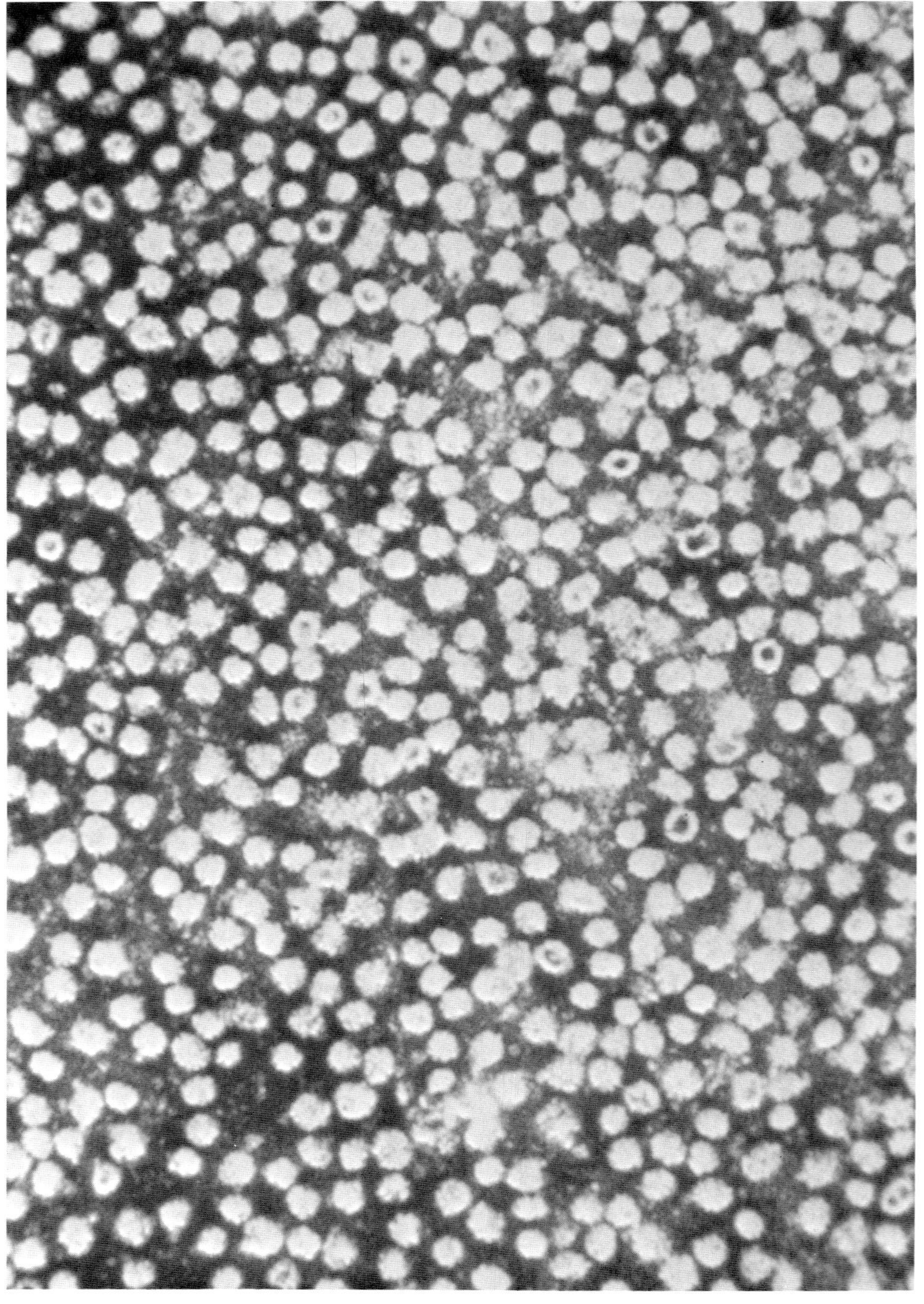

HBsAg-containing plasma is drawn in U.S.-licensed plasmapheresis establishments according to existing federal regulations for obtaining source plasma (Table V includes a list of federal regulations applicable to various steps in the manufacture of plasma-derived HBsAg particle vaccines). Once obtained, the vaccine plasma is shipped under regulations relating to etiologic agents. Each unit of plasma is tested for its content of HBsAg, subtyped unless previously established, and individually tested to assure microbial sterility.

The plasma units once tested are pooled (Fig. 3). The *plasma pool* is tested to assure microbial sterility, innocuity in adult and suckling mice, and tested to assure the absence of adventitious agents by inoculating samples into embryonated eggs (allantoic sac and yolk sac) and cell cultures (Vero and WI-38 cells).

The HBsAg particles are purified and inactivated as illustrated in Fig. 1. The *final inactivated vaccine* is evaluated by electron microscopy and inoculated into HBV-susceptible chimpanzees as described earlier. In addition, it is tested for extraneous substances including formaldehyde, thimerosal, and aluminum; and finally it is tested to assure microbial sterility and inocuity.

The *final alum-adsorbed vaccine* (Fig. 4) is tested for potency by a quantitative radioimmunioassay against a reference vaccine (799-2) at the manufacturer and at the Office of Biologics Research and Review, followed by a mouse potency test, which also employs this alum-adsorbed reference vaccine.

The regulation of licensed hepatitis B vaccine that is not of plasma origin will obviously require testing and/or assurances different from and in addition to those applied to plasma-derived HBsAg particle vaccine. Questions concerning sensitization to yeast antigens, concerns regarding cell lines used to produce HBsAg, the HBV gene inserts employed, the promoters used, and the efficacy of the final product at preventing HBV infection by "heterologous" HBV, will have to be addressed and applied where applicable.

References

Alexander, J., Bey, E., Whitcutt, J. M., and Gear, J. H. S. (1976). *S. Afr. J. Med. Sci.* **41**, 89–98.
Alter, H. J., and Blumberg, B. S. (1966). *Blood* **27**, 297–309.

Figure 4. Electron micrograph of purified HBsAg "spheres" (vaccine) prior to adding alum adjuvant (×200,000).

Barin, F., Andre, M., Goudeau, A., Coursaget, P., and Maupas, P. (1978). *Ann. Microbiol. (Paris)* **129B,** 87–100.

Barker, L. F., Maynard, J. E., Purcell, R. H., Hoofnagle, J. H., Berquist, K. R., London, W. T., Gerety, R. J., and Krushak, D. H. (1975). *J. Infect. Dis.* **132,** 451–458.

Blumberg, B.S., Alter, H. J., and Visnich, S. (1965). *JAMA, J. Am. Med. Assoc.* **191,** 541–546.

Blumberg, B. S., Gersley, B. J., and Hungerford, D. A. (1967). *Ann. Intern. Med.* **66,** 924–931.

Bond, H. E., and Hall, W. T. (1972). *J. Infect. Dis.* **125,** 263–268.

Burrell, C. J., Proudfoot, E., Keen, G. A., and Marmion, B. P. (1973). *Nature (London), New Biol.* **243,** 260–262.

Burrell, C. J., Mackay, P., Greenway, P. J., Hofschneider, P. H., and Murray, K. (1979). *Nature (London)* **279,** 43–47.

Centers for Disease Control (1981a). *Morbid. Mortal. Week. Rep.* **31,** 317–328.

Centers for Disease Control (1981b). *Morbid. Mortal. Week. Rep.* **31,** 465–467.

Chairez, R., Steiner, S., and Melnick, J. L. (1973). *Intervirology* **1,** 224–238.

Code of Federal Regulations (1979). Title 21, Part 640. U.S. Gov. Printing Office, Washington, D.C.

Crosnier, J., Jungers, P., Couroucé, A., Laplanche, A., Benhamon, E., Degos, F., Lacour, B., Prunet, P., Cerisier, Y., and Guesry, P. (1981). *Lancet 1,* 455–459.

Dane, D. S., Cameron, C. H., and Briggs, M. (1970). *Lancet 1,* 695–698.

Dreesman, G. R., Hollinger, F. B., Suriano, J. R., Fujioka, R. S., Brunschwig, J. P., and Melnick, J. L. (1972). *J. Virol.* **10,** 469–476.

Francis, D. P., Hadler, S. C., Thompson, S. E., Maynard, J. E., Ostrow, D. G., Altman, N., Braff, E. H., O'Malley, P., Hawkins, D., Judson, F. N., Penley, K., Nylund, T., Christie, G., Myers, F., Moore, J. N., Gardner, A., Doto, I., Miller, J. H., Reynolds, G. H., Murphy, B. L., Schable, C. A., Clark, B. T., Curran, J. W., and Redeker, A. G. (1982). *Ann. Intern. Med.* **97,** 362–366.

Gerber, M. A., and Thung, S. N. (1981). *Fed. Proc., Fed. Am. Soc. Exp. Biol.* **40,** 364 (abstr.).

Gerety, R. J. (1981). *Ann. Intern. Med.* **95,** 229–231.

Gerety, R. J., and Tabor, E. (1982). *JAMA, J. Am. Med. Assoc.* **249,** 745–746.

Gerety, R. J., Tabor, E., Purcell, R. H., and Tyeryar, F. (1979). *J. Infect. Dis.* **140,** 642–648.

Giles, J. P., McCollum, R. W., Berndtson, L. M., Jr., and Krugman, S. (1969). *N. Engl. J. Med.* **281,** 119–122.

Hilleman, M. R., Bertland, A. U., Buynak, E. B., Lampson, G. P., McAleer, W. J., McLean, A. A., Roehm, R. R., and Tytell, A. A. (1978). *In* "Viral Hepatitis" (G. N. Vyas, S. N. Cohen, and R. Schmid, eds.), pp. 525–537. Franklin Inst. Press, Philadelphia, Pennsylvania.

Hitzeman, R. A., Chen, C. Y., Hagie, F. E., Patzer, E. J., Liu, C.-C., Estell, D. A., Miller, J. V., Yaffe, A., Kleid, D. G., Levinson, A. D., and Oppermann, H. (1983). *Nucleic Acids Res.* **11,** 2745–2763.

Hoofnagle, J. H., Gerety, R. J., Tabor, E., Feinstone, S. M., Barker, L. F., and Purcell, R. H. (1977). *Ann. Intern. Med.* **87,** 14–20.

Krugman, S., Ward, R., and Giles, J. P. (1962). *Am. J. Med.* **32,** 717–728.

Krugman, S., Giles, J. P., and Hammond, J. (1967). *JAMA, J. Am. Med. Assoc.* **200,** 365–373.

Krugman, S., Giles, J. P., and Hammond, J. (1970). *J. Infect. Dis.* **122,** 432–436.

Krugman, S., Giles, J. P., and Hammond, J. (1971). *JAMA, J. Am. Med. Assoc.* **218,** 1655–1670.

Krugman, S., Holley, P., Davidson, M., Simberkoff, M. S., and Matsaniotis, N. (1981). *J. Med. Virol.* **8,** 119–121.

LeBouvier, G. L., and Williams, A. (1975). *Am. J. Med. Sci.* **270,** 165–171.

Lu, J. C.-F., Shih, J. W.-K., Mitchell, F. D., Smallwood, L. A., Gerety, R. J., and Ford, E. C. (1984). *In* "Viral Hepatitis and Liver Disease" (G. N. Vyas, J. L. Dienstag, and J. H. Hoofnagle, eds.), p. 659. Grune & Stratton, New York.

McAleer, W. J., Buynak, E. B., Maigetter, R. Z., Wampler, D. E., Miller, W. J., and Hilleman, M. R. (1984). *Nature (London)* **307**, 178–180.

Maupas, P., Goudeau, A., Coursaget, P., Drucker, J., and Bagros, P. (1976). *Lancet 1*, 1367–1370.

Moriarty, A. M., Hoyer, B. H., Shih, J. W.-K., Gerin, L., and Hamer, D. H. (1981). *Proc. Natl. Acad. Sci. U.S.A.* **78**, 2606–2610.

Murray, R., Diefenbach, W. C. L., and Ratner, F. (1954). *JAMA, J. Am. Med. Assoc.* **154**, 1072–1074.

Neefe, J. R., Norris, R. F., and Reingold, J. G. (1954). *JAMA, J. Am. Med. Assoc.* **154**, 1066–1071.

Office of Biologics Research and Review (1977). "Guidelines for the Plasmapheresis of HBsAg Reactive Donors." Bethesda, Maryland.

Okochi, K., and Murakami, S. (1968). *Vox Sang.* **15**, 374–385.

Prince, A. M. (1968). *Proc. Natl. Acad. Sci. U.S.A.* **60**, 814–821.

Purcell, R. H., and Gerin, J. L. (1975). *Am. J. Med. Sci.* **270**, 395–399.

Smith, G. L., Mackett, M., and Moss, B. (1983). *Nature (London)* **302**, 490–495.

Steiner, S., Huebner, M. T., and Dreesman, G. R. (1974). *J. Virol.* **14**, 572–577.

Sukeno, N., Shirachi, R., Yamaguchi, J., and Ishida, N. (1972). *J. Virol.* **9**, 182–183.

Szmuness, W., Stevens, C. E., Zang, E. A., Harley, E. J., and Kellner, A. (1981a). *Hepatology* **1**, 377–385.

Szmuness, W., Stevens, C. E., Harley, E. J., Zang, E. A., Taylor, P. E., Alter, H. J., and the Dialysis Vaccine Trial Group (1981b). *J. Med. Virol.* **8**, 123–129.

Tabor, E., Barker, L. F., and Gerety, R. J. (1980). *J. Med. Virol.* **6**, 279–284.

Tabor, E., Copland, J. A., Mann, G. F., Howard, C. R., Skelly, J., Snoy, P., Zuckerman, A. J., and Gerety, R. J. (1981). *Intervirology* **15**, 82–86.

Tabor, E., Purcell, R. H., London, W. T., and Gerety, R. J. (1983a). *J. Infect. Dis.* **147**, 531–534.

Tabor, E., Buynak, E., Smallwood, L. A., Snoy, P., Hilleman, M., and Gerety, R. J. (1983b). *J. Med. Virol.* **11**, 1–9.

Valenzuela, P., Medina, A., Rutter, W. J., Ammerer, G., and Hall, B. D. (1982). *Nature (London)* **298**, 347–350.

Vyas, G. N., Rao, K. R., and Ibrahim, A. B. (1972). *Science* **178**, 1300–1301.

World Health Organization (1980). Proposed requirements for Hepatitis B Vaccine, WHO/BS 79.1239, pp. 1–20. W.H.O., Expert Committee on Biological Standardization, Geneva.

Zuckerman, A. J. (1979). *Lancet 1*, 547–548.

Chapter 17

Active Immunization/Polypeptide and Newer Hepatitis B Vaccines

ARIE J. ZUCKERMAN
Department of Medical Microbiology
London School of Hygiene and Tropical Medicine
London, England

I. Introduction

Many viral vaccines contain a number of complex antigenic determinants that induce protective humoral and cellular immune responses. Such vaccines are usually prepared from the intact virus or a portion of the virus such as the coat protein or its subunits after growth *in vitro* in cell culture. Such vaccines may also contain contaminating antigenic components, proteins, and other material derived from the virus, the host cell in which the virus has been grown or from the substrate, which are not relevant to protective immunity and which may induce undesirable side effects (Wilson, 1967). Vaccines are, of course, subject to strict manufacturing requirements and control to ensure safety and freedom from contamination and untoward complications.

The failure of numerous investigators to propagate hepatitis B virus in the laboratory *in vitro* has prevented the development of conventional vaccines from this virus grown in cell cultures. Attention has therefore been directed to the use of alternative sources of viral antigen for active immunization, including the use of hepatitis B surface antigen, the non-infectious surplus protein coat of the virus, which is purified from the plasma of asymptomatic human carriers and subsequently subjected to

413

Copyright © 1985 by Academic Press, Inc.
All rights of reproduction in any form reserved.
ISBN 0-12-280672-7

inactivation procedures. Since hepatitis B surface antigen leads to the production of neutralizing or protective surface antibody as shown by serological surveys and experimental transmission studies in human volunteers and chimpanzees susceptible to hepatitis B infection, purified 22-nm spherical surface antigen particles have been developed as vaccines. It is generally accepted that the preparations of the 22-nm particles, when pure, are free of nucleic acid and therefore noninfectious, but the fact that the starting material is human plasma obtained from persons infected with hepatitis B virus means that extreme caution must be exercised to ensure that the preparations of antigen are free of all harmful contaminating material, including host components. Some concern has been expressed about the possible induction of harmful immunological reactions to human host components, including preexisting structures of liver cells, which may be present either as an integral component of the viral surface antigen or be intimately associated with the antigen as a contaminant derived from cells or from plasma (Zuckerman, 1975; Melnick *et al.*, 1976), but neither reactions of this type nor autoimmune responses have been observed with the highly purified 22-nm particle vaccines in chimpanzees and the many individuals immunized (see Chapter 16).

Nevertheless, there are advantages in chemically characterized antigen, since many studies have shown that considerable variation exists between protein analyses of purified hepatitis B surface antigen obtained from different sources and of different serological subtypes (see review by Howard and Burrell, 1976). As another example, the advantages of vaccines based on pure subunit antigen have been demonstrated with influenza A, where a vaccine consisting of the neuraminidase and hemagglutinin subunits has been shown to be adequately immunogenic when given in fewer doses, and it was less reactogenic than the whole killed-virus vaccine.

II. Polypeptide Composition of Hepatitis B Surface Antigen

Preparations consisting of the separated 22-nm particles, which constitute the bulk of the hepatitis B surface antigen material in the sera of most carriers, have been analyzed both chemically and serologically in several laboratories, but with varying results. Although in most studies at least two major polypeptides were found in the molecular weight range of 20,000 to 30,000, variable amounts of larger components were frequently present (see Howard and Zuckerman, 1974; Shih and Gerin,

1975, 1977; Dreesman *et al.*, 1975; Skelly *et al.*, 1978). It is possible that some of these polypeptides represent integral host-coded proteins that may play a role maintaining and preserving surface antigenic reactivity.

Various studies have shown that individual polypeptides are immunogenic after inoculation into guinea pigs. Dreesman *et al.* (1975) prepared antisera to five polypeptides derived by solubilization of hepatitis B surface antigen with sodium dodecyl sulfate (SDS) in the presence of urea. Some variation was found in the responses obtained against individual polypeptides prepared from subtypes **adw** and **ayw.** In each case, however, antibody to the surface antigen was raised in animals inoculated with the 24,000, 35,000, or 40,000 molecular weight polypeptides. Antisera to six or seven polypeptides of molecular weight 23,000 to 97,000, separated from purified surface antigen particles of subtypes **adw** and **ayw,** were raised in guinea pigs by Gold *et al.* (1976). Most or all of the polypeptides stimulated antibodies to the **d** or **y** subdeterminants, and therefore these antigenic determinants are part of the constitutent structure of the polypeptides. Shih and Gerin (1977) found up to seven polypeptides in purified 22-nm particles representing the three major subtypes of the surface antigen (**adw, ayw,** and **adr**). Two polypeptides with molecular weights of 23,000 and 29,500 were found as the major components. The remaining polypeptides varied within each subtype both in number and in relative concentration. Peterson *et al.* (1977) identified two major bands of polypeptides, with molecular weights of 16,000–28,000 and 40,000–90,000.

Purified polypeptides from the 22,000 and 28,000 molecular weight bands had amino acid compositions essentially identical to each other and to the intact surface antigen. The amino-terminal and carboxy-terminal sequences of the amino acids in these two major polypeptides, which accounted for 75% of the total protein, showed that hepatitis B surface antigen with determinants **adw** consists of a single major polypeptide chain or two homolgous polypeptide chains, which differ only in limited areas of their structure. The difference in the molecular weight of these two components is due to the carbohydrate moiety of the glycoprotein of the second band. Inoculation into guinea pigs of the 22,000 molecular weight polypeptide emulsified in Freund's complete adjuvant elicited antibodies to the group specific determinant **a** and to one other of the major subdeterminants **d.** The 28,000 molecular weight polypeptide, however, did not induce an antibody response, and it was suggested that the discrepancy in the immunogenicity of the glycosylated peptides reported in other studies could have been due to contamination of the two major polypeptides.

Shih *et al.* (1978) later studied the immunogenicity of the major polypeptides separated from purified surface antigen using double-antibody radioimmunoprecipitation. Each of three polypeptides (23,000, 29,500, and 72,000 molecular weight, respectively) were trace labeled and used as the radioligand in the assay. Each polypeptide contained both the group-specific determinant and the subtype-specific determinant, as shown by precipitation by antiserum to the native surface antigen and by antisera prepared against the separated polypeptides, thereby indicating a high degree of serological relationship among these three components. Although these findings suggest that each individual polypeptide may contain amino acid sequences that are essential for immunoreactivity, results obtained after separation of components with SDS are difficult to interpret. Renaturation of polypeptides into a native conformation may be inaccurate or incomplete, and since antigenicity in globular proteins is dependent on three-dimensional conformation, the antigenic determinants of such molecules may differ markedly from those of the original state. A further consideration is that substantial losses in protein yield frequently occur when individual polypeptides are extracted from polyacrylamide gels.

Nonionic detergents and bile salts have been used extensively for the dissociation of viruses into soluble complexes that retain biological activity. Simons *et al.* (1973) disrupted the virus envelope of Semiliki forest virus into soluble protein and lipid complexes by treatment with Triton X-100, an alkylpolyethoxy alcohol. The protein and lipid complexes were then separated by density gradient centrifugation in the presence of the detergent. Hayman *et al.* (1973) successfully separated the surface glycoproteins of influenza and mouse mammary tumor viruses by affinity chromatography, using columns of immobilized phytohemagglutinin equilibrated with buffer containing sodium deoxycholate. A considerable advantage in these studies was the retention of the biological activities of the envelope glycoproteins after disruption of the virus. Skelly *et al.* (1979a) disrupted purified hepatitis B surface antigen with 2% Triton X-100 in the presence of salt to yield a product with an estimated sedimentation coefficient of 3.9 S. Fractionation of radiolabeled antigen by passage through columns of immobilized concanavalin A resulted in the separation of three components into two fractions. The first fraction, which did not bind to the lectin, contained exclusively a 64,000 molecular weight polypeptide. This component reacted with serum albumin antibodies and produced peptide maps similar to albumin after treatment with trypsin. The second fraction was obtained by eluting bound material from the immobilized lectin column with α-methyl-D-mannoside, and was found to contain the p28 and p23 polypeptides as the major components. Since p23 was not previously found to be glycosylated, this polypeptide probably remained bound to gp28 by a protein–protein linkage after detergent treatment. The reactivity of this material with antibodies to the surface antigen, in the absence of any detectable reactions with antibodies to normal serum components, indicates that hepatitis B surface antigen reactivity resides with this subunit preparation. Thus the technique of Trition X-100 solubilization followed by affinity chromatography allows the preparation of milligram quantities of immunologically reactive material, which was not possible previously by preparative SDS–polyacrylamide gel electrophoretic techniques.

Although the two major polypeptides of purified hepatitis B surface antigen of molecular weight 22,000–25,000 or 26,000 and glycoprotein of molceular weight 28,000–30,000 have been frequently designated p22 or p23 and gp28, Peterson (1981) proposed these should be more properly designated p25 and gp30, based on the probable true molecular weight of the protein as deduced from the DNA sequence of the viral gene. The two proteins were examined by amino acid analysis, Edman degradations, carboxypeptidase digestion, and peptide mapping after tryptic hydrolysis of polyacrylamide gel electrophoresis (PAGE) in the presence of SDS, two-dimensional thin-layer chromatography and electrophoresis, and high performance liquid chromatography (HPLC). The results showed that p25 and gp30 have the same amino acid composition, the same NH_2-terminal sequence, and the same carboxyl-terminal sequence. Both proteins are cleaved only by trypsin into two large fragments. The fragments corresponding to the NH_2-terminus of each protein are identical. However, the carboxyl-terminal fragments differ in that the fragment from gp30 contains carbohydrate. Digestion after aminoethylation revealed that the carboxyl-terminal fragments of both p25 and gp30 were further digested to yield a number of identical peptides, with the only demonstrable difference being in the large peptide-containing carbohydrate. These results, and the fact that treatment of hepatitis B surface antigen with anhydrous hydrofluoric acid converted gp30 into p25, support the conclusion that these two major proteins differ only by the presence of carbohydrate in gp30. The NH_2-terminal sequence, carboxy-terminal sequence, and the amino acid composition of several internal tryptic peptides were found to be consistent with the protein sequence predicted from the DNA sequence of hepatitis B virus.

III. Hepatitis B Polypeptide Vaccines

The advantages of a polypeptide vaccine derived from any source include precise biochemical characterization, exclusion of genetic material of viral origin, and exclusion of host- or donor-derived substances (Zuckerman, 1975, 1976). The disadvantages of polypeptide vaccines include low yield if strong ionic detergents are used for separation, although the yield has been substantially improved by the use of non-ionic detergents (Skelly *et al.*, 1979a, 1981a). In addition, timing of appearance, titer, and duration of antibody responses need to be studied carefully. Hepatitis B polypeptide vaccines containing hepatitis B specific antigenic determinants associated with a nonglycosylated polypeptide with a molecular weight of 23,000 to 25,000 and a glycosylated polypeptide with a molecular weight of 28,000 to 30,000 have been prepared and tested for safety, immunogenicity, and protective efficacy in susceptible chimpanzees (Dreesman *et al.*, 1981; Tabor *et al.*, 1982).

There are two other published reports on possible approaches to the production of a hepatitis B polypeptide vaccine and a method for the preparation of a minimal antigenic structure containing only the group-specific determinant **a** of the surface antigens. Miashiro *et al.* (1980) purified the spherical 22-nm hepatitis B surface antigen particles, without regard to HBsAg subtypes, from the plasma of asymptomatic carriers (former blood donors) by three cycles of ultracentrifugation. The purified particles were then treated with 1% SDS at 37°C for 2 hr in the absence of a reducing agent (1% v/v 2-mercaptoethanol). This treatment resulted in the solubilization of the outer coat of the particle, yielding a polypeptide with a molecular weight of 49,000. This polypeptide carried the common determinant of the surface antigen, **a**, as well as the four subdeterminants **d**, **y**, **w**, and **r**. This polypeptide was found to be a potent immunogen in mice, even though the recovery of the polypeptide on the basis of optical density at 280 nm was 2% of the starting surface antigen material.

When the 49,000 molecular weight polypeptide was reduced in the presence of 2-mercaptoethanol, it split into two polypeptides with molecular weights of 22,000 and 27,000. These latter two polypeptides were considerably less antigenic and immunogenic. Miashiro *et al.* (1980) proposed that the 49,000 molecular weight polypeptide could be used as a vaccine. Karelin and Zhdanov (1981) searched for a minimal structure that contains only the **a** antigenic determinant for use as a vaccine, rather than employ the 22-nm spherical particles or their antigenic polypeptides. The 22-nm hepatitis B surface antigen particles were purified from the plasma of carrier donors. The purified particles were treated with 0.1% pronase in the presence of 1% SDS at 37°C overnight for self-digestion of the residual proteolytic activity. The resulting antigenic fragments contained the group-specific antigenic determinant **a**, and ~30% or less of subdeterminant activity **y** was also preserved.

The electrophoretic mobility of the fragments referred to as gp12 in SDS–PAGE corresponded to globular proteins with a molecular weight of 12,000 (or less). The antigen gp12 differed from the native hepatitis B surface antigen in its isoelectric point and UV-absorption spectrum. This antigenic material was resistant to heat, but it was inactivated after treatment with neuraminidase free of any other glycosidase activity. It may therefore be assumed that the terminal neuraminic acid residue plays a role in the composition of the **a** antigenic determinant. Aggregates of gp12 were immunogenic for guinea pigs, and antibodies to **a** and **y** were produced, but none to proteins of normal human plasma. It was suggested that the differences between the native antigen and gp12 could result from the aggregated state of gp12, which masks a certain portion of the antigen determinants, and that the use of one essential antigenic determinant would be a harmless and effective vaccine.

The purification of viral coat subunits in large quantities presents considerable problems, particularly with viruses possessing a lipoprotein envelope in which the immunogenic components are integral membrane proteins that are highly hydrophobic, insoluble in aqueous media. The extraction of the antigenic polypeptides by the nonionic detergent Triton X-100 resolved one of the problems. However, polypeptides in monomeric solution in high concentrations of detergent are not a suitable vaccine. Consequently, a method of detergent removal that allows the gp28 and p23 complex of hepatitis B surface antigen to reassociate into water-soluble protein micelles was developed (Skelly *et al.*, 1981a). Protein micelles are aggregates of polypeptides arranged so that the hydrophobic regions are sequested in the interior of the particles with the hydrophilic residue on the surface, so that the micelles are water soluble.

The buoyant density of the micelles prepared from chimpanzee carrier plasma in cesium chloride was 1.25 g/ml compared to a density of 1.19 g/ml for intact 22-nm particles, an increase consistent with the removal of most of the lipid by the solubilization procedure. Electron microscopy showed that the micelles were pleomorphic and fluffy in appearance, with diameters in the range of 60 to 200 nm (mean, 120 nm). Polyacrylamide gel electrophoresis showed that both gp28 and p23 were present in similar proportions as in the original detergent extract. These polypeptides together constituted 40% of the total protein of the purified 22-nm particles used as starting material. Ninety percent of the gp28–p23 complex was recovered from a concanavalin-A-Sepharose column, and the final yield of the two polypeptides in micelle form was estimated to be 60–70% of the amount originally present in the intact 22-nm particles.

The micelles competed effectively with intact 22-nm surface antigen particles for surface antibody in a radioimmunoprecipitation test. Their

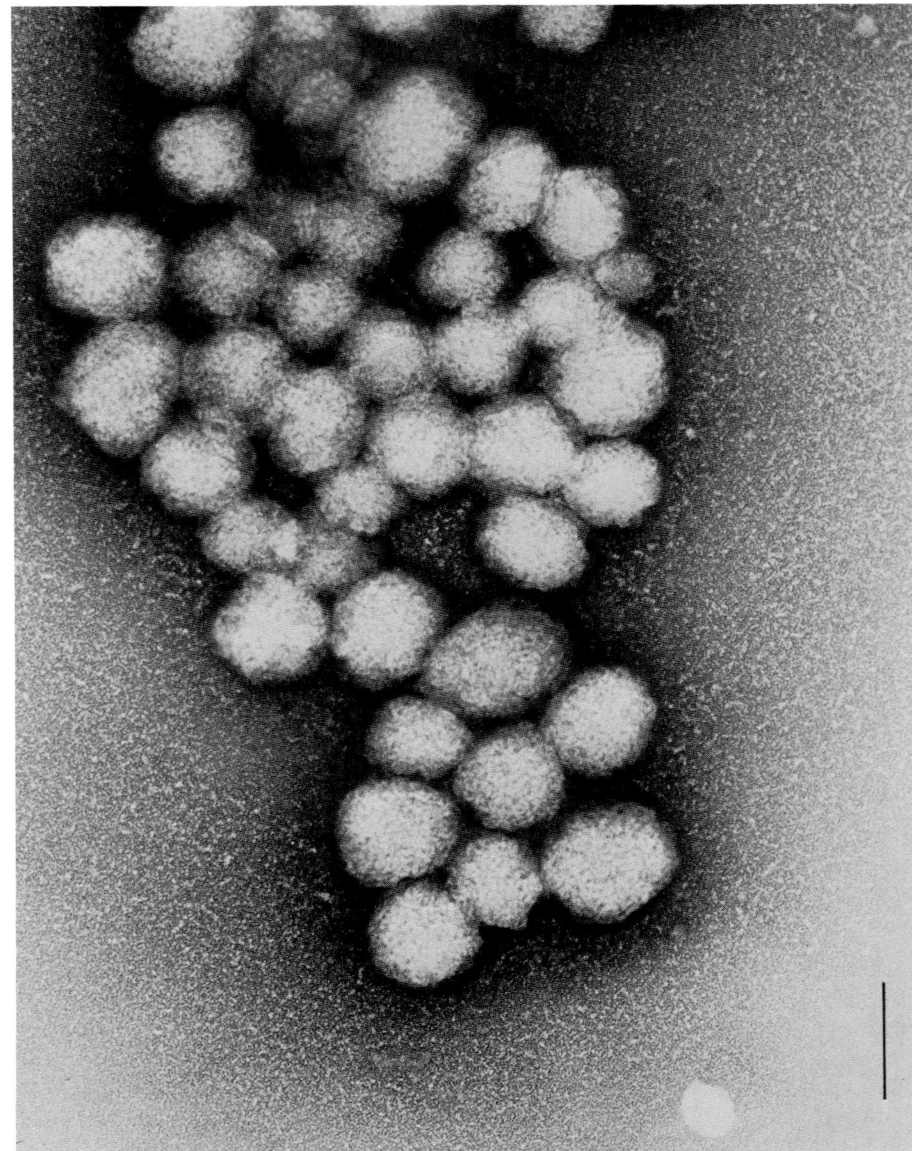

immunogenicity was compared in a mouse potency test, since the serological response in mice has been a useful indicator of the immunogenic potential of candidate hepatitis B vaccines (see Chapter 16). Consistently higher levels of antibody (anti-HBs) were induced in animals receiving micelles, possibly also with a higher affinity than those elicited by native HBsAg. Several factors may, singly or in combination, account for the greater immunogenicity of the micelles, including their large size, altered distribution of antigenic sites, or the absence in them of host-derived serum proteins such as albumin. Young *et al.* (1982) prepared polypeptide micelles from hepatitis B surface antigen purified from plasma pooled from asymptomatic human carriers. The buoyant density in sucrose was 1.24 g/ml, and electron microscopy showed the micelles to be spheroidal particles in the range of 140 to 250 nm (mean diameter, 200 nm), with the surface of the particles being composed of discrete globular and stranded units (Fig. 1).

The antigenic activity of the polypeptides, as determined by radioimmunoassay, was preserved throughout solubilization and reassociation. The results showed that the antigenic complex of gp28 and p23 can be readily isolated in high yield from intact 22-nm particles, and that this complex can be reassociated into a micellar form as has been described for other viral envelope proteins. The chemical purity, specific serological activity, and immunogenicity of the micelles, taken together with the ease of their preparations on a large scale, strongly favor their development as an alternative "second-generation" hepatitis B vaccine.

Formaldehyde is widely used for the inactivation of viral vaccines, yet there is little published information on the effects of formaldehyde on hepatitis B surface antigen. Skelly *et al.* (1981b) reported that treatment with formaldehyde under conditions generally used for viral inactivation had little effect on the antigenicity or immunogenicity of the intact 22-nm surface antigen particle or on that of the protein micelles. Pretreatment with formaldehyde had no effect on the ability of Triton X-100 to disrupt the particles, nor did it alter the behavior of the disrupted material in affinity chromatography. Polypeptides in a micellar form may also be a suitable preparation of vaccines from antigenic proteins produced by the expression of cloned hepatitis B virus DNA in prokaryotic and eukaryotic cells and from peptides produced by chemical synthesis (Howard *et al.*, 1982).

Figure 1. Electron micrograph of negatively stained micelles prepared from hepatitis B surface antigen of human origin. The scale bar represents 200 nm. (From a series by P. Young, C. R. Howard, and A. J. Zuckerman).

IV. Vaccines from "Antigen-Producing" Cell Lines

Antigen sources from other than human carriers of markers of hepatitis B virus are becoming available from heteroploid surface antigen-secreting cells derived from hepatocellular carcinoma (see, Aden *et al.*, 1979; Skelly *et al.*, 1979b; Copeland *et al.*, 1980; Das *et al.*, 1981; Wen *et al.*, 1981). The surface antigen is non-infectious (Tabor *et al.*, 1981); it is of relatively simple biochemical composition, the cell lines can be characterized, techniques are available to ensure freedom from contaminating nucleic acid, and potent inactivating agents are available. However, the cell lines are transformed and show heterotransplantibility, and therefore development of such vaccines must proceed with great caution. This topic has been recently discussed and reviewed by Mann *et al.* (1982) (see also Chapter 16).

V. Application of Recombinant DNA Techniques to the Development of Hepatitis B Vaccines

Particularly attractive sources of antigenic material would be prokaryotic cells expressing hepatitis B surface antigen proteins as a result of cloning of fragments of hepatitis B virus DNA and propagation in *Escherichia coli* using plasmids and derivatives of λ bacteriophages as vectors (Burrell *et al.*, 1979; Edman *et al.*, 1981; Charnay *et al.*, 1979, 1980; MacKay *et al.*, 1981). This resulted in the determination of the nucleotide sequence of the viral DNA and the organization of the viral genome (Valenzuela *et al.*, 1979; Galibert *et al.*, 1979; Pasek *et al.*, 1979). Although *E. coli* has generally been used as the host cell for expressing cloned genes (Sninsky *et al.*, 1979; Sninsky and Cohen, 1982), there are advantages in using other bacteria such as *Bacillus subtilis* for the production of viral and other polypeptides. For example, *B. subtilis* is nonpathogenic and does not produce endotoxin, and it excretes several extracellular proteins in large amounts. Furthermore, *Bacillus* strains are widely used commercially for producing antibiotics and enzymes, and in Japan *B. subtilis* (natto) is used as a source of food for human consumption. Recently, hepatitis B core antigen and the major antigen of foot-and-mouth disease virus have been produced in *B. subtilis* after the insertion of the appropriate viral DNA into a plasmid vector (Hardy *et al.*, 1981).

Expression of hepatitis B proteins in eukaryotic cells has also been achieved in mutant mouse LM cells (Dubois *et al.*, 1980) and in HeLa cells (Hirschman *et al.*, 1980; Hirschman and Garfinkel, 1982), but transformed heterotransplantable cell lines have not yet been licensed for vaccine production. The genome of simian virus 40 (SV-40) has been used as a vector by attachment of a fragment of hepatitis B virus DNA carrying the surface antigen gene and the surface antigen was expressed in monkey kidney cells (Moriarty *et al.*, 1981). Expression of hepatitis B surface antigen has also been obtained in yeast cells. The antigen has similar morphology, sedimentation coefficient, and buoyant density as the 22-nm spherial particles found in human plasma (Valenzuela *et al.*, 1982), and this preparation represents an important source for development of a vaccine against hepatitis B.

VI. Chemically Synthesized Vaccines

The prospect of synthetic vaccines is an important development offering many advantages in attaining the ultimate goal of chemically produced, pure, uniform, and safe multivalent vaccines to replace many current bacterial and viral vaccines, which often contain a large number of irrelevant microbial antigenic determinants, proteins, and other materials that contaminate the essential immunogen and may lead to untoward side effects. Sela (1975) noted that as a result of work in progress since 1966, the conceptual way to synthetic vaccines was open, since the feasibility for such an approach had been demonstrated in studies with tobacco mosaic virus after the identification of an antigenic determinant and its amino acid sequences responsible for the immunogenic activity of the virus. Such amino acid moieties can be synthesized, and when coupled to a carrier protein induce the production of neutralizing antibody in experimental animals. Subsequently, it was also shown that it is possible to use a synthetic macromolecule for eliciting antibodies reacting exclusively with a specific region of a native egg white lysozyme. This was achieved by synthesizing a particular segment of the enzyme from its amino acid components, attaching the peptide to branched poly-DL-alanine as carrier, and using the conjugate for immunization. The resulting antibodies reacted with native lysozyme via a unique region that is conformation dependent.

In 1976, the neutralization of a bacterial virus was accomplished by Langbeheim *et al.* with antibody elicited by a synthetic antigen. The following are more recent examples of synthetic peptides that have been shown to be immunogenic in laboratory animals, illustrating the feasibility of using this approach for the ultimate production of chemically synthetic vaccines.

Diptheria toxin is a single polypeptide chain of 62,000 molecular weight with two disulfide bridges. There is evidence that the loop of 14 amino acids subtended by the disulfide bridge near the NH_2 terminus is implicated both in the toxicity and the immunological specificity of the molecule. A synthetic tetradecapeptide linked covalently to two different carriers by Audibert *et al.* (1981) elicited antibodies in guinea pigs that bind specifically with the toxin and neutralize its dermonecrotic and lethal effects. This is believed to be the first example of successful active immunization against a bacterial toxin using a synthetic antigen. Another example is the induction of type-specific protective immunity by Beachey *et al.* (1981) using a synthetic peptide of *Streptococcus pyogenes* M protein that contained only 12 amino acid residues. The immunogenicity of such small peptides indicates a way to the development of safe vaccines against streptococcal infections which cause rheumatic fever and rheumatic heart disease. The efficacy of very small peptides would permit the disposal of a large portion of the protein molecule, and therefore should reduce the chances of eliciting immunological cross-reactions against host tissues.

Similar approaches to the development of chemically synthesized hepatitis B vaccines were described a few years ago by several investigators (Rao and Vyas, 1973; Anonymous, 1973; Zuckerman and Howard, 1973, 1975; Zuckerman, 1975), and current progress suggests that such synthetic peptide vaccines are within reach (Zuckerman, 1982a,b). Valenzuela *et al.* (1979) and others identified an 892-base pair region along the DNA strand of hepatitis B virus with the **adw** determinants using cloned DNA fragments, and the full sequence of the 226 amino acids constituting the 23,000–25,000 molecular weight polypeptide of hepatitis B surface antigen was predicted. The corresponding sequence for the **ayw** subtype suggested a variation of 16 amino acids (Galibert *et al.*, 1979). Employing a computer program that had been used to predict the internal and external residues of proteins with known structure, Lerner *et al.* (1981) chemically synthesized 13 peptides corresponding to amino acid sequences predicted from the nucleotide sequence for hepatitis B surface antigen. Seven of 13 free or protein carrier-linked synthetic peptides elicited an antipeptide response in rabbits. Where used, the carrier protein was keyhole limpet hemocyanin in complete and subsequently in incomplete Freund's adjuvant. Antisera against four of the six soluble peptides, which ranged from 10 to 34 amino acid residues, reacted with the native antigen and also precipitated the 25,000 and 30,000 molecular weight major polypeptides of hepatitis B surface antigen. Hopp and Woods (1981) also used a computerized analysis of the amino acid sequences of the surface antigen protein of hepatitis B virus to predict a putative dominant epitope, the sequence of Lys-Pro-Thr-Asp-Gly-Asp, corresponding to positions 141–146 of the surface antigen. They then synthesized a tetradecapeptide containing residues 138–149 of the surface antigen plus two glycine residues at its COOH terminal. The four cystein residues were replaced by α-aminobutryic acid in order to prevent polymerization and other side reactions common to sulfhydryl-containing peptides.

The prediction that the synthetic peptide contains a major epitope of hepatitis B surface antigen was confirmed. It was also demonstrated that this sequence of amino acids contains the group-specific determinant **a** and the subdeterminant **d**, but not the epitope of subdeterminant **y** or that of albumin. When the peptide was attached to aldehyde-stabilized human erythrocytes and injected into mice, it induced the formation of antibody to the hepatitis B surface with and without the use of Freund's complete adjuvant (Prince *et al.*, 1982). Vyas (1981) previously reported that a synthetic oligopeptide of 13 amino acids in the sequence 136–147 represented a partial analog of the a determinant of the hepatitis B surface antigen.

Dreesman *et al.* (1982) reported the results of a study also using a computer analysis of the amino acid sequence of a 25,000 molecular weight HBsAg polypeptide to predict two hydrophilic regions of the surface antigen molecule. Two cyclic peptides containing disulfide bonds in the region between amino acid sequences 117 and 137 were synthesized. The two synthetic peptides with sequences 117–137 and 122–137 were incorporated into several adjuvants including Freund's complete adjuvant, alum, and multilamellar liposomes with and without muramyl dipeptide. Groups of BALB/c mice were immunized intraperitoneally with each of the preparations. Antibody to HBsAg was induced 7–14 days after inoculation in ~50% of the mice in each group, and in four or five of six mice when the immunizing preparation of the 117–137 peptide was emulsified with Freund's complete adjuvant. On day 21, however, the peak levels of antibody decreased in most groups of mice. It should be noted that antibody response was elicited in mice after a single injection without covalent linkage to a carrier protein. Further studies with synthetic hepatitis B peptides are in progress.

An immune response to an intact strain of type A human influenza virus using a synthetic peptide has also been described more recently (Muller *et al.*, 1982). A peptide analogous to sequence 91–108 of the hemagglutinin of type A H3N2 influenza virus was synthesized by the

Merrifield solid-phase method, and the peptide was covalently linked to several macromolecular carriers. The conjugate with tetanus toxoid was used for the immunization of rabbits and mice with the production of specific antibodies, which were protective against infection with a relatively low viral challenge in mice with the A/Texas/77 mouse-adapted influenza virus. The preliminary results thus also indicate the potential of synthetic material for eliciting antiviral immunity against an important and common pathogen.

Synthetic peptides may well be employed in due course as vaccines, although mixtures of more than one of the peptides may be required. Of the many questions that remain to be answered, the critical issues are whether antibodies induced by synthetic immunogens will be protective and whether protective immunity will persist. Some of the carrier proteins and some of the adjuvants that had been linked to the synthetic molecules cannot be used in man, and it is therefore essential to find acceptable and safe materials for covalent linkage, or alternatively to synthesize sequences that do not require linkage. It is clear that we are entering the era of antigen and antibody engineering, and the prospect of multivalent synthetic vaccines against a variety of microbial agents appears to be within reach.

Acknowledgments

The work on hepatitis in progress at the London School of Hygiene and Tropical Medicine is supported by generous grants from the Medical Research Council, the Department of Health and Social Security, the Wellcome Trust, and the World Health Organization. The hepatitis B vaccine development project is generously supported by the Department of Health and Social Security, the British Technology Group (formerly the National Research Development Corporation), the Wellcome Trust, and by the Commission of the European Economic Community.

References

Aden, D. P., Fogel, A., Plotkin, S., Damjanov, I., and Knowles, B. B. (1979). *Nature (London)* **282**, 615–616.
Anonymous (1973). *Nature (London)* **241**, 499.
Audibert, F., Jolivet, M., Chédid, L., Alouf, J. E., Boquet, P., Rivaille, P., and Siffert, O. (1981). *Nature (London)* **289**, 593–594.
Beachey, E. H., Seyer, J. M., Dale, J. B., Simpson, W. A., and Kang, A. H. (1981). *Nature (London)* **292**, 457–459.

Burrell, C. J., MacKay, P., Greenaway, P. J., Hofschneider, P. H., and Murray, K. (1979). *Nature (London)* **279**, 43–47.

Charnay, P., Pourcel, C., Louise, A., Fritsch, A., and Tiollais, P. (1979). *Proc. Natl. Acad. Sci. U.S.A.* **76**, 2222–2226.

Charnay, P., Gervais, M., Louise, A., Galibert, F., and Tiollais, P. (1980). *Nature (London)* **286**, 893–895.

Copeland, J. A., Skelly, J., Mann, G. F., Howard, C. R., and Zuckerman, A. J. (1980). *J. Med. Virol.* **5**, 257–264.

Das, P. K., Nayak, N. C., Tsiquaye, K. N., and Zuckerman, A. J. (1981). *Br. J. Exp. Pathol.* **61**, 648–654.

Dreesman, G. R., Chairez, R., Suarez, M., Hillinger, F. B., Courtney, R. J., and Melnick, J. L. (1975). *J. Virol.* **16**, 508–515.

Dreesman, G. R., Hollinger, F. B., Sanchez, Y., Oefinger, P., and Melnick, J. L. (1981). *Infect. Immun.* **32**, 62–67.

Dreesman, G. R., Sanchez, Y., Ionescu-Matiu, I., Sparrow, J. T., Six, H. R., Peterson, D. L., Hollinger, F. B., and Melnick, J. L. (1982). *Nature (London)* **295**, 158–160.

Dubois, M. F., Pourcel, C., Pousset, S., Chany, C., and Tiollais, P. (1980). *Proc. Natl. Acad. Sci. U.S.A.* **17**, 4549–4555.

Edman, J. C., Hallewell, R. A., Valenzuela, P., Goodman, H. M., and Rutter, W. J. (1981). *Nature (London)* **291**, 503–506.

Galibert, F., Mandart, E., Fitoussi, F., Tiollais, P., and Charnay, P. (1979). *Nature (London)* **281**, 646–650.

Gold, J. W. M., Smith, J. W.-K., Purcell, R. H., and Gerin, J. L. (1976). *J. Immunol.* **117**, 1404–1406.

Hardy, K., Stahl, S., and Kupper, H. (1981). *Nature (London)* **293**, 481–483.

Hayman, M. J., Skehel, J. J., and Crumpton, M. J. (1973). *FEBS Lett.* **29**, 185–188.

Hirschman, S. Z., and Garfinkel, E. (1982). *Hepatology* **2**, (Suppl.), 79–84.

Hrischman, S. Z., Price, P., Garfinkel, E., Kristman, J., and Acs, G. (1980). *Proc. Natl. Acad. Sci. U.S.A.* **77**, 5507–5511.

Hopp, T. P., and Woods, K. R. (1981). *Proc. Natl. Acad. Sci. U.S.A.* **78**, 3824–3828.

Howard, C. R., and Burrell, C. J. (1976). *Prog. Med. Virol.* **22**, 36–103.

Howard, C. R., and Zuckerman, A. J. (1974). *Intervirology* **4**, 31–44.

Howard, C. R., Skelly, J., Tabor, E., Gerety, R. J., Kremastinou, J., Tsiquaye, K. N., and Zuckerman, A. J. (1982). *In* "Viral Hepatitis" (W. Szmuness, H. J. Alter, and J. E. Maynard, eds.), pp. 411–423. Franklin Inst. Press, Philadelphia, Pennsylvania.

Karelin, V. P., and Zhdanov, V. M. (1981). *Mol. Virol.* **18**, 237–244.

Langbeheim, H., Arnon, R., and Sela, M. (1976). *Proc. Natl. Acad. Sci. U.S.A.* **73**, 4636–4640.

Lerner, R. A., Green, N., Alexander, H., Liu, F.-T., Sutcliffe, G., and Shinnick, T. M. (1981). *Proc. Natl. Acad. Sci. U.S.A.* **78**, 3403–3407.

MacKay, P., Pasek, M., Magazin, M., Kovacic, R. T., Allet, B., Stahl, S., Galibert, W., Schaller, H., Bruce, S., and Murray, K. (1981). *Proc. Natl. Acad. Sci. U.S.A.* **78**, 4510–4514.

Mann, G. F., Copeland, J. A., Skelly, J., Howard, C. R., and Zuckerman, A. J. (1982). *In* "Viral Hepatitis" (W. Szmuness, H. J. Alter, and J. E. Maynard, eds.), pp. 69–80. Franklin Inst. Press, Philadelphia, Pennsylvania.

Melnick, J. L., Dreesman, G. R., and Hollinger, F. B. (1976). *J. Infect. Dis.* **133**, 210–229.

Miashiro, S., Imai, M., Takahaski, K., Machida, A., Gotanda, T., Miyakawa, Y., and Mayumi, M. (1980). *J. Immunol.* **124**, 1589–1593.

Moriarty, A. M., Hoyer, B. H., Shih, J. W.-K., Gerin, J. L., and Hamer, D. H. (1981). *Proc. Natl. Acad. Sci. U.S.A.* **78,** 2606–2610.
Muller, G. M., Shapira, M., and Arnon, R. (1982). *Proc. Natl. Acad. Sci. U.S.A.* **79,** 569–573.
Pasek, M., Goto, T., Gilbert, W., Zink, B., Schaller, H., Mackay, P., Leadbetter, G., and Murray, K. (1979). *Nature (London)* **282,** 575–579.
Peterson, D. L. (1981). *J. Biol. Chem.* **256,** 6975–6983.
Peterson, D. L., Roberts, I. M., and Vyas, G. N. (1977). *Proc.Natl. Acad. Sci. U.S.A.* **74,** 1530–1534.
Prince, A. M., Ikram, H., and Hopp, T. P. (1982). *Proc. Natl. Acad. Sci. U.S.A.* **79,** 579–582.
Rao, K. R., and Vyas, G. N. (1973). *Nature (London), New Biol.* **241,** 240–241.
Sela, M. (1975). *In* "Antiviral Mechanisms" (M. Pollard, ed.), pp. 91–98. Academic Press, New York.
Shih, J. W.-K., and Gerin, J. L. (1975). *J. Immunol.* **115,** 634–639.
Shih, J. W.-K., and Gerin, J. L. (1977). *J. Virol.* **21,** 347–357.
Shih, J. W.-K., Tan, P. L., and Gerin, J. L. (1978). *J. Immunol.* **120,** 520–525.
Simons, K., Helenius, A., and Garoff, H. (1973). *J. Mol. Biol.* **80,** 119–133.
Skelly, J., Howard, C. R., and Zuckerman, A. J. (1978). *J. Gen. Virol.* **41,** 447–457.
Skelly, J., Howard, C. R., and Zuckerman, A. J. (1979a). *J. Gen. Virol.* **44,** 679–689.
Skelly, J., Copeland, J. A., Howard, C. R., and Zuckerman, A. J. (1979b). *Nature (London)* **282,** 617–618.
Skelly, J., Howard, C. R., and Zuckerman, A. J. (1981a). *Nature (London)* **290,** 51–54.
Skelly, J., Howard, C. R., and Zuckerman, A. J. (1981b). *J. Virol. Methods* **3,** 51–59.
Sninsky, J. J., and Cohen, S. N. (1982). *Hepatology* **2** Suppl., 725–785.
Sninsky, J. J., Siddiqui, A., Robinson, W. S., and Cohen, S. N. (1979). *Nature (London)* **279,** 346–348.
Tabor, E., Copeland, J. A., Mann, G. F., Howard, C. R., Skelly, J., Snoy, P., Zuckerman, A. J., and Gerety, R. J. (1981). *Intervirology* **15,** 82–86.
Tabor, E., Howard, C. R., Skelly, J., Snoy, P., Goudeau, A., Zuckerman, A. J., and Gerety, R. J. (1982). *J. Med. Virol.* **10,** 65–74.
Valenzuela, P., Gray, P., Quiroga, M., Zaldivan, J., Goodman, H. M., and Rutter, W. J. (1979). *Nature (London)* **280,** 815–819.
Valenzuela, P., Medina, A., Rutter, W. J., Ammerer, G., and Hall, B. D. (1982). *Nature (London)* **298,** 347–350.
Vyas, G. N. (1981). *INSERM Symp.* **18** 227–236.
Wen, Y.-M., Copeland, J. A., Mann, G. F., Howard, C. R., and Zuckerman, A. J. (1981). *Arch. Virol.* **68,** 157–163.
Wilson, G. S. (1967). "The Hazards of Immunization." Athlone Press, London.
Young, P., Vaudin, M., Dixon, J., and Zuckerman, A. J. (1982). *J. Virol. Methods* **4,** 177–185.
Zuckerman, A. J. (1975). *Nature (London)* **255,** 104–105.
Zuckerman, A. J. (1976). *Lancet* **1,** 1396–1397.
Zuckerman, A. J. (1982a). *Nature (London)* **295,** 98–99.
Zuckerman, A. J. (1982b). *Br. Med. J.* **284,** 686–688.
Zuckerman, A. J., and Howard, C. R. (1973). *Nature (London)* **246,** 445–447.
Zuckerman, A. J., and Howard, C. R. (1975). *Bull. N. Y. Acad. Med. [2]* **51,** 491–500.

Chapter 18

New Technologies

J. WAI-KUO SHIH*
Hepatitis Branch
Office of Biologics Research and Review
Food and Drug Administration
Bethesda, Maryland

I. Introduction

Ever since the discovery of hepatitis B surface antigen, the focus of interest has been on its immune reactivity. This reactivity has provided the basis for antigen detection, antigen subtyping, measurements of immune responsiveness, and vaccine development. By contrast, structural analysis of the antigen has been complicated by the complexity of the components of HBsAg, and the functional analysis of HBsAg as a

*Present address: Department of Transfusion Medicine, Clinical Center, National Institutes of Health, Bethesda, Maryland

429   Copyright © 1985 by Academic Press, Inc.
All rights of reproduction in any form reserved.
ISBN 0-12-280672-7

whole and identification of individual polypeptides in particular have been impaired by the lack of a practical infectivity assay system. Analyses of the physicochemical structure and the biological function of HBsAg have concentrated primarily on elucidation of its antigenicity and evaluation of its immunogenicity. The experience obtained in studing model protein–antigens led to the conclusion that the antigenicity is, in large part, conformation dependent. Amino acids that are spatially distant in linear sequence can be brought into proximity by secondary or tertiary structure to form an antigenic site (Crumpton, 1974; Atassi, 1975). Although short segments of amino acid sequence were identified on the proteins as antigen sites, the importance of conformational arrangement in the native antigen cannot be underestimated.

Previous approaches to defining antigenic determinants were primarily divided into two categories: isolation and characterization of immunologically active fragments and comparison of the native antigen with the molecule after specific modification. However, each approach imposed its own particular difficulty when applied to the study of an antigen with the complexity of HBsAg. The definition and assessment of purity of serum-derived particulate HBsAg antigen were difficult. HBsAg was recognized as a particularly stable particle resistant to most fragmenting treatments, probably because of its high content of lipids and hydrophobic polypeptides. It was found to be resistant to a variety of modifications designed to elucidate its antigenic activity. The immunogenicity of a particulate antigen composed of essentially identical subunits of polypeptide such as HBsAg provided a unique model for the study of immune response to this kind of antigen. Researchers were able to dissociate the particle into its constitutent polypeptides and to demonstrate that the dissociated subunits were identical to the native particles in antigenic composition, but far less immunogenic (Shih and Gerin, 1975). Investigators were also able to approximate the particulate nature of HBsAg by forming liposomes (Sanchez *et al.*, 1980) or micelles (Skelly *et al.*, 1981). Incorporation of HBsAg polypeptides into liposomes or micelles restored their immunogenicity.

Between the discovery of Australia antigen in the late 1960s and the licensing of the first hepatitis B vaccine in 1982, an enormous amount of information on the immune reactivity of HBsAg was accumulated. This information not only contributed to the basic understanding of the antigen and the virus from which the antigen was derived, but also to vaccine development and immunization practices. Kohler and Milstein (1975) opened a new era in immunology by introducing "hybridoma" technology for preparing unlimited amounts of monoclonal antibodies to specific antigens. At the same time, recombinant DNA research established itself both in basic molecular biology and in the application of this technology for resolving difficult biological research problems. Investigators have quickly employed both technologies in hepatitis B research, and the resulting information has had a substantial impact on our understanding of HBV. In this chapter, I shall review our understanding of the structure–function relationships of HBsAg in terms of immune reactivity and summarize the contribution of new technologies to this field.

II. Conventional Approaches to the Elucidation of Structure–Function Relationships

A. Stability of HBsAg

The stability of the antigenic activity of HBsAg was demonstrated very early. Kim and Bissell (1971) reported that using a double-diffusion precipitation assay, the immune reactivity of the hepatitis-associated antigen (HBsAg) was stable to heat (up to 6 hr at 56°C), to repeated freezing and thawing, to acid (pH 2–5, 3 hr, 37°C) or alkali (pH 9–10, 3 hr, 37°C) and to most commonly used proteolytic enzymes. The antigen was partially susceptible to digestion by subtilisin or subtilopeptidase A. They also showed that the antigen was stable in 8 M urea and that this solution did not increase the susceptibility of the antigen to proteolytic enzymes. In the same study, Kim and Bissell showed that immune reactivity was affected by treatment with 1% (or higher concentration) sodium dodecyl sulfate (SDS). Using a quantitative radioimmunoprecipitation (RIP) assay, we have shown that 0.1, 0.5, or 1.0% SDS will reduce the antigenic activity of HBsAg by 20, 35, and 55%, respectively (J. Shih, unpublished data). The complete extraction of lipid with diethyl ether did not affect antigenicity. This suggested that the antigenic determinant(s) of HBsAg was protein. This stability of HBsAg can be attributed to its being an exceedingly hydrophobic molecule with a high content of disulfide bridges, proline, and tryptophan residues (Sukeno et al., 1975; Shih and Gerin, 1977b; Peterson, 1981). The high lipid content, ~25% of the total mass of the particle (Steiner et al., 1974; Takahashi, 1975; Gavilanes et al., 1982), may also contribute to its resistance to enzymatic modification.

B. Effects of Reduction and Alkylation on Antigenic Activity

The importance of disulfide bridges in maintaining the antigenic activity and particulate structural integrity of HBsAg was first demonstrated by Sukeno *et al.* (1972). They showed that the titer of purified HBsAg was reduced from 1:1024 to 1:4 in the immunoelectroosmophoresis (IEOP) assay after reduction of the antigen by dithiothreitol (DTT) in 8 M urea. About 80% of the original activity was recovered after dialysis in saline phosphate buffer; electron microscopic observations showed that reconstituted particles were 18 nm in diameter, compared to the 22-nm native particle. Alkylation of reduced particles with iodoacetamide resulted in total loss of both antigenicity and morphologically intact particles. Vyas *et al.* (1972) also reported that reduced and alkylated HBsAg could induce a delayed-type hypersensitivity response in guinea pigs but did not elicit humoral antibody, suggesting the importance of disulfide bond-dependent conformation in stimulating the humoral antibody response. In a similar study by Dreesman *et al.* (1973), it was shown that reduction and alkylation destroyed antigenicity either in the presence or the absence of urea. In contrast, loss of morphological integrity occurred only after treatment with DTT and iodoacetamide in 8 M urea. Treatment with iodoacetamide alone did not alter antigenic activity, which suggested that free sulfhydryl groups do not play a major role in determining the chemical nature of the antigenic determinants.

Imai *et al.* (1974) found that a part of the HBsAg antigenic activity was relatively resistant to reduction and alkylation. This common antigenic determinant(s) of HBsAg that is resistant to reduction and alkylation was designated as AuRe, in contrast to AuS (antigenic determinants which are sensitive to the treatment). This AuRe is possessed by different samples of untreated HBsAg, irrespective of their antigenic subspecificities. AuRe is considered to constitute a part of the common antigenic structure of HBsAg, but it can be distinguished from the reduction sensitive **a** determinant as defined by the polyclonal group-specific anti-**a** reagent in common use.

The result of an experiment designed to demonstrate the reactivation of antigenic activity of reduced HBsAg by oxidation and the presence of reduction–alkylation-resistant antigenic determinant(s) is shown in Table I. The totally reduced HBsAg retained ~10% of the original antigenic activity, and quickly regained its antigenic activity upon air oxidation. However, only ~60% of the original activity was recovered after oxidation at low pH for 18 hr. Aliquots of the reduced material were

TABLE I

Reduction and Reoxidation or Alkylation of HBsAg

Treatment	Antigenicity[a] RIA (S/N)	Immunogenicity[b] PHA titer (anti-HBs)
Control[c]	29.3	1:256,000
Reduction[c]	4.9	1:32
Reduction Reoxidation[d]		
t_0	5.1	
t_{15} min	8.3	
t_{60} min	11.9	
t_{18} hr	20.1	1:1,024
Reduction–alkylation[e]	4.4	1:512
Reduction–alkylation twice[f]	4.3	

[a]Antigenicity was determined by anti-HBs as determined by RIA with sera at the same dilution. Control sera were in the linear portion of the titration curve.

[b]Immunogenicity was determined by immunizing each of four guinea pigs with 6 μg of antigen in complete Freund's adjuvant and boosting them 1 month later with the same amount of antigen. Sera were tested for anti-HBs 2 weeks after the booster dose.

[c]HBsAg was reduced in 8 M urea, pH 8.6, with 0.14 M 2-mercaptoethanol under N_2 for 4.5 hr. For the reduced HBsAg preparation, the sample was dialyzed against H_2O with bubbling N_2 for 18 hr; the pH was then adjusted to 3.0 with HCl.

[d]The above dialyzed sample (footnote c) was made to contain 6 mM cysteine and 0.6 mM cystine in 25 mM Tris–HCl, pH 8.6, and incubated at 37°C. At the designated time, aliquots were taken and diluted with PBS for RIA.

[e]The reduced HBsAg was alkylated with 0.16 M iodoacetamide in the dark and then dialyzed against H_2O for 18 hr.

[f]The above reduced and alkylated HBsAg (footnote e) was retreated by the reduction–alkylation procedure described.

further alkylated with iodoacetamide in 8 M urea. When this reduction and alkylation procedure was repeated once more on the prereduced and alkylated HBsAg, minimum reduction of antigenic activity was observed as compared to the sample after reduction alone. Substantial reduction of antigenic activity was noted after treatments, but significant activity remained detectable for all forms of modified antigens. This confirmed the observation of Imai *et al.* (1974) regarding the presence of reduction- and alkylation-resistant determinant(s) on HBsAg. The immunogenicity of modified HBsAg was examined by immunizing guinea pigs; the results are shown in Fig. 1. Antibodies against the native particle were elicited by all modified antigens. Reoxidized HBsAg apparently possessed the most immunogenic activity, and alkylated antigen was more immunogenic than the totally reduced form.

In 1980, Neurath and Strick developed radioimmunoassay (RIA) procedures specifically for the determination of antibodies to the reduction–

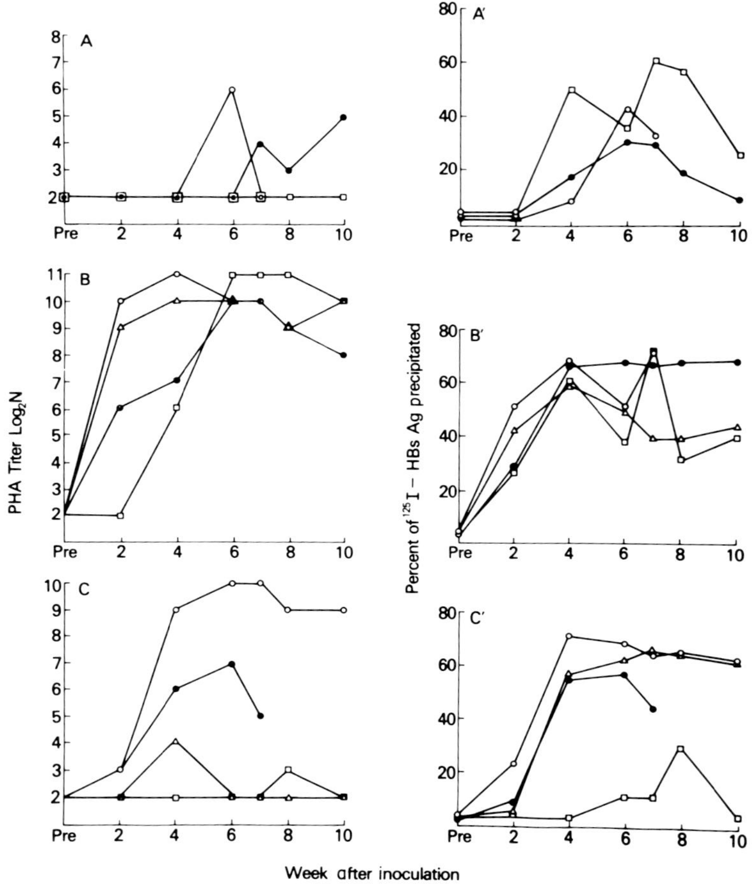

Figure 1. Immune responses to reduced, reoxidized, or reduced and alkylated HBsAg. Guinea pigs were immunized with 6 μg of modified HBsAg/**adw** in complete Freund's adjuvant at day 0 and again during the fourth week. The kinetics for production of anti-HBs by each animal was determined by PHA in Fig. 1 A–C for reduced, reoxidized, and reduced and alkylated HBsAg, respectively. The corresponding antibodies specific for the group determinant **a** from each guinea pig were also examined by RIP with ^{125}I-HBsAg/ayw at a 1 : 50 dilution, and are shown in Figs. 1A′, 1B′, and 1C′.

alkylation resistance determinant in both humans and in experimental animals. They observed the appearance of additional antigenic determinants after treatment, and suggested that those antibodies specific for denatured HBsAg (Shih *et al.*, 1978) would be useful tools to study HBV-specific polypeptides *in vitro*.

C. Modification by Enzymatic or Chemical Treatments

Kim and Bissell (1971) observed that in the absence of any dissociating agent, the antigenic activity of HBsAg was resistant to digestion by enzymes. Subsequently, Neurath *et al.* (1975) showed that treatment of the antigen with *Vibrio cholera* neuraminidase (EC 3.2.1.18) resulted in the release of sialic acid and the consequent increase of the isoelectric point from pH 4.35 to 5.45. The *in vivo* life span of the desialylated antigen in rabbit serum was reduced 10- to 20-fold. This increased rate of removal was attributed to the fact that the desialylated HBsAg induced a greater humoral antibody response than the untreated antigen. J. Shih, H. Swiderska, and J. L. Gerin (unpublished data) also investigated neuraminidase treatment of HBsAg. In their study, purified HBsAg was digested with neuraminidase or phospholipase A2 and phospholipase C in the presence of 0.2% Triton X-100. Antigen incubated in buffer served as a control. The antigens were repurified and the antigenicity compared by titration in RIA. Identical titers were observed for the control and the neuraminidase-treated antigens, whereas HBsAg treated with Triton X-100 and phospholipases had $\sim$100-fold lower titer (Fig. 2). The immu-

TABLE II

Guinea Pig Potency Test of Modified HBsAg

Treatment	Dilution[a]	Ratio[b]	Log_{10} ID_{50}[c]
None	10^0	4/4	-2.5
	10^{-1}	4/4	
	10^{-2}	4/4	
	10^{-3}	0/4	
Neuraminidase	10^0	4/4	-2.5
	10^{-1}	4/4	
	10^{-2}	4/4	
	10^{-3}	0/4	
Phospholipase A+	10^0	3/4	-0.8
Phospholipase C+	10^{-1}	2/4	
Triton X-100	10^{-2}	0/4	
	10^{-3}	0/4	

[a]Single IM inoculation of 0.2 ml diluted in 0.1% pre-serum. Undiluted (10^0) dose contains 4 μg of HBsAg protein.

[b]Number positive/number negative; positive means $P/N \geq 2.1$ in Ausab (Abbott Laboratories) test without dilution of the test sera. All pre-sera were negative.

[c]ID_{50}, 50% immunizing dose.

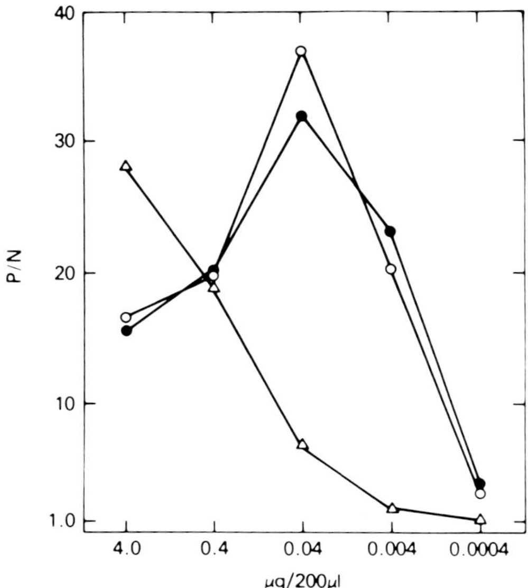

Figure 2. The antigenicity of modified HBsAg. HBsAg preparations of 2 mg/2.5 ml each were treated with 50 units of neuraminidase (O—O) or 0.2% Triton X-100, 23 units of phospholipase A2, and 12.5 units of phospholipase C (△—△) at 37°C for 6 hr. Antigen alone incubated under the same conditions and the mixture of the enzymes and detergents were used as the normal control (●—●) and the reagent blank, respectively. The modified antigens were pelleted through sucrose and resuspended in 0.1% normal guinea pig serum before the determination of antigenic activity by RIA (Ausria II). P/N is the ratio of positive counts above the mean of the negative controls. The abscissa is the dilution of antigens tested.

nogenicity of the modified antigen was examined by an immunological potency test in guinea pigs (Table II). There was a 50-fold difference in the immunizing dose of HBsAg treated with Triton X-100 and phospholipases and those treated in other various ways.

Neurath *et al.* (1978) showed that HBsAg could be delipided with either chloroform–methanol (2 : 1, v/v) or 1,1',3,3'-tetramethyl urea without affecting either the morphological integrity of the particles or their antigenicity. The delipided antigen had a buoyant density of 1.27–1.31 g/ml in CsCl as compared with 1.18–1.20 g/ml for intact HBsAg. However, Sugimoto and Toyoshima (1981) reported that even though a variety of detergents, including deoxycholate, SDS, Triton X-100, and cetyltrimethylammonium bromide did not cause a significant inactivation of HBsAg, N-cocodyl-L-arginine ethyl ester (CAE), a cationic detergent, was a potent inactivator of HBsAg. Treatment of HBsAg with 0.25% CAE resulted in total loss of antigenic activity and an increase in buoyant density to 1.29 g/ml. All attempts to reactivate the antigenic activity and to restore the original morphological forms failed. A stable aggregate of the denatured HBsAg–CAE complex was formed. Burrell *et al.* (1973) reported a progressive loss of HBsAg serological activity after oxidation with 0.01 *M* periodate, suggesting that the integrity of the carbohydrate moiety was necessary for antibody binding.

Shiraishi *et al.* (1978) showed that antigenic determinants **a** and **d** were especially sensitive to treatment with periodate, whereas determinants **r** and **w** were found to be quite stable. They also prepared monospecific antibodies, anti-**r** and anti-**w**, by using premodifed HBsAg as an immunogen in guinea pigs. However, Neurath *et al.* (1981) showed that addition of tunicamycin to PLC/PRF/5 cell culture media did not affect the production of antigenically active HBsAg. Alexander *et al.* (1982) also reported that glycosylation was not required for continued synthesis and export of the antigenic HBsAg particles produced by the hepatoma cell line PLC/PRF/5. These results and the production of fully antigenic particles by prokaryotic cells with cloned HBV DNA suggested that the carbohydrate moiety of HBsAg is not essential for its immunological activity. The earlier observation of the alteration of activity after modification may have resulted from the reaction between periodate and tryptophan, methionine, or tyrosine in the protein (Atassi, 1967).

Various chemical modifications performed in an attempt to elucidate the antigenic determinants of HBsAg were reported by Neurath *et al.* (1981). Reagents considered specific for the amino acid residues lysine, methionine, cysteine, arginine, tyrosine, tryptophan, glutamic acid, and aspartic acid were used to treat purified HBsAg particles. Based on observed alterations of HBsAg antigenic activity and the known amino acid sequence of the HBsAg polypeptide, an antigenic determinant was postulated to lie within amino acid residues 135–155.

D. Isolation of Active Fragments

Experiments designed to isolate antigenically active fragments containing defined HBsAg antigenic sites were performed by many investigators; only limited data were obtained. Rao and Vyas (1973), after ultrasonication treatment of HBsAg in the presence of 8 *M* urea and 2-mercaptoethanol, isolated a 6000-dalton peptide that retained a low level of HBsAg serological activity in a PHA assay. However, no data were presented on the affinity of antibody binding by this material, or whether it contained only group-specific, subtype-specific, or multiple determinants. Dreesman *et al.* (1973) reported the release of a fragment from

HBsAg after treatment with 8 M urea and 0.1 M dithiothreitol, followed by 0.3 M HCl. It had a molecular weight of 4,000–12,000 and was active in competitive RIA. Further characterization has not been reported.

Burrell *et al.* (1976) showed that the combined treatment of HBsAg with 0.1% SDS and 0.1% trypsin would release antibody-binding material of 5,000–15,000 daltons. By competitive RIP assay, it was shown that this carbohydrate-containing material represented the bulk of the group-specific determinant(s) **a**. Combined treatment with SDS and chymotrypsin (1 mg/ml) converted HBsAg particles of **ad** subtype into fragments with molecular weights <10,000 (Neurath *et al.*, 1978). These carbohydrate-containing fragments had both the group-specific determinant **a** and the subtype-specific determinant **d**. In the same study, Neurath *et al.* (1978) reported that a lower concentration of chymotrypsin (0.1 mg/ml) or trypsin would not digest HBsAg into low molecular weight fragments, whereas treatment with subtilisin or pronase in the presence of SDS resulted in fragmentation without retaining antigenic activity. HBsAg of subtype **ay** appeared to be resistant to proteolytic cleavage by chymotrypsin.

Machida *et al.* (1982) reported the isolation of a glycopolypeptide from purified gp29 of HBsAg after digestion with Nagarase and Pronase P. This glycopeptide contained 15 amino acid residues; its amino-terminal sequence was determined to be Lys-Pro-Thr-Asp-Gly-Asn. The polysaccharide moiety contained 5 mol of N-acetylglucosamine, and was connected with Asn at the sixth position from the NH_2 terminus. Antibodies against HBsAg were raised in mice injected with either isolated peptide or its ovalbumin conjugate. The anti-HBs activity was blocked by each of the p23 preparations isolated from HBsAg particles of **adw, adr,** or **ayw** subtypes. This suggested that the sequence of 15 amino acids, not the polysaccharide moiety, constituted a common antigenic determinant of HBsAg.

E. Antigenicity of Isolated Polypeptide Fractions

Since the particulate nature of HBsAg was established and was shown to consist of multiple components (Gerin, 1972), one of the major approaches to analyzing the structure–function relationship has been the isolation of antigenically active polypeptides. Using polyacrylamide gel electrophoresis (PAGE), it was noted that purified HBsAg could be dissociated into its polypeptide components only in the presence of the anionic detergents, SDS, or sodium sarkosyl (J. Shih, unpublished data). Chaotropic reagents, high concentrations of urea or guanidine–HCl, alone or in combination with nonionic detergents such as Nonidet P-40,

Triton X-100, or Tween 80 in the presence of 2-mercaptoethanol all failed to dissociate particles into their constituent polypeptides. When purified HBsAg preparations were analyzed in SDS–PAGE, 5–7 Coomassie blue staining bands were observed. These were designated P-1 through P-7 (P = polypeptide); their molecular weights were found to be 23,000, 29,500, 36,000, 41,500, 53,500, 72,000, and 97,000, respectively (Shih and Gerin, 1977a; Gerin and Shih, 1978).

To analyze the antigenicity of HBsAg and its constituent polypeptides (Shih and Gerin, 1973, 1975; Shih *et al.*, 1978), individual polypeptide fractions were isolated by extracting gel slices containing the peptide of interest. The purity of the polypeptide in each fraction was confirmed by reelectrophoresis in analytical SDS–PAGE. The isolated fractions exhibited no antigenicity in the standard PHA or sandwich RIA designed to detect particulate HBsAg. Antibodies to these polypeptide fractions were therefore prepared by immunizing guinea pigs with gel slice extracts (Shih and Gerin, 1975). Polypeptide P-2 was much more immunogenic than other polypeptides; it induced a rapid antibody response characterized by high titers of antibody. Anti-HBs activity was induced by P-6 only after repeated immunizations. In a competitive RIP assay using radioiodinated HBsAg as ligand, the avidities of antibodies against P-2 and P-6 were found to be 15-fold higher than antibodies against P-1 (Gerin *et al.*, 1975; Shih and Gerin, 1975). Antibodies to polypeptide fractions of both **ad** and **ay** subtype were analyzed for their reactivity against native particulate HBsAg. Antibody activities to both group-specific (**a**) and subtype-specific (**d** or **y**) determinants were detected by PHA (Gold *et al.*, 1976).

The polypeptide isolation procedure was subsequently improved with preparative SDS–PAGE, and larger quantities of purified polypeptides were obtained. A representative preparative SDS–PAGE elution profile is shown in Fig. 3. When each of the purified polypeptides, which were radioiodinated with ^{125}I, reacted as ligand with antibodies against polypeptides in a double antibody RIP assay, interesting and significant results were obtained. The polypeptide from each fraction was precipitable not only by the antibody induced by that fraction but also by antibodies induced to other fractions. This result suggested that all polypeptides from HBsAg shared common antigenic determinants (Shih *et al.*, 1978). In the same report, it was shown that P-2 prepared from one HBsAg **adw** subtype was precipitated by antibodies against P-1 of two other HBsAg **adw** and one HBsAg **ayw** preparation. Each of the polypeptides (P-1, P-2, and P-6) contained both group and subtype determinants, as shown by specific reaction with isolated monospecific antibodies, and induced antibodies against both kinds of determinants.

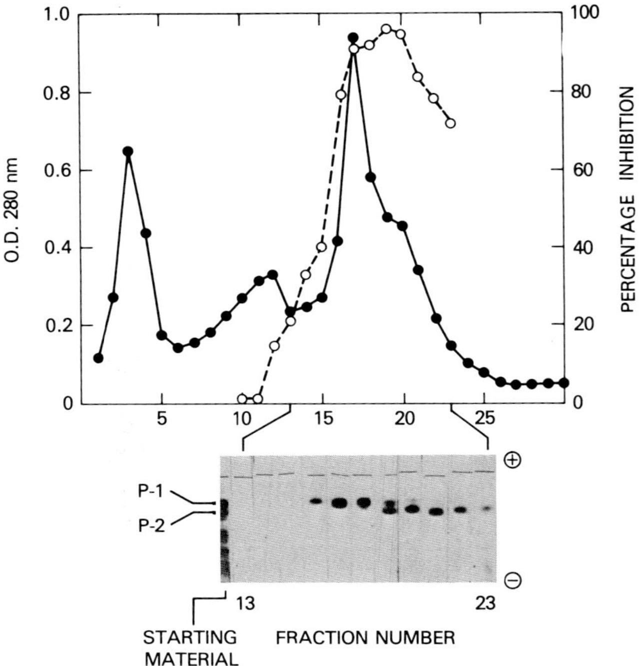

Figure 3. Preparative gel electrophoresis of HBsAg polypeptides. Two mg of purified HBsAg was solubilized at 60°C for 10 min in 1% SDS and 1% 2-mercaptoethanol, and electrophoresed in a preparative 7.5% acrylamide gel (20 × 150 mm); the electrophoretic buffer was 0.1% SDS in 0.1 M Tris–glycine buffer, pH 8.4, and bromphenol blue (BPB) was the tracking dye. The anode is on the left of the figure for the preparative gel. An aliquot (150 μl) of each 1.5-ml fraction was electrophoresed on an analytical gel of the same system and compared with the pattern of the starting material on the far left. The corresponding fraction numbers of two gel systems are indicated. Another aliquot (10 μl) of each fraction was assayed in the competitive inhibition radioimmunoassay (O- - -O). In this double antibody competitive inhibition assay, ^{125}I-P-2 was the ligand, and guinea pig anti-P-2 was the antibody; rabbit anti-guinea pig IgG was used as the second antibody.

These data were especially pertinent to polypeptides P-1 and P-2, since these two peptides were shown to have identical amino acid compositions (Shih and Gerin, 1977b). Polypeptide P-2 and P-5 were shown to exist as glycopeptides (Shih and Gerin, 1977a; Chairaz *et al.*, 1975). Figure 4 shows the result of an experiment carried out with [125]I P-2. After the digestion of this peptide with endoglycosidase H, all remaining material had the molecular weight of P-1. This observation supported the conclusion that P-2 is the glycosylated counterpart of P-1. This was confirmed by Peterson *et al.* (1977), who showed that P-1 and P-2 had identical amino acid sequences at their amino and carboxy terminals.

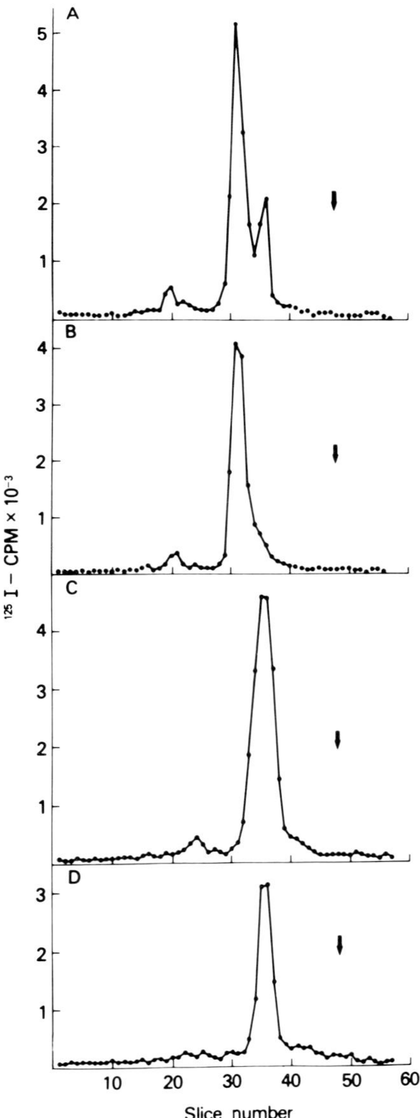

Figure 4. Conversion of gp29 to p23 by endoglycosidase. Purified and radioiodinated individual HBsAg polypeptide gp29 and p23 were mixed (A) and electrophoresed in SDS–PAGE for comparison with gp29 alone (B) or with samples of gp29 (C) and p23 (D) predigested with proteinase-free *Pseudomonas* endoglycosidase (kindly provided by G. Gilbert Ashwell of NIAMDD, NIH). Cylinder gels of 7.5% acrylamide were run and cut into 1-mm slices for counting. The arrow indicates the center of the tracking dye.

Peterson (1981) later reported the structural analysis of these two polypeptides in detail.

Production of antibody to individual polypeptide fractions derived from purified HBsAg was also reported by Dreesman *et al.* (1975). In contrast to the results reported by Shih and Gerin (1975), some of the polypeptide fractions elicited only subtype-specific antibodies, and some of the polypeptide fractions did not induce any anti-HBs activity. Cabral *et al.* (1978) also showed that guinea pigs immunized with HBsAg polypeptides P-1 and P-2 developed cell-mediated immunity, as determined by the macrophage migration inhibition assay. The humoral immune reponse to either of the polypeptides, as measured by RIA, was substantially lower than that observed in animals immunized with the same amount of protein in the form of intact particles (Cabral *et al.*, 1978). The sharing of similar antigenic determinants by different HBsAg polypeptides was also demonstrated by Sanchez *et al.* (1981), who reported cross-reaction of polypeptides with antibodies made against other peptide fractions.

The immunogenicity of purified polypeptides obtained from disrupted and reduced HBsAg particles was intrinsic to each peptide fraction. This activity was governed by amino acid sequences, and the conformation assumed after isolation. However, the activity of an individual peptide could be enhanced by improving its "nativeness" through the use of the thiol–disulfide-exchange procedure described by Saxena and Wetlaufer (1970). Figure 5 illustrates an experiment. When polypeptide P-1 (p23) or P-2 (gp29) was incubated with 8×10^{-3} M cysteine and 4×10^{-4} M cystine at 37°C for 90 min, a 10-fold increase of antigenic activity was observed for both polypeptides in a competitive inhibition assay (J. W.-K. Shih and J. L. Gerin, unpublished data).

Skelly *et al.* (1979) disrupted purified HBsAg with 2% Triton X-100 in the presence of salt to obtain a fraction with a much lower sedimentation rate than that shown by the native particle in a sucrose gradient. A purified fraction consisting of P-1 and P-2 was then isolated using a concanavalin A column.

An interesting and potentially important observation relating to polypeptide fractions was reported by Mishiro *et al.* (1980a). When purified HBsAg was treated with SDS in the absence of reducing agents, a polypeptide with a molecular weight of 49,000 (designated as P49) was isolated by gel filtration on Sephadex G-200. This P49 consisted of 2% of the input protein based on absorbance at 280 nm. It apparently represented a structural unit of the surface of the HBsAg particle, since it bore all common (**a, Re**) and subtype (**d, r**) determinants. On the basis of specific activity, this polypeptide had the same antigenic porency as the 22-nm

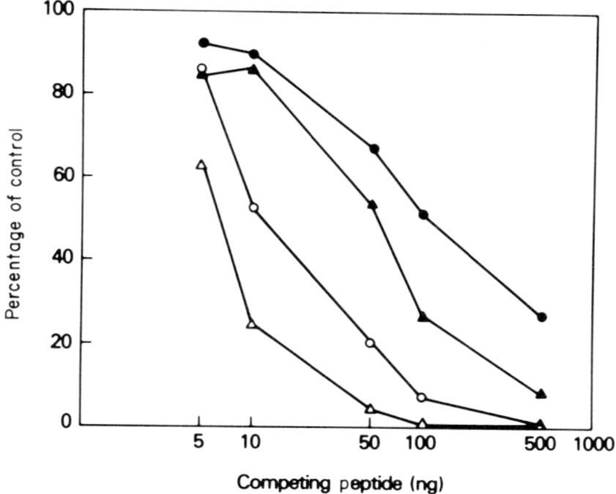

Figure 5. Activation of isolated HBsAg polypeptides by thiol–disulfide exchange. Individual HBsAg polypeptide p23 or gp29 isolated by preparative SDS–PAGE was dialyzed against 8 × 10^{-3} M cysteine and 4 × 10^{-4} M cystine in 25 mM Tris–glycine buffer, pH 8.6, at 37°C for 90 min (peptide concentration, 3 μg/ml). The activity was measured by competitive inhibition RIA; in the system, ^{125}I-gp29 was used as ligand, and guinea pig anti-gp29 was the binding antibody. The indicated amount of competing polypeptide, p23 (circle) or gp29 (triangle), was added to the reaction mixture prior to the addition of antibody. Filled symbols are for controls; open symbols are for the treated samples.

HBsAg particle and was equally immunogenic, judging from the induction of corresponding antibodies in mice. When the 49,000-dalton polypeptide was reduced with 2-mercaptoethanol, it cleaved into 22,000- and 27,000-dalton polypeptides with a drastic decrease in both antigenicity and immunogenicity. Mishiro *et al.* (1980b) also suggested that on the removal of this P49 outer coat of HBsAg, a nucleus of HBsAg was exposed. The tubular forms of hepatitis B surface antigen, rather than the Dane particles or 22-nm spherical forms, were specifically bound to the nucleus of HBsAg. The biological significance of this binding and of the tubular forms themselves has not been established. The possibility of tubular forms of HBsAg being useful as pathological or epidemiological markers of HBV infection deserves further consideration.

F. Involvement of Serum Proteins

The involvement of host components in the structure of hepatitis B surface antigen has been the subject of much controversy. In the beginning, it was suggested that HBsAg particles might be modified serum proteins (Millman *et al.*, 1971). Host proteins were the intrinsic components of the particles, formed during HBV infection. Later, the association of host components, either liver derived or serum derived, with HBsAg was thought likely to elicit adverse effects in recipients of vaccine preparations (Zuckerman, 1975).

Several serum protein components, such as prealbumin, albumin, apolipoproteins C and D, and the α chain of immunoglobulin G were reported to be constituent components of HBsAg (Neurath *et al.*, 1974). The particles were subjected to affinity chromatography on columns of insolubilized antibodies to normal human plasma. Prior exposure of the particles to 8 M urea, 5 M KI, pH 2.2, detergents, organic solvents, or proteolytic enzymes failed to prevent their adsorption to the immunoadsorbents. Goudeau *et al.* (1974) pointed out that nonspecific adsorption of HBsAg to immunoadsorbents could contribute to misleading conclusions. However, Burrell (1975) found that traces of normal serum components tightly bound to the particles gave low affinity immunoprecipitation reactions with antisera to several serum proteins. After testing antiserum to normal human liver in reactions with HBsAg, Burrell (1975) concluded that no antigenic determinants present in human liver cells were integral to the structure of HBsAg particles. Using highly purified radioiodinated HBsAg in an RIP assay, Shih *et al.* (1980b) showed that a subpopulation of HBsAg particles contained human albumin (HSA). Among different preparations of both **adw** and **ayw** subtypes, 20–40% of HBsAg particles were precititated by anti-HSA antibodies. When the isolated polypeptide fractions were individually examined by precipitation with 19 different rabbit anti-human protein sera, only P-6 was found to react significantly with anti-HSA. By competitive-inhibition assay, Shih *et al.* (1980b) also demonstrated that both HSA- and HBsAg-specific polypeptides of 68,000–72,000 daltons coexisted in the polypeptide P-6 fraction, but on separate molecules. Since the amount of P-6 varied in each preparation of HBsAg, as shown by SDS–PAGE, and in view of the observation that P-6 was released into the supernatant after prolonged storage, an experiment was designed to assess the exchange of released P-6 with the P-6 component of the particles (J. L. Gerin and J. W.-K. Shih, unpublished data). Polypeptide P-6 fraction and HBsAg were radioiodinated and each was mixed with the other unlabeled material. After various intervals P-6 and HBsAg were reisolated and the exchange of radioactivity into the unlabeled fraction was measured. No significant exchange was observed. This suggested that the 22-nm HBsAg particles were the finite product and that the serum protein components were contaminants that were not required for the integrity of the particles.

Imai *et al.* (1979) demonstrated the presence of a receptor for polymerized human albumin on HBV particles as well as on 20-nm HBsAg particles isolated from plasma. This receptor was species specific and protein in nature. An RIA for albumin-binding sites associated with HBsAg was described by Neurath and Strick (1979). Other investigators found that these receptor sites could be detected in either HBeAg or anti-HBe-positive sera (Hansson and Purcell, 1979). Receptors for polymerized albumin were reported to occur on HBsAg-containing hepatocytes and the PLC/PRF/5 hepatoma cell line (Ionescu-Matiu *et al.*, 1980; Thung and Gerber, 1981), as well as on isolated individual HBsAg polypeptides (Ionescu-Matiu *et al.*, 1980). Explaining the significance of this polymerized albumin receptor will require further study.

III. Hybridoma Technology

A. Production of Monoclonal Antibodies to HBsAg

The hybridoma technology introduced by Kohler and Milstein (1975) has been applied by many investigators, resulting in the production of monoclonal antibodies to HBsAg, HBeAg (Imai *et al.*, 1982), and HBcAg. These monoclonal antibodies have been utilized to elucidate the antigenic structure of HBV components, to delineate the antigenic determinants, and to develop diagnostic reagents. Their potential use as reagents for therapy and affinity chromatography have also been explored.

By fusion of either HBsAg/**adw**, or HBsAg/**ayw**, primed BALB/c mouse spleen cells with either P3x63-Ag8 or P3-NS1/1-Ag4-1 (NS-1) mouse myeloma cell lines, Shih *et al.* (1979, 1980a) produced hybridomas secreting anti-HBs. Six anti-HBs-producing cell lines have been established; BX182, BX259, BX248, CN324, DN238, and DN296. All six monoclonal antibodies are of the IgG1 subclass with κ light chains. Each clone showed a characteristic pattern of reactivity in RIA, when tested against solid phases coated with antigens of different subtypes, followed by either ^{125}I-HBsAg or ^{125}I-goat anti-mouse IgG probes. The pattern of reactions for each clone was stable through generations of cell culture *in vitro* and in passages as ascites in mice. The specificity of anti-HBs from each clone was examined by its reaction with ^{125}I-HBsAg of several subtypes in an RIP assay. Four types of reactions could be identified and related to the conventional serological subtyping definitions; they were anti-**a** (BX259 and CN324), anti-**d** (BX128), and possibly anti-**w** (BX248 and DN296) and anti-**y** (DN283). However, in subsequent experiments with a direct binding assay, more complex and less readily explained reaction patterns were observed. The results are shown in Table III.

TABLE III
Subtyping Murine Monoclonal Anti-HBs[a]

HBsAg subtype	BX 259	BX 182	CN 324	BX 248	DN 296
adr	+	+	−	−	−
adw	+	+	+	+	+
adw$_4$	+	+	+	−	−
ayr	+	−	−	−	−
ayw$_1$	+	−	+	−	−
ayw$_2$	+	+	+	+	+
ayw$_3$	+	−	−	+	+

[a]Equivalent amounts of HBsAg from different subtypes were used to coat Ausria II (Abbott Lab.) beads, followed by incubation with the testing monoclonal anti-HBs antibodies. The bound anti-HBs was determined by radioiodinated goat anti-mouse IgG.

Binding of monoclonal antibodies to HBsAg particles occurred irrespective of the conventional serological definition. This could be interpreted as a reflection of the fine specificity possessed by the monoclonal antibodies, or conversely, the heterogenity of epitopes on the surface of HBsAg among the different individual antigens.

Present *et al.* (1980) reported the production of murine monoclonal anti-**a**, anti-**d** antibodies using the NS-1 parental myeloma. These monoclonal antibodies had affinity constants ranging from 10^8 to $>10^{10}$. (Subsequently, these antibodies became commercially available through Hybritech Incorporated, La Jolla, California.)

A large number of murine monoclonal antibodies to HBsAg were obtained by Wands and Zurawski (1981) using NS-1 parental myeloma cells. They investigated the effect of the route of immunization, the interval between primary and secondary immunizations, and the immunizing antigen concentration on the production of monoclonal antibodies. Several high-affinity monoclonal antibodies of IgM and IgG isotype-producing cell lines were established. These antibodies have been utilized in the construction of solid-phase "sandwich" RIA (Wands *et al.*, 1981). Wands *et al.* (1980) showed that one of the ^{125}I-HBsAg polypeptides isolated by SDS–PAGE was precipitated by monoclonal antibodies specific for **adw** subtype or for both **adw** and **ayw** subtypes. Shorey *et al.* (1981) investigated a number of monoclonal anti-HBs antibodies in solid-phase RIA against a panel of 510 HBsAg-positive plasma samples. These samples had previously been subtyped with RIA using conventional antisera, and included HBsAg types **adw2, adw4, adr,**

aywl, ayw2, ayw3, ayw4, and **ayr.** The monoclonal antibodies used in the experiment were shown to recognize different determinants, as demonstrated by the lack of competitive inhibition in the antigen binding study. The results of 17,850 assay determinations indicated that two monoclonal anti-HBs reacted with every subtype of HBsAg. Another anti-HBs identified all but two specimens. In contrast, four monoclonal anti-HBs showed selective binding to certain subtypes, and they were able to identify subsets of antigen present in **adw2, ayw2,** and **ayw3** subtypes. Quantitative differences of binding to the particles by monoclonal antibodies were also observed by these investigators.

Goodall *et al.* (1981) reported the establishment of several monoclonal anti-HBs cell lines, designated RF-HBs-1 through RF-HBs-7. To produce these antibodies the mice had been immunized with purified HBsAg with NS-1 myeloma cells as the fusion partner. The RF-HBs-1 cell line has been shown to produce anti-HBs that reacts with all HBsAg particles tested, whereas most of the other clones produced antibody with limited specificities.

Kennedy *et al.* (1983) generated 17 monoclonal anti-HBs cell lines by fusing NS-1 myeloma cells with spleen cells from mice immunized with the **ayw** subtype of HBsAg. Eleven of these antibodies had specificity against the group-specific **a** determinant of HBsAg; two demonstrated antibody activity against the **w** HBsAg subtype; one was directed against human albumin, the three against human IgG. All of these monoclonal antibodies were of the IgG class.

B. Mapping the Antigenic Determinants

One important and useful purpose of monoclonal antibodies is to delineate antigenic determinants to understand their structure–function relationships. Monoclonal antibodies provide the means to analyze antigenic function in terms of epitopes. Neither well-adsorbed monospecific polyclonal antiserum nor direct fragmentation of antigen polypeptide has been able to achieve this. Stone and Nowinski (1980) developed a competitive antibody-binding assay for topological mapping of viral surface proteins. Gerhard *et al.* (1981) constructed an antigenic map of influenza virus hemagglutinin (HA) by comparative antigenic analysis of different mutants with a panel of selected monoclonal anti-HA antibodies. They noted that a single amino acid substitution could induce considerable change in antibody binding. Based on information obtained through their topological mapping of antigenic sites on hemagglutinin with monoclonal antibodies, Lubeck and Gerhard (1982) were able to detect conformational changes of the HA molecule induced by the binding of monoclonal antibody at topologically distinct antigenic sites. More importantly, topographical analysis of viral epitopes accomplished using monoclonal antibodies has provided an understanding of the mechanism of viral neutralization (Massey and Schochetman, 1981).

Monospecific polyclonal antisera prepared by cross-adsorption (Holland, 1976), affinity chromatography (Miyakawa *et al.*, 1975), or induction of anti-**y** in a chimpanzee carrier of HBsAg **adw** subtype (Tabor *et al.*, 1976) have provided valuable information on the antigenic composition of HBsAg (Holland, 1976) and the distribution of antigenic determinants on HBsAg constituent polypeptides (Shih *et al.*, 1978). They have been useful in demonstrating subtype-specific determinants on the surface of HBV particles (Hess *et al.*, 1979), and for development of reagents for subtyping both HBsAg and anti-HBs (Hoofnagle *et al.*, 1977). However, since HBsAg contains only one primary amino acid sequence and none of the constitute polypeptides has known biological function, without a realistic means for assay of the infectivity by HBV *in vitro* only limited structural analyses on the distribution of HBsAg antigenic sites have been performed, without attempting to elucidate its function.

The cumulative understanding is that HBsAg is a large particle with a diameter between 16 and 27 nm. It is composed of two major polypeptides with the same primary amino acid sequence and several minor polypeptides with different modifications, such as glycosylation or polymerization into dimer or higher molecular weight molecules, and possibly contains host serum proteins and other unidentified primary gene products. By conventional serological identification, a common cross-reacting antigenic determinant called group-specific determinant (**a**), which is probably a composite of many epitopes, and two mutually exclusive allelic determinants (**d** or **y** and **w** or **r**), called type-specific determinants, were found on the surface of HBsAg particles. This complicated molecular architecture obviously contributes to the complexity encountered in defining HBsAg epitopes with monoclonal antibodies. With the limited experience stated in the previous section, several investigators have observed both quantitative and qualitative differences in epitope distribution and its quantitative presence during HBsAg of the same subtype from different sources.

David *et al.* (1981), using a competitive antibody-binding assay, obtained interesting information regarding the relative proximities of one of the **a**-specific antigenic determinants. The epitope defined by monoclonal anti-HBs/**a**, HYB-259, appeared to be spatially very close to that recognized by anti-HBs, HBI-456, which also recognized group-specific **a** determinants but was only partially inhibited by the third monoclonal anti-HBs/**a**, HYB-410. This suggested the existence of at least two sterically distinct antigenic determinants that do not show subtype specificity. The HYB-410 determinant is sterically adjacent to the subtype-specific determinants **d** or **y**, as noted by the strong inhibition of binding monoclonal anti-HBs/**d** or anti-HBs/**y**. Data presented by David *et al.* (1981) also indicated that at least two distinct subtype **y** determinants could be detected. However, one must be cautious when designing and interpreting this kind of experiment. Differences in affinities of the antibodies and the possibility of induced conformational change of the testing antigenic molecule are among the points that deserve consideration.

In developing monoclonal antibodies to woodchuck hepatitis virus surface antigen (WHsAg), Cote *et al.* (1982) established a panel of monoclonal antibodies that was divided into three categories. One monoclonal anti-WHs, 101-2, defines a common antigenic determinant (HV/101) among the three mammalian hepadna virus surface antigens, HBsAg, WHsAg, and ground squirrel hepatitis virus surface antigen, GSHsAg. Seven other monoclonal anti-WHs antibodies react with both WHsAg and GSHsAg to various degrees; three monoclonal anti-WHs antibodies bind only to WHsAg. The hepadna virus group-specific antibody (101-2) reacts with HBsAg subtype variants in a group-specific rather than a subtype-specific manner. This finding, plus those obtained with an HBsAg-specific, group-reactive monoclonal antibody (BX259) discussed in the previous section (Section III,A), suggest that there are at least two group-reactive epitopes of HBsAg: one that is virus specific (HBV/259), and one that is common to two other mammalian hepadna viruses (HV/101). Using 11 monoclonal anti-WHs antibodies, Cote and Gerin (1983) were able to map 5 distinct antigenic sites on the surface of WHsAg. One of these sites apparently was the common determinant present on all hepadna viruses studied so far.

C. Applications of Monoclonal Antibodies against HBsAg

Monoclonal anti-HBs antibodies have been successfully applied to clinical diagnosis, immunotherapy in experimental animals, and as reagents in immunoaffinity chromatography. The availability and consistency of monclonal antibodies make them the ideal reagents for all the applications mentioned above, but care should be taken in developing their usage. For example, a monclonal antibody could be so specific that a point mutation within the epitope would abolish its immunological reactivity (Gerhard *et al.*, 1981). On the other hand, by isolation and propagation of a single clone, antibody to a minor determinant could be magnified and lead to cross-reactivity. A few examples of the usages of monclonal anti-HBs antibodies are discussed below.

Wands *et al.* (1981) have used monoclonal IgM antibodies to develop a solid-phase sandwich RIA for the detection of HBsAg. They took advantage of the multivalancy of IgM for binding a multideterminant antigen to achieve high sensitivity. The claimed detection limit of the assay was <100 pg of HBsAg per milliliter of plasma. This is approximately the lower limit of the most sensitive commercial "third-generation" RIA based on polyclonal antibodies. Using this IgM–IgM RIA, Wands *et al.* (1982a,b) subsequently detected high binding activity in the serum of liver disease patients without HBV markers and Australian aboriginals who were negative for HBsAg by conventional RIA. The same samples, however, were usually negative when tested by monoclonal IgG anti-HBs or by an assay that used monoclonal IgM anti-HBs on the solid phase only. Shafritz *et al.* (1982) reported that by using the same monoclonal anti-HBs antibodies they could detect HBsAg determinants in human serum when this antigen was present in immune complexes, and that a significant proportion of selected sera that are positive by the monoclonal anti-HBs RIA but negative by polyclonal anti-HBs RIA contain complementary HBV DNA sequences by molecular hybridization analysis. Care should be taken in interpreting detection results obtained by using monoclonal antibodies, since monoclonal antibodies has been shown repeatedly to possess cross-reactivity to unrelated materials. Sera contaminated with bacteria could also give false signals in the nucleic acid hybridization test with probes containing plasmid sequences. It is interesting to note that the monoclonal IgM anti-HBs (5D3) studied by Wands *et al.* (1981) showed 10- to 100-fold greater reactivity toward **ay** subtype than **ad** subtype in the samples tested. This monoclonal IgM anti-HBs was used only on the solid phase in a commercial RIA for the detection of HBsAg. The radioactive probe consisted of two monoclonal IgG anti-HBs antibodies. This assay was developed by Centocor Inc. (Malvern, Pennsylvania) as the first Food and Drug Administration-licensed monoclonal antibody diagnostic kit, and is marketed by Nuclear Medical Laboratories (Dallas, Texas).

In an attempt to develop a diagnostic reagent with the monoclonal anti-HBs antibodies described by Present *et al.* (1980), David *et al.* (1981) encountered difficulty in defining the nature of antibody specificity for a complex antigen such as HBsAg. Even the affinity constants measured for a given monoclonal antibody were different when tested against HBsAg samples that had identical HBsAg subtypes but were from different sources. In the development of an RIA, one should recognize that an antibody that shows high affinity for antigen when measured in the fluid phase may not react more strongly than a low-affinity antibody on the solid phase. Combinations of monoclonal antibodies for use in an assay, even when they have been shown to recognize different epitopes, may not improve the efficiency of binding. These authors also raised the concern of the "too specific" nature of monoclonal antibodies for use as immunodiagnostics.

The successful application of three murine monoclonal antibodies in a solid-phase RIA for HBsAg was described by Goodall *et al.* (1981). Monoclonal anti-HBs antibodies RF-HBs-1, RF-HBs-2, and RF-HBs-4 were shown to detect 7.0, 0.5, and 2.0 ng/ml of HBsAg, respectively. The combination of all three monoclonal anti-HBs had a limit of detection of 0.5 ng/ml with the same ^{125}I-RF-HBs-1 as tracer. The combined monoclonal anti-HBs assay was able to detect all 247 known HBsAg-positive sera as defined by two separate conventional RIAs, yet with a single monoclonal antibody on the solid phase, 0.8 to 13.8% of the HBsAg-positive serum samples would have been undetected in the assay.

Some potential therapeutic uses of monclonal anti-HBs were illustrated by the experiments of Shouval *et al.* (1982a,b). They showed that monoclonal anti-HBs IgM (clone 5D3), IgG2a (clone 5C3), and IgG1 (clone 2C6), developed by Wands *et al.* (1981), could attach to the surface of the human hepatocellular carcinoma cell line PLC/PRF/5, which synthesizes and secretes HBsAg. In the presence of complement, both the IgM and the IgG2a but not the IgG1 lysed PLC/PRF/5 cells in culture. Human hepatoma cell lines SK-Hep 1 and Mahlavu, which do not synthesize HBsAg, did not undergo complement-mediated cell lysis in the presence of these monoclonal anti-HBs antibodies. These authors also demonstrated the anti-HBs effect in athymic nude mice injected with PLC/PRF/5 cells (Shouval *et al.*, 1982b). Monoclonal anti-HBs IgM (5D3) not only suppressed tumor growth but also prevented tumor formation in some of the mice injected with tumor cells. Monoclonal anti-HBs IgG2a (5C3) produced some suppression of tumor growth, whereas the IgG1 (clone 2C6) had no effect on tumor growth. The variable effect of these monclonal antibodies on tumor growth in nude mice has not yet been correlated with differences in their avidity for HBsAg or their ability to recognize different HBsAg epitopes. Since the tumorogenecity of the PLC/PRF/5 cell line has not been directly linked to the HBV genome or to its capability for HBsAg production, the interpretation of the modification of tumor growth by monoclonal anti-HBs remains unclear.

Application of monoclonal anti-HBs antibodies as immunoaffinity chromatographic reagents has been evaluated by Lu *et al.* (1984) in comparison to standard centrifugation techniques. Comparable yields and purity of HBsAg preparations were obtained by affinity chromatography on monoclonal antibody columns in a relatively short time. Antigen prepared by such procedures also showed immunogenicity comparable to that of conventional preparations, as measured by mouse potency tests.

IV. Recombinant DNA Technology

A. Production of Antigenically Active Particles

Since the successful cloning of HBV DNA (Charnay *et al.*, 1979; Burrell *et al.*, 1979; Sninsky *et al.*, 1979) and the establishment of its nucleotide sequence (Valenzuela *et al.*, 1979; Galibert *et al.*, 1979; Pasek *et al.*, 1979), numerous investigators have performed experiments to induce the expression of cloned HBV DNA to produce its encoded proteins (Mackay *et al.*, 1981). Attempts to express the HBsAg gene directly in *Escherichia coli* were unsuccessful. The speculations were that HBsAg protein was toxic to the host bacteria, or that the newly synthesized HBsAg protein was quickly degraded. Small amounts were produced only when the S gene was fused with the β-galactosidase gene carried by λ phage (Charnay *et al.*, 1980) or with the β-lactamase gene carried by a constructed plasmid, ptrpL1 (Edman *et al.*, 1981). When the cellular extract was made, newly synthesized protein with an estimated molecular mass equivalent to the sum of HBsAg (23,000 daltons), and the mass of the expected fusion protein was precipitated by anti-HBs.

Expression of the HBsAg gene in yeast was much more successful. Valenzuela *et al.* (1982) reported that they synthesized HBsAg in the yeast *Saccharomyces cerevisiae* by using an expression plasmid that employed the 5'-flanking region of yeast alcohol dehydrogenase I as a promoter to transcribe surface antigen-coding sequences. The amount of HBsAg protein produced from 200 ml of yeast culture was 2–5 μg, calculated from RIA detection of HBsAg. The protein synthesized in yeast was assembled into particles having properties, such as buoyant density in CsCl, sedimentation rate in a sucrose gradient, and morphological characteristics by electron microscopy, similar to those of the 22-nm particles secreted by a human hepatoma cell line. The fact that HBsAg proteins synthesized in yeast were assembled into particulate form suggested that this probably is the intrinsic nature of the HBsAg polypeptide. However, only polypeptide p23, not the glycosylated gp29 form, was synthesized in the yeast system.

Miyanohara *et al.* (1983) placed the *S* gene of HBV under the control of the repressible acid phophatase promoter of the yeast *S. cerevisiae* in a plasmid capable of autonomous replication in both yeast and *E. coli*. Yeast transformed by this plasmid synthesized up to 5×10^5 molecules of immunologically active HBsAg polypeptide per cell. The HBsAg polypeptides produced in the yeast cells were assembled into 20-nm spherical particles, and were immunogenic in guinea pigs. This and the results of Valenzuela *et al.* (1982) supported the earlier suggestions that glycosylation of HBsAg is not essential for its immunological activities. However, detailed analysis of the effects of glycosylation of HBsAg immune reactivity would require direct quantitative comparison of the glycosylated form of antigen with its unglycosylated conterpart derived from the same DNA clone.

Several investigators have reported the expression of the HBsAg gene in mammalian cell culture systems. Dubois *et al.* (1980) used a derivative plasmid of pBR322 containing two HBV genomes in tandem to cotransform a mutant mouse L cell deficient in thymidine kinase with the cloned herpes simplex virus thymidine kinase gene. HBsAg was synthesized by all of the 15 clones examined. The HBsAg, in contrast to that produced in yeast, was secreted into the cell culture medium as particles having the same characteristics as those found in human serum. It was estimated that $2–4 \times 10^4$ particles were produced per mouse cell per 24 hr. Moriarty *et al.* (1981) constructed a simian virus 40 recombinant carrying a 1350-bp *Bam*HI fragment of DNA from HBV. Cultured monkey kidney cells infected with this recombinant produced HBsAg. The antigen was secreted into the culture medium as 22-nm particles with the same physical properties, antigenic composition, and constituent polypeptides as those found in HBsAg in sera. Approximately 2.5 µg of antigen was produced per 1×10^7 cell per 72 hr. An HBsAg preparation purified from this cell culture fluid has been used to immunize two chimpanzees, thereby demonstrating its applicability as an alternative antigen source for vaccine (Gerin *et al.*, 1984). Liu *et al.* (1982) developed a special SV 40-based vector for efficient direct expression of foreign genes. *Eco*RI and *Bam*HI restriction fragments of HBV genome containing the surface antigen gene were inserted, and the synthesis of HBsAg protein was observed in monkey cells infected with this vector. Again, 22-nm particles were secreted into the culture medium and were shown to be indistinguishable from those formed by the hepatoma cell line. Later Crowley *et al.* (1983) showed that the expression of HBsAg did not require an intact copy of the SV 40 72-bp repeat, suggesting that the hepatitis genome itself contains an enhancer element. They also were able to adapt the vector to COS cells for production of HBsAg. In these cells, synthesis continued for up to 3 weeks at a level of 1×10^8 molecules of HBsAg per cell per day.

B. Prediction of the Immunogenicity of HBsAg Fragments on the Basis of Nucleotide Sequence

The nucleotide sequence encoding the HBsAg gene was localized on the cloned HBV genome by identifying the sequence coding for the 19 amino acids present in the amino-terminal region of HBsAg polypeptides p23 and gp29 (Peterson *et al.*, 1977). This reading frame terminated downstream after 226 amino acids. Peterson (1981) confirmed this conclusion, that is, that the protein sequence predicted from the DNA sequence was indeed that of the isolated protein, by determining the amino acid sequence of 30 residues at the amino terminus and 3 residues at the carboxy terminus, and by peptide mapping of the middle portion of the HBsAg protein.

Recombinant DNA cloning and sequence determination have greatly facilitated the accumulation of knowledge concerning the structure and biological functions of the proteins of HBV. However, to assign a specific function to an unknown protein by prediction from the DNA sequence would be difficult. Lerner (1982) suggested that a solution could be approached by preparing specific antibodies against chemically synthesized polypeptides with primary structures selected according to the corresponding DNA sequence. These antibodies could then be used for defining the function of the gene product in question. For developing this approach, HBsAg and hemagglutinins of influenza virus were the first two proteins chosen. HBsAg and HA were selected for their unique hydrophobicity and known crystallographic structure, respectively. Peptides encompassing the majority of the protein were synthesized, and the corresponding antibodies produced (Lerner *et al.*, 1981; Green *et al.*, 1982). The results of both studies indicated that the strategy was workable and supported the general concept that chemically synthesized peptides representing various domains of the predicted protein could be prepared on the basis of the nucleotide sequence, the corresponding antibodies raised, and finally that these antibodies would react with the native protein. A few "rules" for recognizing the most likely immunogenic amino acid sequences and the minimum size requirement for the peptides were also determined (Lerner, 1982).

Recognizing the fact that antigenic determinants are usually on the surface of the protein, projected into the medium, and composed of charged amino acids with hydrophilic side chains, Hopp and Woods (1981) developed a method for locating protein antigenic determinants by analyzing amino acid sequences in order to find the points of greatest local hydrophilicity. This method was developed by using 12 proteins for which extensive immunochemical analyses had been accomplished, and was subsequently used to predict antigenic determinants of many proteins of interest. Amino acid residues 141–146 were found to have the greatest average hydrophilicity of the HBsAg protein; a 12-residue polypeptide containing this region was synthesized and shown to be antigenically active. A computer program written for this method of predicting the locations of protein antigenic determinants and a demonstration of its application (with the influenza HA as an example) were published by Hopp and Wood (1983).

C. Activities of Chemically Synthesized HBsAg Polypeptides

Initially Lerner *et al.* (1981) chemically synthesized 13 peptides corresponding to amino acid sequences predicted from the nucleotide sequence of the HBsAg gene. Antisera against 4 of the 6 soluble peptides longer than 10 amino acids were reactive with native antigen, and specifically precipitated the 23,000- and 28,000-dalton components from detergent-disrupted HBV particles. The 4 peptides were those corresponding to amino acid residues 2–16, 22–35, 48–81, and 95–109. All peptides except for that representing residues 48–81 were coupled to carrier protein [keyhole limpet hemocyanin (KLH)] for immunization. The elicited antibodies were shown to remove DNA polymerase activity from HBV-containing sera (Gerin *et al.*, 1983). Subsequently, the peptides equivalent to amino acid residues 110–137, as predicted from DNA sequences of the cloned HBV genome of both **ad** (Valenzuela *et al.*, 1979) and **ay** (Charnay *et al.*, 1979) subtypes, were synthesized. Analyses of antibodies against peptides 110–137 and the additional 4 described above showed that at least three nonoverlapping sequences contain epitopes contributing to the common cross-reacting antigenic determinant, designated as the group-specific **a** determinant. A relatively hydrophilic region of the surface antigen protein, spanning amino acid residues 110–137, specified the major **d** and **y** subtype system (Gerin *et al.*, 1983). The **d/y** subtype appears to depend upon changes in one or more amino acids at positions 127, 131, and 134 of the HBsAg protein. This region contained a high level of amino acid substitutions, as shown by nucleotide sequences (Charnay *et al.*, 1979; Pasek *et al.*, 1979; Valenzuela *et al.*, 1979) and direct amino acid sequencing (Peterson *et al.*, 1982), suggesting that this is an antigenically important area of the protein. A peptide consisting of amino acid residues 110–137 of **y** subtype HBsAg protein, when coupled to a carrier protein and adjuvanted, stimulated a brisk anti-**y** response in chimpanzees. The results offered promise for the eventual application of chemically synthesized peptides as vaccines against hepatitis B.

A peptide corresponding to residues 138–149 of HBsAg protein was chemically synthesized by Hopp and Woods (1981) and was found to bind specifically to antibodies against HBsAg (Hopp, 1981). This peptide was also shown to have antigenic specificities **a** and **d**, but not **y**, when tested by passive hemagglutination inhibition with monospecific antisera (Prince *et al.*, 1982). When the peptide was conjugated to human erythrocytes and injected into mice, it induced the formation of Anti-HBs whether Freund's adjuvant was used or not.

Dreesman *et al.* (1982) synthesized a peptide containing 16 amino acid residues (122 through 137 of the sequence for p23 of **ayw** subtype reported by Charnay *et al.*, 1979). To mimic the native conformation, a disulfide bridge was introduced between cysteine residues 124 and 137. The resulting cyclic peptide was designated SP1. The immunogenicity of this cyclic peptide, aggregated in micelles or covalently coupled to tetanus toxoid, was assessed in mice (Sanchez *et al.*, 1982). Antibodies against HBsAg were induced by both preparations, administered either in saline or adsorbed on alum adjuvant. A common human anti-HBs idiotype–antiidiotype reaction was partially inhibited by this SP1 peptide (Kennedy and Dreesman, 1983). The disulfide bond was critical; this inhibitory effect was abolished upon reduction and aklylation. The epitopes associated with this peptide, both the cyclic and the linear form, were characterized by a panel of monoclonal antibodies with defined specificity for the cross-reactive group **a** antigenic determinant(s) and for the **y** and **w** subtypes (Ionescu-Matiu *et al.*, 1983). The cyclic, but not the linear, form of SP1 reacted with 5 of 14 anti-**a** monoclonal antibodies, demonstrating that the cyclic peptide contained a conformation-dependent **a** epitope. Only one anti-**a** antibody reacted with both cyclic and linear forms of SP1. Both cyclic and linear SP1 reacted with all three anti-**y** monoclonal antibodies, indicating that a sequential **y** epitope was also present on SP1; no **w** reactivity was detected. Ionescu-Matiu *et al.* (1983) also used monoclonal antibodies to analyze the idiotype association. They showed that antibodies that bound cyclic SP1 also inhibited the binding of a common human anti-HBs idiotype with its rabbit anti-idiotype serum, whereas a monoclonal antibody that did not react with the cyclic SP1 also failed to inhibit the idiotype–antiidiotype reaction. Thus, the conformational **a** epitope present on the cyclic SP1 appears to contain the major determinant recognized by human antibodies elicited following natural HBV infections.

Seven overlapping peptide analogues corresponding to residues between 122 and 158 were chemically synthesized by Bhatnagar *et al.* (1982) according to the nucleotide sequence of a cloned HBsAg/**adw** gene (Valenzuela *et al.*, 1979). The immunological reactivity of these synthetic peptides was studied by immunization of rabbits after coupling them to KLH. Results indicated that the nonapeptide sequence 139–147 represented all, or at least an essential part of, the **a** determinant of HBsAg.

Neurath *et al.* (1982b), on the basis of their previous chemical modification experiments (Neurath *et al.*, 1981) predicted the localization of a major HBsAg determinant within residues 135–155. They synthesized a peptide with this sequence, linked it to macromolecular carriers, and used it to immunize rabbits. A heterogeneous population of IgG and IgM antibodies reacting with peptide 135–155 was elicited, but only IgM antibodies reacted with HBsAg. The equilibrium constant for the reaction of these antibodies with HBsAg was approximately two orders of magnitude lower than that for the reaction with peptide 135–155 and or for the reaction between HBsAg and anti-HBs. Preimmunization with peptide did not result in an enhanced response to subsequent immunization with HBsAg. The results stressed the need for critical evaluation of the immunological response(s) elicited by synthetic peptides both at humoral and cellular levels, and indicated that sophisticated mimicking of conformational determinants of the HBsAg protein may be required for synthetic vaccine production.

Shih *et al.* (1984) have examined the immunogenicity of synthetic peptide fragments corresponding to HBsAg protein residues 1–20, 21–47, 48–81, and 156–185. These peptides, with the exception of peptide 48–81, are insoluble in aqueous medium and were used as immunogens without being coupled to a carrier protein. Three rabbits were each inoculated with 100 μg of each synthetic peptide in complete Freund's adjuvant, and booster immunizations of 100 and 50 μg each, respectively, were administered in incomplete Freund's adjuvant at 2-week intervals. With the exception of one rabbit that received peptide 21–47, all the rabbits produced significant amounts of anti-HBs after the second booster. Rapid and strong antibody responses were seen in some of the rabbits immunized with peptides 1–20 or 48–81. The antibody concentrations equivalent to 9375 and 6250 mIU/ml were determined 9 weeks postimmunization in some of the rabbits that received peptide 1–20 or 48–81, respectively. Anti-HBs at titers of 1 : 625 were maintained between week 6 and 12 by these animals. Immune responses were therefore easily elicited to short peptide fragments that were not coupled to carrier protein. The insolubility of these peptides could be the basis for this result. However, antibodies induced in this series of studies were all of the IgM subclass. Even after repeated immunization, there was no conversion to IgG subclass or any anamnestic responses, despite the fact that the animals were monitored for 16 weeks and longer.

The antibodies produced by rabbits inoculated with these HBsAg peptide fragments showed intriguing reaction patterns with HBsAg of known subtypes. Table IV shows the result of subtyping the antibody activities elicited to these peptides as determined by blocking RIA (Hoofnagle *et al.*, 1977). With the exception of anti-peptide 21–47, which reacted with all HBsAg samples tested and could be defined as anti-group determinant **a**, the antibodies were not definable according to the conventional serological classification. The results also reflected the heterogeneity of the distribution of antigenic sites among HBsAg particles and suggested the need for redefining the antigenic determinants in terms of epitopes. The clear-cut reaction between individual HBsAg preparations and rabbit antisera against peptide fragments indicated the potential usefulness of reagents prepared this way in the elucidation of the antigenic determinants of macromolecules.

V. Future Prospects

The intensive research on the immunological reactivity of HBsAg has brought us some basic understanding of the structure of the antigen, and has contributed to the development of an effective, modern vaccine for use against one of the most important diseases in the public health arena. However, through these studies we have also come to understand the complexity of this virus and its surface antigen. In the absence of a cell culture system to replicate HBV, detailed analyses of the structure and biological function of HBV and HBsAg were severely impaired. The recent technological revolution in biological research, including molecular cloning and monoclonal antibody production, has permitted breakthroughs in the characterization of HBV and its associated antigens.

Analysis of the antigenic epitopes of HBsAg with monoclonal antibodies has revealed that the heterogeneity of HBsAg particles is much more extensive than was previously suspected (Shorey *et al.*, 1981). The identification of nonoverlapping multiple monoclonal antibodies to specific determinants defined by conventional serology supports the notion that more than one antigenic site is involved in either group- or type-

TABLE IV

Specificity of Rabbit Antibodies to Insoluble Synthetic HBsAg Fragments

Rabbit number	8202	8206	8208	8211
Amino acid residues	1–20	21–47	48–81	156–185
Blocking HBsAg subtype	Percent inhibition (reactivity)			
aywl[a]	93.8(+)	72.3(+)	97.9(+)	97.6(+)
ayw2[a]	102 (+)	76.1(+)	98.3(+)	11.2(−)
ayw3[a]	0 (−)	63.3(+)	4.0(−)	0 (−)
ayr[a]	15.0(−)	71.1(+)	15.0(−)	2.3(−)
adw[a]	100 (+)	90.2(+)	94.4(+)	100 (+)
adw4[a]	0.7(−)	51.9(+)	27.8(−)	2.3(−)
adr[a]	0 (−)	59.4(+)	8.4(−)	75.8(+)
adw[b]	101 (+)	98.2(+)	99.3(+)	100 (+)
ayw[b]	100 (+)	80.2(+)	18.9(−)	0.5(−)
adr[b]	14.8(−)	75.5(+)	4.2(−)	0 (−)

[a]HBsAg-positive sera subtyped at the First International Workshop, Paris, 1975.
[b]HBsAg-positive sera subtyped in our laboratory.

specific determinants (Shih *et al.*, 1978). The nucleotide sequences deduced from cloned HBV DNA enhanced the determination of the amino acid sequence of HBsAg (Peterson, 1981). Similarly, the availability of the nucleotide sequences for both **ad** and **ay** HBsAg subtypes enable us to localize and synthesize the corresponding peptides and to demonstrate their antigenicity (Gerin *et al.*, 1983). In combination with the utilization of antiidiotypic antibody produced against human anti-HBs antibodies, monoclonal antibodies with defined specificity, and synthetic HBsAg peptides, Inoescu-Matiu *et al.* (1983) demonstrated a procedure for investigating antigenic determinants within convalescent antisera appearing during recovery from hepatitis B infections.

Large quantities of HBsAg particles have been synthesized with cloned HBV DNA in several expression systems. New generations of vaccine can be expected from recombinant DNA and chemical synthetic procedures. The experiences obtained in the studies with synthetic peptides as immunogens stressed the need for critical evaluation of immune responses to such an antigen at both humoral and cellular levels. The usefulness of such responses in protection of the host remains to be seen. For the practical purpose of developing a vaccine composed of synthetic peptides, many considerations will be required. The selection of an appropriate and effective carrier protein for the short peptide fragments could pose difficulties. The new generation of adjuvants such as dimuramyl peptide-related compounds could be explored in combination or direct linkage with synthetic peptides. Large peptide could be synthesized by linking short, well-defined synthetic fragments. Semisynthetic molecules obtained by chemically combining peptides produced by chemical syntheses and biochemical engineering techniques might provide critical comformational requirements.

These are examples to illustrate the direct contributions of new technologies to the elucidation of structure–function relationships of HBsAg. However, these new technologies are still in their infancy insofar as practical usage is concerned. Novel ideas and procedures are needed for analyzing the immune response of the host to HBsAg at both humoral and cellular levels in terms of epitopes, and establishing the structural features of HBsAg that are essential for inducing protective antibodies. Genetically engineered mutants with point mutations, deletions, or additions can be produced to localize the structures involved in immunogenicity and other biological functions. Libraries of monoclonal antibodies with known specificities can be prepared and used to detect conformational alterations, and to identify specific epitopes in the native and denatured antigen. One can predict that the combined utilization of molecular cloning products and monoclonal antibodies will lead to the identification of all the antigenic determinants of HBsAg particles. "Super antigens" containing only the essential determinants gathered from different subtypes may thus be capable of being produced for diagnostic and prophylactic use.

Acknowledgments

The author would like to thank Dr. John S. Finlayson of the Office of Biologics Research and Review, FDA, for his review of the manuscript and Dr. John L. Gerin of Georgetown University for his continuous encouragement.

References

Alexander, J. J., Van Der Merwe, C. F., Saunders, R. M., McElligott, S. E., and Desmyter, J. (1982). *Hepatology* **2**, 92s–96s.
Atassi, M. Z. (1967). *Biochem. J.* **102**, 478–487.
Atassi, M. Z. (1975). *Immunochemistry* **12**, 423–438.
Bhatnagar, P. K., Papas, E., Blum, H. E., Milich, D. R., Nitecki, D., Karels, M. J., and Vyas, G. N. (1982). *Proc. Natl. Acad. Sci. U.S.A.* **79**, 4400–4404.
Burrell, C. J. (1975). *J. Gen. Virol.* **27**, 117–126.

Burrell, C. J., Proudfoot, E., Keen, G. A., and Marmion, B. P. (1973). *Nature (London) New Biol.* **243**, 260–262.

Burrell, C. J., Leadbetter, G., Mackay, P., and Marmion, B. P. (1976). *J. Gen. Virol.* **33**, 41–50.

Burrell, C. J., Mackay, P., Greenaway, P. J., Hofschneider, P. H., and Murray, K. (1979). *Nature (London)* **279**, 43–47.

Cabral, G. A., Marciano-Cabral, F., Funk, G. A., Sanchez, Y., Hollinger, F. B., Melnick, J. L., and Dreesman, G. R. (1978). *J. Gen. Virol.* **38**, 339–350.

Chairez, R., Hollinger, F. B., Brunschwig, J. P., and Dreesman, G. R. (1975). *J. Virol.* **15**, 182–190.

Charnay, P., Mandart, E., Hampe, A., Fitoussi, F., and Tiollais, P. (1979). *Nucleic Acids Res.* **7**, 335–346.

Charnay, P., Gervais, M., Louise, A., Galibert, F., and Tiollais, P. (1980). *Nature (London)* **286**, 893–895.

Cote, P. J., Jr., and Gerin, J. L. (1983). *J. Virol.* **47**, 15–23.

Cote, P. J., Jr., Dapolito, G. M., Shih, J. W.-K., and Gerin, J. L. (1982). *J. Virol.* **42**, 135–142.

Crowley, C. W., Liu, C.-C., and Levinson, A. D. (1983). *Mol. Cell. Biol.* **3**, 44–55.

Crumpton, M. J. (1974). *In* "The Antigens" (M. Sela, ed.), Vol. 2, pp. 1–78. Academic Press, New York.

David, G. S., Present, W., Martinis, J., Bartholomew, R., Desmond, W., and Sevier, E. D. (1981). *Med. Lab. Sci.* **38**, 341–348.

Dreesman, G. R., Hollinger, F. B., McCombs, R. M., and Melnick, J. L. (1973). *J. Gen. Virol.* **19**, 129–134.

Dreesman, G. R., Chairez, R., Suarez, M., Hollinger, F. B., Courtney, R. J., and Melnick, J. L. (1975). *J. Virol.* **16**, 508–515.

Dreesman, G. R., Sanchez, Y., Ionescu-Matiu, I., Sparrow, J. T., Six, H. R., Peterson, D. L., Hollinger, F. B., and Melnick, J. L. (1982). *Nature (London)* **295**, 158–160.

Dubois, M., Pourcel, C., Rousset, S., Chany, C., and Tiollais, P. (1980). *Proc. Natl. Acad. Sci. U.S.A.* **77**, 4549–4553.

Edman, J. C., Hallewell, R. A., Valenzuela, P., Goodman, H. M., and Rutter, W. J. (1981). *Nature (London)* **291**, 503–506.

Galibert, F., Mandart, E., Fitoussi, F., Tiollais, P., and Charnay, P. (1979). *Nature (London)* **281**, 646–650.

Gavilanes, F., Gonzalez-Ros, J. M., and Peterson, D. L. (1982). *J. Biol. Chem.* **257**, 7770–7777.

Gerhard, W., Yewdell, J., and Frankel, M. E. (1981). *Nature (London)* **290**, 713–717.

Gerin, J. L. (1972). *In* "Hepatitis and Blood Transfusion" (G. N. Vyas, H. A. Perkins, and R. Schmid, eds.), pp. 205–219. Grune & Stratton, New York.

Gerin, J. L., and Shih, J. W.-K. (1978). *In* "Viral Hepatitis" (G. N. Vyas, S. N. Cohen, and R. Schmid, eds.), pp. 147–153. Franklin Inst. Press, Philadelphia, Pennsylvania.

Gerin, J. L., Shih, J. W.-K., and Kaplan, P. W. (1975). *Am. J. Med. Sci.* **270**, 115–121.

Gerin, J. L., Alexander, H., Shih, J. W.-K., Purcell, R. H., Dapolito, G., Engle, R., Green, N., Sutcliffe, J. G., Shinnick, T. M., and Lerner, R. A. (1983). *Proc. Natl. Acad. Sci. U.S.A.* **80**, 2365–2369.

Gerin, J. L., Purcell, R. H., and Lerner, R. A. (1984). *In* "Modern Approaches to Vaccines: Molecular and Chemical Basis of Virus Virulence and Immunogenicity" (R. M. Chanock and R. A. Lerner, eds.), pp. 121–125. Cold Spring Harbor Laboratory, Cold Spring Harbor, New York.

Gold, J. W. M., Shih, J. W.-K., Purcell, R. H., and Gerin, J. L. (1976). *J. Immunol.* **117**, 1404–1406.

Goodall, A. H., Miescher, G., Meek, F. M., Janossy, G., and Thomas, H. C. (1981). *Med. Lab. Sci.* **38**, 349–354.

Goudeau, A., Houwen, B., and Dankert, J. (1974). *Lancet 2*, 1325.

Green, N., Alexander, H., Olson, A., Alexander, S., Shinnick, T. M., Sutcliffe, J. G., and Lerner, R. A. (1982). *Cell* **28**, 477–487.

Hansson, B. G., and Purcell, R. H. (1979). *Infect. Immun.* **26**, 125–130.

Hess, G., Shih, J. W.-K., Arnold, W., Gerin, J. L., and Meyer zum Bushenfelde, K.-H. (1979). *J. Immunol.* **123**, 1189–1194.

Holland, P. V. (1976). *In* "HBs Antigen Subtypes" (A. M. Couroucé, P. V. Holland, J. Y. Muller, and J. P. Soulier, eds.), p. 19. Karger, Basel.

Hoofnagle, J. H., Gerety, R. J., Smallwood, L. A., and Barker, L. F. (1977). *Gastroenterology* **72**, 290–296.

Hopp, T. P. (1981). *Mol. Immunol.* **18**, 869–872.

Hopp, T. P., and Woods, K. R. (1981). *Proc. Natl. Acad. Sci. U.S.A.* **78**, 3824–3828.

Hopp, T. P., and Woods, K. R. (1983). *Mol. Immunol.* **20**, 483–489.

Imai, M., Gotoh, A., Nishioka, K., Kurashina, S., *et al.* (1974). *J. Immunol.* **112**, 416–419.

Imai, M., Yanase, Y., Nojiri, T., Miyakawa, Y., and Mayumi, M. (1979). *Gastroenterology* **76**, 242–247.

Imai, M., Nomura, M., Gotanda, T., Sano, T., Tachibana, K., Miyamoto, H., Takahashi, K., Toyama, S., Miyakawa, Y., and Mayumi, M. (1982). *J. Immunol.* **128**, 69–72.

Inoescu-Matiu, I., Sanchez, Y., Hollinger, F. B., and Melnick, J. L. (1980). *J. Med. Virol.* **6**, 175–178.

Inoescu-Matiu, I., Kennedy, R. C., Sparrow, J. T., Culwell, A. R., Sanchez, Y., Melnick, J. L., and Dreesman, G. R. (1983). *J. Immunol.* **130**, 1947–1952.

Kennedy, R. C., and Dreesman, G. R. (1983). *J. Immunol.* **130**, 385–389.

Kennedy, R. C., Inoescu-Matiu, I., Adler-Storthz, K., Henkel, R. D., Sanchez, Y., and Dreesman, G. R. (1983). *Intervirology* **19**, 176–180.

Kim, C. Y., and Bissell, D. M. (1971). *J. Infect. Dis.* **123**, 470–476.

Kohler, G., and Milstein, C. (1975). *Nature (London)* **256**, 495–497.

Lerner, R. A. (1982). *Nature (London)* **299**, 592–596.

Lerner, R. A., Green, N., Alexander, H., Liu, F.-T., Sutcliffe, G., and Shinnick, T. M. (1981). *Proc. Natl. Acad. Sci. U.S.A.* **78**, 3403–3407.

Liu, C.-C., Yansura, D., Levinson, A. D. (1982). *DNA* **1**, 213–221.

Lu, J. C-F., Shih, J. W.-K., Mitchell, F. D., Smallwood, L. A., Gerety, R. J., and Ford, E. C. (1984). *In* "Viral Hepatitis and Liver Disease" (G. N. Vyas, J. L. Deinstag, and J. H. Hoofnagle, eds.), p. 659. Grune & Stratton, Orlando, Florida.

Lubeck, M., and Gerhard, W. (1982). *Virology* **118**, 1–7.

Machida, A., Kishimoto, S., Ohnuma, H., Miyamoto, H., Baba, K., Oda, K., Nakamura, T., Funatsu, G., Miyakawa, Y., and Mayumi, M. (1982). *Mol. Immunol.* **19**, 1087–1093.

Mackay, P., and Burrell, C. J. (1976). *J. Gen. Virol.* **33**, 181–191.

Mackay, P., Pasek, M., Magazin, M., Kovacic, R. T., Allet, B., Stahl, S., Gilbert, W., Schaller, H., Bruce, S. A., and Murray, K. (1981). *Proc. Natl. Acad. Sci. U.S.A.* **78**, 4510–4514.

Massey, R. J., and Schochetman, G. (1981). *Virology* **115**, 20–32.

Millman, I., Hutanen, H., Merino, F., and Bauer, M. E. (1971). *Res. Commun. Chem. Pathol. Pharmacol.* **2**, 667–686.

Mishiro, S., Imai, M., Gotanda, T., Takahashi, K., Sano, T., Yoshizawa, H., Miyakawa, Y., and Mayumi, M. (1980a). *J. Med. Virol.* **6**, 269–278.

Mishiro, S., Imai, M., Takahashi, K., Machida, A., Gotanda, T., Miyakawa, Y., and Mayumi, M. (1980b). *J. Immunol.* **124**, 1589–1593.

Miyakawa, Y., Imai, M., and Mayumi, M. (1975). *J. Immunol.* **114,** 1135–1137.

Miyanohara, A., Toh-E, A., Nozaki, C., Hamada, F., Ohtama, N., and Matsubara, K. (1983). *Proc. Natl. Acad. Sci. U.S.A.* **80,** 1–5.

Moriarty, A. M., Hoyer, B. H., Shih, J. W.-K., Gerin, J. L., and Hamer, D. H. (1981). *Proc. Natl. Acad. Sci. U.S.A.* **78,** 2606–2610.

Neurath, A. R., and Strick, N. (1979). *Intervirology* **11,** 128–132.

Neurath, A. R., and Strick, N. (1980). *J. Med. Virol.* **6,** 309–322.

Neurath, A. R., Prince, A. M., Lippin, A. (1974). *Proc. Natl. Acad. Sci. U.S.A.* **71,** 2663–2667.

Neurath, A. R., Hashimoto, N., and Prince, A. M. (1975). *J. Gen. Virol.* **27,** 81–91.

Neurath, A. R., Strick, N., and Huang, C. Y. (1978). *Intervirology* **10,** 265–275.

Neurath, A. R., Strick, N., and Oleszko, W. R. (1981). *J. Virol. Methods* **3,** 115–125.

Neurath, A. R., Strick, N., Baker, L., and Krugman, S. (1982a). *Proc. Natl. Acad. Sci. U.S.A.* **79,** 4415–4419.

Neurath, A. R., Kent, S. B. H., and Strick, N. (1982b). *Proc. Natl. Acad. Sci. U.S.A.* **79,** 7871–7875.

Pasek, M., Goto, T., Gilbert, W., Zink, B., Schaller, H., Mackay, P., Leadbetter, G., and Murray, K. (1979). *Nature (London)* **282,** 575–579.

Peterson, D. L. (1981). *J. Biol. Chem.* **256,** 6975–6983.

Peterson, D. L., Roberts, I. M., and Yvas, G. N. (1977). *Proc. Natl. Acad. Sci. U.S.A.* **74,** 1530–1534.

Peterson, D. L., Nath, N., and Gavilanes, F. (1982). *J. Biol. Chem.* **257,** 10414–10420.

Present, W. A., King, M. P., Bland, A. F., and Allen, V. G. (1980). *Fed. Proc., Fed. Am. Soc. Exp. Biol.* **39,** 929.

Prince, A. M., Ikram, H., and Hopp, T. P. (1982). *Proc. Natl. Acad. Sci. U.S.A.* **79,** 579–582.

Rao, K. R., and Vyas, G. N. (1973). *Nature (London), New Biol.* **241,** 240–241.

Sanchez, Y., Ionescu-Matiu, I., Dreesman, G. R., Kramp, W., Six, H. R., Hollinger, F. B., and Melnick, J. L. (1980). *Infect. Immun.* **30,** 728–733.

Sanchez, Y., Ionescu-Matiu, I., and Dreesman, G. R. (1981). *Virology* **114,** 71–84.

Sanchez, Y., Ionesco-Matiu, I., Sparrow, J. T., Melnick, J. L., and Dreesman, G. R. (1982). *Intervirology* **18,** 209–213.

Saxena, V. P., and Wetlaufer, D. B. (1970). *Biochemistry* **9,** 5015–5022.

Shafritz, D. A., Lieberman, H. M., Isselbacher, K. J., and Wands, J. R. (1982). *Proc. Natl. Acad. Sci. U.S.A.* **79,** 5675–5679.

Shih, J. W.-K., and Gerin, J. L. (1973). *Abst. Annu. Meet. Am. Soc. Microbiol.,* p. 220.

Shih, J. W.-K., and Gerin, J. L. (1975). *J. Immunol.* **115,** 634–639.

Shih, J. W.-K., and Gerin, J. L. (1977a). *J. Virol.* **21,** 347–357.

Shih, J. W.-K., and Gerin, J. L. (1977b). *J. Virol.* **21,** 1219–1222.

Shih, J. W.-K., Tan, P. L., and Gerin, J. L. (1978). *J. Immunol.* **120,** 520–525.

Shih, J. W.-K., Cote, P. J., Jr., and Gerin, J. L. (1979). *Transfusion* **19,** 637.

Shih, J. W.-K., Cote, P. J., Jr., Dapolito, G. M., and Gerin, J. L. (1980a). *J. Virol. Methods* **1,** 257–273.

Shih, J. W.-K., Tan, P. L., and Gerin, J. L. (1980b). *Infect. Immun.* **28,** 459–463.

Shih, J. W.-K., Gerety, R. J., Liu, D. T.-Y., Yajima, H., Fujii, N., Nomizu, M., Hayashi, Y., and Katakura, S. (1984). *In* "Modern Approaches to Vaccines: Molecular and Chemical Basis of Virus Virulence and Immunogenicity" (R. M. Chanock and R. A. Lerner, eds.), pp. 127–132. Cold Spring Harbor Laboratory, Cold Spring Harbor, New York.

Shiraishi, H., Shirachi, R., Sekine, T., and Ishida, N. (1978). *J. Gen. Virol.* **38,** 363–367.

Shorey, J., Brown, R. D., and Wands, J. R. (1981). *Hepatology* **1,** 546.

Shouval, D., Shafritz, D. A., Zurawski, V. R., Jr., Isselbacher, K. L., and Wands, J. R. (1982a). *Nature (London)* **298**, 567–569.

Shouval, D., Wands, J. R., Zurawski, V. R., Jr., Isselbacher, K. L., and Shafritz, D. A. (1982b). *Proc. Natl. Acad. Sci. U.S.A.* **79**, 650–654.

Skelly, J., Howard, C. R., and Zuckerman, A. J. (1979). *J. Gen. Virol.* **44**, 679–689.

Skelly, J., Howard, C. R., and Zuckerman, A. J. (1981). *Nature (London)* **290**, 51–54.

Sninsky, J. J., Siddiqui, A., Robinson, W. S., and Cohen, S. N. (1979). *Nature (London)* **279**, 346–348.

Steiner, S., Hubner, M. T., and Dreesman, G. R. (1974). *J. Virol.* **14**, 572–577.

Stone, M. R., and Nowinski, R. C. (1980). *Virology* **100**, 370–381.

Sugimoto, Y., and Toyoshima, S. (1981). *Antimicrob. Agents Chemother.* **20**, 120–127.

Sukeno, N., Shirachi, R., Yamaguchi, J., and Ishida, N. (1972). *J. Virol.* **9**, 182–183.

Sukeno, N., Shiraishi, H., and Ishida, N. (1975). *Tohoku J. Exp. Med.* **116**, 179–182.

Tabor, E., Gerety, R. J., Smallwood, L. A., and Barker, L. F. (1976). *J. Immunol.* **117**, 2038–2040.

Takahashi, T. (1975). *J. Jpn. Med. Assoc.* **73**, 225.

Thung, S. N., and Gerber, M. A. (1981). *Infect. Immun.* **32**, 1292–1294.

Valenzuela, P., Gray, P., Quiroga, M., and Zaldivar, J. (1979). *Nature (London)* **280**, 815–816.

Valenzuela, P., Medina, A., Rutter, W. J., Ammerer, G., and Hall, B. D. (1982). *Nature (London)* **298**, 347–350.

Vyas, G. N., Rao, K. R., and Ibrahim, A. B. (1972). *Science* **178**, 1300–1301.

Wands, J. R., and Zurawski, V. R., Jr. (1981). *Gastroenterology* **80**, 225–232.

Wands, J. R., Carlson, R. I., and Zurawski, V. R., Jr. (1980). *Abstr. Am. Assoc. Study Liver Dis. 1980*, p. 1063.

Wands, J. R., Carlson, R. I., Schoemaker, H., and Isselbacher, K. J. (1981). *Proc. Natl. Acad. Sci. U.S.A.* **78**, 1214–1218.

Wands, J. R., Bruns, R. R., Carlson, R. I., Ware, A., Menitore, J. E., and Isselbacher, K. J. (1982a). *Proc. Natl. Acad. Sci. U.S.A.* **79**, 1277–1281.

Wands, J. R., Marciniak, R. A., Isselbacher, K. J., Varghese, M., Don, G., Halliday, J. W., and Powell, L. W. (1982b). *Lancet 1*, 977–980.

Zuckerman, A. J. (1975). *Nature (London)* **255**, 104–105.

Index